OXFORD MEDICAL PUBLICATIONS

Medical
Psychotherapy

Oxford Specialist Handbooks published and forthcoming

Oxford Specialist Handbooks in Psychiatry
Medical Psychotherapy

Edited by

Jessica Yakeley

Fellow of the British
Psychoanalytical Society,
Consultant Psychiatrist in
Forensic Psychotherapy, Portman
Clinic, Director of Medical
Education and Associate Medical
Director, Tavistock and Portman
NHS Foundation Trust, London
UK; Editor of Psychoanalytic
Psychotherapy, UK

Gwen Adshead

Consultant Forensic Psychiatrist
and Psychotherapist, Southern
Health Foundation Trust, UK

Laura Allison

Consultant Psychiatrist, South
London and Maudsley NHS
Foundation Trust, London, UK

James Johnston

Consultant Psychiatrist in
Psychotherapy, Leeds and York
Partnership NHS Foundation
Trust, Leeds, UK; British
Psychoanalytic Council Registered
Member, North of England
Association of Psychoanalytic
Psychotherapists (NEAPP),
UK; Visiting Lecturer, Tavistock
and Portman NHS Foundation
Trust, London, UK; Chair, Royal
College of Psychiatrists Medical
Psychotherapy Faculty Education
and Curriculum Committee
2011–2015; Member of the
Association for Psychoanalytic
Psychotherapy in the NHS, UK

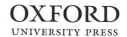

OXFORD
UNIVERSITY PRESS

OXFORD
UNIVERSITY PRESS

Great Clarendon Street, Oxford, OX2 6DP,
United Kingdom

Oxford University Press is a department of the University of Oxford.
It furthers the University's objective of excellence in research, scholarship,
and education by publishing worldwide. Oxford is a registered trade mark of
Oxford University Press in the UK and in certain other countries

Published in the United States of America by Oxford University Press
198 Madison Avenue, New York, NY 10016, United States of America

British Library Cataloguing in Publication Data

Data available

Library of Congress Control Number: 2015955009

ISBN 978–0–19–960838–6

Printed and bound in China by
C&C Offset Printing Co., Ltd.

Foreword

This book comes to birth at a propitious moment. Its cradle, to use the authors' metaphor borrowed from Bevan's founding vision for the NHS, is beset by a series of interlinked crises, affecting medicine, psychiatry, and indeed books themselves. For all its spectacular advances—to some extent a product of them—medicine is increasingly fragmented and super-specialized. The role of the physician with a synoptic and on-going relationship with her patient—a deep knowledge of the strengths and vulnerabilities of the individual in a family and social context—is evanescent. Even in a free at the point of access service, consultation is increasingly viewed as a quasi-commercial transaction, in which the patient is a 'customer' for whom doctors proffer a 'service'—rather than an attachment relationship based on security, sensitivity, continuity, and epistemic trust. There is a consequent plague of over-diagnosis and over-treatment. Prevention and health promotion are downgraded and starved of funds. The pervasiveness of chronic illness is unmatched by appropriate theory and practice.

Psychiatry has not been immune to these changes. Lip service is played to continuity of care, but the reality is a plethora of teams, professions, and special interests. Patients move—are passively 'moved'—from one clinical encounter to another, with little acknowledgement of the specificity of the attachment relationship, or the inevitability of grief on separation. Flanked by the rival disciplines of neurology/neuroscience and clinical psychology, psychiatry struggles to define its unique role. A life-course, developmental perspective fades in a culture that favours fiscal 'illness-episodes' over the uniqueness of the individual. The protesting user's voice is increasingly heard, but responses are typically superficial and dismissive.

Medical psychotherapy—psychotherapeutic psychiatry—has suffered its own wounds in this maelstrom. Psychotherapy services have become marginalized within the psychiatric family, depicted as 'soft', 'Freudian' (i.e. antediluvian), and lacking an evidence base. Without a clearly identifiable client group (the claim that psychotherapy is relevant to *all* aspects of psychiatric work merely provokes all-things-to-all-men dismissal), managers cut psychotherapy and psychotherapists with impunity, betting that protest will be muted and can be dubbed as self-interest. Some wounds have been self-inflicted. Compared with the USA and Germany, UK medical psychotherapists have been slow to engage in research or penetrate academe; psychoanalytic psychotherapists, the majority of the workforce, have been at best ambivalent about admitting their CBT and systemic colleagues into the fold; the need for free and respectful communication with other psychiatric colleagues has been neglected; cases cherry-picked; the cabal of true believers has sometimes perversely celebrated marginalization rather than facing up to its weaknesses.

But, as this book so brilliantly exemplifies, crisis also equates to opportunity. Here, I believe, spelt out in magnificent detail, lies the psychiatry, not just the medical psychotherapy, of the future. Its practitioners claim legitimacy through triple expertise in medicine, psychiatry, and psychotherapy. Developmental perspectives and doctor–patient collaboration come as second nature. The individual life-history is paramount. Psychological therapies' robust evidence base equals or surpasses that of pharmacotherapy, and has remarkable 'sleeper' effects which mean that its benefits accrue well beyond therapy completion. Internecine wars—Freud's 'narcissism of minor differences'—finally overcome, the different schools of psychotherapy work respectfully together. Medical psychotherapy has an essential role in helping people suffering from personality disorders. Consultation-liaison and group therapy skills, together with a specialized understanding of developmental processes, mean that medical psychotherapy can contribute directly or indirectly (through staff support) to the entire spectrum of psychiatric illnesses.

Finally, Gutenberg outlives its obituarists: there is confirmation here of the extraordinary staying-power, virtue, and value of 'the book'. This future Bible for psychiatric trainees comprehensively brings together in-depth theoretical exposition, amusing cartoons, exam-friendly lists, touching case histories, and fluid communication amongst psychotherapeutic modalities and psychiatric specialisms. All this is done in encyclopaedia format in which the four editors and 56 contributors remain individually anonymous, yet speak with a collective voice of reason, authority, and hope. This lovely volume is a true phoenix, and one which all psychiatrists and psychotherapists should and will have open on their desks for a generation.

Jeremy Holmes, MD FRCPsych,
Visiting Professor,
School of Psychology,
University of Exeter, UK

Preface

Listening with medicine in mind

The *Oxford Specialist Handbook of Medical Psychotherapy* aims to evoke the experience of listening to patients with medicine in mind. What do medicine and mind have in common? What do doctors and psychotherapists have in common? Why is it helpful to be a medically qualified professional when working with psychological distress?

In this book, we will argue that the medical approach to studying the body and its disorders has much in common with the psychotherapist's approach to the study of mind and psychological distress, and vice versa. In general practice, it is well known that the psychological is closely related to the physical; general physicians and even surgeons are now accepting that the study of the mind is crucial to working with the body. Psychotherapists too need to pay close attention to diagnosis and symptoms, and to the careful exercise of technical skill in helping people recover.

The common values of medicine and psychotherapy lie in trying to understand a patient's problems within the limitations imposed by the ailment and the patient's own capacities. The therapeutic medical attitude is not unique to the practice of psychotherapy— it is the quotidian medical skill of the doctor, within the doctor–patient relationship, which defines psychotherapeutic medicine.

When a doctor can move from their skill in the identification of the medical or psychiatric problem to identification with the person with the problem, not being bound in this identification or spellbound by the problem, moving in mind reflexively between the external and internal problem, they are embodying psychotherapeutic medicine. Psychotherapeutic medicine is the guiding principle of this book, with medical psychotherapy expressing the integration of the values of the importance of the doctor–patient relationship and psychotherapeutic psychiatry. The *OSH of Medical Psychotherapy* connects psychiatrists and therapists with medical psychotherapy, exemplifying the relationship between the body of medicine, the mind of psychiatry, and the spirit of psychotherapy.

Who is this book for?

The book is a unique compendium of psychotherapies commonly delivered in the NHS by medical psychotherapists, psychotherapists, psychologists, and psychiatrists. It is aimed at the 'cradle to grave' range of nascent, newly qualified, training, and senior doctors—an audience of medical students, foundation year doctors, core and advanced psychiatry trainees, consultant psychiatrists, GPs, specialty doctors in psychiatry, and academics. It will also be of interest to professionals from other disciplines practising within the fields of health and social care such as nurses, psychologists, counsellors, child psychotherapists, social workers, and many others, as well as carers, patients, and service users, many of whom may have experienced some form of talking therapy first-hand.

What we hope will connect all of the patients, doctors, professionals, and members of the public who read this book will be an interest in contemporary psychotherapies and seeking to learn about their distinctive, and their overlapping, theories, concepts, training, and research evidence, and how the therapies are applied in practice, illustrated by anonymous case vignettes. The *OSH of Medical Psychotherapy* is written by therapeutic specialists in their fields in a house style which aims to be succinct, accessible, and evocative—an echo of what a therapist might try to offer the person or people with whom they seek to communicate.

Why is this book important?

The importance of the *OSH of Medical Psychotherapy* lies in its attempt to offer an overview of psychotherapies under the umbrella of the ontology of medical psychotherapy. It provides a link between different professions and ways of thinking about the problems of being human, without synthesis and without becoming a Tower of Babel with a confusion of tongues. Each therapy is given its own voice, and the reader is invited to hold in mind, and to integrate, the disparate array of myriad ways of healing minds. The illustrations by James Johnston, introducing and linking the twelve chapters of the Handbook, aim to be emotionally evocative, drawing from life in ways which echo the text they mirror.

Origins of this Handbook

The book has had a long gestation—from James Johnston's initial idea of the book in 2008 conceived in the confluence of a past comforting memory in anxious moments of the need for the *Oxford Handbook of Clinical Medicine* in his white coat pocket as a house officer and present extinction anxiety about the disappearance of medical psychotherapy, another vital vade mecum needed in uncertain times . . .

The *OSH of Medical Psychotherapy* would not exist without the receptivity to its conception by the Oxford University Press Commissioning Editor Chris Reid who was unfamiliar with the world of medical psychotherapy, more used to publishing the work of other medical specialists, including anaesthetists. James joked that perhaps his welcome support for this book was because he was used to doctors who work with the unconscious.

The first editorial group led by James (Gwen Adshead, Chess Denman, Chris Mace, and Stirling Moorey) was reduced to James and Gwen, following Chris's untimely death in 2010. After Chess and Stirling stepped down, Gwen's experienced tenacity helped keep the idea of the book alive, inspiring James to form a new editorial group with Jessica Yakeley as a tireless and thoughtful lead editor and Laura Allison as an editor representing the vitality of younger and more recently qualified consultant medical psychotherapists. The OUP staff Pete Stevenson and Lauren Dunn reassured us that this long gestation is not unusual—as a symbol of the survival of medical psychotherapy, we hope the book inspires therapeutic development in psychiatrists, other doctors, and others.

We are indebted to our sixty contributors who have written the individual sections which make up each of the 12 main chapters of the Handbook. Many of our authors are senior specialists in their fields, but others, of equal importance, are higher trainees in medical psychotherapy who represent the voices of the future.

The *OSH of Medical Psychotherapy*, like therapy, like life, like the cradle to grave career of a doctor, is a work in progress. It reflects the human diversity in which there can be no way of settling on a consensus of what makes for a good life or a good therapy. We hope that readers will find it useful in their work as psychotherapists, wherever they are, and that they will contribute to future editions.

JY, JJ, GA, LA, 2016

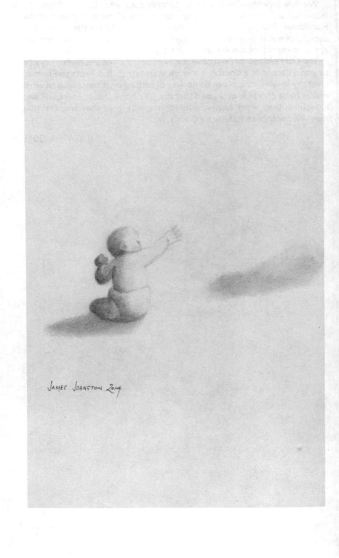

JAMES JOHNSTON 2014

Contents

Contributors

Gwen Adshead
Consultant Forensic Psychiatrist
and Psychotherapist, Southern
Health Foundation Trust, UK
*Chapter 2: Group therapy and
group analysis*
*Chapter 5: Group therapy and
group analysis*
*Chapter 8: Theories of personality
development*
Chapter 9: Ethics and boundaries

Laura Allison
Consultant Psychiatrist, South
London and Maudsley NHS
Foundation Trust, London, UK
Chapter 6: Problems through life

Penelope Aspinall
Head of Counselling, University
of Bradford, UK
Chapter 2: Counselling
Chapter 5: Counselling

Jina Barrett
Adult Psychotherapist and
Organisation Consultant, The
Tavistock and Portman NHS
Foundation Trust, Portman Clinic,
London, UK
Chapter 6: Older adults
Chapter 7: Dementia

Dinesh Bhugra
Professor of Mental Health and
Cultural Diversity, Section of
Cultural Psychiatry, Institute of
Psychiatry, London, UK
Chapter 7: Sexual dysfunction

Jan Birtle
Consultant Psychiatrist, Medical
Psychotherapy Tutor, and
Associate Medical Director,
Worcestershire Health and Care
Trust, Malvern, UK; Honorary
Senior Lecturer, University of
Worcester, UK
*Chapter 5: Therapy in clinical
practice*
*Chapter 12: Rehabilitation and
social psychiatry: psychotherapies,
applications, and research*

Julia Bland
Consultant Psychiatrist in
Psychotherapy, Maudsley
Hospital, London, UK
*Chapter 2: Systemic family and
couple therapy*
*Chapter 5: Systemic family and
couple therapy*

Jane Blunden
Consultant Psychiatrist
in Psychotherapy and
Psychotherapy Tutor, Sussex
Partnership NHS Foundation
Trust, Sussex, UK
Chapter 2: Cognitive analytic therapy
Chapter 5: Cognitive analytic therapy

Luigi Caparrotta
Fellow British Psychoanalytical
Society, Consultant Psychiatrist
in Psychotherapy, Camden &
Islington Psychodynamic
Psychotherapy Service,
Camden and Islington Foundation
Trust, St Pancras Hospital,
London, UK
Chapter 6: Problems through life
*Chapter 7: Psychotherapy and
medication; Anxiety and anxiety
disorders*

Anne Cooper
Consultant Psychiatrist in CBT,
Leeds and York Partnerships
Foundation Trust, Leeds, UK
*Chapter 2: Cognitive behavioural
therapy*
*Chapter 4: Cognitive behavioural
assessment and formulation*
*Chapter 5: Cognitive behavioural
therapy*

Sandra Evans
Consultant Psychiatrist/Senior
Lecturer in Psychiatry, East
London Foundation NHS Trust,
Vice Chair, Faculty of Old Age
Psychiatry, Royal College of
Psychiatrists, London, UK;
Associate Dean for Psychiatry
and Deputy Dean for Students,
Barts & the London SMD,
London, UK
*Chapter 12: Psychiatry of old age:
psychotherapies, applications, and
research*

Gearóid FitzGerald
Consultant Psychiatrist in
Psychotherapy, Leeds and York
Partnerships NHS Foundation
Trust, Leeds, UK
Chapter 10: Balint groups

Christian Foerster
Charité – Universitätsmedizin
Berlin, Germany
Chapter 7: Sexual dysfunction

Rachel Gibbons
Consultant Psychiatrist in
Psychiatry and Psychotherapy,
Complex Care Service,
Halliwick, St Ann's Hospital,
Barnet Enfield & Haringey MHT,
London, UK
*Chapter 10: Teaching
psychotherapy to mental
health professionals*

Catherine Goodwin
Dramatherapist, Avon and
Wiltshire Mental Health
Partnership NHS Trust, Secure
Services LDU, Bristol, UK;
Visiting Lecturer, Dramatherapy
MA, Department of Psychology,
University of Roehampton,
London, UK
Chapter 2: Drama therapy
Chapter 5: Drama therapy

Else Guthrie
Consultant in Psychological
Medicine and Honorary Professor
of Psychological Medicine,
Manchester Mental Health and
Social Care Trust, Manchester
Royal Infirmary, Manchester, UK
*Chapter 2: Psychodynamic
interpersonal therapy*
*Chapter 5: Psychodynamic
interpersonal therapy*
*Chapter 12: Liaison psychiatry:
psychotherapies, applications,
and research*

Rex Haigh
Consultant Psychiatrist in Medical
Psychotherapy, Berkshire
Healthcare NHS Foundation
Trust, Bracknell, UK; Professor
of Therapeutic Environments
and Relational Health, School
of Sociology and Social Policy,
Nottingham University, UK
*Chapter 2: Therapeutic
communities*
*Chapter 5: Therapeutic
communities*

Az Hakeem
Consultant Psychiatrist and Medical
Psychotherapist, The Priory
Hospital Roehampton, London,
UK; Visiting Professor of Psychiatry
and Applied Psychotherapy,
University of Bradford, UK
*Chapter 7: Gender dysphoria and
intersex conditions*

Rob Hale
Honorary Consultant
Psychotherapist, Portman Clinic,
Tavistock and Portman NHS
Foundation Trust, London, UK
Chapter 6: Suicide and self-harm

Donna Harrison
Forensic Psychologist in
Training, Partnerships in Care,
Nottinghamshire, UK
*Chapter 2: Dialectical behaviour
therapy*
*Chapter 5: Dialectical behaviour
therapy*

Angela Hassiotis
Professor of Psychiatry of
Intellectual Disability, UCL
Division of Psychiatry, London,
UK; Consultant Psychiatrist,
Camden Learning Disability
Service, London, UK
Chapter 7: Intellectual disability
*Chapter 12: Psychiatry of intellectual
disability: psychotherapies, applica-
tions, and research*

Nick Hayman
Music Psychotherapist, Avon
and Wiltshire Mental Health
Partnership NHS Trust,
Bristol, UK
Chapter 2: Music therapy
Chapter 5: Music therapy

Kevin Healy
Consultant Psychiatrist in Medical
Psychotherapy, New Dawn NHS
England Commissioned Inpatient
Tier 4 Assessment, Treatment
and Consultation Service for
Women with a Diagnosis of
Severe Personality Disorders,
Cygnet Healthcare, Ealing, UK;
Independent Practitioner in
Private Practice, London, UK
*Chapter 11: Neuroscience and
psychotherapy*

Jason Hepple
Chair of the Association for
Cognitive Analytic Therapy,
Consultant Psychiatrist in
Psychological Therapies,
Somerset Partnership NHS
Foundation Trust, UK
*Chapter 2: Cognitive analytic
therapy*
*Chapter 5: Cognitive analytic
therapy*

Jeremy Holmes
Visiting Professor, School of
Psychology, University of
Exeter, UK
Foreword

James Johnston
Consultant Psychiatrist in
Psychotherapy, Leeds and
York Partnership NHS
Foundation Trust, Leeds, UK;
British Psychoanalytic Council
Registered Member, North
of England Association of
Psychoanalytic Psychotherapists
(NEAPP), UK; Visiting
Lecturer, Tavistock and
Portman NHS Foundation
Trust, London, UK; Chair,
Royal College of Psychiatrists
Medical Psychotherapy Faculty
Education and Curriculum
Committee 2011–2015;
Member of the Association for
Psychoanalytic Psychotherapy in
the NHS, UK
*Chapter 1: Psychotherapeutic
medicine: thinking cradle to
grave*
Chapter 4: Consultation
*Chapter 7: Integrating
psychotherapy in psychiatry*
*Chapter 10: Reflective practice
groups*
*Chapter 12: General adult
psychiatry: medical psychotherapies,
applications, and research*

William Rhys Jones

Consultant Psychiatrist, Yorkshire Centre for Eating Disorders, Leeds and York Partnership NHS Foundation Trust, Seacroft Hospital, Leeds, UK
Chapter 7: Eating disorders

Ian Kerr

Honorary Consultant Psychiatrist and Psychotherapist, NHS Lanarkshire, Coathill Hospital, Coatbridge, Scotland
Chapter 2: Cognitive analytic therapy
Chapter 5: Cognitive analytic therapy

Wale Lagundoye

Clinical Director and Consultant Addiction Psychiatrist, Sheffield Health & Social Care NHS Foundation Trust, Sheffield, UK
Chapter 7: Substance misuse
Chapter 12: Psychiatry of addictions: psychotherapies, applications, and research

Roslyn Law

Consultant Clinical Psychologist, IPT Lead, Anna Freud Centre, London, UK; Assistant Director of Psychology and Psychotherapies, South West London and St George's Mental Health NHS Trust, Springfield Hospital, London, UK
Chapter 2: Interpersonal psychotherapy
Chapter 5: Interpersonal psychotherapy

Alessandra Lemma

Professor of Psychological Therapies, Tavistock and Portman NHS Trust/Essex University, UK; Visiting Professor, Psychoanalysis Unit, University College London, UK
Chapter 2: Dynamic interpersonal therapy
Chapter 5: Dynamic interpersonal therapy

Kath Lovell

Managing Director, Emergence CIC, London, UK
Chapter 10: Service user involvement

Vikram S Luthra

Consultant Psychiatrist, Becklin Centre, Leeds, UK; Hon. Lecturer, University of Leeds, Leeds, UK
Chapter 4: Is my patient suitable for psychotherapy?

Paul MacAllister

Consultant Psychiatrist in Forensic Psychotherapy, Wells Road Centre for Community Forensic Psychiatry, Nottingham, UK
Chapter 8: Personality disorder services

Brian Martindale

Consultant Psychiatrist, Nuffield Health Newcastle upon Tyne Hospital, Newcastle-upon-Tyne, UK
Chapter 7: Psychoses

Tristan McGeorge

Consultant Forensic Psychiatrist, Central and North West London NHS Foundation Trust, London, UK
Chapter 8: Psychological therapy in secure settings

Anuradha Menon

ST8 Dual Trainee in Psychoanalytic Psychotherapy and General Adult Psychiatry, Leeds and York Partnerships NHS Foundation Trust, Department of Psychotherapy, Leeds, UK; Department of Liaison Psychiatry, Leeds General Infirmary, Leeds, UK
Chapter 3: General therapeutic competencies

Marilyn Miller

Art Psychotherapist, Complex
Psychological Interventions Team,
Bristol Mental Health, Avon and
Wiltshire NHS Mental Health
Trust, Bath, UK
Chapter 2: Art psychotherapy
Chapter 5: Art psychotherapy

Sue Mizen

Consultant Psychiatrist in
Medical Psychotherapy Devon
Partnership NHS Trust, Wonford
House Hospital, Exeter, UK;
Chair of the Psychotherapy
Faculty Exec., Royal College of
Psychiatrists, UK
Chapter 8: Personality disorders

John Morgan

Consultant Psychiatrist, Yorkshire
Centre for Eating Disorders,
Leeds, UK; Senior Lecturer in
Eating Disorders, St George's
University of London, UK
Chapter 7: Eating disorders

Lou Morgan

Executive Director, Emergence
CIC, London, UK
*Chapter 10: Service user
involvement*

Mary Murphy-Ford

Consultant Child and Adolescent
Psychiatrist, Tavistock and
Portman NHS Foundation Trust,
London, UK; Locum Consultant
Psychiatrist and Psychotherapist
in Perinatal and Parent-Infant
Mental Health Service, Chelsea
and Westminster Hospital,
Central and North West
London NHS Foundation Trust,
London, UK
Chapter 6: Problems through life
*Chapter 12: Child and adolescent
psychiatry: child and adolescent
psychotherapies, applications, and
research*

Shari Mysorekar

Consultant Forensic Psychiatrist
and Medical Psychotherapist,
Stockton Hall Hospital, York, UK
*Chapter 3: General therapeutic
competencies*

Anton Obholzer

Emeritus Consultant, Tavistock
and Portman NHS Foundation
Trust, London, UK; Senior
Faculty, INSEAD French
International Business School
Global Leadership Centre,
Fontainebleau, France
*Chapter 10: Psychotherapeutic
understanding of organizational
processes*

Phil Osborne

Consultant Psychiatrist in
Medical Psychotherapy,
Specialist Psychotherapy Service,
Stockton-on-Tees, Tees Esk and
Wear Valleys NHS Foundation
Trust, UK
Chapter 4: Formulation

Zoe Otter

Forensic Psychologist in
Training, Partnerships in Care,
Nottinghamshire, UK
*Chapter 2: Dialectical behaviour
therapy*
*Chapter 5: Dialectical behaviour
therapy*

Aleksandar M Pavlovic

Higher Trainee in Medical
Psychotherapy and General
Adult Psychiatry, Leeds and York
Partnership NHS Foundation
Trust, Leeds Psychology and
Psychotherapy Service,
Leeds, UK
*Chapter 4: What type of therapy?,
Assessing the course of therapy,
Assessing the outcome of therapy*

Giovanni Polizzi

Consultant Psychiatrist in Medical
Psychotherapy, South London
and Maudsley NHS Foundation
Trust, London, UK
*Chapter 2: Mentalization-based
treatment*
*Chapter 5: Mentalization-based
treatment*

Ruta Rele

Consultant Psychiatrist in
Substance Misuse, Sheffield
Health and Social Care NHS
Foundation Trust, Sheffield, UK
Chapter 7: Substance misuse
*Chapter 12: Psychiatry of
addictions: psychotherapies,
applications, and research*

Florian Ruths

Consultant Psychiatrist & Cognitive
Therapist, South Lambeth
Assessment and Treatment Team,
Mood, Anxiety & Personality
Clinical Academic Group,
London, UK
*Chapter 2: Schema therapy,
Mindfulness-based interventions
and therapies*
*Chapter 5: Schema therapy,
Mindfulness-based interventions
and therapies*

Anna Seymour

Senior Lecturer in Dramatherapy,
Department of Psychology,
University of Roehampton,
London, UK
Chapter 2: Dramatherapy
Chapter 5: Dramatherapy

Eman Shweikh

Specialist Registrar (ST5) in
Forensic Psychiatry, Barnet,
Enfield and Haringey Mental
Health NHS Trust, London, UK
*Chapter 8: Psychological therapy
in secure settings*

Dinesh Sinha

Consultant Psychiatrist in
Psychotherapy, East London NHS
Foundation Trust, London, UK
*Chapter 10: Planning psychotherapy
services within psychiatric care,
Psychotherapy and management*

Gail Skillington

Consultant Forensic Psychologist,
Partnerships in Care,
Nottinghamshire, UK
*Chapter 2: Dialectical behavioural
therapy*
*Chapter 5: Dialectical behavioural
therapy*

Julian Stern

Consultant Psychiatrist in
Psychotherapy, Adult Dept,
Tavistock and Portman NHS
Trust, London, UK
*Chapter 7: Medically unexplained
symptoms*

Jo Stubley
Consultant Psychiatrist in Psychotherapy, Adult Dept, Tavistock and Portman NHS Trust, London, UK; Clinical Lead, Adult Trauma Services, Tavistock and Portman NHS Trust, London, UK; Member British Psychoanalytic Society, UK
Chapter 7: Trauma-related conditions

Kristy Summers
Forensic Psychologist in Training, Partnerships in Care, Nottinghamshire, UK
Chapter 2: Dialectical behaviour therapy
Chapter 5: Dialectical behaviour therapy

David Taylor
Visiting Professor, Psychoanalysis Unit, Research Department of Clinical, Educational & Health Psychology, University College London, UK; Honorary Consultant Psychotherapist, Tavistock and Portman NHS Foundation Trust, London, UK
Chapter 7: Affective disorders

Antonio Ventriglio
Section of Psychiatry, University of Foggia, Department of Clinical and Experimental Medicine, Foggia, Italy
Chapter 7: Sexual dysfunction

Jessica Yakeley
Fellow of the British Psychoanalytical Society, Consultant Psychiatrist in Forensic Psychotherapy, Portman Clinic; Director of Medical Education and Associate Medical Director, Tavistock and Portman NHS Foundation Trust, London UK; Editor of Psychoanalytic Psychotherapy, UK
Chapter 1: Medical psychotherapy: what is it?
Chapter 2: Concepts and models: introduction, Psychoanalytic psychotherapy
Chapter 4: Psychodynamic assessment and psychotherapy
Chapter 5: Psychoanalytic psychotherapy
Chapter 6: Violence and aggression
Chapter 7: Paraphilias
Chapter 8: Antisocial personality disorder, Narcissistic and histrionic personality disorders
Chapter 11: Research in psychotherapy
Chapter 12: Forensic psychiatry: forensic psychotherapies, applications, and research

Symbols and abbreviations

£	pound sterling
$	dollar
AAI	Adult Attachment Interview
ACAT	Association for Cognitive Analytic Therapy
ACT	acceptance and commitment therapy
ADHD	attention-deficit/hyperactivity disorder
A&E	accident and emergency
AIS	androgen insensitivity syndrome
AMT	analytical music therapy
AN	anorexia nervosa
APA	American Psychiatric Association
APT	adaptive pacing therapy
ASC	altered state of consciousness
ASD	acute stress disorder
ASPD	antisocial personality disorder
AvPD	avoidant personality disorder
BAAT	British Association of Art Therapists
BABCP	British Association of Behavioural and Cognitive Psychotherapies
BACP	British Association for Counselling and Psychotherapy
BADth	British Association of Dramatherapists
BAMT	British Association of Music Therapists
BCT	behavioural couples therapy
BDD	body dysmorphic disorder
BDNF	brain-derived neurotropic factor
BED	binge eating disorder
BMGIM	Bonny Method of Guided Imagery and Music
BMI	body mass index
BMT	behavioural music therapy
BN	bulimia nervosa
BPA	British Psychoanalytic Association
BPAS	British Psychoanalytical Society
BPC	British Psychoanalytic Council

BPD	borderline personality disorder
BPF	British Psychotherapy Foundation
BPSD	behavioural and psychological symptoms of dementia
CAH	congenital adrenal hyperplasia
CAMHS	child and adolescent mental health services
CAT	cognitive analytic therapy
CBT	cognitive behavioural therapy
CBTp	cognitive behavioural therapy for psychosis
CCRT	Core Conflictual Relationship Theme
CCT	Certificate of Core Training; Certificate of Completion of Training
CFS	chronic fatigue syndrome
CM	contingency management
CMHT	community mental health team
COPP	Commission on Psychotherapy by Psychiatrists
CORE	Centre for Outcomes Research and Effectiveness; Clinical Outcomes in Routine Evaluation
CORE-OM	Clinical Outcomes in Routine Evaluation–Outcome Measure
CPA	Care Programme Approach
CPD	continuing professional development
CPN	community psychiatric nurse
CRM	comprehensive resource model
CROM	clinician-rated outcome measure
DANOS	Drug and Alcohol National Occupational Standards
DBT	dialectical behavioural therapy
DEXA	dual-energy X-ray absorptiometry
DIP	Drug Intervention Programme
DIT	dynamic interpersonal therapy
DLB	dementia with Lewy bodies
DNA	deoxyribonucleic acid
DPD	dependent personality disorder
DRA	differential reinforcement of alternate behaviour
DRI	differential reinforcement of incompatible behaviour
DRO	differential reinforcement of other behaviour
DSM-5	*Diagnostic and Statistical Manual of Mental Disorders*, fifth edition

DSPD	Dangerous and Severe Personality Disorder
DZ	dizygotic
EBD	emotional and behavioural difficulties
EBP	evidence-based practice
EFT	energy-focused therapy
EMDR	eye movement desensitization and reprocessing
EPR	embodiment–projection–role
FPS	Forensic Psychotherapy Society
FSS	functional somatic syndromes
GA	group analysis
GAD	generalized anxiety disorder
GET	graded exercise therapy
GIM	guided imagery and music
GLM	Good Lives Model
GMC	General Medical Council
GMP	*Good Medical Practice*
GP	general practitioner
GPSQ	Gender Preoccupation and Stability Questionnaire
HCPC	Health and Care Professions Council
HPC	Health Professions Council
HPD	histrionic personality disorder
IAFP	International Association for Forensic Psychotherapy
IAPT	Improving Access to Psychological Therapies
IBS	irritable bowel syndrome
ICATA	International Cognitive Analytic Therapy Association
ICD	International Classification of Diseases
IDD	intellectual and developmental disorder
IDTS	Integrated Drug Treatment System
IGA	Institute of Group Analysis
IPA	International Psychoanalytic Association
IPAF	interpersonal affective pattern
IPP	Imprisonment for Public Protection
IPT	interpersonal therapy
IQ	intelligence quotient
JCHPT	Joint Committee on Higher Psychiatric Training
kcal	kilocalorie
kg	kilogram

KUF	Knowledge and Understanding Framework
LHRH	luteinizing hormone-releasing hormone
LPPU	London Pathways Progression Unit
LTC	long-term condition
m	metre
MA	Master of Arts
MAPPP	multi-agency public protection panels
MBCT	mindfulness-based cognitive therapy
MBI	mindfulness-based interventions
MBRP	mindfulness-based relapse prevention
MBSR	mindfulness-based stress reduction
MBT	mentalization-based treatment
MBT-ASC	MBT adherence and competence scale
MCI	mild cognitive impairment
mg	milligram
MHA	Mental Health Act
MI	motivational interviewing
mRNA	messenger ribonucleic acid
MSc	Master of Science
MSSM	multiple self-states model
MUS	medically unexplained symptoms
MZ	monozygotic
NCD	mild neurocognitive disorder
NHS	National Health Service
NICE	National Institute for Health and Care Excellence
NMDA	*N*-methyl-*D*-aspartate
NMT	neurologic music therapy
NPD	narcissistic personality disorder
OCD	obsessive–compulsive disorder
OMPFC	orbitomedial prefrontal cortex
OPCD	obsessive–compulsive personality disorder
OSAP	Offender Substance Abuse Programme
OSFED	other specified feeding or eating disorder
OT	occupational therapy/therapist
PBE	practice-based evidence
PCL-R	Psychopathy Checklist-Revised

PCPCS	Primary Care Psychotherapy and Consultation Service
PET	positron emission tomography
PFC	prefrontal cortex
PhD	Doctor of Philosophy
PICU	psychiatric intensive care unit
PIPE	Psychologically Informed Planned Environment
PIT	psychodynamic interpersonal therapy
PPD	paranoid personality disorder
PROM	patient-reported outcome measure
PRU	pupil referral unit
PSI	psychosocial interventions
PSQ	Personality Structure Questionnaire
PTSD	post-traumatic stress disorder
QALY	quality-adjusted life-year
RCT	randomized controlled trial
RMO	resident medical officer
RNR	risk–need–responsivity
RR	reciprocal role
RRP	reciprocal role procedure
SCIE	Social Care Institute for Excellence
SCM	structured clinical management
SD	somatization disorder
SDR	sequential diagrammatic reformulation
SFT	solution-focused therapy
SIG	Special Interest Group
SIGN	Scottish Intercollegiate Guidelines Network
SMC	specialist medical care
SMI	serious mental illness
SOTP	Sex Offender Treatment Programme
SPD	schizoid personality disorder
SSRI	selective serotonin reuptake inhibitor
StPD	schizotypal personality disorder
TC	therapeutic community
tf-CBT	trauma-focused cognitive behavioural therapy
TFP	transference-focused psychotherapy
TPP	target problem procedure

UK	United Kingdom
UKCP	United Kingdom Council for Psychotherapy
USA	United States
USP	unique selling point
VBP	values-based practice
VCM	vulnerable child mode
VRAG	Violence and Risk Appraisal Guide
WEMSS	Women's Enhanced Medium Secure Services
WFMT	World Federation of Music Therapy
WMA	World Medical Association
WPF	Westminster Pastoral Foundation
YSQ	Young Schema Questionnaire
ZPD	zone of proximal development

Introduction

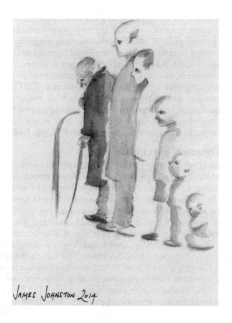

James Johnston 2014

Medical psychotherapy: what is it?

(See ➲ General adult psychiatry: medical psychotherapies, applications, and research in Chapter 12, pp. 544–50.)

Medical psychotherapy is one of the six psychiatry higher specialties approved by the General Medical Council (GMC) for specialist registration. Specialists in medical psychotherapy work with others to assess, manage, and treat people with mental health difficulties, using talking therapies and applied psychotherapeutic techniques in supervision, consultation, and reflective practice. Although the professional title *medical psychotherapist* is commonly used, consultant psychiatrist in psychotherapy, consultant psychiatrist in medical psychotherapy, and consultant medical psychotherapist are titles also used by psychiatrists trained as psychotherapists with a Certificate of Completion of Training (CCT) in medical psychotherapy.

Medical psychotherapy is a small medical specialty, with around 50 higher trainees nationally at any one time, and around 140 consultant medical psychotherapists (RCPsych survey 2015), many of whom are in less than full-time National Health Service (NHS) consultant medical psychotherapy posts. Currently, medical psychotherapy training involves 3 years in core psychiatry training, followed by a further 3 years of higher specialty training for a single CCT in medical psychotherapy alone, or 5 years for a dual CCT in medical psychotherapy and another psychiatric specialty. Accredited dual training programmes for medical psychotherapy and forensic psychiatry (forensic psychotherapy) were initiated nationally in 1999, and dual training programmes for medical psychotherapy and general adult psychiatry have become increasingly popular in the past decade and are now offered by most deaneries in the United Kingdom (UK). All higher psychotherapy trainees are required to achieve competencies in the three major modalities of psychoanalytic psychotherapy, cognitive behavioural psychotherapy (CBT), and family (systemic) therapy, and to choose one in which to 'major' or specialize. This is usually psychoanalytic psychotherapy, although a few trainees may choose cognitive behavioural therapy as their major modality (see ➲ Training in medical psychotherapy in Chapter 12, pp. 548–9).

History of medical psychotherapy

How did psychotherapy emerge as a separate specialty within psychiatry? Until the First World War, psychiatry in the UK was primarily concerned with the treatment of mentally ill patients within large mental hospitals or asylums. At the beginning of the last century, Ernest Jones, a psychiatrist, became interested in psychotherapy and psychoanalysis, travelled to Vienna to work with Freud, and, in 1924, founded the Institute of Psychoanalysis in London. During the First World War and the presentation of many of its survivors with shell shock, there was increasing interest in neurotic, or non-psychotic, disorders. This led to the founding of the Tavistock Clinic and the Cassel Hospital in London, both institutions that were interested in investigating and developing psychoanalytic ideas. During the Second World War, this interest continued and developed into group and therapeutic community treatments, stimulated by the work of psychiatrists such as Wilfred Bion, Tom Main, and Siegmund Heinrich Foulkes. In 1948, the NHS was formed; some institutions, such as the Cassel Hospital, the Portman Clinic, and the Tavistock Clinic, all elected to become part of the NHS, whereas the Institute of Psychoanalysis chose to remain independent. Psychoanalytic therapy, both in the private sector and within the NHS, remained predominantly based in London, although a few outposts began to form in cities such as Edinburgh, Leeds, and Newcastle, and a few training organizations were founded outside of London such as the Scottish Institute of Human Relations.

Meanwhile, medical doctors treating psychiatric patients were still known as physicians in psychological medicine, and psychiatry was seen as a branch of medicine and neurology. It was not until 1971 that the Royal College of Psychiatrists was founded, and, in 1975, psychotherapy was recognized by the then Department of Health and Social Security as a separate specialty within psychiatry, along with general psychiatry, child and adolescent psychiatry, forensic psychiatry, and psychiatry of mental handicap (now psychiatry of intellectual disability). The Joint Committee on Higher Psychiatric Training (JCHPT) was established in the 1970s to oversee the higher training programmes in each of the psychiatric specialties. The number of higher training posts in psychotherapy increased over the 1980s and 1990s to its current level and has remained relatively stable, despite several changes in the commissioning and delivery of postgraduate medical education since then. The number of consultant posts in medical psychotherapy also increased to reach a peak of almost 100 full-time equivalent posts nationally in 2006 but has subsequently reduced to its current levels, and remains under threat of further reduction with the recent decommissioning of psychoanalytic psychotherapy services and the perception that all psychological treatments can be as effectively delivered by less expensive, non-medically trained therapists.

Medical psychotherapy in the NHS has been predominantly psychoanalytic in orientation and, until recently, has been delivered in psychotherapy departments underpinned by psychoanalytic principles, based in psychiatric (or sometimes medical) hospitals or, more recently, mental health trusts, and led by consultant medical psychotherapists. These psychotherapy departments remained relatively separate from departments of psychology, which tended to be based in universities and other academic institutions, and which trained psychologists in behavioural and cognitive, rather than psychoanalytic, models. Moreover, a close interrelationship existed between psychotherapy in the NHS and the private sector, particularly in matters of training. Until a little over a decade ago, almost all medical psychotherapists were additionally trained in psychoanalysis or in psychoanalytic psychotherapy at private training institutions such as the Institute of Psychoanalysis, the (then) British Association of Psychotherapists and the Scottish Institute of Human Relations, and the North of England Association for Psychoanalytic Psychotherapists.

In recent years, with an increasing emphasis on commissioning only 'evidence-based' treatments, CBT and other briefer forms of therapy more successfully demonstrating their clinical effectiveness in empirical studies than psychoanalytic psychotherapy, and the growth of alternative government-funded psychological therapy services such as Improving

Access to Psychological Therapies (IAPT) in primary care, traditional psychotherapy departments with a more long-term psychodynamic focus have been under threat. Some, such as the therapeutic community, the Henderson Hospital, have been forced to close altogether, whilst others have been reduced in size and decentralized, encouraged to move into community mental health teams (CMHTs) and to provide a range of briefer therapies, including CBT, and to use outcome measures on a regular basis. Others have been reconfigured into specific services for more complex conditions such as personality disorders or medically unexplained symptoms, rather than continuing to treat patients with a range of problems, including anxiety, depression, and less well-defined difficulties in their lives and relationships, who are increasingly being seen within primary care. Not surprisingly, these changes have created anxieties and tensions, resulting in more psychoanalytic psychotherapists leaving their NHS work to go into full-time private practice, and concerns about the future of psychoanalytic psychotherapy within the public sector.

Why *medical* psychotherapy?

Psychotherapy today, both within the NHS and in the private and voluntary sectors, encompasses a vast field offering numerous different therapeutic treatment modalities, practised by a multidisciplinary workforce with different core professional backgrounds and varying levels of specialist psychotherapy training. Moreover, the boundary between counselling and psychotherapy is not clear-cut; the development of psychotherapeutic competencies may be thought of as incorporating increasing levels of complexity, depth, and expertise, from a basic psychotherapeutic stance and supportive attitude that all practitioners in mental health should demonstrate to the sophisticated knowledge and application of theories and techniques of the trained psychotherapist. However, the idea of levels may be too simplistic; some might argue that supportive therapy is the most difficult and requires the most training, and there are many experienced and gifted counsellors who offer a carefully thought-out integration of different therapeutic approaches appropriately tailored to the needs of the individual.

Within the multi-professional psychotherapy workforce, medically trained psychotherapists comprise only a small minority. Most talking therapies available within the NHS are now delivered by clinical psychologists and therapists from other core disciplines, including nursing, social work, and child psychotherapy. However, the tripartite training and qualifications as doctor, psychiatrist, and specialist psychotherapist (whether psychoanalytic, cognitive behavioural, or systemic) place the medical psychotherapist in a distinctive position of bridging the gap between two of the dominant paradigms in the care of the mentally ill—the physical paradigm and the psychological paradigm. As a medical doctor, the medical psychotherapist is trained to understand the structure and function of the body and brain; to take a systematic approach to assessment, formulation, and treatment; and to take on responsibility and leadership roles. As a psychiatrist, the medical psychotherapist has an extensive biopsychosocial training in the assessment, formulation, and treatment of mental disorders; has undergone psychotherapy training in at least three different therapeutic modalities, and is expert in at least one; and takes a developmental perspective on mental life which affords integration of past with present in planning the patient's pathway and care process. The medical psychotherapist is therefore able to integrate physical and psychological perspectives and offer a bridge between psychiatry, psychotherapy, general practice, and allied mental health professions, championing the development of a psychotherapeutic psychiatry and ensuring that high-quality, therapeutically informed services are maintained. By being a doctor of body, brain, and mind, the medical psychotherapist is conversant with the latest research in neuroscience and treatment efficacy, yet remains aware of the central therapeutic value of relationships and, as such, is able to offer a range of approaches and therapeutic interventions that produce effective and meaningful outcomes for patients and their families.

What does the medical psychotherapist do?

The consultant in medical psychotherapy holds an essential role in both the clinical and training spheres within mental health, as well as being active within management, leadership, academia, and research.

- Clinical—this is manifest in both direct and indirect contributions to their organizations:
  - Direct clinical role: undertaking assessments and delivering treatment (therapy) for individuals with severe and/or complex psychopathology, e.g. personality disorder, dual diagnosis, medically unexplained symptoms, eating disorders
  - Indirect clinical role: interventions in helping mental health providers to support staff teams and professionals from different disciplines through supervision, consultation, and reflective practice.
- Training (see → Psychotherapeutic medicine: *thinking cradle to grave* in Chapter 1, pp. 8–12)—within medicine and psychiatry, the medical psychotherapist promotes therapeutic professional development from medical school through foundation, core, advanced, and post-membership years for psychiatrists in mental health:
  - Medical psychotherapists are leading the development of medical school psychotherapy schemes and Balint groups for medical students across the UK, in which the exposure of medical students to reflection on their relationship with patients enhances their interpersonal insight and skills for their future as doctors and contributes to a more therapeutically aware medical workforce.
  - Consultant psychiatrists in medical psychotherapy also have an essential role in ensuring that the curriculum requirements for postgraduate psychotherapy training in core and advanced psychiatry are met. Within psychiatry, trainees are required to demonstrate competency in psychotherapy during their core psychiatry training, and are expected to continue to develop these competencies as they progress through advanced psychiatry training. The crucial role of the consultant psychiatrist in psychotherapy in leading psychotherapy training in psychiatry was evidenced in the first Royal College of Psychiatrists' Medical Psychotherapy survey of psychotherapy training in psychiatry in 2012, which showed that the College curriculum was more likely

to be fulfilled if the Psychotherapy Tutor possessed a medical psychotherapy CCT. The GMC undertook a quality assurance review of medical psychotherapy in 2012, and their findings replicated those of the Medical Psychotherapy survey, which led to an action plan, including the requirement that all core psychotherapy training in psychiatry should be led by a consultant psychiatrist in psychotherapy. This medical psychotherapy leadership role was incorporated in the core curriculum in March 2015.
  - Medical psychotherapists also contribute to the continuing professional development (CPD) of consultant psychiatrists and other professionals in health, social care, criminal justice, education, and other fields through teaching, supervision, consultation, and reflective practice.
- Management and leadership:
  - Designing and delivering effective psychological therapy services that will be commissioned in the current evidence-based rationed health economy
  - Ensuring robust clinical governance frameworks for psychological therapy services regarding safety, quality, and effectiveness of services
  - Developing and maintaining psychological, social, and cultural health in institutions
  - Promoting public understanding of mental health.
- Academic and research:
  - Promoting practice-based evidence: evidencing the effectiveness of treatment services via the meaningful monitoring of therapeutic outcomes and patient experience
  - Promoting evidence-based practice: knowing and disseminating the evidence base for the effectiveness of psychological therapies
  - Involvement in formal research projects both quantitative, e.g. empirical studies of treatment effectiveness, and qualitative, e.g. studies of patient experience of treatment
  - Links with other research fields, e.g. attachment, neuroscience, infant and child development
  - Developing and refining research paradigms to address the complexity of psychotherapeutic experience.

Layout of the handbook

The book comprises 12 main chapters, each divided into sections. The first chapter introduces medical psychotherapy as a distinct psychiatric specialty and describes the development and nurturance of a psychotherapeutic attitude within medicine and psychiatry in all stages of a doctor's career from medical student to senior clinician.

The next four chapters comprehensively cover both the generic and specific principles of the medical psychotherapy modalities that we have chosen as being most representative of those delivered within mental health services in the UK. Chapter 2 starts with an overview of the theoretical and philosophical debates regarding the proliferation of different models of psychotherapy within the field and is followed by separate sections for each psychotherapy modality, describing their theoretical frameworks, concepts, trainings, and research evidence. Chapter 3 details the general therapeutic competencies that are needed across all of the modalities, focusing on the development of the therapeutic alliance and engaging the patient, handling emotions, dealing with breaks and endings, assessing and managing risk, and using clinical supervision. Chapter 4 covers the many different aspects of assessment in psychotherapy, with particular focus on the two main modalities of psychodynamic treatment and CBT, and includes guidance on how to assess patient suitability, choosing the most appropriate and available psychotherapy, how to complete a psychotherapeutic formulation, and what constitutes a consultation in psychotherapy. Chapter 5 mirrors Chapter 2 in consisting of sections for each specific psychotherapy modality, describing the different components of treatment: the key techniques and competencies, how these specific interventions effect change, the clinical populations treated, and two clinical vignettes, the first describing the treatment of a more straightforward case and the second detailing a more complex case. All of the clinical examples in the book are based on real cases, but the details are sufficiently disguised and altered to protect patient confidentiality.

Chapter 6 gives an account of human life through a psychodynamic lens, from a developmental view of the lifespan from infancy to old age; through the lived experience of interpersonal relationships, gender, sexuality, ethnicity, and culture; to an exploration of the disruptions and traumas that may puncture and alter our existence in fundamental ways. Although this chapter exposes the psychoanalytic bias of its editors, it also reveals universal life themes and challenges the boundary between what might be considered normal and what might be considered pathological within the wide and diverse spectrum of human experience.

Although, in general, we espouse a more dimensional than categorical approach to psychiatric nosology, Chapters 7 and 8 are organized according to diagnostic categories in line with contemporary psychiatric classifications of mental disorders. Diagnostic terms and criteria are those of the *Diagnostic and Statistical Manual of Mental Disorders*, fifth edition (DSM-5), with additional reference to International Classification of Diseases (ICD)-10 when indicated. Chapter 7 describes the main psychotherapeutic approaches and interventions used in the full range of mental conditions, developmental disorders, and intellectual disabilities encountered within psychiatric practice, and promotes an integrative approach that reflects a true implementation of the biopsychosocial model. The important topic of personality disorder has been allowed a chapter to itself in Chapter 8; this not only allows space to describe the wealth of exciting advances in the understanding of the aetiology of these conditions which have informed the development of more effective treatments for disorders which many believed were untreatable, but also this is because we believe medical psychotherapists are uniquely qualified to treat people with personality disorders, for whom a therapeutic approach encompassing considerations of body, mind, emotions, behaviours and relationships with self and other is critical.

Chapters 9, 10, and 11 cover topics that are relevant to all clinical practice and demonstrate the value of a psychotherapeutic perspective. Key issues regarding the ethics and boundaries of medical and psychiatric care, including legal and moral considerations, are explored in Chapter 9. Chapter 10 describes the application of psychotherapeutic principles and services within the wider health care system, focusing on management, teaching and consultation, organizational dynamics, and, most importantly, the meaningful involvement of patients and service users in the planning and delivery of services. Chapter 11 summarizes the historical and current findings and trends in the rapidly advancing field of psychotherapy research and its links with neuroscience, now encompassing a substantive body of empirical studies that demonstrate the treatment efficacy of specific therapeutic interventions and the neurobiological correlates of mechanisms of psychic change.

Finally, Chapter 12 explores the relationship between medical psychotherapy and the other specialties and trainings within psychiatry, from general adult psychiatry to the smaller psychiatric sub-specialties of child and adolescent, forensic, intellectual disability, old age, addictions, liaison, and rehabilitation and social psychiatry. Each section in this chapter addresses the clinical applications, research evidence, and trainings involved in the psychotherapeutic interventions within each respective psychiatric specialty, revealing the central role that medical psychotherapy plays within the discipline of psychiatry.

As with other books in the *Oxford Specialist Handbooks in Psychiatry* series, we have tried to keep the text concise and to the point (as much as is possible for psychotherapists!), highlighting key facts and topics, sometimes at the expense of fuller detail and discussion. This is because the series consists of handbooks for clinicians that promote brevity and ease of reference, rather than comprehensive textbooks. Referencing has therefore been kept to a minimum and has been replaced by recommended reading lists at the end of each section or chapter. Because there is some overlap between different parts of the book, topics are cross-referenced within all of the chapters and their sections.

Recommended reading

General Medical Council. *Small Specialties Thematic Review: Quality Assurance Report for Medical Psychotherapy 2011–2012.* Available at: ℗ http://www.gmc-uk.org/Medical_psychotherapy—report—FINAL.pdf_51696150.pdf.

Pedder J (1996). Psychotherapy in the British National Health Service: a short history. *Free Associations* 6(1): 14–27.

Royal College of Psychiatrists (2006). *Council Report CR139: Role of the Consultant Psychiatrist in Psychotherapy,* Royal College of Psychiatrists: London.

Royal College of Psychiatrists and Royal College of General Practitioners (2008). *College Report CR151: Psychological Therapies in Psychiatry and Primary Care (2008).* Royal College of Psychiatrists: London.

Psychotherapeutic medicine: *thinking cradle to grave*

The cradle and the grave that the reader is invited to think about in the title refer both to the history and personal development of the patient and to the professional development of the doctor. In relation to the patient, the cradle and the grave represent the developmental extremes of life and the depth of potential disturbance arising from these extremes.

The doctor is, of course, being human, also exposed to the same cradle to grave extremes of potential disturbance. The *cradle* signifies primitive developmental states of mind, and the *grave* signifies the gravity of facing death or mourning loss and the anxiety about death which can arise out of unbearable states of mind. In psychiatry, the *cradle* signifies confronting the sometimes devastating impact of primitive emotional disturbance and the anxieties that surround the *grave* emanating from the risk of death.

Socrates observed that the unexamined life is not worth living. It might be said that the unexamined mind is borne from the feeling that life is not worth living. The vicissitudes of living contribute to, and maintain, mental pain. The doctor who approaches the person in physical pain will recall the medical phrase 'on examination.' The reflective doctor approaching another in mental pain will also consider their own emotional responses, so that the examined mind becomes a reflexive process which includes the doctor's examination and use of their responses to understand the patient.

Psychotherapeutic medicine involves a *therapeutic attitude* which validates the emotional experience of the doctor as a source of learning about the emotional experience of the person who presents to them. A therapeutic attitude would not be a state of peace and calm, because it reflects engagement in the challenges of being alive; it involves feelings across the human range and being involved in the problems of being human. If a therapeutic attitude is idealized as seeking a state of stillness, contemplation, and self-reflection in a meditative state, then the ordinary struggle of being alive is missed. Live emotional contact with the person beyond the presenting problem includes emotional contact for the doctor with their own mind, and this is the aim of the self-reflective practice intended learning outcome ('ILO-19') which was included in the core curriculum of training for all psychiatrists in 2014. The inclusion of self-reflective practice is one of the strategic aims of the Medical Psychotherapy Faculty Education and Curriculum Committee, embodied in its *Thinking Cradle to Grave* strategy which aims toward the development of psychotherapeutic medicine and psychiatry (Johnston 2015). An idea central to this aim is that being a doctor involves emotional work for the doctor in order to remain engaged with the emotional life of the patient, and this requires recognized and protected space for self-reflective practice.

Because a therapeutic attitude is integral to the development of the doctor, this self-reflective capacity needs to be nurtured at medical school (the cradle) and to continue to be developed throughout the doctor's career, all the way to retirement (the grave). As a spiral curriculum of emotional work, there can be a developing therapeutic attitude as the leitmotif of the core human threads of illness, disease, and dying is encountered and explored at a different developmental level from undergraduate to postgraduate levels.

Undergraduate therapeutic attitude

The emotional demands on a medical student may be in holding on to the recollection of what they brought with them in their vocation to train as a doctor, retaining a sense of the whole person's humanity, rather than 'the abdomen in bed eight.' The past in the present for the emerging doctor would be in recalling the ordinary uncertainties in the midst of extraordinary technical knowledge.

Postgraduate therapeutic attitude

In the postgraduate years, the student learns to become a doctor, and the struggle in this early phase of development will be in beginning to consciously and unconsciously sift positive and negative identifications between different mentors, as the student finds a professional mind of their own. The doctor who does not seek refuge in a scientific attitude or pursue the medical carapace of defensive practice, but is prepared to remain open to therapeutic risk in emotional terms and interested in meeting each patient as an individual, would be showing signs of emotional resilience and the possibility of growth.

In the early years as a consultant psychiatrist, the doctor grapples with their place as a leader, as well as learning to bear responsibility, risk, and uncertainty with patients, relinquishing reliance on systems of certainty from training and seniors. In the later years, the emotional demands of maintaining and developing creative interest in the work without despair and cynicism, which are not associated with the patient but, more commonly, the employing institution and management, are features of resilience in the mature consultant psychiatrist. Mature ambivalence and therapeutic literacy in a consultant psychiatrist may be revealed in their openness to continuing to learn from their work and remaining, in some way, still passionate about what they do, whilst cognizant of the limitations of what they personally can bear.

Medical psychotherapeutic attitude

One of the contributions of medical psychotherapists is to try to embody a therapeutic attitude in their institutions in their contacts with colleagues and managers. Their struggles in doing so within their context will, in their self-reflective practice, include trying to work to maintain an open mind. A closed mind is one in which curiosity is inhibited or deadened and reflection paralysed, otherwise known as 'burnout'. An open mind, in which curiosity remains possible and a cynical state of mind does not overwhelm a balanced outlook, can be very hard to maintain. Potent leadership does not deny, but recognizes, the challenges of fear and demoralization in systems in which there is increasing pressure to reduce resources, particularly where economic limitations take priority over cognizance of emotional limitations.

The three Rs

The three Rs for psychiatry, thinking in cradle to grave terms, are recruitment, renewal, and revalidation. A therapeutic attitude is pivotal to success in the three Rs, paradoxically by accommodating failure.

Recruitment

For psychiatry to attract doctors, it has to become more therapeutically minded. Psychiatry is not the place to begin; the beginning is in the other specialties of medicine and surgery, when the student first encounters patients. In the Royal College of Psychiatrists Medical Student Psychotherapy Schemes, the aim of introducing Balint groups (see ➲ Balint groups in Chapter 10, pp. 484–96) across all UK medical schools is being established, before psychiatry placements are undertaken by students. The aim is to develop psychotherapeutic medicine, and some of these student doctors may, as a side effect of this reflective practice, choose a career in psychiatry. The paradoxical failure here is that, whilst the schemes may not always be successful in recruiting doctors to psychiatry, more therapeutically minded doctors beyond psychiatry will be helped to develop.

Renewal

For those medical students who are inspired to become psychiatrists because they enjoy reflection and want to develop a psychotherapeutic attitude to patients, a renewal of psychotherapeutic psychiatry is vital to ensure it *retains* therapeutically minded psychiatrists. The paradoxical failure in this instance would be that, in the success of recruitment to psychiatry of therapeutically minded psychiatrists, psychotherapeutic psychiatry itself has failed to develop, and disillusioned new recruits leave, with a professional ratchet effect of loss further inhibiting renewal. Failure to mitigate this loss for psychiatry could foster a wake-up call for psychotherapeutic renewal to retain the therapeutically minded doctors.

Revalidation

The CPD of psychiatrists reflects their role as parental figures in training, who carry the culture for trainees. Their willingness to engage in developing their therapeutic attitude to psychiatry, for example, in participating in consultant psychiatrist Balint groups, would embody the need to feed the parents, in order to ensure recognition of the needs for a therapeutic feed in those who succeed them. Failure to accommodate the therapeutic grave for the seniors could help to write the obituary for the therapeutic cradle for the students and trainees who are the next generation of psychiatrists.

Psychotherapeutic psychiatry

The development of psychotherapeutic psychiatry involves recognition that the majority of people suffering from mental illness, personality disorder, mental pain, or mental deadness will not see medical psychotherapists, but many will see psychiatrists. A robust medical psychotherapeutic training that parallels and equals the potency of biological training is necessary for all psychiatrists, because it is necessary for all of their patients. This is not to suggest that all psychiatrists need to train as medical psychotherapists. We suggest that, for psychiatrists (and all mental health professionals) to be able to develop and maintain a capacity to bear and think with people suffering extreme mental disturbance, they need to sustain a clinical routine of protecting reflective space in which to examine their own emotions in response to the people who come to them.

The future of medical psychotherapy

Following the 2013 GMC requirement for medical psychotherapy leadership in core psychotherapy training schemes filtering through the zeitgeist, there are signs across the UK that some deaneries and local education training boards are appointing consultant psychiatrists in psychotherapy for the sole purpose of fulfilling the psychotherapy training for core psychiatry trainees. A strategic tension lies in the appointment of medical psychotherapy CCT holders solely to deliver psychotherapy training without a clinical context. The acceptance of this would, over time, erode the specialty of medical psychotherapy, as, without a clinical infrastructure, the delivery of psychotherapy training would take place in a psychiatric vacuum. This is not an adaptive response to extinction anxiety.

The GMC requirement that all medical psychotherapists and non-medical psychotherapists are in active practice is a welcome support to ensure that those who train psychiatrists practise what they teach. It is vital to maintain and develop psychotherapeutic psychiatry clinically, since, without this clinical context, psychotherapy training for psychiatrists becomes a marginal activity which defeats its purpose by reinforcing the peripheral position of psychotherapy in psychiatry as an activity fit for purpose solely in the Ivory Tower. Without psychotherapy, the profession of psychiatry is impoverished; the disappearance of medical psychotherapy would reinforce a prejudicial view of psychiatry as offering a reductionist medical model narrowly defined as being heavy on biology, but light on the social, cultural, and the psychotherapeutic.

However, psychotherapy inevitably evokes ambivalence in psychiatry, as it does in individuals, because it involves emotional work and making contact with painful realities. Giving a place for affective subjectivity in developing psychotherapeutic medicine challenges the professional pressure towards a reductive medical model by including the feelings of the doctor about their relationship with their patients. Medical psychotherapists represent this discomforting position within psychiatry, subverting the attraction towards a settled view of a patient in medical terms which disavows the ordinarily human perspective. The loss of a meaningful medical psychotherapy contribution in the robust clinical development of psychotherapeutic psychiatry would therefore contribute to the demise of psychiatry as a profession. Turning a blind eye to the cradle of thought in early development could lead to a grave risk of losing the therapeutic heart of psychiatry.

Recommended reading

General Medical Council. *Small Specialties Thematic Review: Quality Assurance Report for Medical Psychotherapy 2011–2012*. Available at: ℛ http://www.gmc-uk.org/Medical_psychotherapy—report—FINAL.pdf_51696150.pdf.

Hinshelwood R (2004). *Suffering Insanity: Psychoanalytic Essays on Psychosis*. Routledge: Hove and New York.

Johnston J (2015). *Thinking Cradle to Grave: Developing Psychotherapeutic Medicine and Psychiatry, iteration XIV*. Therapeutic Education Strategy of the Royal College of Psychiatrists Medical Psychotherapy Faculty Education and Curriculum Committee. ℛ https://www.rcpsych.ac.uk/pdf/Thinking%20Cradle%20to%20Grave%20final%20iteration%20XIV%2016th%20July%202015.pdf.

Main T (1989). Some medical defences against involvement with patients. In: John J, ed. *The Ailment and Other Psychoanalytic Essays*. Free Association Books: London.

Shoenberg P and Yakeley J (eds) (2014). *Learning about Emotions in Illness. The Role of Psychotherapeutic Teaching in Medical Education*. Routledge: London.

Concepts and models

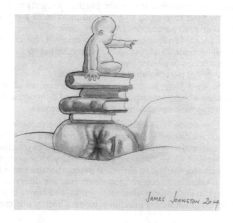

Concepts and models: introduction

Historical context

A broad historical overview of the psychotherapy movement might show that psychoanalysis dominated the first half of the twentieth century, to be gradually challenged by the rise of the cognitive behavioural and humanistic traditions from the 1970s onwards, the first major split occurring between psychoanalysis and behaviourism. However, from the inception of the psychoanalytic movement, theoretical disagreements occurred within the original Freudian model, resulting in professional rivalries, splits, and schisms, and the emergence of many different theoretical schools within psychoanalysis alone. This proliferation of differing models has continued throughout the psychotherapy field, so that, whilst in the 1950s only 36 different therapeutic approaches had been identified, by 1980, this had risen to around 250, and, by the end of the twentieth century it was estimated that there were over 400 named therapeutic modalities, and there is no indication that this rate of increase has abated.

The development of different therapeutic models has tended to be based less on scientifically accountable grounds, and more on marked differences in the theoretical opinions, professional and cultural identities, and the personalities of the, often charismatic and inspirational, founders of new therapies. This has led to a confusing, and arguably untenable, therapeutic landscape, in which modalities compete with each other in 'therapy wars' and which critics highlight as evidence that the field lacks scientific credibility and is more driven by the fame or profit-seeking motives of rivalrous leaders.

Models of therapy

Historically, specific models of psychotherapy tended to be thought of as primarily related to specific psychological theories of personality, rather than methods of treatment. Moreover, psychotherapists consciously or unconsciously tend to choose to train and practise in a model that is compatible with their personality and world view.

Horton has identified four basic elements that will constitute any particular model or modality of counselling or psychotherapy:

- Basic assumptions or philosophy
- Formal theory of personality and development
- Clinical theory defining goals, principles, and processes of change, and providing a cognitive map, giving a sense of direction and purpose
- Related therapeutic operations, skills, and techniques.

Therapeutic modalities are often classified under three main groupings or 'major modalities'—psychodynamic, cognitive behavioural, and humanistic/existential—reflecting the three main psychotherapeutic traditions that have emerged over the past century. However, this classification may be more suited to individual psychotherapy and is less helpful when one takes into account treatments that are delivered to more than one person in the form of couple, group, and family therapies, or those delivered to whole organizations. Indeed, both group therapy and family or systemic therapy may be considered to be psychotherapy traditions in their own right, within which different approaches from all of the aforementioned cognitive behavioural, psychoanalytic, and humanistic traditions have been incorporated. More recently, integrative therapies have emerged which combine specific elements from therapies from different traditions, as well as emphasize the effective ingredients or 'common factors' that are present in all therapies such as the therapeutic alliance or relationship.

Monism versus pluralism

A more global analysis of the state of the psychotherapeutic endeavour reveals theoretical antitheses between the paradigms of monism, purism, and specificity on the one hand, and of pluralism, eclecticism, and universality on the other.

Therapeutic monism or *purism* proposes that therapeutic modalities are differentiated by their own unique qualities, therapeutic approaches, and techniques and will have superior effects, compared to other methods or modalities, often related to specific diagnoses, e.g. CBT for obsessive–compulsive disorder (OCD). Limitations to this approach include the risks of minimizing the importance of therapeutic factors common to all psychotherapies, offering the patient only one choice of treatment which may not be appropriate to that individual's problem or personality, and destructive divisions and rivalries within the wider psychotherapy profession.

The monistic or purist approach tends to be allied with a model of *psychotherapeutic specificity*, based on a natural science paradigm in which, under defined circumstances, specific interventions will result in specific effects. Most outcome studies of psychotherapy are based on a specificity paradigm, in which one psychotherapeutic approach is compared to another, often for a well-defined pathological condition or diagnosis. This has led to a list of 'empirically supported' or 'evidence-based' psychotherapy treatments, of which the superiority to other treatment methods has been demonstrated by carefully designed studies, the gold standard methodology being the randomized controlled trial (RCT).

However, although there is some evidence that therapists who stick to one model obtain better results than those who use elements of different models, a consistent finding in psychotherapy research is that of the outcome equivalence of different therapies, in that no specific therapy has been shown to have greater efficacy than any other. This has been referred to as the '*Dodo effect*', based on the conclusion of the dodo in Lewis Carol's *Alice in Wonderland* that 'Everybody has won and all must have prizes'.

Pluralism, in contrast to monism, recognizes the value of many different perspectives or, in the case of psychotherapy, therapeutic models, and seeks to hold unity and diversity in balance. Pluralism embraces *universality*, as well as specificity, in highlighting the healing effects of universal or '*common factors*' that are not specific to particular approaches but form a basis to all psychotherapies, e.g. aspects of the therapeutic relationship such as warmth or empathy. A pluralistic therapist might work primarily within a specific model and would incorporate therapeutic concepts and methods from other models where they thought appropriate.

Eclecticism is less encompassing than pluralism in emphasizing the selecting out of techniques from a number of different approaches, without adhering to any particular model. It is a pragmatic and empiricist approach that is interested in identifying what works for each individual under specific circumstances. Pluralism and eclecticism have been criticized for being atheoretical, unscientific, and syncretic.

Integration

In practice, the majority of psychotherapists appear to occupy a middle ground between the purists and the pluralists, although it is difficult to gain an accurate picture, as many therapists who identify themselves publicly with a particular theoretical orientation or psychotherapeutic school may in private consciously and unconsciously draw from other therapeutic models in their clinical work. Some therapists, however, avow amalgamation explicitly and make a conscious effort to integrate therapeutic approaches, reflecting a trend within the contemporary psychotherapy field in general towards greater dialogue and cross-fertilization between researchers, theoreticians, and clinicians from different therapeutic orientations, but also resulting in a specific therapeutic modality termed 'psychotherapy integration'.

Norcross and Newman have identified three main routes towards integration:

- *Common factors* (see ➜ Common factor research, pp. 519–22): this approach highlights the non-specific factors that appear to be effective across all therapeutic modalities. The common factor approach, as originally conceptualized by Jerome Frank, sees psychotherapy as a socially constructed healing process, in which the adoption by the therapist of a credible theory is only one factor amongst other common factors that will contribute to change. More recently, Laska *et al.* (2014) have defined these necessary common factors as:
  - An emotionally charged bond between the patient and therapist
  - A confiding healing setting in which therapy takes place
  - A therapist who provides a psychologically derived and culturally embedded explanation for emotional distress
  - An explanation of therapy that is adaptive and accepted by the patient
  - A set of procedures that is engaged by the patient and therapist that leads the patient to enact something positive, helpful, or adaptive.
- *Technical eclecticism*: here therapists select out and combine empirically supported techniques, skills, and strategies from a range of approaches, without completely adopting the theoretical model behind the intervention. Examples include Beutler's systematic eclectic therapy and Larzarus's multimodal therapy.
- *Theoretical integration*: this approach focuses on theories, not just interventions, seeking to find the points of convergence between different theoretical approaches to produce a more comprehensive,

coherent, and effective treatment. Examples include cognitive analytic therapy (CAT) (see ➔ Cognitive analytic therapy in Chapter 2, pp. 47–52, and in Chapter 5, pp. 194–202), psychodynamic interpersonal therapy (PIT) (see ➔ Psychodynamic interpersonal therapy in Chapter 2, pp. 56–61, and in Chapter 5, pp. 207–14), and dynamic interpersonal therapy (DIT) (see ➔ Dynamic interpersonal therapy in Chapter 2, pp. 61–63, and in Chapter 5, pp. 215–20).

Medical psychotherapy modalities

Clearly, of the vast array of different therapy modalities identified in the literature and clinical practice, we are only able to present a small fraction, which we propose may be grouped under the category of 'medical psychotherapy modalities'. These include the major modalities—psychoanalytic/ psychodynamic, cognitive behavioural, systemic and group therapies—in which all medical psychotherapists receive intensive training, as well as other modalities that have emerged from one or more of these traditions originally for the treatment of specific diagnostic categories, such as depression or personality disorder, such as IPT, CAT, dialectical behavioural therapy (DBT), or mentalization-based treatment (MBT). We have tried to include the modalities that are most commonly available in the NHS, representing those that medical psychotherapists would be expected to encounter or are able to refer to in their clinical practice.

To some extent, the selection in this first edition of the book reflects a bias towards the psychoanalytic tradition, which historically was the primary therapeutic orientation of the majority of medically qualified psychotherapists, who trained as psychoanalysts and applied psychoanalytic ideas into the development of psychodynamic psychotherapies at institutions such as the Tavistock Clinic and Cassel Hospital in London after the Second World War, and subsequently founded psychotherapy departments within the NHS in other parts of the UK. By contrast, the development and practice of CBT in the UK has tended to remain dominated by clinical psychologists. However, all medically qualified psychotherapists, whether or not their primary orientation is psychodynamic, must also be trained in CBT, which today represents the commonest modality available within the NHS, due to both the greater strength of its evidence base and its shorter-term nature than psychoanalytic and other psychotherapies.

In a rationed managed care system, treatments in general are increasingly having to demonstrate their effectiveness, and psychotherapy has perhaps had to prove its case more strongly than biomedical interventions. Therapies which lack a credible evidence base are less likely to be commissioned, and patients, policy makers, and society in general rightly want to know that treatments work. We strongly believe that all psychotherapists should also be curious as to whether and how the therapy they are offering is safe and effective, and be open to changing their theories and techniques when there is evidence that they may be ineffective or even harmful. We have therefore highlighted the importance of research throughout this book, and all of the chapters in this section describe the evidence base for each psychotherapy modality.

We have omitted the somatic experiencing therapies such as senso-rimotor therapy, energy-focused therapy (EFT), and the comprehensive resource model (CRM) that have been developed for the treatment of trauma and its sequelae. Eye movement desensitization and reprocessing (EMDR) is also not included as a distinct section. This is because these therapies are not practised extensively by medically trained psychother-apists, psychiatrists, or non-medical psychotherapists in the NHS at the time of writing the book. However, in the context of an ambivalent, but increasing, rapprochement between neuroscience and psychotherapy, it is possible that the neurological body/brain basis of the ego Freud rec-ognized will be reflected in more use of these so-called body therapies. Freud's abandoned Project for a Scientific Psychology (1950 [1895]) was his first attempt to offer a neurological basis for psychology. It is of inter-est, given the focus on early affective experience in development, that these recent body therapies do not refer to their Freudian antecedent though use some of his earlier techniques, e.g. tapping on a patient's forehead and face, with its echo of his trials of a forehead 'pressure technique' which Freud relinquished, along with hypnosis. A limitation in the focus on the somatic brain may reflect the scientific privilege of mat-ter over meaning, with a movement from symbol to symbolic equation where brain changes are equated with psychic changes as a form of 'body armour' to defend the science of psychotherapy which has a different view about the meaning of what the matter is.

Our choice of modalities also reveals a bias towards excluding thera-pies from the humanistic-existential tradition such as person-centred therapy, existential therapy, gestalt therapy, and transactional analysis. We have also omitted therapies from other approaches, such as the inte-grative and pluralistic, and those derived from systemic and constructiv-ist views such as solution-focused and narrative therapies.

Whilst we acknowledge that many counsellors and psychotherapists are increasingly offering these therapies, they are mostly only available in the private sector and tend to have less of an evidence base to date than those from the psychodynamic, and particularly the cognitive behav-ioural stable.

This reveals a leaning towards the monism/specificity model of psy-chotherapy, aligned with a natural science paradigm described above, in which the term 'medical psychotherapy' fits more comfortably with a medical model and, as such, may be more integrated within the dis-cipline of psychiatry. However, we also are aware of the limitations of the positivistic paradigm that has dominated British psychiatry with its emphasis on empiricism and objectivity, and would argue that more nuanced qualitative, subjective, and holistic approaches, drawing from the social sciences and humanistic traditions, are also necessary for the psychotherapeutic study of the multitude of psychic processes, cogni-tive, emotional, and somatic states, and modes of relating that make up human nature.

Training in medical psychotherapies

All psychiatrists must complete training in the major psychotherapy modalities, as part of their core curriculum set by the Royal College of

Psychiatrists, and a consultant psychiatrist in medical psychotherapy will have received a further three to five years of formal specialist and intensive training leading to a Certificate of Core Training (CCT) in Medical Psychotherapy (see ➜ Chapter 12). Similarly, all clinical psychologists will receive formal training in CBT and other modalities. However, many psychotherapists do not have a core medical or psychology discipline background, and there has been wide variance in the standard and quality of trainings in counselling and psychotherapy in general in the UK over the years.

Marked differences between trainings exist regarding qualification at entry requirements, length of training, requirements for personal therapy and supervision, number of hours of supervised clinical practice, and the theoretical content of courses. Statutory regulation of the psychotherapy profession, despite being on the political agenda for many years, has to date not been realized beyond assured voluntary regulation. This contrasts sharply with the well-established regulation of doctors and medical education by the GMC. Psychotherapy and counselling are therefore regulated on a voluntary basis by professional bodies with overlapping membership with varied ethical structures and complaint and fitness to practise procedures in place.

The main UK psychotherapy organizations are the British Association for Counselling and Psychotherapy (BACP), the United Kingdom Council for Psychotherapy (UKCP), the British Psychoanalytic Council (BPC), and the British Association of Behavioural and Cognitive Psychotherapies (BABCP), all of which act as accrediting bodies by overseeing the quality of the trainings and course programmes of their member psychotherapy organizations, ensuring they meet the relevant minimum standards, as well as ensuring that their qualified members meet fitness to practise requirements.

Maintaining high-quality and transparent training standards is important, not just to produce competent therapists, but also for research in knowing what is expected to be delivered for any particular therapy that is being studied. Following the lead from CBT, there is a trend amongst psychotherapy in general towards competency frameworks for individual therapies (detailing what skills therapists should be able to deliver), which may be used to inform manualized treatments (detailing how therapists should deliver that therapeutic approach) with measures developed to ensure therapeutic adherence to that model.

Although the psychoanalytic and humanistic therapies find it more problematic to manualize from the myriad dynamics of the therapeutic relationship which is prioritized as the focus of intervention and vehicle of change, frameworks for psychodynamic and humanistic competences have been developed in the last few years.

All of the sections in this chapter give details of the training required in the particular modality under discussion. General therapeutic competences common to all psychotherapies are described in ➜ Chapter 3, and the key techniques and competences for each specific psychotherapeutic modality are described in detail in the respective sections of ➜ Chapter 5. Although the therapeutic modalities that we have included under the group of 'medical psychotherapies' vary in the nature of their trainings and defined skills and competences, they are all united in their endeavour to ensure that their particular therapy is identifiably and consistently delivered to a high quality.

Recommended reading

Fonagy P and Lemma A (2012). Does psychoanalysis have a valuable place in modern mental health services? Yes. *BMJ*, 344, e1211.

General Medical Council. *Small Specialties Thematic Review: Quality Assurance Report for Medical Psychotherapy 2011–2012*. Available at: ℬ http://www.gmc-uk.org/Medical_psychotherapy—report—FINAL.pdf_51696150.pdf.

University College London. *Competence Frameworks. Supervision of Psychological Therapies*. Available at: ℬ https://www.ucl.ac.uk/pals/research/cehp/research-groups/core/competence-frameworks/Supervision_of_Psychological_Therapies.

Psychoanalytic psychotherapy

Key concepts

Psychoanalytic psychotherapy, sometimes called psychodynamic or exploratory psychotherapy, is based on the principles and methods of psychoanalysis. Although psychoanalysis has evolved considerably since Freud, many of his basic tenets remain central to contemporary theory and practice. Key concepts include unconscious mental activity, psychic determination, the role of conflict in creating psychic disturbance, transference, resistance, and a developmental perspective in which childhood experiences are critical in shaping the adult personality.

The talking cure

Psychoanalysis was founded by *Sigmund Freud* (1856–1939), a Viennese neurologist, who invented the 'talking cure' as a treatment for hysteria in the late nineteenth century. Freud first experimented with hypnosis to discover the power of 'abreaction', a technique of hypnotic suggestion that enabled the patient to recover repressed memories of childhood traumatic events. Through verbalizing the feelings associated with the original trauma, Freud discovered that the patient's hysterical symptoms disappeared. This led Freud to conceptualize hysteria as the repression of ideas and wishes that are unacceptable to the conscious mind and expressed through bodily symptoms. Freud, however, soon abandoned this cathartic method, when he found that many patients appeared to be resistant to hypnosis, and replaced it with the technique of 'free association', in which the patient tries to say whatever is on their mind, however painful, shameful, trivial, or seemingly irrelevant—the challenging method of emotional honesty which remains a cornerstone of psychoanalytic psychotherapy today.

The unconscious

Psychoanalytic psychotherapy is underpinned by a theory of mental functioning, in which parts of the mind are conceptualized as being inaccessible and mental processes occur outside of conscious awareness. Although Freud did not discover the unconscious, he made the unconscious arena of the mind into the main object of investigation in psychoanalysis. Although they can never be fully known, the unconscious contents and processes of the mind are revealed through the analysis of dreams, slips of the tongue or writing (*parapraxes*), and patterns of speech, which provide a window into the underlying unconscious feelings, fantasies, and desires that motivate our conscious thoughts and manifest behaviour.

Models of the mind

Freud aspired that psychoanalysis should be a general psychology, embedded in biology, with his theory of the drives or instincts. He continually revised his theories throughout his lifetime and never arrived at a complete and unified model of the mind. Whilst the structural model, containing his final dualistic theory of two opposing instincts—the life instinct (Eros) and the death instinct (Thanatos)—may have been influential and controversial, different aspects of Freud's theories have been emphasized and developed by different psychoanalytic schools, and psychoanalytic psychotherapists today tend to use a blend of selected elements of his theories to inform their clinical practice.

In Freud's *topographical model*, the mind was divided into three systems, separated from each other by censors. In the *system preconscious*, mental contents can easily be brought into the *system conscious* by shifting awareness, whereas the contents of the *system unconscious* are unacceptable to the conscious mind and are therefore kept from conscious awareness by the forces of repression but emerge in the guise of symptoms.

Limitations to Freud's topographical model led him to develop his second model of the mind— the *structural model*, in which the mind is divided into three parts: id, ego, and superego. The *id* is a reservoir of unconscious sexual and aggressive drives, which are morally unacceptable to conscious civilized thought and must be kept at bay. The id operates under the domination of the pleasure principle, in which the primary aim is the avoidance of pain and gratification of instinctual demands. It is governed by primary process thinking, in which opposites coexist, wishes are fulfilled, and there are no contradictions, negatives, or sense of time. The *ego* contains both conscious and unconscious parts and is the executive organ of the psyche, controlling motility, perception, and contact with reality. The *superego* evolves from part of the ego as the outcome of the Oedipus complex, with the internalization of parental standards and goals to establish the individual's moral conscience and censorship. Through defence mechanisms, located in the unconscious, the ego modulates the drives coming from the id and performs a difficult task in attempting to mediate between the conflicting demands of the id, superego, and reality.

Psychic determinism

Freud proposed that, although we may think we have control over our lives and operate through free choice, our conscious thoughts and actions are shaped and controlled by unconscious forces. Moreover, symptoms and behaviours are meaningful and may be 'overdetermined', containing multiple complex meanings which coalesce, serving several functions in responding to the demands of both external reality and the unconscious needs of the internal world.

Developmental approach

Freud emphasized a developmental or historical approach to the individual, that present symptoms were caused by past events, particularly those that occurred in infancy and childhood, which he thought were overwhelmingly important. Moreover, he believed that mental functioning was on a spectrum of normal to abnormal, so that the same psychic mechanisms that operated in the adult neurotic were normal in all of us at an earlier stage of childhood development. He believed that children were influenced by sexual drives and proposed a developmental trajectory in which the early manifestations of infantile sexuality were associated with bodily functions such as feeding and bowel control. Psychosexual development consists of instinctual energy shifting from oral to anal to phallic to genital *erotogenic* zones, respectively, where each corresponding stage of development is characterized by particular functions and objectives but builds upon and subsumes the accomplishments of the preceding stage. Failure to negotiate the emotional demands of each stage is linked to the development of a neurotic complex, the character traits in adult life.

The Oedipus complex

Freud named the Oedipus complex after the Greek tragedy, in which Oedipus unknowingly killed his father and married his mother. Freud proposed that the Oedipus complex was a normal stage of development, occurring between the ages of 3 to 5 years, where the boy is attracted to his mother and develops feelings of rivalry and jealousy for his father. The equivalent constellation in the little girl is called the *Electra complex*. Castration anxiety refers to the boy's fear that his father will castrate him for his desire for the mother. Resolution of the Oedipus complex results in the formation of the superego. Failure to negotiate the Oedipus complex may result in deficits in the capacity to enjoy healthy loving and sexual relationships, and give rise to neurotic illness in adulthood.

Defence mechanisms

Defence mechanisms are unconscious mental processes aimed at the reduction and elimination of anxiety or change liable to threaten the integrity and stability of the individual. They contain interwoven determinants, values and beliefs, and conscious and unconscious elements. They may be individual or interpersonal, form part of the boundary between self and others, and are essential to group and social life. Defence mechanisms may be classified according to a hierarchy from the most immature or pathological to the most mature or healthy (see Table 2.1) and may change over time.

In Freudian theory, defence mechanisms are a function of the ego and defend against impulses and thoughts that are unacceptable to the conscious mind. They resolve conflict between instinctive needs (id), internalized prohibitions (superego), and external reality. Freud believed that neurotic illness was the result of conflict between the instinctual drives and the external world, or between different parts of the mind. This conflict between the ego and id can result in neurotic symptoms, as unacceptable sexual and aggressive thoughts and feelings break through the

Table 2.1 Hierarchy of defence mechanisms

Immature or primitive defences	
Denial: avoiding awareness of painful aspects of external reality by negating sensory data.	**Projection:** perceiving and reacting to one's own unacceptable inner impulses and thoughts as if they were outside the self and attributing them to someone else.
Splitting: compartmentalization and lack of integration between incompatible experiences of polarized aspects of self and other to prevent conflict.	**Projective identification:** attributing unacceptable aspects of the self to someone else (i.e. projection) but going further, in that the target of the projection is unconsciously pressurized to behave, think, and feel in keeping with what has been projected into them.
Dissociation: temporary loss of identity, memory, consciousness, or perception as a way of retaining an illusion of psychological control in the face of helplessness or loss of control.	**Idealization:** attributing perfect or near-perfect qualities to others as a way of avoiding anxiety or negative feelings such as contempt, envy, or anger.
Acting out: expressing an unconscious wish or fantasy impulsively through action as a way of avoiding painful affect.	**Somatization:** converting emotional pain or other affect states into bodily symptoms and focusing concern on somatic, rather than psychic, manifestations.
Regression: returning to an earlier phase of development or functioning to avoid the conflicts and tensions associated with the current stage of development.	**Schizoid fantasy:** Retreating into a private internal fantasy world to avoid anxiety and conflict about interpersonal situations.
Higher-level (neurotic) defences	
Introjection: internalizing the qualities of an object or significant person. This is an essential part of normal development, but, when used defensively, it can be used to avoid the awareness of loss or separation from the object.	**Identification:** also a normal part of development and closely related to introjection, but more permanent. In identification, by internalizing the qualities of another person, they become part of the self, whereas, in introjection, the internal representations still feel like 'other'.
Displacement: shifting feelings associated with one idea or object onto another.	**Intellectualization:** using excessive and abstract ideation and undue focus on the inanimate to avoid difficult feelings; often associated with intimacy and relationships with other people.
Isolation of affect: separating an idea from its associated affect state to avoid emotional turmoil.	

(Continued)

Table 2.1 (*Contd.*)

Higher-level (neurotic) defences	
Rationalization: justification of unacceptable feelings, beliefs, and attitudes to make them tolerable to oneself.	**Sexualization:** endowing an object, significant person, or behaviour with sexual significance to turn a negative experience into an exciting one or to ward off anxiety.
Reaction formation: transforming an unacceptable wish or impulse into its opposite.	**Isolation:** splitting or separating an idea from the affect that accompanies it but is repressed, to avoid emotional turmoil.
Repression: expelling unacceptable ideas or impulses or blocking them from entering consciousness.	**Undoing:** attempting to negate sexual, aggressive, or shameful implications from a previous comment or behaviour by elaborating, clarifying, or doing the opposite.

Mature defences	
Humour: using comedy or irony to distance oneself from painful feelings and thoughts.	**Suppression:** consciously or semi-consciously postponing attention to a particular feeling or idea. It differs from repression or denial in that it is conscious, and discomfort is acknowledged but minimized.
Asceticism: eliminating the pleasurable aspects of experience, because of moral values and internal conflicts produced by that pleasure.	**Altruism:** committing oneself to the needs of others above one's own.
Anticipation: realistically planning and thinking about possible future bad outcomes or worrying in advance about things to dilute the anxiety.	**Sublimation:** transforming socially objectionable or internally unacceptable aims into socially acceptable ones. Feelings, e.g. aggressive or sexual, are acknowledged, modified, and directed towards a socially acceptable goal.

ego's censorship barrier and are converted into substitute compromise formations to prevent them from fully entering consciousness. Conflict between the ego and superego can cause feelings of low self-esteem, shame, and guilt due to the ego's failure to live up to the high moral standards imposed by the superego.

Repetition compulsion

Trauma can overwhelm the ego, breaking through its defences and rendering it helpless and unable to function. Freud coined the term repetition compulsion to describe a person's unconscious tendency in adult life to repeat behaviour associated with past traumatic experiences, in an attempt to resolve feelings of helplessness and conflict. Freud later explained this as a manifestation of the death instinct.

Resistance
Although patients may be consciously motivated to seek psychotherapeutic help for their difficulties, they may be unconsciously opposed to changing engrained internal patterns of thoughts and feelings. Resistance is a defence mechanism that arises during treatment to avoid experiencing the psychic pain associated with previously repressed unpleasant impulses and affects that the therapy is attempting to uncover and explore. Resistances to treatment can take overt and covert forms such as missing appointments, being late to sessions, being silent, or not hearing interpretations.

Transference
In psychoanalysis and psychoanalytic psychotherapy, examination and interpretation of transference is a cornerstone of treatment. The classical Freudian understanding of transference refers to the wishes and feelings that the patient develops towards the analyst, which reflect childhood conflicts and may serve as a resistance to the process of free association. With the growth of the object relations theory, transference has been subsequently conceptualized as the externalization and manifestation of the patient's internal object relations in the relationship with the analyst.

Countertransference
Countertransference describes the unconscious emotional reactions that the therapist has towards the patient, and arises as a result of unresolved conflicts in the therapist interacting with contributions or projections from the patient. As with the transference, Freud originally saw countertransference as a resistance to treatment, but contemporary analysts see it as a valuable source of useful information about the patient and his internal object relations. Countertransference is by definition unconscious, and therefore conscious feelings about a patient may be misleading and disguise more unconscious and less acceptable feelings, e.g. feelings of boredom in the therapist may conceal more unconscious hostile feelings towards the patient.

Key contributors
Psychoanalysis has evolved significantly in both theory and practice since Freud, with the development of different theoretical schools. Overall, contemporary psychoanalytic theorizing has shifted from the 'one-person psychology' of classical Freudian drive theory towards a 'two-person psychology', in which the role of object relations in both normal development and psychopathology, and particularly the importance of the early mother–infant relationship in the pre-Oedipal period, is highlighted.

Anna Freud (1895–1982), Freud's daughter, made significant contributions to psychoanalysis by elaborating on known individual ego defence mechanisms and identifying new ones, e.g. *identification with the aggressor*, a defence mechanism in which the aggressive characteristics of a feared object are internalized, so that they are more under the individual's control. She made seminal contributions to child analysis, particularly focusing on the role of the ego in development, and was instrumental in the development of the school of *ego psychology* in the United States (USA). She founded the Hampstead Clinic in London (now the Anna Freud Centre).

Melanie Klein (1882–1960) also worked with children and developed a form of child psychoanalysis in which children's play was interpreted as the symbolic expression of unconscious processes. She is the originator of *object relations theory*, which has become the predominant theoretical model in contemporary psychoanalytic psychotherapy. She focused on the role of *unconscious phantasies*, which she believed were object-relating and exist from birth as the psychic expressions of the life and death instincts. She developed a theory of internal object relations, focusing on Freud's concept of the death instinct, which she saw as central to the understanding of envy and destructiveness. However, she differed from Freud in postulating that the formation of the superego occurs in the first few months of life via the internalization of the death instinct, and therefore predates the Oedipus complex, rather than being its outcome.

Klein envisaged the infantile mind as being formed through the primitive defence mechanisms of projection, introjection, splitting, and projective identification. The baby's first experiences are dominated by his instinctual aggressive impulses and phantasies, which initially cannot be integrated with pleasurable experiences of the breast but are projected and split between the 'good breast' and 'bad breast'. The baby's projection of aggression and his fear of retaliation cause primitive anxieties of persecution and annihilation, creating a state of mind which Klein called the *paranoid schizoid position*. The *depressive position* develops later when the baby is able to attribute his ambivalent and conflicting feelings towards the same object, and integrate and internalize his experiences so that the good and bad breasts are now seen as aspects of the same person who is able to survive the baby's envious and destructive attacks. The normal adult oscillates between these two states of mind throughout life, but, when primitive anxieties and defences predominate, psychic growth is arrested, and pathological defensive organizations or *psychic retreats* may form by psychotic splitting of the mind into encapsulated and underdeveloped areas.

Wilfred Bion (1897–1979) developed Klein's concept of projective identification in exploring the relationship between mother and baby. Bion introduced the concept of *containment* to describe the function of projective identification in the analytic situation as paralleling the way the baby projects its unbearable distress into the mother. Via her *reverie* or capacity to understand through empathic identification with her baby, the mother can bear the baby's intolerable anxieties, moderate them, and feed them back to her baby in a form which he can tolerate, thus promoting healthy mental and physical development. The analyst's function is analogous—he 'contains' the patient's projections in a state of reverie and responds with appropriate interpretations.

Donald Winnicott (1896–1971) was both a psychoanalyst and paediatrician and one of the central figures in the British Independent Group and object relations theory. Like Klein and Bion, he also recognized the importance of the early mother–infant relationship but focused more on the role of the environment, particularly the more positive aspects such as play and creativity, rather than the role of innate aggression in personality development. In the context of a responsive *holding environment* facilitated by a *good enough mother*, the baby may develop their *true self*. However, where there have been impingements to the baby's developing sense of self through inadequate maternal care, a *false self* develops in which the baby adapts to the conscious and unconscious narcissistic needs of the mother at the expense of development of his true self, which remains hidden. Winnicott also developed the notion of the *transitional object*—a favourite object of a child, such as a blanket or teddy bear, that serves as a soothing substitute for the mother in her absence and facilitates the child's efforts to become separate and independent. The transitional object operates in a *transitional space*, in which more symbolic functioning may gradually develop, which may become the source of art, creativity, and religion.

Michael Balint (1896–1970) was another prominent member of the British Independent Group of object relations theorists. He attributed a central role in psychological development for *primary object love* and proposed that a *basic fault*, or fundamental deficit in internal psychic structure, ensues when there are maternal failures, leading to a sense of something missing in adulthood. He was also influential in setting up groups, now known as *Balint groups*, for medical doctors to discuss psychodynamic and emotional aspects of the relationships with their patients.

john Bowlby (1907–1990) was the founder of *attachment theory* and proposed that the human need for significant relationships was universal and established at a psychobiological level. In contrast to the psychoanalytic theories of his time, Bowlby emphasized the role of the external world and the child's real experiences, as opposed to internal fantasy, in normal development. Influenced by ethology and evolutionary theory, Bowlby and his followers showed how the infant's relationship and proximity-seeking behaviour to his mother or primary object is both instinctual but also determined by the object's behaviour. Attachment research demonstrates how early disruptions in attachment caused by separation, trauma, or loss can produce long-term pathological effects predisposing to mental illness and character abnormalities in adult life.

In North America, *ego psychology*, developed by psychoanalysts, such as Heinz Hartmann (1894–1970) and Erik Erikson (1902–1994), was the predominant psychoanalytic school until the 1970s. Ego psychology focuses on the functions and properties of the ego, including defence mechanisms, the regulation of instinctual drives, relation to reality, and object relationships. Hartmann described autonomous ego functions which are primary and develop independently of conflict and include perception, learning, intelligence, language, thinking, and motility. Erikson built on Freud's concept of psychosexual stages to produce a psychosocial theory of development describing crucial stages in the individual's relationships with the social world across the life cycle.

Heinz Kohut (1913–1981) developed *self-psychology* from his work with narcissistic patients. He proposed that the development and maintenance of self-esteem and self-cohesion was fundamental to character development and that deficits caused by maternal empathic failures, rather than conflicts over aggression and sexuality, lay at the core of all psychopathology. By contrast, **Otto Kernberg**, a prominent object relations theorist in the USA who was influenced by Melanie Klein's theories and worked with patients with borderline personality disorder (BPD), emphasized the role of aggression and splitting of the ego in personality pathology. In more recent years, a number of post-modern schools, such as the *relational, intersubjectivist*, and *constructivist*, have emerged from within North America, which all emphasize the two-person nature of psychoanalytic treatment and that knowledge or 'truth' does not reside with the therapist but is co-constructed in the interaction between patient and therapist.

What is the evidence base?

The evidence base for psychoanalytic psychotherapy has lagged behind that of other forms of psychotherapy, particularly CBT. This is due to the methodological challenges in conducting outcome research into longer-term exploratory therapy such as the randomization of patients, manualization of treatment, recording sessions, measuring changes in deeper personality structures, rather than symptom remission, and the fear by some therapists that these research procedures may interfere with the patient's treatment.

Nevertheless, there is an accumulating body of high-quality empirical evidence supporting the efficacy of psychoanalytic psychotherapy, which suggests that scepticism regarding the scientific nature of psychoanalytic psychotherapy is not justified and may reflect biases in the dissemination of research findings. Recent meta-analyses that pool the results of many different independent studies, including RCTs of long-term psychoanalytic psychotherapy, show that the effect sizes for psychoanalytic psychotherapy are as large as those reported for other evidence-based therapies, such as CBT, for a large range of disorders, including depression, anxiety, panic disorders, somatoform disorders, substance misuse, personality disorders. Moreover, patients who receive psychoanalytic psychotherapy maintain therapeutic gains and continue to improve after cessation of treatment. The results of these outcome studies have gone some way in challenging the 'equivalence paradox' or 'Dodo effect'—the finding in psychotherapy research that no one therapy has consistently been found to be more effective than another, leading to the assumption that 'common factors' to all psychotherapies, such as providing hope, the offering of a relationship with a therapist, and providing a rationale and set of activities accounted for improvements, rather than any modality-specific strategy (see ➔ Common factor research in Chapter 11, pp. 519–22).

Qualitative process research has looked at specific concepts and techniques within psychoanalytic psychotherapy and attempted to correlate different interventions with outcome. The Core Conflictual Relationship Theme (CCRT), a measure of key unconscious personal themes identified through studying the process notes of psychotherapy sessions, provided one of the first scientific and objective measures of the concept of transference and demonstrated that individuals have only a few basic transference patterns, that these derive from early parental relationships, and that these patterns may gradually change during the course of therapy. These findings have been corroborated by research using the Adult Attachment Interview (AAI), a psychodynamically informed assessment interview that produces a narrative measure of the person's attachment experiences and relational disposition. The AAI has been used to track changes in psychoanalytic psychotherapy to show how patients can move from pathological attachment patterns to more secure attachment patterns as therapy progresses.

Research into psychological defences and their interpretation in treatment includes studies that assess patients' defences on a moment-to-moment basis and shows that defences and defensive functioning improve with treatment. This research also elucidates the role of defences in mediating treatment by improving symptoms and investigates how therapeutic interventions lead to changes in defensive functioning within and across sessions. Studies examining the effects of transference interpretations indicate that a moderate quantity of transference interpretations may mediate an increase in insight, leading to better outcomes in longer-term therapy, but a high frequency of transference interpretations may be counterproductive, particularly with more disturbed patients who have personality pathology, as it may serve to increase their hostility and resistance by fortifying their defences to ward off perceived attacks.

Psychoanalytic psychotherapy training

In the UK, the BPC is the professional association and voluntary regulator of the psychoanalytic psychotherapy profession, accrediting psychoanalytic psychotherapy trainings and publishing a register of practitioners who are required to follow their ethical code and meet fitness-to-practise standards. Formal clinical training in psychoanalytic psychotherapy tends to last over several years and ranges from the most intensive psychoanalytic trainings accredited by the International Psychoanalytic Association (IPA), such as the British Psychoanalytic Society (BPAS) and the British Psychoanalytic Association (BPA) involving seeing patients four or five times per week, through three-times-a-week psychotherapy trainings offered by, for example, the British Psychotherapy Foundation (BPF), to less intensive psychodynamic trainings involving once- or twice-weekly therapy with organizations such as the Westminster Pastoral Foundation (WPF).

Most psychoanalytic psychotherapy trainings are based on a tripartite model of education comprising a personal training psychotherapy or analysis, theoretical and clinical seminars, and the treatment of individual patients under supervision. Many psychotherapy trainings also include a course in infant observation, in which the psychotherapy trainee observes a mother and baby in the family home. This offers the experience of being an involved or 'participant' observer of the unfolding emotional relationship between the mother and child, which facilitates the development of observational skills, and containing emotional attitudes essential to the therapeutic relationship with patients, as well as learning to apply theories of child development to what is observed in practice.

Psychotherapists may come from a variety of core clinical professional disciplines, including medicine, psychology, social work, and nursing. Medical psychotherapy is a small sub-specialty of psychiatry that involves three years of higher psychiatry training leading to a CCT in medical psychotherapy (see ➲ Chapters 1 and 12). Psychotherapists may also come from non-clinical backgrounds such as academia or teaching. In these cases, some exposure to clinical work, e.g. an honorary clinical placement on a psychiatric ward for six months, is usually deemed necessary, before the trainee therapist is allowed to commence seeing his or her own individual patients.

Most psychotherapy trainings are offered by training institutes run as private enterprises or charities, which train therapists to work primarily as private practitioners; however, a few trainings, such as higher training in medical psychotherapy in psychiatry or the Interdisciplinary Training in Adult Psychotherapy at the Tavistock and Portman NHS Foundation Trust, are based within the NHS and aimed at training therapists to work in the public sector. In the UK, psychoanalytic psychotherapy institutes have historically offered training mostly in London; however, in recent years, trainings have been actively developed in other areas of the country such as Leeds.

Recommended reading

Bateman A and Holmes J (1995). *Introduction to Psychoanalysis*. Routledge: London.
Lemma A (2003). *Introduction to the Practice of Psychoanalytic Psychotherapy*. Wiley: Chichester.
Levy KN, Meehan KB, Temes CM, and Yeomans FE (2012). Attachment theory and research: implications for psychodynamic psychotherapy. In: Levy RA, Ablon JS, and Kachele H, eds. *Psychodynamic Psychotherapy Research: Evidence-Based Practice and Practice-Based Evidence*. pp. 401–16. Humana Press: New York.
Sandler J, Dare C, and Holder A (1992). *The Patient and the Analyst*. Karnac Books: London.
Shedler J (2010). The efficacy of psychodynamic psychotherapy. *American Psychologist*, **65**, 98–109.

Cognitive behavioural therapy

Key concepts

The model

CBT is based on several principles, which together constitute the cognitive model:

- It is not the event that causes problems but how we view or appraise it
- For every event we have a set of thoughts, feelings, behaviours and physiology and each of these domains can affect the others
- How we appraise situations is dependent on our earlier and subsequent experiences, the views we have of ourselves, the world, others and the future
- Behaviour can impact strongly on how we think and feel.

For example when Mick's wife came home late from work, he **thought**, *'Poor thing, she really is working too hard at the moment' and* **felt** *compassion for her. He has had a fairly straightforward life with no major tragedies, and he believes that the world is an OK place to live in. He started preparing* **(behaviour)** *the tea. Meanwhile, Paul's wife was also late home from work, and he started to* **think**, *'Oh no! What if something has happened to her on the way home?' which made him* **feel** *quite anxious, led to palpitations and nausea* **(physiology)**, *and led to him pacing around the room* **(behaviour)**, *too distracted to carry on preparing the tea he had planned. Paul's first wife was killed in a car crash, and his mother died in a house fire when he was seven. He believes that the world is a dangerous place.*

Therapy helps people learn to make changes in how they appraise situations and address any unhelpful behaviours.

Levels of cognition

The words appraisals, thoughts, or cognitions can be used interchangeably. However, cognitions are traditionally divided into three levels:

- Automatic thoughts: these are the most immediate or accessible cognitions, or streams of thoughts, which pop into our heads in response to any situation. These can be positive or neutral, but CBT is generally directed towards the problematic thoughts, known as 'negative automatic thoughts', where people tend to interpret situations in a negative way.
- Core beliefs: these are the beliefs people develop about themselves, the world, and others as a result of their early and subsequent experiences. Again these may be positive or neutral (e.g. I am OK) or negative (e.g. I am bad; others are untrustworthy; the world is dangerous). They may not be immediately obvious or accessible, unless probed for.
- Rules for living: if you explore further people's negative beliefs, you may uncover the beliefs or rules they have developed to deal with the world or beliefs they have about themselves (e.g. don't get close to others, so they won't realise you are bad; don't trust others, so they can't let you down; be prepared at all times).

Key features

- CBT is generally seen as a brief, focused psychotherapy, anchored in the here and now and based on the cognitive behavioural model.
- It involves defining a problem to work on and developing SMART goals to aim for (specific, measurable, achievable, realistic, time-limited).
- Therapy is driven by the shared formulation or understanding of the problem, which is developed in the first few sessions, and is generally in diagrammatic form. Any interventions are based on this case formulation.
- Therapy is collaborative in nature, using a style of questioning called Socratic questioning and guided discovery (see ➔ 'Socratic questioning and guided discovery' bullet point in Chapter 5, Underpinning competencies, pp. 173–4).
- It is highly structured, with the setting of an agenda at the start of each session.
- It makes use of homework and emphasizes between session activities.

- Feedback at regular intervals is encouraged from the patient, and frequent therapist or patient summaries occur.
- Both relevant standardized (formal, validated measures, e.g. Beck Depression Inventory) and idiographic (developed in therapy) measurements are made at regular intervals regarding the index problem.
- Treatment uses both cognitive change and acceptance techniques, as well as behavioural experiments and other behavioural techniques.
- There is a clear relationship between the science or theory behind CBT and the actual clinical practice, and the therapy is evidence-based. Where evidence suggests that an intervention is unhelpful, e.g. the use of thought stopping in OCD, this is dropped from practice, and conversely helpful treatments are incorporated into therapy, e.g. recent trials suggest that behavioural activation for depression is highly effective, and this treatment is now generally seen as the appropriate first-line treatment for depression.
- For straightforward diagnoses, such as social anxiety and panic disorder, well-validated treatment protocols have been developed and should be incorporated, where applicable.
- A 'continuum principle' applies where mental health problems are seen on a continuum with normal behaviour, and the CBT theory applies to anyone, not just patients.
- Therapy is practical in nature. The use of jargon is discouraged. Talking to patients on the way from the waiting room is not discouraged. Some sessions will necessitate leaving the comfort of the office base and doing home-based exposure sessions or experiments on buses.
- A typical course of therapy with a straightforward problem lasts 12–20 sessions. Broadly speaking, treatment can be divided into three phases—an initial assessment and a formulation phase, lasting 1–6 sessions, a treatment phase lasting 10–20 sessions, and a consolidation phase lasting 2–4 sessions.

Key contributors

CBT in its present form acknowledges roots in both behavioural and cognitive traditions, and the term has come into place to describe an amalgamation of the two.

The science of behaviourism
- This arose partly in response to frustration at the perceived elusiveness of psychoanalysis, with proponents keen to look at the observable part of human nature in a scientific way, identifying target problems, and measuring change in observable behaviour.
- Two schools of behaviour therapy developed in the 1950s, one on each side of the Atlantic.
- The British camp was headed up by **Joseph Wolpe** and **Hans Eysenck**, who were influenced by Pavlovian theory and concentrated their efforts on developing treatments for anxiety disorders, assuming problems arose due to problematic conditioning.
- Meanwhile, the American group of psychologists, including **Ogden R Lindsley**, were more influenced by Skinnerian theory and operant conditioning and tended to work with more chronic mental health patients, including inpatients with schizophrenia. However, diagnoses

were frowned upon, with any disorder being described purely in behavioural terms, such as 'disruptive behaviour', and token economy systems were set up to shape and reward 'good' behaviour.
- Whilst both groups were, in many ways, highly successful, disillusionment arose, partly because of concerns about the loosening of the link between science and clinical practice and partly because of a lack of success in treating depression with purely behavioural means.

Cognitive therapy
- Meanwhile, **Aaron Beck**, an American psychiatrist and originally a psychoanalyst, had developed a new form of therapy—cognitive therapy. The underpinning theory was that an individual's affect and behaviour are largely determined by the way in which he structures the world.
- Similarly, **Albert Ellis**'s rational emotive therapy arose around the same time.
- Both therapies shared the idea that problematic thinking or 'cognitive distortions' led to disturbances in mood, which could be corrected by 'correction of these faulty constructs', i.e. helping people learn to think differently. Both therapies also emphasized the importance of behavioural work, e.g. Beck's cognitive therapy of depression devotes a chapter to behavioural techniques, asserting the importance of helping improve a patient's functioning via, e.g. activity scheduling, before looking at cognition.
- Whilst highly successful clinically, it was noted by prominent cognitive psychologists that the development of cognitive therapy for depression proceeded largely in isolation from basic cognitive science.

Cognitive behavioural therapy
- Ultimately, however, the two therapies merged to become what we know today as CBT, which acknowledges the importance of thoughts and behaviours and maintains the importance of rigorous outcome research.
- Contemporary key contributors include **David Clark**'s influential theory of panic disorder (1986), **Paul Salkovskis**'s model of OCD, **Adrian Well**'s theory of metacognition (2000), and **Anke Ehlers** and **David Clark**'s influential model of post-traumatic stress disorder (PTSD) (2000).

What is the evidence base?
CBT has clear evidence to support its use for the treatment of:
- Depression
- Panic/agoraphobia
- Generalized anxiety disorder
- Specific phobias
- Social phobia
- Obsessional compulsive disorder
- PTSD
- Bulimia
- Some personality disorders.

It has limited support for the treatment of anorexia, schizophrenia, and bipolar disorder.

The UK National Institute for Health and Care Excellence (NICE) produces a number of guidelines for the appropriate treatment of particular disorders, based on a thorough review of available evidence, and concludes that CBT is the treatment of choice in:

- Depression: for those with moderate or severe depression, in combination with antidepressant medication; for those at risk of relapse or with residual symptoms
- Eating disorders: for bulimia nervosa (BN) and binge eating disorder (BED)
- Generalized anxiety and panic
- PTSD: trauma-focused CBT or EMDR
- OCD and body dysmorphic disorder (BDD): group or individual CBT, including exposure and response prevention
- Schizophrenia: CBT should be offered to all.

Cognitive behavioural therapy training

Training opportunities are widely available within the UK. The BABCP is the national body which regulates CBT therapists and training. Although most health-care staff will have access to some very basic CBT training at some point in their training, and many trusts and organizations offer basic courses, to gain accreditation with the BABCP, and hence recognition as a fully trained therapist, requires the completion of a recognized training course, usually to the level of a Postgraduate Diploma level, alongside stipulated requirements for seeing a certain amount of patients under supervision. The recent IAPT initiative (see ➔ Improving Access to Psychological Therapies services in Chapter 10, pp. 463–4) saw the development of several new training centres around the country and the training up of many new therapists to work in primary care, delivering evidence-based therapies in a timely manner for patients with anxiety and depression, who had previously been untreated or forced to wait on secondary care waiting lists for, in some cases, several years for therapy. This initiative has been highly successful in increasing the number of trained therapists nationally.

Recommended reading

Beck AT, Rush AJ, Shaw BF, and Emery G (1979). *Cognitive Therapy of Depression*. Guilford Press: New York.

Rachman S (2015). The evolution of behaviour therapy and cognitive behaviour therapy. *Behaviour Research and Therapy*, **64**, 1–8.

Westbrook D, Kennerley H, and Kirk J (2007). *An Introduction to Cognitive Behaviour Therapy Skills and Applications*. Sage Publications: London.

Systemic family and couple therapy

Systemic therapy is the psychological treatment of families, couples, or individuals, which focuses on interpersonal effects. Therapy attempts to enhance creative and constructive interactions, whilst minimizing the destructive aspects of relationships. The therapeutic stance is characterized by curiosity, uncertainty, and the valuing of diversity.

Key concepts

Focus on relationships

The defining characteristic is the *focus on relationships* as the context in which individual difficulties occur. Unlike most approaches in psychiatry and psychotherapy, the emphasis is not on the individual and intrapsychic, but on the interpersonal. Thus, it is *both* a way of conceptualizing symptoms by contextualizing them, *and* a treatment modality.

Circularity

The assertion is that change in one part of the relational 'system' has reverberating effects within it; the emphasis is on the *circularity* of processes within relationships, rather than linear ones, thus minimizing blame.

A simple clinical example of circularity is the restless baby with an anxious mother, in contrast to a placid mother/infant pair, whereby, in each case, tension or calm is amplified in a circle between the two protagonists.

Social construction of meaning

Lately, the notion of circularity has been expanded and reinforced by the theory of *social constructionism*, the idea of joint construction of meaning between individuals through language and gesture. Put simply, I, the self, varies according to the different others with whom I am relating. So the self is seen not as a core discrete entity, but as a variable and fluidly interdependent construct, endlessly recreated in dialogue with others (or from dialogue between aspects of the self).

Mentalization

Systemic family and couple therapy puts *communication* and miscommunication at the centre of therapeutic work: what is said or done, and how that is understood by others. This is shared with the concept of *mentalization,* a capacity in the individual to recognize that others experience differently and that differences in perception can be thought about, talked about, understood, and tolerated.

Emphasis on resources

Unlike some therapies, there is a particular *emphasis on strengths and resources*, even in bleak situations (as in the 'recovery model' in relation to serious mental illness). The therapeutic stance is that people who present have struggled to resolve problems unsuccessfully, but that there is a reserve of potential motivation for change inherent in even entrenched or despairing couples or families.

This positivity risks ignoring the aggression and destructiveness in many family interactions, but often families benefit from being assumed to be predominantly benign, particularly in the early (joining) phase of therapy, when a strong sense of shame and failure often predominates. Challenging the family to change destructive patterns comes later, when a collaborative therapeutic relationship is established.

Alongside the fostering of the family's conscious awareness of strengths is the relative diminution of the centrality of the therapeutic relationship. *Autonomy and choice* are emphasized and regression discouraged, and spacing of sessions (often 2- to 4-week gaps) reinforces the importance and potential for change in the time lived between sessions and what families can do for themselves.

Pattern recognition

Pattern recognition, within interactions and across generations, is a central ingredient in systemic work, shared with other modalities. The family tree or genogram often elicits repetitive patterns across generations. For example: 'It looks as if noisy fights are quite normal on your side of the family, whereas, on your side, open conflict is banned ... I wonder whether that helps explain why *you* find the current rows so unbearable?'.

Power and diagnostic 'labelling'

Family therapists are interested in *power*, especially uneven power in relationships, including the therapeutic one, and how power differentials affect opportunity, attitude, and behaviour. It is commonplace that socio-economic status determines access to health care, but systemic family therapists pay particular attention to how external disadvantage and prejudice affect families. Care is taken to avoid assumptions about the family's attitudes or experience—an explicitly respectful approach to difference is key.

Compared to both psychoanalytic and cognitive therapies, family therapy may be *more political (with a small p) and egalitarian* in its approach. The stance is not neutral, but positively celebratory of cultural difference, which is explored openly, both within the family and between the family and therapist(s), including those of gender, race, religion, age, class, culture, and sexual orientation. Normative assumptions are avoided. The therapist takes a 'one down' position of curiosity about the family who remain experts on themselves. This attitude sits well with the contemporary cultural shift in health, the growth of patient choice, information, responsibility, participation, and shrinking of paternalism.

Aware of how the wider cultural, political, and professional discourse shapes the therapeutic experience, systemic family therapists are wary of the potentially stigmatizing effect of psychiatric diagnoses. However, access to psychological treatment in a highly managed health-care system is increasingly diagnosis-dependent. Nevertheless, contemporary psychiatrists and psychotherapists need to be aware of ICD and DSM as culturally relative constructs, not absolute truths.

Collaborative therapeutic alliance

A self-reflexive stance is expected in most therapies. The systemic therapist notes their own reactions and may disclose them, when useful. The position is that of a professional temporarily included in the family system, attempting to sustain a collaborative therapeutic alliance, without stimulating dependence. Carmel Flaskas writes of 'conditional pragmatism', meaning a variable degree of intensity of therapeutic involvement by the therapist, titrated against the changes in the family.

Distance regulation

Family therapists are acutely aware of *distance regulation* within families, looking for flexibility or rigidly enmeshed patterns of attachment. Can this family or couple tolerate intimacy, but also allow individuals room to manoeuvre separately? Is the family open to outsiders? Is change and development encouraged or seen as a threat?

Risk management

Family therapists may have expertise in the assessment and management of risk. An initiative in East London (Reclaiming Social Work) has trained social workers in systemic family therapy, with good results. Systemic couple work has also been shown to be a containing and useful model in the management of domestic violence.

Flexibility, breadth, and complexity

A core value in systemic family therapy is *flexibility*. The therapist works with whoever is available, applied to both family members and staff. The style is relatively informal and unhierarchical—younger family members or the inexperienced therapist can offer a useful perspective. Systemic therapists are comfortable working across service boundaries such as that between child and adolescent mental health services (CAMHS) and adult mental health. They take a developmental view of the family from infancy through to older adulthood, with the shape of the family expanding and shrinking over time. Parental mental ill health and its impact on children is an area where family therapists contribute.

The therapist needs a *breadth* of knowledge of adult and child mental health, as well as co-morbidity and the subtle interaction of mental illness and personality, with or without substance misuse. Therefore, systemic family therapists contribute in a wide *range of service settings*, from learning disability to forensic, adult to child mental health, perinatal, older adult services, etc. The systemic therapist is well placed to *manage co-morbidity and complexity*, the interaction of personality and diagnosis, and the challenge of multidisciplinary work with colleagues.

Systemic family therapists are employed in primary care, CMHTs, inpatient settings, schools, social services, and third sector agencies.

They can work singly (with supervision) or in pairs, with or without a reflecting team. The reflecting team process, with live supervision, gives a unique simultaneous experience of treatment, supervision, and teaching. This flexibility contrasts with other therapeutic modalities where consistency of the setting is a key ingredient.

Key contributors

Many of the original family therapists (e.g. Minuchin) were psychoanalysts who became interested in how the family and societal context impacted on individuals. Another strand of family therapy theory began with cybernetics, the study of feedback within biological systems (Bateson). There has always been international cross-fertilization of ideas and an iconoclastic tendency for new ideas to overthrow earlier positions; however, in the last 20 years, the field has matured and now has a solid central theoretical orientation which still encourages innovation and creativity. Most recently, systemic ideas are informing the delivery of mainstream psychiatric care, particularly in relation to psychosis.

Gregory Bateson (1972), a British-born anthropologist and evolutionary biologist, worked in the USA and described circular, recursive causality as characteristic of living forms. He saw the family as a *system*, with reinforcing patterns of feedback, a metaphor of biological or mechanical homeostasis. Bateson also described the '*double-bind*' where different levels of communication in the family are contradictory; thus, the individual may be trapped, unable to respond coherently, and he associated this context with the onset of psychotic symptoms.

Salvador Minuchin (1967, 1978), an Argentinian working in the US, was the originator of *structural family therapy*, with its emphasis on the importance of the generational boundaries between parents and children. He described the family as a social organization, with subsystems (e.g. parental couple), boundaries, alliances, and coalitions. He pointed out '*transgenerational alliances*' (such as mother and anorexic daughter with father distanced or excluded) as unhelpful. He encouraged parents to act consistently together, to maintain clear generational boundaries, and take authority, which he saw as necessary and containing for the development of children. He posited that a disengaged and inconsistent parental response, ranging from inattention to violence, led to children who could not learn rules or internalize any control themselves.

John Bowlby (1988) with his seminal work on attachment has permeated the field of family therapy.

Robin Skynner (1976), group analyst, child psychiatrist, and family therapist, and founder of the Institute of Family Therapy in London, described the well-functioning family in terms of a containing secure base from which the individual can separate and develop.

John Byng Hall (1988) described the unconscious pressures on the individual and family to conform or reject the style of the older generation; he coined the terms '*replicative*' and '*corrective*' scripts. This remains clinically useful when helping families understand their own attitudes and behaviour, particularly using the genogram.

Jay Haley (1976) advocated *strategic family therapy* in the 1970s. This is the most behavioural type of family therapy, the least interested in unconscious processes, and is structured from the beginning, setting goals and focused on 'solving the problem' in the most efficient way. The 'problem' is defined as a type of behaviour that is part of a sequence of acts between people, in the family or couple, but includes the relevant social milieu, psychiatric services, probation, the school, etc. Interventions are aimed at disrupting repetitive, unhelpful sequences (she feels neglected and complains; he avoids her, so she feels more neglected) to allow more creative alternatives to emerge.

Strategic family therapy uses the concept of '*frames*', the way the situation is defined (glass half-full or half-empty), and '*reframing*' is changing the conceptual or emotional view of a situation, thus changing its meaning.

de Shazer described *brief solution-focused therapy*, emphasizing the amplifying of *exceptions* as solutions—if depression is the problem, the solution is to do more of whatever you do when you are less depressed, enhancing the sense of control, with a positive shift in cognition and affect, following behavioural change. He objected to the '*problem-soaked narrative*', observing families as burdened and trapped by a language of hopelessness. The focus is explicitly future-orientated, '*solution talk*', de-emphasizing the past. Simple and specific tasks may be set to support change, e.g. 5 minutes listening to each other's account of their day; they must be reported back on at the next session.

Selvini–Palazzoli, **Cecchin**, **Boscolo**, and **Prata** were Italian psychiatrists and psychoanalysts who constituted *the Milan research group*. Influenced by post-modernism, and with their concepts of hypothesizing, circularity, neutrality, and paradoxical comments, they changed the family therapy field permanently from the 1980s onwards.

Their method involved a pre-session team discussion with *hypothesizing*, then an initial session of assessment by an observed therapist, who then left the room to consult with a team of colleagues, subsequently returning to the family to deliver a '*prescription*' or task. Finally, there was a post-session team discussion. They saw families for about ten sessions at monthly intervals.

They often offered a '*paradoxical*' *comment* by noting how the symptoms of the index patient and the other family members are all inspired by the wish to preserve family cohesion. This was a deliberately mysterious attempt to use the momentum of resistance to effect change.

A *hypothesis* is a suggestion made by the therapist on the basis of available information, before therapy begins. It is not true or false, but more or less useful, and should be easily abandoned when it is shown to be inaccurate by clinical experience. The hypothesis reduces muddle, keeping the therapist actively tracking relational patterns in the family, and must be systemic, including all elements of the family and explaining overall relational functioning.

Circularity is getting family members to comment on other relationships, e.g. to *a*, 'if *x* is irritating *y*, what does *b* do?' *Circular questioning* is when the answer to the first question shapes the next question, leading to a jointly-arrived-at new understanding. Questions are particularly designed to elicit difference and introduce new perspective, and may have embedded suggestions.

Neutrality is the recommended Milan stance of friendly detachment and being curious without taking sides. However, this was challenged in relation to domestic violence and child abuse where therapeutic neutrality was deemed unacceptable.

Over time, the two men in the Milan group Boscolo and Cecchin moved away from the idea of the team delivering a '*perturbing*' message to the family towards *the way of asking questions becoming the intervention*. This *conversation/discourse model* has been called '**post-Milan**', and teams evolved different versions internationally. These included **Karl Tomm** in Calgary, **Lynn Hoffman** in Amherst, **David Campbell** in London, and **Tom Andersen** in Norway. Tom Andersen was the originator of the 'reflecting team' approach where clinicians offer their thoughts to the family in a group conversation, and then the family have an opportunity to comment on the fairness/usefulness or otherwise of the clinicians' ideas. This is a transparent, democratizing, affirming technique, which is appreciated by families and allows trainees to participate actively in therapy.

Elizabeth Kuipers developed a behavioural and psycho-educational family approach, building on earlier work of **Julian Leff** on expressed emotion aiming to improve communication and realistic negotiation in families where one member has schizophrenia—shown to reduce the relapse rate and improves compliance in schizophrenia; recommended in NICE guidelines for schizophrenia.

Monica McGoldrick described the *family life cycle*, a developmental view of families, in which the central underlying process is the expansion, contraction, and realignment of the relationship system to support the entry, exit, and development of family members in a functional way. The family therapist seeks to understand why the family is presenting *now*—often a life cycle transition stresses the system, as it needs to adapt and develop but struggles to do so: the separation of adolescent children, the couple becoming parents, new members as adult children's partners, the empty nest. This model also highlights family events outside the ordinary developmental cycle which challenge the structure such as bereavement, illness, unemployment, divorce, or separation.

Virginia Goldner (1988) was a feminist family therapist who stressed the white male dominance of the family therapy field, mirroring the general inequality of gender opportunity, violence against women, and mother-blaming in therapy. She insisted that gender was not just another 'secondary, mediating variable like race, class, or ethnicity, but rather a fundamental organizing principle of all family systems'. She emphasized the idealization of the family as a place of gender cooperation, in contrast to the outside world where women are 'politically and economically one-down'. In 1990, Goldner and colleagues described couples with repetitive violence of men against women. They unpack the social and intergenerational gender pressures contributing to both the male violence (disowned vulnerability, 'macho' stereotyping) and the female victimization (women caught between the internally sanctioned ideal of the woman who always cares for others and the wish to voice their own views).

Other family therapists at this time became interested in the relationship between the therapeutic process and language, meaning, and narrative, and include **Anderson and Goolishian** (1988), **Michael White** (1990), and **John Burnham** (1992) who utilized social constructionist ideas in his '*Approach—Method—Technique*'.

Jaakko Seikkula (2003), a Finnish psychologist, has described a network-based language approach to psychiatric care, called '*open dialogue*'. This is an approach to first-episode psychosis which reduces the need for hospitalization and medication, and has been successfully fostered in Scandinavia and Northern Europe, much less in the US or UK.

Burbach and **Stanbridge** (2009) are key figures in relation to service implementation in the UK in developing the Somerset model of family-sensitive mainstream services, as well as specific systemic interventions in CMHTs and inpatient wards. The model promotes seeing the patient in their relational context, not as a sick individual, with a genuine collaborative triangle of service user, family, and professionals.

What is the evidence base?

Numerous studies and meta-analyses have demonstrated the effectiveness of systemic family therapy. These include the following:

Carr (2000 and again in 2009) reviewed the evidence for family therapy and systemic intervention in a range of child and adult areas. He concluded that there is evidence of effectiveness for adults in schizophrenia, mood disorders, including major depression and bipolar disorder, anxiety disorders, including OCD, agoraphobia, panic, alcohol abuse, adjustment to chronic physical illness, as well as domestic violence and relationship distress. With children and adolescents, he found evidence for this approach in infancy with sleep, feeding, and attachment difficulties, conduct problems, including attention-deficit/hyperactivity disorder (ADHD), adolescent conduct disorder, drug misuse, emotional problems, including anxiety, school refusal, OCD, depression, grief, bipolar disorder, and deliberate self-harm. Similarly, there is evidence for family therapy in eating disorders (anorexia, bulimia, and obesity) and for somatic problems such as enuresis, encopresis, abdominal pain, poorly controlled diabetes, and asthma.

In the UK, Pilling et al. (2002) did a meta-analysis of family interventions and CBT in schizophrenia and found that family therapy had clear preventative effects on the outcome of psychotic relapse and readmission, in addition to benefits in medication compliance. This study informed the inclusion of family interventions in NICE guidelines for the psychological treatment of schizophrenia.

Shadish et al. (2003) reviewed 20 meta-analyses and found an average effect size of 0.65 after treatment and 0.52 at 6- to 12-month follow-up. They also found a better outcome in 71% of treated families, compared to controls.

Sydow et al. (2010) found that 34 out of 38 RCTs showed systemic treatment as effective and stable at follow-up, up to 5 years, and supported its use in mood disorders, eating disorders, substance misuse, schizophrenia, anxiety disorders, and mental and social factors related to medical conditions.

Julian Leff and his group in the London Depression Intervention Trial found that couple therapy was as effective as antidepressants but had wider benefits.

Russell Crane has also done extensive health economic research on the benefits of intervening in families and couples in terms of subsequent reduced health-care usage.

In deference to the need for evidence of effectiveness in systemic family therapy, a freely available and validated outcome measure for systemic family therapy, the *SCORE 15*, has been developed by the author and colleagues, which has been translated into over ten languages. SCORE 15 is a 15-item quantitative and qualitative self-report measure, giving a snapshot of current family functioning, with dimensions of strengths and adaptability, difficulties, and disrupted communication.

Family therapy training

Family therapy training is normally delivered as a part-time Master of Science (MSc) course, offered to professionals already qualified in psychiatry, psychology, psychiatric nursing, or social work. This is offered in a number of centres across the UK. (For further information, see ♫ http://www.aft.org.uk.)

It is increasingly recognized that shorter trainings (e.g. 1–2 years part-time) can allow systemic skills to develop and contribute to multidisciplinary team-working. There has also been an effort to offer basic training to CMHTs and psychiatric ward staff to enhance 'family-friendly policies' across mental health trusts and reduce staff anxiety about dealing with patients' relatives (see the Somerset model).

Recommended reading

Anderson T (1987). The reflecting team: dialogue and meta-dialogue in clinical work. *Family Process*, **26**, 371–93.

Burbach F and Stanbridge R (1998). Family intervention in psychosis service integrating the systemic and family management approaches. *Journal of Family Therapy*, **20**, 311–25.

Cecchin G (1987). Hypothesising, circularity, and neutrality revisited: an invitation to curiosity. *Family Process*, **26**, 405–13.

Dallos R and Draper R (2000). *An Introduction to Family Therapy: Systemic Theory and Practice.* Open University Press: Buckingham.

McNamee S and Gergen K (1992). *Therapy and Social Construction.* Sage: London.

Group therapy and group analysis

Key concepts

The theory and practice of group therapy and group analysis entail an understanding of:

* How humans interact in groups and the importance of the 'social mind' to the functioning of the human psyche
* How psychological change can be brought about using group processes.

The social mind

Homo sapiens evolved from other primates that live and function in social groups. Robin Dunbar (a social anthropologist) has shown that enhanced neocortical volume in humans is directly related to group size. Humans typically relate to a variety of groups: family/intimate groups (3–15), work groups (10–30), and communities (up to 120). Like other primates, humans who are not connected to groups are at risk of illness and early death; social isolation and exclusion are also associated with violence perpetration and victimization.

Enhanced neocortical volume in humans is associated with language skills which facilitate communication between group members and the development of different kinds of relationships that can be mentally represented across time and distance. Mentalizing skills have evolved in humans that allow group members to 'read' and reflect on the intentions of others, specifically in relation to threat, sexual pair bonding, and care giving. Mentalizing processes play a crucial role in the development of a social mind in children, and lack of secure attachment in childhood is associated with poor mentalizing skills in adulthood and impaired capacity to make social relationships and connect to social groups.

Human flourishing is associated with group membership. Vaillant found that optimal psychological functioning across the lifespan is associated with group affiliation of some sort—whether this is with family groups, clubs, or sports teams. Although it is possible for humans to use groups for malign purposes against other human groups, in general, group processes facilitate human learning, the development of ideas, and good-quality decision-making.

There are a number of processes that have been observed in both human and non-human groups, and which are relevant to *any therapist* running therapy groups. Groups typically form vertical hierarchies in relation to threat from external sources and perceived power/status within groups. There is usually a continual process of competition for higher ranking, although this varies from group to group in terms of the degree of activity, and many groups are stably led for long periods. Human groups typically oscillate between more cooperative periods of function (with flattened hierarchies) and more competitive periods if the group is threatened in some way. Pair bondings can disrupt well-functioning groups by acting as a focus for a split in a group and the formation of a rival group. Anxious groups may pick on one member and bully them, eventually expelling them. Group members who fail to make bonds with others may be expelled from groups and die early.

Psychological change in groups

Psycho-education, training, and psychotherapeutic processes can all be delivered in groups. Earliest examples of using groups for psychological development include religious communities and the self-help groups of Alcoholics Anonymous. Groups can facilitate learning, because members learn from each other and group membership promotes hope and compassion for suffering or distress. Group membership also assists learning, because it counteracts shame and social isolation.

Most forms of psychological therapy can be delivered in group format, making use of the educational and pro-social aspects of groups that facilitate psychological change. Group therapy can be short- or long-term, manualized or member-led, more or less supportive, and more or less focused on changing behaviour or cognitions. Many therapies are delivered in a group format for efficiency, although empirical evaluation becomes harder.

In addition, group analysis (GA) is a body of theory and therapeutic practice that argues that group processes are the medium for psychological change in the members of those groups. GA is not just psychoanalysis delivered in a group form; it is a psychological process of change that emerges from the experience of being a group with others, and the interpersonal dynamics that flow between members, both conscious and unconscious. Participation in group therapy can lead to reduction in the use of immature defences and subjective distress, and amelioration of negative personality traits. Studies of combined group and individual therapy have found that group members can develop enhanced capacity to mentalize, i.e. to reflect on their own mental states and those of others.

Group analysis involves thinking psychologically about:

- The group as a whole and the administration of the group
- The inner world and internal working models of each group member
- The dynamics of the interpersonal interactions between members, including defences within the group
- The experience of the conductor.

In addition to group therapies and group analysis, therapeutic change can also be effected through membership of a community of others with similar goals. The beneficial aspects of joining a community have been known since mediaeval times, but specifically therapeutic communities (TCs) were developed in the 1950s and 1960s (see ➜ Therapeutic communities in Chapter 2, pp. 75–80, and in Chapter 5, pp. 243–50).

Most people are wary of joining a new group of any sort; this anxiety is probably instinctual and an aspect of mammalian genetic heritage. However, the benefits of group therapy are profound and long-lasting. Group interventions should be offered to all patients who are not acutely disturbed or paranoid as part of a recovery and rehabilitation programme. These interventions may be educational and supportive, or promote changes in mentalizing or affect regulation; typically group interventions include all these aspects.

Group analysis can also be applied to organizations and social systems that themselves can become 'disordered' (see ➜ Psychotherapeutic understanding of organizational processes in Chapter 10, pp. 471–5). Group analysts address work teams as systems that have pathologies and defences, and so contribute to organizational management and development.

Key contributors

Group therapy and group analysis built on the work of psychodynamic theorists generally.

In the UK, **SH Foulkes** was a psychoanalyst who proposed that group analysis was analysis of the group, by the group, including the conductor. He used Freudian ideas in thinking about psychological change in groups but was also influenced by sociologists such as Norbert Elias, and anthropological studies of the development of mind. Foulkes emphasized the positive therapeutic potential of groups through the development of what he called 'the Matrix', a virtual set of relationships that is built up of the interactions between group members across time. Foulkes believed that psychological change takes place at different levels of the mind—a conscious level and a transferential level—but also a 'primordial level' reflecting our ancient roots as group animals. More recent group analytic thinkers (such as **Farhad Dalal** and **Morris Nitsun**) have challenged what they see as Foulkes's idealization of group processes and described how groups may enact antisocial and destructive impulses such as racism and scapegoating.

Wilfred Bion (see ➜ Key contributors in Chapter 2, pp. 25–8) was a psychoanalyst who applied analytic thinking to work groups, based on his experience of working with soldiers with neurotic dysfunction during the Second World War. He set up the 'Northfield experiment', which applied analytic thinking to work groups. Bion described dysfunctional processes (which he called *basic assumptions*) that groups develop that prevent them from carrying out their primary task; these include getting into pairs that undermine whole group participation, dropping out of groups altogether, and taking up a passive dependent relationship towards the group conductor. Bion's thinking about work groups was later built on, and developed by, **Isobel Menzies Lyth** in relation to the caring professions. She described how both workers and institutions consciously develop strategies and behaviours that unconsciously defend staff from awareness of negative feelings about their primary task, especially if that task generates anxiety, fear, or disgust (see ◗ Psychotherapeutic understanding of organizational processes in Chapter 10, pp. 471–5).

In the USA, **Irvin Yalom** developed an approach to group therapy that combined both analytic and existential thinking in therapy. Based on research with both outpatient and inpatient groups, Yalom described a number of group processes that were therapeutic and led to positive psychological change. Yalom's work has been highly influential in the USA and is the basis for most group therapy practised there. His textbook on group psychotherapy is now in its sixth edition.

What is the evidence base?

Group psychotherapies are complex to evaluate for a variety of reasons. First, each group contains as many variables as there are members; group members are not homogenous and do not experience a group intervention identically. Second, there is a vital empirical distinction between the delivery of a therapeutic technique (e.g. DBT) in a group format and the effectiveness of group therapy as an agent of psychological change in its own right. Third, it is hard to ensure that the therapists are delivering the same intervention; developing manuals for therapy represents an attempt to make therapists more homogenous but risks replacing therapy with taught courses of therapist-led instruction, which does not include attention to group processes of social cohesion and interpersonal relating.

Despite these obstacles, there have been many empirical studies of group therapies over the last decade. In the USA, Canada, and Europe, there is now an extensive body of evidence-based therapeutic experience of psychodynamic group therapy with many different populations and diagnostic problems. Psychodynamic group therapy is offered to patients with personality disorders, addictions, eating disorders, mood disorders, traumatic experiences, pathological grief, and offenders, with and without mental disorders. Key researchers in the field of psychodynamic group therapy (especially what works in group therapy) include **Morris Lesczc** (building on the work of Yalom), **Gary Burlingame**, **Steinar Lorentzen**, and **Roel Verheul**. Recent work by **Peter Fonagy** and **Anthony Bateman** has demonstrated the efficacy of combined group and individual work for individuals with chronic suicidal feelings and self-harming behaviours (see ◗ Mentalization-based treatment in Chapter 2, pp. 66–70, and in Chapter 5, pp. 229–34).

A UK-wide systematic review by Blackmore (2009) of published studies of group effectiveness found five high-quality RCTs of group therapy, with effect sizes ranging from 0.2 to 0.74. Conditions treated with group therapy included pathological grief, binge eating, personality disorders, mixed diagnoses, and aggression in men. Blackmore's review concludes that group therapy is more effective than either waiting list or case-controlled supportive therapies, and as effective as individual therapy. Subsequent studies by Lorentzen's group in Norway, and Bateman and

Fonagy in the UK, found that both outpatient and inpatient group psychotherapy are effective for people with personality disorders of varying types. In addition, there is evidence that therapies delivered in group formats are effective, e.g. DBT which has a weekly group component (see ➔ Dialectical behavioural therapy in Chapter 2, pp. 63–6, and in Chapter 5, pp. 220–9) and MBCT (see ➔ Mindfulness-based interventions and therapies in Chapter 2, pp. 73–5, and in Chapter 5, pp. 239–43) which is delivered as an 8-week group. The group format makes for economic efficiencies in terms of the cost-effectiveness of therapist time.

Group therapies typically last between 12 and 36 months; there is some evidence that, for complex psychopathology, most change is effected in the first 12–18 months of therapy. Group therapy seems especially effective for disorders and problems that have a social component to them such as social anxiety or cluster B personality disorders. Group therapies are also helpful in helping to shape pro-social attitudes so are increasingly used with antisocial populations such as criminal offenders.

Contraindications
There is very little in the way of an evidence base with respect to contraindications for group therapy. It is usually assumed that any contraindications will be similar to those for individual work, e.g. low intelligence quotient (IQ) or brain damage, inability to see experience in psychological terms, profound passive aggression or narcissism ('It's not my problem, it's someone else's'), dishonesty, and denial. People who are actively paranoid, suicidal, or addicted may also struggle to engage in therapy that encourages them to explore difficult feelings. However, in the history of psychodynamic therapy, there have been many patient groups or symptoms where it has been said that psychodynamic therapy is contraindicated, but where subsequent research has disproved this. For example, group analysts used to say that personality disorders or offenders could not be treated in psychodynamic therapy or only with great difficulty, which has been clearly disproved.

This is not to say that patients in group therapy may not have periods of distress and disturbance during the process of therapy (as happens in individual therapy). Some therapists ask patients to make contracts in respect of self-harm or suicide, whilst they are in therapy, because they anticipate that there may be periods of increased risk. The major risk in group therapy is that patients drop out of therapy when it gets difficult, and so do not have the experience of learning more about the operation of their minds and different ways of relating to their distress. Group therapy may also be complicated by overt acting out, such as verbal or even (rarely) physical aggression, which the therapist will need to manage. Most disturbances in group therapy arise from a combination of negative factors interacting together: in the individual patient, in the group process, and in the therapist. Co-therapy and supervision are helpful when groups become disturbed, and are essential from the start with groups of patients with complex needs.

There is no empirical evidence base that group therapies are contraindicated for any particular symptom or diagnosis; rather, each person's presentation and potential response to therapy have to be assessed individually, in light of the evidence (just as consultant surgeons do). Disturbance and therapeutic ruptures of disturbance may be a sign that therapy is working, rather than the opposite. Psychological change is usually painful and anxiety-provoking, and this needs to be explained to potential group members at the assessment stage as part of the preparation. This is why it is crucial at the assessment stage to ascertain whether the patient really wants to change their minds about themselves and others. People who do not want to change their minds may be better off with supportive therapy for distress or therapies that are largely psycho-educational.

Group therapy and group analysis training

In the UK, Europe, and Australia, formal trainings in group analytic therapy are available, e.g. via the Institute of Group Analysis (IGA) and the WPF. Formal training takes 3–4 years and includes running a therapy group under supervision, attendance at regular theory seminars, and participation in a therapy group as a patient. The IGA offers Diploma level courses in group work practice and a Master's level qualifying course.

However, gaining basic skills in running therapy groups is harder to find. The IGA runs introductory and foundation courses across the UK, which are popular and offer an experiential group experience. Details can be found on the IGA website (∂ http://www.groupanalysis.org/).

Like other psychodynamic trainings, group therapists train using a mixture of theoretical and experiential learning. Group analysts typically have training in both individual and group therapy. Most recognized trainings involve attendance at theory seminars, supervision groups, and participation as a patient in a therapy group. Group analysts need to be comfortable with challenging environments and working with other people. Most trainings include theoretical attention not only to psycho-analytic thought, but also sociology, anthropology, and evolutionary psychology.

Recommended reading

Dalal F (1998). *Taking the Group Seriously*. Jessica Kingsley: London.

Foulkes SH (1984). *Therapeutic Group Analysis*. Karnac Books: London.

Nitsun M (1996). *The Anti-Group: Destructive Forces in the Group and their Creative Potential*. International Library of Group Analysis: London.

Schermer V and Pines M (1994). *Ring of Fire: Primitive Affects and Object Relations in Group Psychotherapy*. Routledge: London.

Yalom ID and Leszcz M (2005). *The Theory and Practice of Group Psychotherapy*. Basic Books: New York.

Cognitive analytic therapy

CAT is an integrative model of psychotherapy initially devised by Anthony Ryle and subsequently further extended by both Ryle and others. CAT was formally named in 1984. The model stresses the internalized relational and social factors fundamental to most mental disorders. CAT adopts a proactive, 'doing with', collaborative style, characterized by an overtly compassionate stance, along with an emphasis on clear description of problems, their apparent origins, and of inviting change. This is achieved through early, jointly constructed, written, and diagrammatic 'reformulations' which are understood as 'psychological tools'. The approach is further characterized by a focus on time limits and on 'ending well'.

Importantly, CAT focuses on working non-judgementally with problematic relational patterns evident in the client's life and arising in therapy between therapist and client, including 'difficult', self-destructive, or even antisocial patterns of thoughts, feelings, and behaviour. This work would always be undertaken in a non-critical or non-judgemental way and would assume that these patterns essentially represent the client trying to survive or cope in the way they have learnt, given their formative experiences and circumstances. Consequently, a major strength of CAT is its ability to engage 'difficult' or 'hard to help' clients and to create a strong therapeutic alliance and higher levels of engagement. CAT has been further developed for use as both an individual and group-based therapy for a range of mental health problems in settings from primary care through to multidisciplinary teams in institutional settings which work with more complex problems such as 'personality'-type disorders related to childhood abuse and trauma, eating disorders, bipolar disorder, substance abuse, medical illness and medically unexplained symptoms, OCD, and gender identity disorders, and in forensic and learning disability settings. CAT is also being used as a consultancy tool for teams and services working with 'difficult' clients, making use of extended 'contextual' reformulations. As such, CAT has by now developed into a mature time-limited integrative psychological therapy and a relational model of human development and its relationship to mental disorder.

Key concepts

Concept of self

CAT is founded on a well-defined concept of a self that is fundamentally socially formed and located, although understood to be determined also by individual genetic endowment and temperament. CAT understands human psychological development (and so also mental disorders or 'psychopathology') to be rooted in, and profoundly influenced by, the early experience of semiotically mediated human relationships in a particular sociocultural context. The model has evolved further in the light of advances in developmental and infant psychology, notably form the work of Colwyn Trevarthen, Vasu Reddy, and Daniel Stern. These have stressed the actively intersubjective nature of developing infants and their predisposition and need for play, collaboration, meaning making, and 'companionship'. Psychological development is understood to occur, in large part, through a process of 'internalization' enabled by our capacity for empathy and intersubjectivity. The process of internalization, following the Russian psychologist Lev Vygotsky, is seen as one that is transformative. This implies that the psychological structures which enable internalization are themselves changed by it. This results in a self that is subjectively and 'objectively' fundamentally different and diverse, depending on formative interpersonal and cultural experiences. This developmental process also generates our values and beliefs and our very 'felt sense' of individual self and of relations to others. CAT therefore also stresses the importance of social and cultural factors (e.g. cultures of abuse, oppression, and inequality) in contributing to mental disorders and also in possibly limiting the outcome of treatment. From this perspective, it is understood that, in an important sense, there can be no such thing as an individual; just as Winnicott postulated with regard to the nursing mother and baby (see ➋ Psychoanalytic psychotherapy in Chapter 2, pp. 20–30). Rather, the individual is seen as a dynamic fragment of a social whole, and correspondingly individual mental health and well-being can only be considered as part of that overall sociocultural context.

Reciprocal roles

The CAT model is also based on the understanding that it is the experience of whole relationships that is internalized. This generates a repertoire of (formative) *reciprocal roles*. A reciprocal role (RR) is a CAT-specific term referring to a relational position between self and other. An internalized (formative) reciprocal role is understood to comprise both poles of that subjective experience (i.e. child-derived and parent/culture-derived). A reciprocal role comprises an implicit (often unconscious) relational memory (which may be traumatic) and also the emotions, cognitions (including cultural values and beliefs), behaviours, and even the body language associated with it. It may be associated with clear specific or general dialogical 'voices'. The latter may represent an important focus of therapy. These formative RRs are understood to determine and underlie our sense of self, of self in relation to others, and also the repertoire of responsive or coping patterns we subsequently develop. These are described as *reciprocal role procedures* (RRPs). An RRP is a CAT-specific term referring to an aim-directed coping or 'responsive' pattern of thoughts, feelings, and behaviours arising out of the experience of formative RR(s). RRPs are usually long-standing, often unconscious and highly resistant to change. They may be highly maladaptive, symptomatic, and self-reinforcing. RRPs may be enacted in both 'external' interpersonal situations and also in 'internal' self-management. They may be described as *traps* (which confirm negative assumptions), *snags* (mistrust of good things), or *dilemmas* (false polarities), depending on their configuration. Such RRPs are enacted both in relation to other people in the 'here and now' (including of course, importantly, in therapy) and also in self-management (in 'self-to-self' role procedures). These may be mediated through a clear internal (e.g. 'critical') dialogic voice. Common reciprocal roles range from, e.g. '*properly caring for–properly cared for*' at one extreme to '*neglecting and abusing–neglected and abused*' at the other. Importantly, enactment of a reciprocal role always anticipates, or attempts to elicit, an expected reciprocal reaction from a historic or current other.

Multiple self-states model

CAT offers a dimensional approach, the *multiple self-states model* (MSSM), to the conceptualization of more severe and complex damage to the self (as in 'borderline'-type disorders), occurring as a result of chronic developmental trauma/emotional adversity, partly due to repeated experiences of dissociation in the context of neurobiological vulnerability. This results in a damaged self, prone to 'switch' or 'flip' into different extreme *self-states* (each characterized by an RR) with greatly reduced ability to self-reflect and cope adaptively. Impulsive enactments of extreme, disconnected RRs within different self-states may, in turn, provoke extreme and unhelpful reciprocal reactions from others, including the therapist, staff team, or family members.

Therapeutic stance

CAT is characterized by a proactive, collaborative therapeutic style and by an overtly compassionate stance which is seen theoretically as important both in engaging clients and generating a robust alliance. This benign relational experience will also gradually in itself be internalized. The CAT theory stresses the importance of clear, early, joint reformulation of presenting problems and of their developmental background. CAT also emphasizes the need to engage with the client in a way that is accessible and usable by each individual, and at a pace each can deal with. This is described, following Vygotsky, as working within the 'zone of proximal development' (ZPD).

Reformulation

Reformulation in CAT refers to the collaborative creation, early in therapy, of an agreed description of presenting (or 'target') problems and their apparent origins, particularly in terms of formative relational and social experiences. Both a *written narrative reformulation* (in the form of a letter) and a *sequential diagrammatic reformulation* (SDR or 'map') will be constructed. Both attempt to describe in a non-judgmental manner the patterns of difficulties with which the client presents and their background origins, and also, as therapy progresses, possible ways of moving forward ('aims' or 'exits') are added to the SDR. These serve as 'route maps' for therapy and also as a means of making sense of, and repairing, possible problematic role enactments not only with others, but also between client and therapist.

Cognitive analytic therapy principles

Although CAT offers an overall structure with a sequence of stages and use of psychological tools, it does not prescribe a detailed manualized treatment and overall adopts a whole person approach. CAT can be seen as being conducted on the basis of a set of ten principles, flexibly and creatively applied in the context of the individual client. Adherence to the CAT model is measured, using an adherence tool called 'C-CAT'. The ten domains of competency for CAT are:

(1) Phase-specific tasks (such as engagement skills in early sessions)
(2) Making theory–practice links
(3) CAT tools (such as narrative reformulation)
(4) Boundaries
(5) Common factor skills
(6) Collaborative climate
(7) Assimilation of warded-off or problematic states
(8) Making links and hypotheses
(9) Managing threats to the therapeutic alliance
(10) Awareness and management of therapist's own reactions/feelings.

Similarly, CAT does not focus principally on symptoms, behaviours, or diagnostic labels, although these may form an important part of the overall picture (e.g. in reformulations) and may require active treatment at some point. As with other relational therapies, this more holistic approach does not fit easily with the way treatments are appraised for use in public services, which can be overly focused on diagnostic labels and symptom reduction, and does not take into account the diversity and overlapping nature of real clinical populations.

Ending well

CAT sees 'ending well' as an important aim in itself. This would be conceptualized as sharing the experience of ending openly and without resorting to old coping patterns (RRPs) and to communicate authentic feelings as they arise. These could include disappointment, anxiety, or anger at the therapist for ending. Not ending well risks generating either unhelpful dependency or may also result in an equally unhelpful, mutually gratifying, and admiring relationship which may perpetuate previous RRPs and undermine attempts at change.

Key contributors

CAT was developed over several decades by **Anthony Ryle** in an attempt to integrate the valid and effective elements of the different, but often contradictory, models of the time. These included behaviourism, early cognitive psychology (notably George Kelly's personal construct theory), and various schools of psychoanalysis (particularly object relations theory and the work of Donald Winnicott and Thomas Ogden). It also represented an effort to develop a brief 'good enough' package in NHS settings for increasing numbers of clients. As such, the model arose, in part, out of a sense of social awareness and responsibility which still characterizes CAT today. CAT has been further transformed by **Lev Vygotsky**'s activity theory and concepts of a 'dialogical' self, deriving from Mikhail Bakhtin—notably through contributions from **Mikael Leiman** in Finland. CAT is also being used to reconceptualize a range of clinical problems and 'disorders' from different psychiatric settings such as later life (**Jason Hepple** and **Laura Sutton**), forensic settings (**Philip Pollock**), and learning disability (**Julie Lloyd** and **Phil Clayton**), and as an organizational consultancy tool (**Ian Kerr** and **Stephen Kellett**).

What is the evidence base?

CAT is acknowledged as an effective, pragmatic, flexible, and integrative approach, popular with clients and therapists, and is accruing a body of research evidence for its effectiveness. The evidence base includes RCTs and outcome studies for mixed and emerging personality disorder in clinical settings, as well as various level studies in a range of common mental and physical disorders such as bipolar disorder, anxiety, depression, anorexia, and diabetes. In a recent review of CAT outcome studies, the effect size for CAT was shown to be moderate to large over a range of studies involving clients with complex disorders. The model is recognized increasingly in treatment guidelines, particularly for more complex or treatment-resistant clients (e.g. CAT is mentioned in NICE guidance for BPD and anorexia, and is a specialist psychological therapy in the IAPT-SMI personality disorder competency framework (see ➲ Improving Access to Psychological Therapies services in Chapter 10, pp. 463–4). In addition, CAT fulfils all the criteria recognized as important in terms of common factors for effective psychotherapies (notably its focus on the therapeutic alliance) and with regard to the so-called 'equivalence paradox'. The latter describes the phenomenon of comparable outcomes for a wide range of 'different' 'brand name' models with considerable (implicit) commonalities (see ➲ Concepts and models: introduction in Chapter 2, pp. 14–20).

Cognitive analytic therapy training

Training in the UK is accredited by the Association for Cognitive Analytic Therapy (ACAT). The International Cognitive Analytic Therapy Association (ICATA) gives guidance for equivalence across a range of trainings available in different member countries, notably Finland, Greece, Italy, Spain, Australia, and India. ACAT is moving towards a formal modularized training portfolio, including 6-month CAT skills trainings in individual CAT practice and, in contextual CAT, a 1-year foundation course in CAT practice, a 2-year CAT practitioner training leading to accreditation as a CAT therapist or practitioner, and a supervisor training programme and a 2-year advanced training leading to UKCP registration as a CAT psychotherapist.

Recommended reading

Clarke S, Thomas P, and James K (2013). Cognitive analytic therapy for personality disorder: randomized controlled trial. *British Journal of Psychiatry*, **203**, 129–34.

Ryle A (1997). *Cognitive Analytic Therapy and Borderline Personality Disorder. The Model and the Method*. John Wiley & Sons: Chichester.

Ryle A and Kerr IB (2002). *Introducing Cognitive Analytic Therapy: Principles and Practice*. John Wiley & Sons: Chichester.

Ryle A, Kellett S, Hepple J, and Calvert R (2014). Cognitive analytic therapy at 30. *Advances in Psychiatric Treatment*, **20**, 258–68.

Wilde McCormick E (2012). *Change for the Better: Self-Help Through Practical Psychotherapy, fourth edition*. Sage: London.

Further information and materials about CAT may be accessed through the website of ACAT (℗ http://www.acat.me.uk/page/home) or of ICATA (℗ internationalcat.org/).

Interpersonal psychotherapy

Key concepts

IPT is a time-limited (typically 16-weekly sessions), interpersonally focused therapy, originally developed to treat depression and now also used with eating disorders. Its efficacy in the treatment of depression and BN has been clearly established, and there is growing evidence supporting its application with a range of other clinical disorders.

IPT works primarily with current interpersonal difficulties. It integrates social and medical models of depression, and explicitly understands depression in the interpersonal context (see Fig. 2.1).

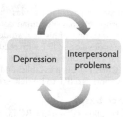

Fig. 2.1 Understanding the relationship between depression and current interpersonal problems.

IPT mainly focuses on the most recent episode of depression and highlights opportunities for interpersonal and symptomatic change in that context. Four interpersonal problem areas are used to focus the work:

- Adjusting to changes in significant roles, e.g. relationship breakdown or redundancy
- Resolving persistent conflict, e.g. between partners or work colleagues
- Learning to live with the loss following a major bereavement, e.g. of a parent or a child
- Struggling to establish and maintain significant relationships.

During the initial 3–4 sessions, a timeline of the current depressive episode is created, diagnosis is explicitly agreed, and psycho-education about depression is discussed. An inventory of current significant relationships is built up to identify resources and difficulties and to place depression in context. These tasks are used to identify the most relevant focus for the remaining sessions. During the middle eight sessions, the agreed target problem is examined in detail to clarify the ways in which the interpersonal difficulties and depression are maintained and to identify opportunities to improve communication and to use or develop interpersonal support to resolve the difficulty. The final sessions of IPT focus on preparing for the end of therapy, reviewing progress, and relapse prevention planning.

Key contributors

IPT is derived from the work of **Adolf Meyer**, **Harry Stack Sullivan**, **John Bowlby** and research on the psychosocial aspects of depression. **Sullivan** (1953) saw interpersonal relationships as the primary means by which to understand the individual and stressed the importance of working with observable and recurrent patterns in day-to-day living. **Meyer** (1957) highlighted the protective and vulnerability factors that arise from the interaction of our biological, social, and psychological make-up. **Bowlby**'s (1969) work on attachment and **Michael Rutter**'s subsequent work on resilience (1972) confirmed the social foundations of an individual's well-being and an individual's capacity to learn and recover from poor early experience through later reparative relationships, adaptive social and communication skills, and problem-solving.

The late **Gerald Klerman**, a psychiatrist, was the principle author of IPT. His wife and co-author **Myrna Weissman** continued to publish on IPT, following his death, with one of his final students **John Markowitz**. **Ellen Frank** and colleagues developed IPT with recurrent depression and bipolar disorder, and **Laura Mufson** extended the reach of IPT to adolescents with depression. **Chris Fairburn** established IPT as a treatment for BN, and **Denise Wilfley** modified IPT to be delivered in a group format.

What is the evidence base?

IPT has been empirically validated in many RCTs. It is recommended by NICE and many other international treatment guidelines as a first-line intervention for depression and BN, and there is a growing body of evidence supporting its application with other conditions. In a meta-analysis of seven major psychological therapies for mild to moderate depression, IPT was the only treatment found to be more efficacious than the others.

The first trials of IPT supported its use as a maintenance treatment for depression and as a treatment for acute depression, with and without medication. Evidence for IPT as an effective maintenance treatment for recurrent depression was replicated with both working age adults and older adults.

In the first trial of IPT combined with antidepressant medication, combined treatment was superior to either treatment alone in reducing depressive symptoms, and IPT resulted in significantly greater improvement in the quality of relationships than medication over 1-year follow-up. Blom et al. (2007) also found combined treatment to be superior to antidepressant medication alone in reducing depressive symptoms, but not to IPT alone. Subsequent studies examining combined treatment have shown that introducing antidepressant medication when IPT alone does not achieve significant change within the first weeks of treatment results in significantly higher recovery rates (79% versus 66%) than combined treatment from the outset. The package of individual or combined treatment required to achieve remission must be continued after treatment to maintain well-being.

IPT has been compared to CBT for depression and BN. In the first trial for depression, few differences were found between the psychological therapies. This finding was replicated by Luty et al. (2007). These studies produced inconsistent findings on the role of baseline severity in determining outcome, with one finding in favour of IPT and the other finding in favour of CBT.

IPT and CBT for BN produce comparable long-term outcomes. CBT produced greater global improvement by the end of treatment, but outcomes were equivalent 4–8 months after treatment ended. Subsequent studies, which have placed fewer restrictions on IPT by allowing interventions common to both approaches, have shown enhanced effectiveness for IPT. Group format IPT and CBT have also been used to treat BED and have been shown to be equivalent in reducing binge eating, eating pathology, and general psychopathology in the short and long term.

IPT has been adapted as a treatment for depressed adolescents and has been shown to be more effective than no treatment or standard school counselling in five RCTs. Controlled comparisons between IPT and CBT for depressed adolescents have produced mixed results, with the first study reporting comparable outcomes in reduction in depressive symptoms and superior outcome of self-esteem and social adaptation for IPT, and the later study reported good outcomes for both treatments, but more favourable results for CBT.

Recent research has looked more closely at the role IPT may have in treating anxiety disorders. Co-morbid generalized anxiety disorder (GAD) does not have a detrimental impact on outcome, whilst co-morbid panic disorder does. When used as a treatment for social anxiety disorder, IPT has demonstrated comparable outcomes to supportive dynamic therapy and CBT. IPT for PTSD, which does not focus on exposure to traumatic reminders, but rather to the interpersonal sequelae of trauma and affect dysregulation, has been evaluated in several open trials and one RCT with different trauma populations. These studies have shown a reduction greater than in no-treatment controls in PTSD and depressive symptoms following IPT.

Interpersonal therapy training

Training opportunities in IPT have developed significantly in recent years, particularly in the UK where it is included in the evidence-based therapies delivered for IAPT services for adults and as part of the service transformation in CAMHS services (CYP IAPT) in England (see ➔ Improving Access to Psychological Therapies services in Chapter 10, pp. 463–4). A map of IPT competencies was developed, and these formed the basis for a national training curriculum and competency-based supervision protocol (see ℘ www.iapt.nhs.uk). Introductory training is conducted over 9–12 months, with 6 training days and subsequent weekly supervision on four cases to complete practitioner accreditation. Accreditation requirements and details of accredited training courses and supervisors are available on the IPT UK website (℘ iptuk.org). More recently, training has been developed for IPT supervisors, which again runs over a series of training days with additional supervised casework as a practitioner and as a supervisor.

IPT practitioners are qualified mental health professionals with prior experience of delivering psychological therapy. IPT is not offered as a first training for novice therapists. IPT practitioners come from a wide range of professional backgrounds, including psychologists, psychiatrists, mental health nurses, and counsellors, and work in primary care, in specialist and secondary services, and in private practice.

Recommended reading

Cuijpers P, Geraedts AS, van Oppen P, Andersson G, Markowitz JC, and van Straten A (2011). Interpersonal psychotherapy for depression: a meta-analysis. *American Journal of Psychiatry*, 168, 581–92.
Frank E (2005). *Treating Bipolar Disorder. A Clinician's Guide to Interpersonal and Social Rhythm Therapy*. Guilford Press: New York.
Markowitz JC and Weissman MM (eds) (2012). *Casebook of Interpersonal Psychotherapy*. Oxford University Press: New York.
Mufson L, Dorta KP, Moreau D, et al. (2004). *Interpersonal Psychotherapy for Depressed Adolescents*, second edition. Guilford Press: New York.
Weissman MM, Markowitz, JC, and Klerman GL (2000). *Comprehensive Guide to Interpersonal Psychotherapy*. Basic Books: New York.

Psychodynamic interpersonal therapy

Key concepts

PIT is also known as the *conversational model of psychotherapy*, and the latter is the preferred term for many clinicians who practise the model. It is a psychotherapy that can be delivered in a variety of different formats, including short-term and long-term treatments.

The general approach is one of *personal problem-solving*, i.e. solving personal problems, and of solving problems in a personal way. Difficulties in personal relationships are brought alive in the therapy, understood, and explored, and solutions tested. There is an emphasis upon getting to know someone, rather than getting to know a lot of facts about them.

The therapeutic process involves developing a particular kind of '*conversation*' with the client, which encourages the development of a feeling language, a conversation in which feelings are experienced and shared, as opposed to being talked about. Problems are directly expressed, presented, or enacted in the 'here and now'. New possibilities for actions and acts are generated between the client and therapist, which can then be tested out and generalized to other settings.

There are three important concepts. The first is '*forms of feeling*', which is crucial to the conversational model approach. Feeling in this context does not mean a faculty of emotion; it refers to a form of 'emotional knowing' or imaginative emotion related to an idea. This requires a different thought process to an intellectual way of thinking about problems and requires a form of creative imaginative or symbolic attitude which links together feeling states, symbols, memories, and experiences.

The second is the notion of '*bodily experience*'. All feeling states are felt within the body as bodily experiences, but they are often talked about as being in the 'mind'. This disconnect encourages a distancing from emotion and a way of processing experience which splits it into separate cognitive, emotional, and somatic domains. By focusing upon bodily experience in the 'here and now' and staying with that experience, it becomes possible to reconnect different domains, so experience is felt as a whole and as a creation of people's past and present interpersonal interactions.

The third is '*minute particulars*'. This is a micro-, as opposed to meta- or macro-, approach. It involves a constant consideration of the subtle, nuanced interactions between the client and therapist. What is going on between two people *right now*?

The model works primarily with interpersonal difficulties. It hypothesizes that human distress (symptomatology) arises and persists from inappropriate ways of dealing with current and past interpersonal hurts, especially those involving loss and separation. Ways of avoiding pain develop, but these often result in actions, which hamper personal growth, independence, and the ability to develop close, trusting relationships. Problem-solving is impaired, whilst problem-avoiding is perpetuated.

Clients are encouraged to focus upon feeling states/bodily experiences in the 'here and now' and to stay with these feelings. This leads to a deeper level of exploration and the association of feelings and experiences to images, impressions, and memories, which, in turn, link to key relationship experiences. Ways of avoiding or warding off hurt or distress are revealed and overcome in a gradual, stepwise, and collaborative process, contingent upon the client's feedback. This process occurs on a cyclical basis throughout the therapy.

The therapy has a psychodynamic component in that there is an assumption that difficult feelings or experiences are warded off and may not be immediately accessible to the client. Bringing experiences and difficult feelings into the here and now is therefore a key aspect of the therapeutic process. A detailed examination of the theoretical basis of the model has been developed by Meares, who draws upon self psychology as basis for the core approach.

In its brief format, the model follows traditional structures for short-term therapies with a focus upon one or two problem areas. The therapist is supportive and collaborative. Ending is acknowledged as being a significant and potentially difficult transition phase for the client. A goodbye letter is given to the client, which seeks to capture the essence of the meetings between the client and therapist, focusing upon positive change and future problem-solving.

Key contributors

The conversational model was developed in the 1960s in the UK by **Robert Hobson** and **Russell Meares**. Their essential idea was that people's primary fundamental disturbance was a disruption or stunting of the ordinary experience of personal existing. They viewed 'self' not as an isolated system, but as part of a larger social organism, which was formed and constantly reformed via interpersonal interactions with others.

Hobson published his thoughts about a new approach to psychotherapy in 1971 in a paper entitled *Imagination and Amplification in Psychotherapy*, and this was followed by a preliminary account of some of the features of the model in *The Pursuit of Intimacy* by Meares in 1977. Hobson then published a fuller account of the therapeutic approach in his book *Forms of Feeling* in 1985.

Frank Margison worked with Robert Hobson to develop teaching tapes on the model in the 1980s and to evaluate the ability to teach the model to psychiatrists in training. **David Shapiro** carried out the first independent evaluations of the efficacy of the model in the late 1980s. **Michael Barkham** and **Gillian Hardy** have also been closely involved in evaluations of the model. **James Moorey** and **Eileen Brierly** have been responsible for delivering training in the model in the UK over the last 20 years.

Russell Meares has further elaborated and developed the theoretical underpinning of the model in relation to BPD. A full exposition of his work has been published recently, and a psychotherapeutic manual for delivering the conversational model for people with BPD is also available. **Anthony Korner** and **Joan Haliburn** have worked closely with Russell Meares and contributed to further development of the model.

Hobson and Meares cited many influences of their work, including Pierre Janet, Hughlings Jackson, Carl Gustav Jung, Jan Vigotsky, Martin Buber, John Bowlby, Miller Mair, Suzanne Langer, and Ludwig

Wittgenstein. They also both stressed the importance of artistic influences in understanding the nature of human experience. Hobson was particularly influenced by the Lake Poets (William Wordsworth and Samuel Taylor Coleridge), William Shakespeare, and William Blake.

Hobson preferred to use the common language of 'men' (or women) to describe people's problems, rather than psychodynamic terminology. Therapists using the model therefore try to capture the essence of people's problems and difficulties using everyday language or concepts, rather than psychodynamic models.

What is the evidence base?

The first evaluations of PIT compared its efficacy for the treatment of depression with a form of CBT. The first study by Shapiro and Firth, published in 1987, involved a cross-over design in which eight sessions of PIT followed by eight sessions of CBT were compared with eight sessions of CBT followed by eight sessions of PIT. There was broad equivalence between the outcomes of the two therapies, and approximately 60% of clients achieved a good outcome.

Two further studies compared 8-session PIT and CBT with 16-session PIT and CBT therapy for clients with depression. There was broad equivalence in outcome between the two treatments on most measures, with CBT showing a better outcome on the Beck Depression Inventory, and PIT showing a better outcome for clients with more severe depression. The group also evaluated a very brief form of PIT and CBT therapy (2 + 1) for treatment of subclinical depression, which involved two sessions of either PIT or CBT, 1 week apart, followed by a follow-up session some weeks later. Both therapies performed well and had better outcomes than wait-list controls.

PIT has been evaluated as a treatment for medically unexplained symptoms in five RCTs. Four of the studies focused upon patients with severe and persistent symptoms, who had not responded to conventional treatments and who had not been helped by specialist medical care.

The first study was published in 1991 and recruited 102 patients with severe and intractable irritable bowel syndrome (IBS). PIT was found to be superior to supportive therapy, both in terms of the reduction of bowel symptomatology and psychological distress. The improvement in outcome was maintained over 12 months. The second study involved patients with severe and retractable functional dyspepsia. Patients in this study were randomized to PIT versus supportive therapy. The outcome showed that PIT was superior to the supportive condition both at the end of treatment and at follow-up 6 months later.

The cost-effectiveness of PIT for the treatment of severe and intractable IBS was evaluated by Creed and colleagues in a large multicentre trial of 257 patients. PIT was compared with antidepressant treatment and usual care. Both PIT and antidepressant treatment resulted in significantly improved outcomes at 12 months post-treatment in relation to both physical and mental health. Only PIT, however, was associated with a significant reduction in health-care use in the 12 months post-treatment, compared with patients who received usual care. The average savings per patient over 12 months were approximately £1000, and, for patients with the most severe symptoms, cost savings were between £2000 and £3000 per annum per patient. These savings included the costs of the therapy.

PIT has been compared to enhanced medical care for patients with persistent multisomatoform disorder, which is characterized by severe and disabling bodily symptoms, of which pain is the commonest symptom. This study was a large multicentre trial conducted in six different cities in Germany, involving over 200 patients. The main findings were that patients who received PIT showed significantly greater improvement in physical and mental health function, compared with the control group, over the course of the study.

Elements of PIT have been incorporated into a group format in a primary care setting for patients with medically unexplained symptoms (MUS). Positive improvements in mental health were found in comparison to usual care following the treatment, but there were no major effects on physical health status.

There has been one RCT which has evaluated PIT as a treatment for self-harm. In this study, 119 patients who had presented to a UK emergency department after an episode of self-poisoning were randomized to four sessions of home-based PIT, in comparison with usual treatment. The therapists in the study were mental health nurses who were trained to deliver PIT but did not have any formal psychotherapy qualification or prior training.

Participants who received PIT had a significantly greater reduction in suicidal ideation at 6-month follow-up, compared with those in the control group. They were much more satisfied with their treatment and much less likely to report further self-harm during the 6-month follow-up period than participants who received usual care. This study showed that nurses with good interpersonal skills could be trained to deliver PIT for self-harm and deliver this treatment effectively.

PIT has also been evaluated as a treatment for distressed high service users. Patients who received PIT, in comparison with controls, reported a reduction in psychological symptoms, an improvement in health status, and a reduction in health-care costs during the 6 months post-treatment. Patients who received PIT required less inpatient treatment, medication, general practitioner (GP) time, and nurse practitioner time in the 6 months post-treatment than controls.

There have been two major evaluations of PIT for patients with BPD, and there is one RCT currently in progress which is comparing PIT with DBT (personal communication from Drs Bendit and Walton, Centre for Psychotherapy, Newcastle, New South Wales, Australia).

Stevenson and Meares reported the treatment and outcome of 30 patients with BPD treated with PIT for 12 months with two sessions per week. These patients showed significant improvements in mental health function over the year and marked improvement on seven behavioural measures, which included self-harm behaviour, violence towards others, use of drugs (both legal and illegal), and number of hospital admissions. The patients who received therapy were compared with a matched group of 30 patients with BPD who were referred to the same clinic where the trial was based, but no therapist was available, so they remained on the waiting list for 1 year. In comparison with this matched group, the patients who received PIT showed significantly greater improvements in mental health function, which was maintained for 5 years. In a further analysis of costs, the use of health care of the 30 patients treated with PIT was examined for the year prior to treatment and the year post-treatment. This showed a saving of $670000 (Australian dollars), compared to a cost of the psychotherapy of $130000, giving a net saving of $540000 or $18000 per patient. Most of the cost savings were in terms of reductions in hospital admissions.

The same team recently carried out a replication study, in which clients with BPD were allocated to treatment or wait-list, depending upon the availability of a therapist. This was not an RCT. The results were very similar to the first study, with significant improvements in the treatment group, in comparison with matched wait-list controls.

Shaw and colleagues carried out an evaluation of inexperienced therapists using the PIT model with patients referred to an NHS psychotherapy service. Patients were randomized to either psychotherapy or wait-list control. Significant improvement was demonstrated in those patients who completed therapy, and there was a non-significant trend towards greater improvement in the immediate treatment group, in comparison to wait-list controls.

Burns and colleagues assessed whether PIT could benefit cognitive function and affective symptoms in patients with Alzheimer's disease. There was, however, no evidence of improvement on the main outcome measures.

Psychodynamic interpersonal therapy training

Several different evaluations of training methods in PIT have been undertaken. The model is easy to learn, and health professionals without prior experience of, or training in, psychodynamic therapy can be taught to use the model effectively.

Experience and knowledge of mental health problems and basic therapeutic skills are essential. PIT training can be undertaken by qualified mental health professionals, including psychologists, psychiatrists, mental health nurses, and counsellors. Training consists of a 5-day course, followed by 12 weeks of supervised practice. A map of PIT competencies has been developed and is available to download.

PIT training is now also offered on several Doctor of Philosophy (PhD) clinical psychology courses, as the second therapy to CBT.

A basic form of the model (PIT:CORE) has also been developed and is being used to enhance and develop the skills of therapists who deliver low-intensity interventions in IAPT services.

Recommended reading

Creed F, Fernandes L, Guthrie E, et al. (2003). North of England IBS Research Group. The cost-effectiveness of psychotherapy and paroxetine for severe irritable bowel syndrome. *Gastroenterology*, **124**, 303–17.

Guthrie E, Kapur N, Mackway-Jones K, et al. (2001). Randomised controlled trial of brief psychological intervention after deliberate self-poisoning. *BMJ*, **323**, 135–8.

Guthrie E, Moorey J, Margison F, et al. (1999). Cost-effectiveness of brief psychodynamic-interpersonal therapy in high utilizers of psychiatric services. *Archives of General Psychiatry*, **56**, 519–26.

Sattel H, Lahmann C, Gündel H, et al. (2012). Brief psychodynamic interpersonal psychotherapy for patients with multisomatoform disorder: randomised controlled trial. British Journal of Psychiatry, 200, 60–7.

Shapiro DA, Rees A, Barkham M, et al. (1994). Effects of treatment duration and severity of depression on the maintenance of gains following cognitive-behavioural therapy and psychodynamic-interpersonal therapy. Journal of Consulting and Clinical Psychology, 63, 378–87.

Dynamic interpersonal therapy

Key concepts

DIT is a short-term (16 sessions) individual psychodynamic therapy protocol for the treatment of mood disorders (specifically depression and anxiety). The protocol was designed in 2008 on the basis of the work of the UK Department of Health-commissioned Expert Reference Group on psychoanalytic psychotherapy competencies drawn from manualized psychoanalytic/dynamic therapies that yielded good results in psychotherapy outcome studies.

DIT's starting point is rooted in the common clinical observation that patients who present as depressed and/or anxious invariably also present with difficulties and distress about their relationships. Although the patient may well experience his problem as 'I cannot sleep and concentrate', the DIT therapist reframes the symptoms as a manifestation of a relational disturbance, which the patient cannot understand or understands in a distorted way, attributing to himself and others motivations which are unlikely or unhelpful. Once the patient is helped to make some changes in the way he approaches his relationship difficulties, depressive symptoms are typically alleviated.

The aims of the therapy are to:

- Identify an attachment-related problem with a specific relational emotional focus that is felt by the patient to be making them depressed
- Work with the patient collaboratively to create a mentalistic picture of interpersonal issues raised by the problem
- Encourage the patient to explore the possibility of alternative ways of feeling and thinking ('playing with a new internal and external reality'), actively using the transference relationship to bring to the fore the patient's characteristic ways of relating
- Ensure the therapeutic process (of change in self) is reflected on
- Near the end of treatment, present to the client a written summary, which they can keep, of the collaboratively created view of the person and the selected area of unconscious conflict, to reduce the risk of relapse.

Key contributors

DIT was developed in 2009 by **Alessandra Lemma**, **Mary Target**, and **Peter Fonagy**—all three clinical psychologists and psychoanalysts—as a collaboration between two key UK institutions that have championed psychoanalytic work within the public health and voluntary sectors, respectively, the Tavistock and Portman NHS Trust and the Anna Freud Centre.

DIT draws on a range of psychoanalytic traditions, most notably object relations theory, Sullivan's interpersonal psychoanalysis, and attachment theory. In particular, Kernberg's integration of object relations theory with ego psychology in the theoretical frame of transference-focused psychotherapy is very close to the heart of DIT's theoretical basis and way of formulating a focus for the intervention.

Bearing in mind these influences, several core assumptions underpin DIT:

- The social origins and nature of individual subjectivity
- The importance of attachments as the building blocks of the mind and as the context for developing crucial social cognitive capacities
- The impact of internalized, unconscious 'self', and 'other' representations on current interpersonal functioning
- The importance of the capacity to mentalize experience, without which the individual is more vulnerable to developmentally earlier modes of experiencing internal reality which, in turn, undermine the capacity to resolve interpersonal difficulties.

What is the evidence base?

DIT is a comparatively new protocol, such that, at the time of writing, the results of the first trial are not yet available. The only published results to date refer to two small-scale pilot studies. In the first, Lemma, Fonagy, and Target (2011) set out to test DIT's acceptability and compatibility with session-by-session monitoring as a prelude to the ongoing RCT. Sixteen consecutively referred depressed patients (aged 20–53) were offered 16 sessions of DIT. Patient outcomes were collected pre-post and on a session-by-session basis, using the PHQ-9 and GAD-7. Therapist and supervision feedback indicated that this structured psychodynamic treatment could be effectively taught and that the key competences involved were acquired and demonstrated in the clinical work supervised. Patients found the treatment acceptable and relevant to their problems. The treatment appeared compatible with session-by-session monitoring of symptoms of anxiety and depression. DIT was associated with a significant reduction in reported symptoms in all but one case, to below clinical levels in 70% of the patients. The results suggested that DIT was promising in its acceptability and effectiveness with an unselected group of primary care patients, and was easily acquired by psychodynamically trained clinicians.

The second published study by Lemma and Fonagy in 2012 focused on a pilot of an 8-session adaptation of DIT in a group format and delivered online. Twenty-four participants were randomly assigned to three groups. Participants in Condition A ($N = 8$) took part in an online DIT group, with self-help materials, facilitated by a therapist. Participants in Condition B ($N = 8$) were given access to a closed virtual group space where they could interact with each other and were supplied with the same self-help materials used by participants in Condition A, but without online therapist facilitation. Participants in Condition C ($N = 8$) received no instructions or facilitation, but had access to an online mental well-being site where they could meet virtually in a large, open, moderated virtual group space to discuss their psychological difficulties. This feasibility study was underpowered to detect significant differences in rates of change between facilitated and unfacilitated provision of material, but decline in symptoms appeared to be superior to control only for the facilitated group when the groups were considered separately. The response of the combined treated groups against the control suggested that the DIT self-help materials may be helpful and appear to support the process of change. Further work is clearly required.

Dynamic interpersonal therapy training

The training programme for DIT provides psychoanalytically/dynamically trained practitioners with a structure within which to conduct a time-limited (16 sessions), manualized psychodynamic therapy. It is intended as a CPD course to hone the skills of already established and qualified psychodynamic practitioners (defined as equivalent to a Diploma level qualification), so as to enable them to deliver an effective brief psychodynamic intervention for the treatment of mood disorders. The training consists of a 4-day course, followed by weekly supervision of two cases for 16 sessions each, and the completion of a case study in order to reach practitioner status.

Pre-entry and accreditation requirements are available on the DIT website (℘ www.d-i-t.org). The training is accredited in the UK by the BPC.

Established training teams now also offer trainings in Holland, Belgium, Denmark, and Italy.

Recommended reading

Lemma A and Fonagy P (2013). Feasibility study of a psychodynamic online group intervention for depression. *Psychoanalytic Psychotherapy* 30: 367–80.

Lemma A, Fonagy P, and Target M (2010). The development of a brief psychodynamic protocol for depression: dynamic interpersonal therapy. *Psychoanalytic Psychotherapy: Applications, Theory and Research* 24: 329–46.

Lemma A, Fonagy P, and Target M (2011). The development of a brief psychodynamic intervention (dynamic interpersonal therapy) and its application to depression: a pilot study. *Psychiatry: Biological and Interpersonal Process* 74: 41–8.

Dialectical behaviour therapy

Key concepts

DBT is an integrative and comprehensive cognitive behavioural treatment, originally developed for chronically suicidal and parasuicidal individuals with a diagnosis of BPD (see ➜ Borderline personality disorder in Chapter 8, pp. 390–6), with the ultimate goal of helping clients to build a life worth living. DBT developed from the failure of standard CBT protocols for chronically suicidal clients due to three main difficulties. First, the focus on change procedures was often perceived as invalidating by the client, often leading to withdrawal from therapy; second, teaching new skills was difficult, whilst treating the client's ongoing suicidality; and third, clients with BPD often unwittingly reinforced the therapist for ineffective treatment and punished them for effective treatment strategies. These difficulties were addressed by modifying the standard cognitive behavioural approach by integrating four other aspects: a focus on acceptance and validation, emphasis on treating therapy-interfering behaviours, an emphasis on the therapeutic relationship, and a focus on the dialectical process.

DBT combines the basic strategies of behaviour therapy with eastern mindfulness practices, residing within an overarching dialectical world-view that emphasizes the synthesis of opposites. The fundamental dialectic in DBT is between validation and acceptance of the client, as they are within the context of simultaneously helping them to change.

DBT is founded on the biosocial theory of personality functioning. The main premise is that BPD is mainly a dysfunction of the emotion regulation system caused by acute emotional vulnerability and emotion modulation difficulties, combined with certain dysfunctional environments.

Emotional vulnerability is characterized by:
• Hypersensitivity to emotional stimuli: the individual reacts quickly and has a low threshold for an emotional reaction
• Intense emotional reactivity: emotional reactions are extreme, e.g. what would cause slight embarrassment for another may cause deep humiliation; annoyance may turn to rage
• Slow return to emotional baseline: reactions are long-lasting.

Emotion modulation refers to the ability to experience and identify emotions, and to then attune to strong emotional stimuli, in order to regulate emotional and behavioural after-effects. Failure to modulate emotions effectively is hypothesized to result in problems with:
• Inhibition of inappropriate behaviour in the presence of intense affect
• Self-soothing—reducing physiological arousal
• Refocusing attention
• Achievement of external, non-mood-dependent goal-directed behavior.

Crucially, BPD develops due to the interaction and transaction between emotion dysregulation and an individual's experience of an invalidating environment. The invalidating environment refers to the experiences (initially encountered during childhood), in which the individual's emotion regulation difficulties are perpetuated and exacerbated by the responses of others. These invalidating responses tend to be disproportionate and inappropriate reactions to the individual's thoughts, beliefs, sensations, and experiences.

DBT is based on a combined capability deficit and motivational model of BPD which acknowledges the effect of the difficulties emerging from the emotional vulnerability and the invalidating environment by focusing on the skills deficits of the borderline individual and enhancing the skills to manage extreme emotionality and reduce maladaptive mood-dependent behaviours, as well as the skills of learning to trust and validate one's own emotions, thoughts, and activities. A major part of DBT is to teach four sets (or modules) of skills:
• *Interpersonal effectiveness*: skills to increase management of conflict situations, obtaining interpersonal objectives, whilst maintaining healthy relationships and self-respect

- *Emotion regulation*: to increase management of emotions, such as fear, anger, sadness, or depression, in the face of actual or perceived negative emotional situations
- *Distress tolerance*: skills to survive and tolerate crisis situations, without increasing the likelihood of negative consequences through impulsive behaviour and reactions
- *Mindfulness*: meditation techniques to enable the individual to experience emotions and avoid emotional inhibition.

DBT serves five main functions:
- Enhances behavioural capabilities
- Improves motivation to change
- Assures that new capabilities generalize to the natural environment
- Structures the treatment environment to support client and therapist capabilities
- Enhances therapist capabilities and motivation to treat clients effectively.

These functions are met through different modes of therapy delivery, including individual psychotherapy, group skills training, phone consultation, and therapist consultation team.

Key contributors

DBT was developed by **Marsha Linehan** and her team for the treatment of chronically suicidal individuals for whom standard CBT was unsuccessful. It has been further developed by Linehan and colleagues into a treatment for multi-disordered individuals with BPD and for other disorders involving emotional dysregulation, including substance dependence in individuals. **Christy Telch** and colleagues have developed the programme for binge eating, and **Alec Miller** and Jill Rathus developed the programme for depressed, suicidal adolescents. **Tom Lynch** has also developed DBT for the depressed elderly.

What is the evidence base?

A summary of research data has been compiled which includes details of published RCTs, published quasi-experimental studies, unpublished quasi-experimental studies, and uncontrolled trials, incorporating elements of DBT.

The first DBT randomized clinical trial, by Linehan and colleagues, compared DBT to a treatment-as-usual (TAU) control condition. This study found that participants in DBT were significantly less likely to attempt parasuicide during the treatment year, reported fewer parasuicide episodes at each assessment point, and had less medically severe parasuicides over the year. DBT was more effective than TAU to limiting treatment dropout, which was the most serious therapy-interfering behaviour. The participants in DBT tended to enter psychiatric units less often, had fewer inpatient psychiatric days per client, and improved more on scores of global, as well as social, adjustment.

Another study by Koons found that women with BPD who participated in DBT had greater reductions in parasuicide acts and in depression scores than those assigned to TAU, as well as significant improvements in suicidal ideation, hopelessness, anger, hostility, and dissociation. Further studies have demonstrated the efficacy of DBT in substance abuse, bulimia, binge eating, and depression in the elderly. There have also been developments within a variety of settings, including inpatient and partial hospitalization, and forensic settings.

The NICE guidelines for BPD developed by the National Collaborating Centre for Mental Health recommend the consideration of the implementation of DBT within services for women for whom the reduction of self-harm and suicidal behaviour is a priority.

Dialectical behavioural therapy training

There is a range of training opportunities offered by the Linehan Institute: Behavioral Tech based in Seattle USA, and the British Isles Training team. There are DBT Basics workshops which introduce core components of the treatment and are appropriate for all levels of experience. More intensive training is offered which involves a minimum of a team of four professionals, preferably with a previous cognitive behavioural background, to attend two individual weeks of training. These individual weeks are normally 6 months apart, in order to implement the programme after the first week and then to return to discuss implementation issues and further coaching. There is separate training for individuals who wish to join an existing team.

Recommended reading

Linehan MM (1993). *Cognitive Behavioral Treatment of Borderline Personality Disorder.* Guilford Press: New York.

Linehan MM (1993). *Skills Training Manual for Treating Borderline Personality Disorder.* Guilford Press: New York.

Linehan MM, Dimeff L, Koerner K, and Miga EM (2014). *Research on Dialectical Behavior Therapy: Summary of the Data to Date.* The Linehan Institute: Seattle.

National Collaborating Centre for Mental Health (2009). *Borderline Personality Disorder: Treatment and Management.* NICE clinical guideline 78. Available at: ℬ http://www.nice.org.uk/guidance/CG78.

Mentalization-based treatment

Key concepts

MBT is a coherent, evidence-based model of psychotherapy for BPD, originally derived from a psychoanalytic model, but also incorporating cognitive and relational elements. Its coherence relates to a developmental model of BPD, based on attachment theory research and empirical evidence.

The term '*mentalization*' originated in the French psychoanalytic school of psychosomatics, and it was later used in research on the 'theory of mind' of autistic patients. More recent developments, linked to a developmental theory and a clinical model of psychotherapy, for BPD will be illustrated here.

Mentalization refers to the fundamental psychological process of engagement with the task of representing oneself and others' mental states and all their manifestations. These would include behaviours, needs, feelings, beliefs, goals, purposes, and reasons. Mentalizing also stresses the active engagement with the task, in perceiving and interpreting behaviour as conjoined with intentional mental states.

Mentalization is universally present in humans. Its capacity is not acquired at birth but is a process which depends on both constitutional and developmental factors, made possible through an early interaction with a facilitating environment, in the context of an attachment relationship.

Mentalizing as a stable, context-dependent, reliable function of one's agentive self would ideally be implicitly available and readily evoked, when required. In real life, however, the process is opaque and linked to idiosyncrasies, so that everyone suffers some subjective variation in their ability to mentalize, given different interpersonal circumstances and emotional responses. Attending to the task requires some tolerance, a trust in its potential, and acceptance both in personal and relational terms of its possible failures. Trauma and other environmental failures can disrupt the development of one's capacity for mentalizing.

The concept is closely linked to other concepts such as mindfulness, which is an enhanced attention to, and awareness of, current experience and reality (see ➜ Mindfulness-based interventions and therapies in Chapter 2, pp. 73–5, and in Chapter 5, pp. 239–43). In mentalizing, the emphasis is less on the current subjective experience and more on the social, interactive nature of the process, its broader applicability to past and future events, and its reflective nature. Fostering a 'mentalizing capacity' to observe and evaluate one's experience is a focus of other therapeutic approaches.

The normal development of mentalization is dependent on the intersubjective process of emerging psychological awareness between the child and his primary caregivers in the context of a secure attachment. Early attachment figures provide an environment where affect regulation can be mastered and which fosters the development of the self. Attachment provides a lasting psychological connectedness between human beings. There are different aspects to attachment, including protection, the regulation of arousal, and the fostering of a personal exploration of the world, which includes mentalizing as an active engagement and curiosity about exploring one's own and others' minds (see ➜ Theories of personality development: attachment theory in Chapter 8, pp. 380–1).

In normal development, the caregiver (who is usually the mother) provides a 'marked mirroring' of the child's emotions, which involves recognizing the child's affective states and the possibility of tolerating, as well as gradually representing and regulating, them. Chronic discontinuities in caregiving and experiences of trauma and abuse result in an inhibition of this process, leading to a failure to regulate affective responses and a fragmented sense of one's self, which are also core features of BPD. In the lack of a continuity of mirroring, the self initially obviates the fragmentation with a passive internalization of the caregiver. This generates the experience of an 'alien self'—a lack of coherence in one's sense of identity—and attempts to externalize the incongruous aspects of the internal experience in new relationships triggering the attachment system. In BPD, this process can rapidly result in uncontrollable changes or surges of emotion and a failure of mentalizing, or *'prementalizing mode'*. This can manifest as 'not thinking', e.g. a bare statement of 'I don't know' or 'it doesn't matter', in the face of reality events that challenge the subject. The failure of mentalization can also manifest as a re-emergence of more primitive modes of thinking or acting out which predate mentalizing. These are present as modes of organizing subjective experience in normal early childhood development, but persist and predominate as deficits in mentalization in people with certain personality disorders, such as BPD, and include:

- *Psychic equivalence*: rigid, paranoid, and concrete thinking where no different, alternative perspectives are possible, what one feels inside equals what is outside, and thoughts cannot be symbolized. In psychic equivalence, an irritable 'I know' stance leaves little room for sharing the task of attributing meaning to oneself or someone else's mental state
- *Pretend mode*: here, mental states are detached from reality. This will become evident in incongruous affective responses, contradictory beliefs, and inconsequential, elaborated talk of thoughts and feelings or **'pseudomentalization'**, mainly experienced by the listener as inaccurate, avoiding gaps and uncertainty, and disconnected from any meaningful context
- *'Teleological mode'*: a mode of thinking in which changes in mental states and the motivations of others are interpreted according to the presence of observable physical actions. For example, impulsive, goal-directed actions or behaviours, such as self-harm, are the only way to express subjective states of mind through recourse to concrete acts.

The development of MBT was originally linked to specific features of BPD, and a failure of mentalizing capacity is a core aspect of the model of BPD proposed. Over recent years, there has been a broadening of the scope of mentalizing outside of this specialist area. Other formats and modifications of MBT aimed at different groups, such as adolescents who self-harm, families, eating disorders, and antisocial personality disorder (ASPD), have been developed and are currently being researched.

Key contributors

The development of MBT originates in attachment theory and John Bowlby's seminal work.

The main contribution to the scientific understanding of mentalization is the work of **Peter Fonagy** and his group. Fonagy's book *Affect Regulation, Mentalization, and the Development of the Self* (2002) is a landmark exploration in the basic concepts of MBT and combines developmental psychology, attachment theory, and psychoanalytic therapy. He has co-authored most of the existing publications on MBT.

Anthony Bateman led the first RCT of MBT. He has worked in close collaboration with Peter Fonagy in the development of the clinical model and its diffusion through numerous publications, and the organization of training, both in the UK and internationally.

Other eminent contributors in the field, which is rapidly growing, include Mary Target and Jon G Allen.

What is the evidence base?

There have been a number of RCTs of MBT demonstrating its efficacy in BPD:

- The first RCT of MBT was published in 1999, in which 44 patients with a diagnosis of BPD were allocated to MBT in a regime of partial hospitalization (MBT-PH) ($N = 19$) or treatment as usual ($N = 19$).
- After 6 months, reduced suicidality, self-harm, depressive symptoms, days in hospital, and improved social and interpersonal functioning were statistically significant in the MBT group. The benefits were maintained and increased in the MBT group at the end of 18 months of follow-up. At 8-year follow-up, patients treated with MBT-PH showed better results in decreased suicidality, service use, use of medication, global function, and vocational status than the control group. Only 13% of these patients still satisfied criteria for BPD, against 84% in the treatment-as-usual group.
- In 2009, an RCT of MBT in a different outpatient setting was published, in which 134 patients were randomly allocated to MBT or to a control group using structured clinical management. Treatment included one individual session and one group session a week for 18 months in the MBT group. Both groups improved. The MBT group had additional benefits in areas of self-reported and clinically significant problems, including suicide attempts and hospitalization.
- An RCT of MBT for self-harm in 80 adolescents was published in 2012, showing a better outcome in reduction of BPD traits, self-harm, and depressive features in the MBT group versus treatment as usual.

Mentalization-based therapy training

The enthusiasm generated by the new availability of an effective treatment for BPD led to a broad diffusion of its general principles, initially through a core training organized by Bateman and Fonagy, consisting of 3 days of intensive lectures and experiential learning at the Anna Freud Centre in London (for more information, visit ✆ http://www.annafreud. org/training-research/mentalization-based-treatment-training/). Currently, there are three components to training: a basic training course, supervision, and a certificate course for practitioner level.

Training requires some pre-existing familiarity with work with BPD patients. Professionals who can train include qualified health workers such as mental health nurses, occupational therapists, clinical/counselling psychologists, psychiatrists, psychotherapists, and social workers.

A detailed account of the theory and practice of MBT was published in 2004, followed by a practical manual of MBT for BPD in 2006. More recently, these basic texts were followed by a *Handbook of MBT* and a *Handbook of Mentalizing in Mental Health Practice*.

The growth of interest and studies, together with the stringent requirements of research protocols, led to the development of an advanced training course for MBT and the production of a quality manual, currently available on the Anna Freud Centre website (✆ http://www.annafreud.

org/training-research/mentalization-based-treatment-training/quality-manual-for-mbt/). The manual introduces a quality system aimed at establishing, monitoring, and improving consistency and adherence to the MBT model. It spells out the levels of competency in the clinical work for the different levels of practitioners, including therapists, supervisors, teams, and programmes.

The recent development of an MBT Adherence and Competence Scale (MBT-ASC) has offered a tool to assess the therapist's stance and intervention, and is now an essential part of the curriculum for therapists' training.

Recommended reading

Allen J, Fonagy P, Bateman A (2008). *Mentalizing in Clinical Practice*. American Psychiatric Publishing: Washington DC.

Bateman A and Fonagy P (2006). *Mentalization-Based Treatment for Borderline Personality Disorder. A practical guide*. Oxford University Press: Oxford.

Bateman A and Fonagy P (eds) (2012). *Handbook of Mentalizing in Mental Health Practice*. American Psychiatric Publishing: Washington DC.

Fonagy P, Gergely G, Jurist EL, and Target M (2002). *Affect Regulation, Mentalization and the Development of the Self*. Other Press: New York.

Karterud S, Pedersen G, Engen M, *et al.* (2013). The MBT Adherence and Competence Scale (MBT-ACS): development, structure and reliability. *Psychotherapy Research*, **23**, 705–17.

Schema therapy

Key concepts

Schema therapy was developed by the psychologist Jeffrey Young during the 1990s and is considered to be a variation of CBT (see ➔ Cognitive behavioural therapy in Chapter 2, pp. 30–4; and in Chapter 5, pp. 172–84). Because of Young's observation of certain patients not responding to classic CBT, Young modified CBT, looking at characterological features and targeting patients with personality problems. Recently, a treatment programme around the treatment of BPD has arisen out of Young's groundbreaking work (see ➔ Borderline personality disorder in Chapter 8, pp. 390–6).

Schema therapy arising out of an aetiological system of unmet childhood needs

Young hypothesized that patients with characterological difficulties showed typical difficulties that could be traced back to unmet needs during childhood or childhood trauma. Young defines five domains of core childhood needs:

• Secure attachment to others with safety, stability, nurture, acceptance, and meeting of basic needs like food and shelter
• Autonomy, competence, and sense of identity
• Freedom to express valid needs and emotions
• Spontaneity and play
• Realistic limits and self-control.

More than classic CBT and overlapping with other developmental psychological models like gestalt therapy and psychodynamic thinking, schema therapy matches unmet childhood needs and/or childhood trauma to the current problems of the patient. It views these unmet needs as key in understanding the patient's characterological problems leading to mental health problems.

Role of schemas in schema therapy

Young observed patterns in the patients' abnormal responses to often unobtrusive triggers. He called these responses *schemas*. Schemas are broad, pervasive themes or patterns in the patient's presentation. They are made of memories, emotions, cognitions, and associated body sensations, referring to oneself and one's relationship with others. They are developed during childhood and adolescence, and elaborated throughout lifetime.

Schemas are always considered dysfunctional to a significant degree and impairing the patients' physical, emotional, and social well-being. Young proposed 18 schemas that could be matched onto domains of unmet childhood needs.

Modes

In order to simplify this heuristic system, the concept of *modes* has gained more clinical relevance in the later developments of schema therapy. Whilst schemas are viewed as more trait-like, somewhat dormant remnants of unmet childhood needs and childhood trauma, modes are seen as states arising out of acute schema activation. Pertinent to the patients' emotional distress are the *child modes*, namely the *vulnerable child* (VC) mode, the *angry child* (AC) mode, and the *demanding parent* (DP) mode. These modes lead to an activation of strong emotionally aversive states. In order to downregulate the overwhelming emotions associated with the above highly emotional and painful childhood modes, the patient uses *coping modes*. The patient copes by avoiding painful states, trying extra hard to counterbalance them (overcompensation) or giving in to the overwhelming sense of defeat (surrender).

Coping modes are associated with more manageable emotions or not experiencing any emotion. The main coping modes are the *compliant surrender mode*, the *avoidant protector mode*, and the *overcompensating mode*. Frequently, these are compared to the three responses to overwhelming threat: *freeze* (compliant surrender), *flight* (avoidant protector), and *fight* (overcompensating modes).

During times of childhood deprivation or abuse, coping modes are instrumental to keeping the child somewhat emotionally and physically protected. In adulthood though, these modes are considered unhelpful and keep the adult stuck in disabling patterns of schema activation and mode '*flipping*'. This mode flipping may lead to the severely disabling symptoms associated with the diagnosis of a personality disorder.

The ultimate aim of schema therapies is to strengthen the *healthy adult mode* (HAM). With the help of modelling healthy adult functioning and healing unmet childhood needs through emotion-focused techniques, the patient is gently taught how to look after his or her activation of childhood modes better and more effectively. The patient learns not to resort to unhelpful coping. Instead the patient is empowered to test and practise healthier and more adult ways of responding to interpersonal challenges, associated with mode activation.

Key contributors

Jeffrey Young can be considered as the founder of schema therapy. Young trained with Aaron Beck, the founder of CBT (see ➲ Cognitive behavioural therapy in Chapter 2, pp. 30–4). Through careful observation of patients with personality disorder and their response to cognitive therapy, Young was able to devise a heuristic system, which he called schema therapy.

Subsequently, a Dutch group around **Arnoud Arntz** from Maastricht developed the treatment manual developed by Young. Their main contribution lies in the conduction of RCTs, which confirms the clinical efficacy and cost-effectiveness of schema therapy.

Ida Shaw and **Joan Farrell** from Minneapolis have more recently completed a trial of a group schema therapy, a combination of group and individual schema sessions. This is particularly exciting, as BPD can be conceptualized as an 'interpersonality disorder'. BPD, as well as other personality disorders, are characterized by recurrent challenges arising in the patient's interaction with other people. Patients find it difficult to mediate and regulate the emotions triggered by relationships with other persons and their individual personality. A group format is therefore seen as the ideal environment to tolerate unpleasant emotions and to experiment and learn new ways of dealing with interpersonal interactions and difficulties.

What is the evidence base?

Schema therapy has a strong evidence base for emotionally unstable BPD in both inpatients and outpatients. It has been shown to be more effective than transference-focused therapy in reducing borderline traits. Schema therapy was found to be cost-effective in a large Dutch study and to lead to discernable changes in brain functioning. Thirty sessions of group schema therapy have been shown to produce even stronger effect sizes, when compared to treatment as usual, with significant reductions of all symptoms specific to BPD and improvement of global functioning scores. Preliminary studies show promising results for other forms of mental health issues, including depression, anxiety, and personality problems.

Schema therapy training

Training in schema therapy is an exciting new therapeutic option. Nonetheless, schema therapy training has a range of challenges; it involves an intimate familiarization with the therapist's own schematic beliefs and receiving supervision with regard to meeting and resolving the therapist's own unmet childhood needs. Personal therapy for a therapist is not mandatory. In schema therapy training, some supervision sessions are used to compassionately attend to the therapist's own emotional challenges in schema therapy terms. If this is insufficiently done, there is a danger that there might be collusion between the patient and the therapist's schema (e.g. the therapist's self-sacrifice schema leading to insufficient boundary setting to the patient's excessive demands).

The use and modelling of the *authentic self* in schema therapy requires the therapist to be emotionally stable, in order not to be overwhelmed by the emotional demands going along with the committed patient–therapist relationship. The therapeutic relationship in schema therapy goes beyond the usual boundaries of the therapeutic relationship—the therapist is asked to go 'the extra mile' to serve as a partially re-parenting figure in the patient's life.

Information about training opportunities can be provided by visiting ℬ http://isstonline.com/home.

Recommended reading

Arntz A and Jacob G (2012). *Schema Therapy in Practice: An Introductory Guide to the Schema Mode Approach*. Wiley-Blackwell: Chichester.

Farrell JM, Reiss N, and Shaw IA (2014). *The Schema Therapy Clinician's Guide*. Wiley-Blackwell: Chichester.

Young JE and Klosko JS (1993). *Reinventing Your Life*. Penguin: New York.

Mindfulness-based interventions and therapies

Key concepts

Mindfulness is a concept that is not easily explained. The spirit of mindfulness-based interventions is about experiencing mindfulness through practical exercises, as it cannot be grasped through verbal descriptions only. The most well-known definition of mindfulness was given by Jon Kabat-Zinn:

> '*Mindfulness means paying attention in a particular way: on purpose, in the present moment, and non-judgementally.*'

Bishop et al. described mindfulness as a continuum of mental processes that serves to understand how functional and dysfunctional feelings and behaviours arise. The goal is to strengthen the former and attenuate the latter. They propose an operational definition of mindfulness based on two components. The first component concerns the self-regulation of attention, directing attention at sensory experiences and mental events arising in the present moment. The second component describes an orientation to openly inviting experiences—every thought, feeling, and physical sensation is accepted without expressing intentional judgement and without wishing to change it.

'*Putting the mind where the body already is . . .*' can be a simplified version of the above. The body and the breath are always in the present moment. The mind tends to oscillate between thoughts about the future (worry), thoughts about the past (rumination), or negatively judging the present (rather than experiencing it). Directing friendliness and kindness towards oneself, whilst observing whatever is in the field of present awareness, is a key ingredient to process that is difficult to put into words.

The creation of scientific evidence for the effectiveness of meditation-based interventions for both physical and mental well-being has led to a wider public interest. Mindfulness-based interventions are nowadays used beyond the health services in other areas of public interest, including education, the criminal justice system, work-related stress, and improving working conditions.

Key contributors

The annexation of Tibet by China in the 1950s triggered a mass exodus of Tibetan monks into exile in India. Enthusiasts from the West returning from India, after having studied with Tibetan refugees, created a renewed interest in Buddhist philosophy and meditation practices in the 1960s and 70s.

In 1979, **Jon Kabat-Zinn**, a committed meditator, gave up his career in molecular biology, in order to introduce secular mindfulness through the Stress Reduction Clinic at the University of Massachusetts in Worcester. His aim was to introduce the practice of meditation to treat clinical populations and make meditation accessible to scientific investigation. Kabat-Zinn developed an 8-week programme, teaching a range of meditation practices to patients with both mental and physical chronic illnesses. He called his intervention *mindfulness-based stress reduction* (MBSR) and conducted clinical trials about its efficacy, in order to reduce distress, both physical and psychological.

With the arrival of CBT as a treatment for depression in the 1980s and 90s (see ➲ Cognitive behavioural therapy in Chapter 2, pp. 30–4; and in Chapter 5, pp. 172–84), it was recognized that the pandemic of depression would not be treatable solely with the help of individual therapy. **John Teasdale**, **Mark Williams**, and **Zindel Segal** adapted the MBSR programme to clinical populations, in order to provide an intervention for relapse prevention of depression. They called their 8-week programme *mindfulness-based cognitive therapy* (MBCT). The publication of their RCT of MBCT in 2000 was the starting point of *mindfulness-based interventions* (MBI) being used in almost all areas of mental health care.

Kabat-Zinn has always been open about the Buddhist roots of mindfulness interventions. He and others propose an hourglass model where Buddhist psychology is informing scientific models, and Western models are feeding back into Buddhist thinking about psychological and physical suffering.

Kabat-Zinn, with the development of MBSR, as well as Teasdale and Williams, with the adaptation of MBSR to MBCT, are the pioneers of MBI in medicine and psychology. Elements of mindfulness have been adapted and integrated in other forms of cognitive behavioural interventions, including acceptance and commitment therapy (ACT), as taught by **Stephen Hayes**, as well as DBT developed by **Marsha Linehan** (see ➲ Dialectical behavioural therapy in Chapter 2, pp. 63–6; and in Chapter 5, pp. 220–9). There is now an explosion of interest in MBI and their research. MBI are nowadays used widely across almost all mental health disorders and for a range of chronic physical illnesses.

What is the evidence base?

MBI are being intensely researched. There are several well-controlled RCTs, mainly for MBCT and depression. MBCT for relapse prevention of depression was included in the NICE guidance of depression in 2005.

In mental health care, good evidence has been created for the efficacy of MBI in many different mental disorders, including depression, bipolar disorder, and eating disorders. A recent meta-analysis was performed by Khoudry (2013) of a total of 12145 patients that were involved in MBI for a variety of psychological problems. Across studies for different disorders, the results indicated an overall medium effect size. However, more specifically, MBI were shown to have large and clinically important effects on patients suffering from depression and anxiety. These effects were maintained at follow-up.

Mindfulness-based therapies and interventions training

Training in MBI starts with a personal meditation practice. For this purpose, self-directed meditation practice can suffice, in order to get a sense of what mindfulness can achieve. In order to train as an MBCT facilitator, personal meditation practice of 3 years is recommended.

Although there is no formal recognized title as an MBI facilitator, a network of qualified teachers already exists. Recommended qualification criteria included personal participation with the mindfulness-based course curriculum and in-depth personal experience of all the core meditation practices of this mindfulness-based programme, and completion of an in-depth, rigorous mindfulness-based teacher training programme or supervised pathway over a minimum duration of 12 months. Practitioners should have a professional qualification in mental or physical health care, education or social care, or equivalent life experience, recognized by the organization or context within which the teaching will take place, and knowledge and experience of the populations to whom the mindfulness-based course will be delivered, including experience of teaching, or therapeutic or other care provision with UK Mindfulness-Based Teacher Trainer Network. Further details can be found at ℘ www.mindfulnessteachersuk.org.uk.

Recommended reading

Kabat-Zinn J (1990). *Full Catastrophe Living: How to Cope with Stress, Pain and Illness Using Mindfulness Meditation*. Bantam Dell: New York.

Keng SL, Smoski MJ, and Robins CJ (2011). Effects of mindfulness on psychological health: a review of empirical studies. *Clinical Psychology Review*, **31**, 1041–56.

Khoury B, Lecomte T, Fortin G, *et al*. (2013). Mindfulness-based therapy: a comprehensive meta-analysis. *Clinical Psychology Review*, **33**, 763–71.

Therapeutic communities

Key concepts

Certain beliefs about human relationships and the nature of therapy are central to TCs:

- Staff are not completely 'well', and residents are not completely 'sick'. There is a basic equality as human beings between staff and residents, who share many of the same psychological processes and experiences.
- Whatever the symptoms or behaviour problems, the individual's difficulties are primarily in his or her relationships with other people.
- Therapy is essentially a learning process, both in the sense of learning new skills—how to relate to others or deal more appropriately with distress—and learning to understand oneself and others.

From anthropological work in the 1950s, Rapaport identified four principles of TC treatment: *democratization, permissiveness, communalism,* and *reality confrontation*:

- *Democratization*: every member of the community should share equally in the exercise of power in decision-making about community affairs
- *Permissiveness:* all members should tolerate from one another a wide degree of behaviour that might be distressing or seem deviant by ordinary standards
- *Communalism*: there should be tight-knit intimate sets of relationships, with sharing of amenities (dining room, etc.), use of first names, and free communication
- *Reality confrontation*: residents should be continuously presented with interpretations of their behaviour, as it is seen by others, in order to counteract their tendency to distort, deny, or withdraw from their difficulties in getting on with others.

More recently, the necessary emotional experiences of being in a TC have been described developmentally in broader terms of universal human development. This outlines how all individuals undergo '*primary emotional development*', which is more or less satisfactory; those who suffer environmental failure with traumas, such as deprivation or abuse, are particularly likely to need an opportunity to repair the damage through a process of '*secondary emotional development*'. The requirements of primary development are modulated by constitutional and physical factors. A TC offers a specific programme for secondary emotional development.

These concepts are based on a wide range of psychological theories:

- *Attachment*: feeling connected and belonging—as developed from the ethological theories of Bowlby
- *Containment*: feeling safe—as in the psychoanalytic theories of Bion and Winnicott
- *Communication*: feeling heard, in a culture of openness—as in Main's 'culture of enquiry'
- *Inclusion*: feeling involved, as part of the whole—based on the group analytic theory of Foulkes and Elias
- *Agency*: feeling empowered with an effective sense of self—based on the theory of Stack Sullivan, existential therapist and critical theorist.

A few other theoretical models have been elaborated specifically for TCs. Those with some face validity include *systemic* (where the TC is viewed as a system having specific interactions with superordinate systems), *social learning theory* (where new patterns of behaviour in relationships are learnt), and *post-modern* (in which an atheoretical collection of elements are juxtaposed in an effective way). The critical theories from the 1960s and 70s of Laing, Szasz, and Illich continue to have relevance to the work, and the newer ones of Bracken and Thomas's '*post-psychiatry*' have much in common. The sociological narrative which questions professional legitimacy in terms of 'actor networks' is also relevant.

It is worth noting that those admitted to a TC for treatment are usually referred to as members, residents, or clients, rather than as patients.

It is most unlikely that one model or theoretical framework will ever capture the essential ingredients of the TC. They have developed as an untidy human endeavour to meet problems of alienation, deviance, and overwhelming distress across numerous settings and times. Any attempt to 'tidy them up' into an operationalized treatment modality is likely to hamper the creativity and spontaneity they need to form, grow, and survive. The mechanisms of natural selection are probably more relevant—the communities that are best adapted to their environment are the ones that are most likely to survive, and those that are ill-adapted or resist change are likely to die.

Key contributors

Despite the recent identification of TCs as a specific entity, their theoretical, practical, and philosophical origins go back much earlier. *'Mentally afflicted pilgrims'* attended the shrine of St Dymphna at Geel in Flanders in the mid-thirteenth century, and some commentators identified this as the first recognizable format reflecting the principles and practices of TCs.

The next documented and identifiable strand of TC ideas emerged in *'moral treatment'* in the eighteenth century. **William William Tuke** founded the Retreat Hospital in York in 1796, based on the development of his ideas on moral treatment. Tuke's particular approach was to treat the insane as closely as possible to how one would treat 'normal' people. Moral treatment is also particularly identified with **Philippe Pinel**, who referred to *'treatment through the emotions'*, and practised at the Salpêtrière in Paris in the early nineteenth century. These ideas crossed the Atlantic, and, in 1817, a hospital was founded in Pennsylvania modelled on the Retreat by the Pennsylvanian Quakers.

Northfield Military Hospital, where many battle-shocked soldiers were received, was the site of two important experiments in military psychiatry between 1943 and 1945. The first was led by the psychoanalysts **Wilfred Bion** and **John Rickman**, and involved a daily parade for men to observe how they worked together and the opportunity to set up numerous activity groups for which they were responsible themselves. Although ostensibly successful, it only lasted 6 weeks. This is probably because it had insufficient support from senior officers and posed too much of a challenge to military procedure. The second Northfield experiment was led by **SH Foulkes**, **Tom Main**, and **Harold Bridger**, and built on the principles of the first but developed them in a more gradual way, with a wider base of support in the Army hierarchy. It treated many men throughout the rest of the war.

An unrelated wartime experiment was taking place under **Maxwell Jones**, a respiratory physiologist, at Mill Hill hospital in North London. He was treating soldiers with 'effort dyspnoea' in groups of about 100. He lectured them about how their symptoms were related to physiological processes and was surprised when new recruits to his programme started to gain much benefit from discussions with those who had been there for some time. A didactic delivery of information had become an emotional sharing of meaning between those who had similar experiences, and it seemed very effective. Jones further developed the method at Mill Hill and used it at Belmont after the war to treat socially excluded individuals with non-psychotic conditions. This programme became the Henderson Hospital and set the scene for the emergence of 'social psychiatry' in the 1950s.

These two pioneers of TCs Tom Main and Maxwell Jones defined them as follows:

> 'An attempt to use a hospital not as an organization run by doctors in the interests of their own greater technical efficiency, but as a community with the immediate aim of full participation of all its members in its daily life and the eventual aim of the resocialisation of the neurotic individual for life in ordinary society.
>
> What distinguishes a therapeutic community from other comparable treatment centres is the way in which the institution's total resources, staff, patients, and their relatives, are self-consciously pooled in furthering treatment. That implies, above all, a change in the usual status of patients.'

The first direct descendant of the wartime experiments was the Henderson Hospital, and its techniques were widely replicated across the world as part of the 1950s and 1960s Social Psychiatry movement. This included the establishment of the first prison TC at HMP Grendon Underwood in Buckinghamshire in 1962. This is a whole prison TC, with six wings of 40 men, each run as a separate clinical unit. Several other TCs in different British prisons have also been established since, including the world's only prison democratic TC for women at HMP Send in Surrey.

In 1958, a new kind of TC was created in America by the forceful personality of its originator **Chuck Dederich**. He started by setting up a weekly group for helping ex-Alcoholics Anonymous members and ex-addicts in his own flat, based around free association, confrontational 'reality attack' encounter groups, and educational seminars, particularly based on philosophical ideas. This was the beginning of Synanon, and it was the first of what came to be known as 'concept-based', 'hierarchical', 'behavioural', or 'programmatic', and, more recently, 'addiction' TCs. In the USA and some areas of Europe, this type of TC is much commoner than the 'democratic TCs' on which this chapter focuses, although there is increasing common ground and growth of mixed models.

Another TC tradition which evolved independently is the field of therapeutic education for children. Bridgeland described residential therapeutic education as 'a first attempt at combining psychotherapeutic ideas with participatory democracy'. **Homer Lane** set up the 'Boys Republic' between 1907 and 1912 in Chicago for deprived urban children. He imported the idea into the UK in 1913 and set up the 'Little Commonwealth' in Dorset, also for disturbed youngsters. In 1924, **AS Neill** set up Summerhill School which continues to this day as an institution specializing in progressive education. In the twentieth and twenty-first centuries, these models have informed the development of progressive education, social pedagogy, and various models of TCs for children and young people.

There are also a number of communities for people with learning disabilities. The best known of these are the Camphill Communities founded by Karl König, which are based on the ideas of Rudolf Steiner and his 'anthroposophy'. A similar Catholic-based movement, called L'Arche, was founded by Jean Vanier in 1964. These two groups are closer in intention to the thirteenth-century long-term caring communities in Geel than to hospital- or community-based treatment programmes, although the modern regulatory environment is proving challenging for long-term group living arrangements.

What is the evidence base?

TCs have a long tradition of research, going back at least to the mid-twentieth century, although the earlier work was predominantly qualitative and descriptive. A summary of non-randomized longitudinal cost-offset studies from the 1990s aimed to show reduction in psychiatric expenditure, and a compilation of accumulated research evidence was compiled in 2004.

Until recently, there has been little systematic evidence of the efficacy of TCs for treating personality disorders, and disagreement over whether those who did benefit were really suffering from psychopathic or personality disorder. Whilst efficacy in this area is still questioned, the picture has recently become clearer with the publication of the first systematic review of TC treatment for people with personality disorders by Lees et al. in 1999. The authors carried out a full search of TC publications and grey literature, collecting over 8000 references from 38 countries. These were reduced to 29 research studies that met the criteria of RCT design (eight studies) or comparative or controlled studies that reported raw data and used conservative outcome criteria (e.g. reconviction rates, rather than psychological improvement). A meta-analysis found that 19 studies showed a positive effect within the 95% level of confidence, whilst the remaining ten straddled the neutral score. The overall summary log odds ratio was -0.567, with a 95% confidence interval of -0.524 to -0.614. The authors concluded that there is strong evidence for the effectiveness of TCs.

However, they also stated that 'therapeutic communities have not produced the amount or quality of research literature that we might have expected, given the length of time they have been in existence'. Although they were referring to the range of research methods, Pearce points out that the lack of modern randomized approaches to investigating the effectiveness of TCs has become particularly marked. He also gives an analysis of why this might particularly be the case in TCs.

A systematic review published by the Home Office in 2003 assessed evidence for interventions for people with personality disorders in general and for dangerous and severe personality-disordered offenders, and made clear recommendations about the most promising treatment interventions for personality disorders in use or currently in development. The reviewers covered TC programmes; cognitive, behavioural, cognitive behavioural, and psychodynamic psychotherapies; and pharmacological and physical treatments. They concluded that 'the TC model currently has the most promising evidence base in this poor field'.

More recently, there has been an increasing requirement for RCTs as sole evidence of effectiveness, which poses particular methodological, theoretical, and ethical problems for TCs. However, the first such trial, based on a non-residential TC model in Oxford, is currently collecting data in the follow-up phase (Pearce, personal communication).

Therapeutic communities training and experience

Traditionally, the teaching and learning of TC theory has been secondary to a more prominent emphasis on relationships and clinical practice. This may be because of the wide range of theoretical underpinnings that theory which is specific to TCs has been historically sparse, and the method draws on a wide range of theoretical disciplines. In the past, it has sometimes appeared that an understanding of Rapoport's four principles and attention to psychodynamic concepts were considered sufficient for effective TC practice.

More recently, theoretical elements have been included in TC training programmes, and many TCs now include theoretical instruction as part of induction procedures for new staff members.

TC-specific training includes residential workshops which are intensive experiential group relations events over 3 days. The longest running and most popular of these is the regular 'Living Learning Experience'. This is an event for TC staff which runs several times per year, in order to give participants the opportunity to see what it feels like to be members of a TC. It is conducted by group analysts experienced in TC work and includes community meetings, small groups, and self-catering and various social activities, all of which are chosen and agreed by the group itself.

Many TCs supplement specific TC training with training in relevant related areas. These most commonly include training at various levels in group analysis and group dynamic approaches, action methods (psychodrama and drama therapy approaches), humanistic and interpersonal therapies (creative arts, transactional analysis, and gestalt), psychoanalytic theory and practice, and systemic approaches.

Many therapy trainings can bring benefits to TC practice beyond the application of specific techniques in specialist therapy groups. Personal therapy is often a beneficial part of such, and disorder-specific trainings are helpful.

Recommended reading

Haigh R (2013). The quintessence of a therapeutic environment. *Therapeutic Communities*, **34**, 6–16.

Haigh R and Tucker S (2004). Democratic development of standards: a quality network of therapeutic communities. *Psychiatric Quarterly*, **75**, 263–77.

Johnson R and Haigh R (2011). Social psychiatry and social policy for the 21st century—relational health. *Journal of Mental Health and Social Inclusion*, **15**, 57–65.

Jones M (1968). *Beyond the Therapeutic Community: Social Learning and Social Psychiatry*. Yale University Press: New York.

Rapoport R (1960). *Community as Doctor*. Tavistock: London.

Art psychotherapy

Key concepts

Art therapy, or art psychotherapy, is a formal psychotherapy, which offers a visual, as well as verbal, language for communication and the expression of thoughts and feelings. No special art skills in the patient or client are needed, beyond the ability and willingness to make marks or manipulate clay. Art therapy works with a wide population, in diverse settings. It is a reflective discipline and aims to be mindful of race, culture, gender, and age.

There is a triangular relationship between the client, the artwork, and the therapist, within a psychotherapeutic framework (see Fig. 2.2).

The art therapy room provides an outer frame for these relationships and has an important symbolic and containing function.

The artwork can:
- Contain powerful feelings
- Hold multiple meanings
- Provide a visual record of therapy sessions
- Give form to intangible experience
- Symbolize material
- Mediate between inner and outer experience
- Hold and express transference.

Key contributors

Art therapy has developed in the UK since the 1940s, alongside psychological and artistic developments in the USA and Europe.

It draws on the Jungian concept of 'active imagination' where patients made art from feelings and dreams; the exploration of the unconscious by Freud; the interest of artists such as the Surrealists, Dubuffet, and Picasso in 'Outsider Art'; and spontaneous art-making.

The artist **Adrian Hill** shared the benefits of creative activity in convalescence with fellow sanatorium patients during the Second World War. **Edward Adamson** was appointed in 1946 to run an Art Therapy Studio

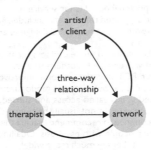

Fig. 2.2 The three-way relationship in art psychotherapy.

at Netherne Psychiatric Hospital. Artists then began to set up Studio-Based Open Groups in NHS psychiatric hospitals. In the USA, **Edith Kramer** and **Margaret Naumburg** were early pioneers of art therapy, and there was much debate on the role of the art therapist, and directive and non-directive approaches.

Art therapy has drawn on psychoanalytic literature, child development, radical psychiatry, philosophy, group work, humanistic approaches, evolutionary theory, anthropology, and science. A non-directive, analytic approach prevailed in the 1990s and 2000s, although practice has since developed evidence-based, condition-specific approaches within clinical guidelines. Art therapists have integrated MBT (see ➔ Mentalization-based treatment in Chapter 2, pp. 66–70, and in Chapter 5, pp. 229–34), CAT (see ➔ Cognitive analytic therapy in Chapter 2, pp. 47–52, and in Chapter 5, pp. 194–202), and DBT (see ➔ Dialectical behaviour therapy in Chapter 2, pp. 63–6, and in Chapter 5, pp. 220–9) approaches in their work, and are also informed by current developments in neuroscience.

The British Association of Art Therapists (BAAT) was established in 1963. The Department of Health recognizes art therapy as part of the NHS.

Psychological therapists and art therapists are registered with the Health Professions Council (HPC). The title of Art Therapist/Art Psychotherapist is a protected one.

What is the evidence base?

There is a substantial body of art therapy literature, nationally and internationally, and an active Art Therapy Research Network. There has been debate about what constitutes the most appropriate form of evidence for art therapy.

NICE guidelines recommend that art psychotherapies are offered to people suffering from psychosis and also to people with dementia. The MultiCenter evaluation of Art Therapy in Schizophrenia: Systematic Evaluation (MATISSE) trial, the largest ever RCT of art therapy, explored the effects of a group interactive art therapy approach with people with a diagnosis of schizophrenia. Quantitative evidence did not show a reduction in outcome measures of negative symptoms or improvements in social or global functioning, although qualitative results indicated social, personal, and interpersonal benefits for service users who had engaged with art therapy and suggested that benefits included greater connection with others, self-expression, reduced social stigma, and enjoyment and satisfaction of creativity.

Findings have also included increased engagement in art therapy amongst people not well engaged in other services.

An earlier smaller RCT had shown some improvement in negative symptoms in schizophrenia, but also that randomization in selection of patients had resulted in increased access and subsequent participation of ethnic minorities, who might not usually be referred for art therapy.

NICE guidelines continue to recommend that art therapies are offered to children and young people with psychosis. Qualitative evidence indicates the efficacy of art therapy much more widely.

Art therapy training

Art therapy training began in the 1960s and is now at Master's level. Trainees will usually be art graduates or, in the case of other disciplines, have a long-standing commitment to art and relevant clinical experience. Training covers psychotherapy, psychology and psychiatry, and studio practice. Trainees take part in experiential art psychotherapy groups and are required to be in personal therapy for the duration of training.

Accredited training courses are shown on the BAAT website.

Art therapists are required to keep abreast of developments in social, cultural, artistic, and psychological thinking, and maintain their own art practice.

Recommended reading

Crawford MJ, Killaspy H, Barnes TR, et al. (2012). Group art therapy as an adjunctive treatment for people with schizophrenia: a randomized controlled trial (MATISSE). Health Technology Assessment, 16, iii–iv, 1–76.

Dalley T (ed) (1987). Art as Therapy. Tavistock: London.

Gilroy A (2011). Art Therapy Research in Practice. Peter Lang: Oxford.

Gilroy A and McNeilly G (eds) (2000). The Changing Shape of Art Therapy: New developments in Therapy and Practice. Jessica Kingsley: London.

Waller D (1991). Becoming a Profession: The History of Art Therapy in Britain. Routledge: London.

Dramatherapy

Key concepts

Dramatherapy is a state-registered profession, regulated by the Health and Care Professions Council (HCPC). The HCPC Standards of Proficiency for Arts Therapists (2003) describes dramatherapy as ' . . . a unique form of psychotherapy in which creativity, play, movement, voice, storytelling, dramatisation, and the performance arts have a central position within the therapeutic relationship.' The British Association of Dramatherapists (BADth) defines dramatherapy as 'having as its main forms the intentional use of the healing aspects of drama and theatre within the therapeutic process. It is a method of working and playing which uses action to facilitate creativity, imagination, learning, insight, and growth.'

The core concepts of dramatherapy derive from the understanding that dramatic processes are part of human growth and development. This is summarized in the developmental paradigm embodiment–projection–role (EPR) which describes three developmental stages:

• *Embodiment*: the sensory physical experience of the relationship with primary carer(s) and the developing of a sense of 'self' through bodily sensation of touch, holding, smell, and sound. The nature of the relationship with primary carers is crucial in developing confidence and security for growth, identity, and independence.

• *Projection*: developing from around 12–14 months, a gradual separation from primary carers, awareness of 'me' and 'not me', beginning to relate to an objective world beyond the body, and

capacity to be in relationship with objects; fashioning and shaping things, e.g. with clay, paint; to control a small world, e.g. by creating 'order' and chaos with bricks, groups of animals; using imagination to create stories with objects which symbolize aspects of the self and others within the story.
- *Role*: overlapping with the projection stage and usually accomplished by age 7, the child takes on the roles formally occupied by objects, is able to manipulate objects imaginatively, incorporate embodied confidence, and is able to explore social relationships, world order, and morality. Through role play, the child explores the limits of their social environment, what is encouraged, and what is sanctioned or ignored.

These phases create a healthy 'vocabulary' of experiences which form an essential core of competencies which support flexibility, resilience, imagination, identity, and the capacity to problem-solve and which are replayed throughout life. The phases overlap and do not follow a rigid pattern.

Key dramatic processes are at work:
- Use of imagination
- Action
- Metaphor and symbol
- Shaping a space for action to take place
- Narrative structures which contain and shape experiences such as telling stories or making plays.

Dramatherapists work with these dramatic structures, as they relate to client need, in order to contain experience in a way which is 'distanced' from everyday reality, but paradoxically in a relationship with it. Within the dramatherapy session, the client can draw on their existing 'vocabulary' to explore how things are and have been, and how they might change. This can be done using methods predicated on how they are in relation to the EPR model, so it can be both a diagnostic tool, as well as a guide to action. The emphasis within a session will be on 'doing' in some form whereby feelings can be concretized through the use of physical action, work with objects and materials, creating stories, and working with 'texts' of different sorts. The aim is to enable the client to explore and 'be with' their distress and social and emotional world in a way that can be manageable, because it is contained within the safety of carefully structured work in the detachment of metaphor. Rituals of time, space, and role are used to create consistency and to enable the client to explore their inner turmoil within an ordered structure. This dramatic construct can be mapped onto cognitive and psychosocial theories of human development, such as those of Piaget, Erikson, and Winnicott, and integrated into any model of therapeutic or educational practice.

Key contributors

In the UK, dramatherapy emerged in the 1970s, alongside theatre practices, which sought to promote participatory drama for individual and social change. **Sue Jennings** and **Gordon Wiseman**, whose orientation was based in theatre, pioneered 'remedial drama', whilst **Marion (Billie) Lindquist** set up the Sesame Institute which focused on movement and drama. Core principles are shared and have remained, but practitioners have developed specialisms from particular aspects of dramatic process or related practices such as storytelling (**Alida Gersie**), role (**Robert Landy**), dramatic text (**Madeline Andersen-Warren, Marina Jenkyns**), spirituality and theatre (**Roger Grainger, Mary Smail**), and ritual (**Sue Jennings, Steve Mitchell**).

What is the evidence base?

Dramatherapy has not been subjected to RCTs or any large-scale research projects. However, there are ample qualitative data to substantiate the effectivity of dramatherapy with a range of client groups in different settings. Research in dramatherapy to date is largely qualitative and case study-based. There is, however, a significant database established by the British Association of Dramatherapists covering evidence-based practice (EBP) and practice-based evidence (PBE) with a range of client groups. There is also a significant body of published literature both in the UK and the USA and two peer-reviewed professional journals *Dramatherapy*, Journal of BADth (Routledge/Taylor and Francis) and *The Drama Therapy Review*, Journal of the North American Drama Therapy Association (Intellect Publishers).

Dramatherapy training

The UK professional body is BADth. Dramatherapists are required to have undertaken an approved course of training to be eligible for registration, to undertake CPD to continue registration, to be in ongoing clinical supervision, and to abide by the codes of ethics of BADth and the HCPC.

In the UK, there are currently five training courses, all delivered at Master of Arts (MA) level and approved by BADth:

• University of Roehampton, London
• Anglia Ruskin University, Cambridge
• Sesame Institute, Central School of Speech and Drama
• Exeter Course, validated by University of Worcester
• University of Derby.

Further information can be obtained at ℰ badth.org.uk.

Recommended reading

Andersen-Warren M and Grainger R (2000). *Practical Approaches to Dramatherapy*. Jessica Kingsley Publishers: London and Philadelphia.

Grainger R (1995). *Drama and Healing: The Roots of Dramatherapy*. Jessica Kingsley Publishers: London and Bristol, Pennsylvania.

Jennings S (1992). *Dramatherapy with Families, Groups and Individuals: Waiting in the Wings*. Jessica Kingsley Publishers: London and Philadelphia.

Jones P (2007). *Drama as Therapy, Theory, Practice and Research*. Routledge: London and New York.

Landy R (1993). *Persona and Performance: The Meaning of Role in Drama, Therapy and Everyday Life*. Jessica Kingsley Publishers: London and Bristol, Pennsylvania.

Pitruzzella S (2004). *Introduction to Dramatherapy, Person and Threshold*. Brunner-Routledge: Hove and New York.

Music therapy

Key concepts

Music therapy is a psychological therapy that works with unconscious process. It does not necessarily require spoken language, verbal intervention, or verbal interpretation. Music therapists may, however, use verbal interventions and interpretation, depending on the client group with which they are working, the individual client, and the music therapist's particular model or approach. Music therapy embraces a rich spectrum of approaches. There is no single definition of music therapy that can adequately describe or fit all of them.

The World Federation of Music Therapy (WFMT) offers this general definition of music therapy:

> 'Music Therapy is the use of music and/or musical elements (sound, rhythm, melody and harmony) by a qualified music therapist with a client or group, in a process designed to facilitate and promote communication, relationships, learning, mobilisation, expression, organization, and other relevant therapeutic objectives, in order to meet physical, emotional, mental, social and cognitive needs. Music therapy aims to develop potentials and/or to restore functions of the individual so that he or she can achieve better intra - and interpersonal integration and, consequently, a better quality of life through prevention, rehabilitation or treatment.'

(WFMT, 1996)

Music therapy settings include:
- Hospitals (NHS and private)
- Preschool specialist nurseries and centres for children
- Special schools for children with learning difficulties
- Mainstream schools
- Residential settings, including care homes
- Nursing homes
- Centres for children and adults with visual or hearing impairments
- Hospices and centres for people living with terminal illness
- Prisons and forensic settings
- Mental health care settings, including CAMHS.

In mental health care settings, music therapists work with people suffering from a range of illness and disorders, including:
- Psychosis
- Anxiety and depression
- Alzheimer's disease and other forms of dementia
- Eating disorders
- BPD
- Bipolar disorder
- Addictions and substance misuse
- Neurodisability.

The British Association of Music Therapists (BAMT) describes music therapy in the field of mental health as:

> 'A psychological intervention, music therapy uses the expressive
> elements of music as the primary means of interaction between
> therapist and client. Attentive listening on the part of the therapist
> is combined with shared musical improvisation using voices and
> instruments so that people can communicate in their own musical
> language, whatever their level of ability. Music therapists work with
> individuals and groups and the methods vary according to the setting
> and the theoretical approach of the music therapist.'

More specific approaches in music therapy include:
- Analytical music therapy
- Music psychotherapy
- Improvisational music therapy
- Creative music therapy (Nordoff–Robbins)
- Guided imagery and music (Bonny method)
- Behavioural music therapy (BMT).

Analytical music therapy
Analytical music therapy (AMT) is an approach to music therapy which is informed by the theories and techniques of psychoanalysis. It involves free musical improvisation between the music therapist and client. One of the aims is to uncover what is going on in the field of transference and countertransference.

Music psychotherapy
Music psychotherapy is informed by psychoanalytic theory and thinking. It incorporates some aspects of verbal psychodynamic psychotherapy where the transference relationship and unconscious processes are in the music, and in the experience of the music, as well as through the traditional types of verbal interactions.

Music psychotherapy involves the following:
- Musical instruments
- Musical improvisation and play
- A developing therapeutic relationship between the music therapist and client
- A triangular relationship involving the musical instruments, the client, and the music therapist
- The transference relationship between the music therapist and client
- The inner world of the client
- The unconscious
- Unconscious processes, as they emerge through sound, music, feelings, thoughts, ideas, and metaphor.

Key contributors
Music therapy has developed from a range of disciplines, including:
- Musical performance and improvisation
- Music psychology
- Psychotherapy

- Psychoanalysis
- General psychology
- Medicine
- Musicology
- Music education
- Special education
- Anthropology
- Anthroposophy.

The broad spectrum of music therapy approaches span from:
- Artistic to scientific
- Musical to psychological
- Behavioural to psychotherapeutic,

There are five main models of music therapy:
- Improvisational music therapy: the Alvin model
- Analytically orientated music therapy: the Priestly model
- Creative music therapy: the Nordoff–Robbins model
- Guided imagery and music: the Bonny method
- BMT: developed by, amongst others, Clifford K Madsen.

Improvisational music therapy
From 1950 to 1980, **Juliette Alvin**, an international concert cellist and pioneer of music therapy, was developing free improvisation therapy, which is now the basis of improvisational music therapy. In this approach, musical improvisation is used in a completely free way, with no musical rules or restrictions. This allows the client to 'let go' on a musical instrument. Alvin perceived music as a potential space for free expression and that, through musical improvisation, aspects of a person's character and personality can be expressed and therapeutic issues addressed. The approach incorporates a range of psychological theories with an orientation towards psychoanalytic theory.

Analytical music therapy
Mary Priestly, an English professional violinist and music therapist, developed AMT in the 1970s. Working with psychiatric clients, Priestly developed a specific theory that underpins her approach of bringing together music therapy and psychoanalysis. The transference relationship is thought about both in terms of psychoanalytic theory and through the experiences of musical improvisation.

Creative music therapy: the Nordoff–Robbins model
Creative music therapy is an improvisational model of music therapy developed between 1959 and 1976 by **Paul Nordoff**, an American composer and pianist, and **Clive Robbins**, who worked in special education. The approach was influenced by:
- Humanistic psychology
- The concepts of Abraham Maslow
- The work of Rudolf Steiner and anthroposophy.

Music is at the centre of the experience, and the client's musical responses are the focus for analysis and interpretation.

Bonny Method of Guided Imagery and Music

Helen Lindquist Bonny, an American music therapist, developed the Bonny Method of Guided Imagery and Music (BMGIM) in the USA through the 1960s and 1970s. BMGIM is a receptive form of music psychotherapy, in which the central procedure is active listening. The client listens to specifically programmed pieces of classical music in a deeply relaxed state, whilst the therapeutic presence of the music therapist or 'guide' supports the client, as imagery is evoked through the listening experience. During listening, the client or 'traveller' is invited to report any images to the therapist/guide. The term 'image' is used to cover a range of experiences: visual images, symbols, feelings, memories, bodily sensations. The therapist's role is to support and witness the imagery process.

Theoretical ideas that inform the BMGIM draw on the work of:
- Abraham Maslow (peak experiences)
- Sigmund Freud (free association)
- Carl Gustav Jung (archetypes and dreams)
- Hanscarl Leuner (guided affective imagery)
- Carl Rogers (client-centred therapy)
- Roberto Assagioli (psychosynthesis).

Behavioural music therapy

BMT was developed in the USA in the 1960s. Notable figures are **Clifford Madsen** and **Vance Cutter**. The aims of BMT involve modification of behaviour. Based on the concept of stimulus–response, music in any form is used to change behaviour or to reduce symptoms of pathology, and not to explore the cause of the behaviour.

Different types of behaviour that can be the focus of the therapy are:
- Psychological behaviour
- Emotional behaviour
- Cognitive behaviour
- Motor behaviour
- Perceptual behaviour.

BMT aims to facilitate:
- Social engagement
- Communication
- Cognitive processes
- Attention and concentration
- Physical activity.

What is the evidence base?

The music therapy profession conforms to the criteria for evidence-based disciplines. Evidence has been collected from a range of RCTs for music therapy, some of which can be located on the *Cochrane Reviews* database. There is a growing body of evidence from RCTs in the following areas:
- Alzheimer's disease and dementia
- Psychosis and schizophrenia
- Depression.

Summary of research findings:
- Music therapy can delay the deterioration of cognitive functions, particularly short-term recall function in dementia patients
- Music therapy can reduce anxiety and depression in patients with mild to moderate Alzheimer's disease
- Music therapy is effective in reducing behavioural disorders in severely demented patients
- Music therapy can reduce agitation disruptiveness and can prevent medication increases in people with dementia
- Individual music therapy is an effective addition to usual care for mental health care clients with low motivation
- Music therapy can improve patients' self-evaluation of their psychosocial orientation and negative symptoms for schizophrenic inpatients needing acute care
- Music therapy can diminish negative symptoms for patients with psychosis and improve interpersonal contact. These positive effects of music therapy may increase the patients' abilities to adapt to the social environment in the community after discharge from the hospital
- Group music therapy can enhance quality of life and spirituality of persons with severe mental illness
- Individual music therapy, combined with standard care, is effective for depression among working-age people.

Music therapy is cited in the UK NICE guidelines for the treatment of dementia and for the treatment of psychosis and schizophrenia, including children and young people with psychosis or schizophrenia. The Nordoff–Robbins Evidence Bank database is a collection of a wide range of references to music therapy, and music and health research papers and other key sources of information.

Music therapy training
Professional music therapy qualifications are at postgraduate MA level in the UK where 'Music Therapist' is a protected professional title.
   The following training courses are recognized by the BAMT and registered by the HCPC:
- MA in Music Therapy—University of South Wales, Newport
- MA in Music Therapy—Roehampton University, London
- MA in Music Therapy—Guildhall School of Music and Drama, London
- MA Music Therapy—University of the West of England
- MA in Music Therapy—Anglia Ruskin University, Cambridge
- Master of Music Therapy (Nordoff–Robbins)—Music, Health and Society, London and Manchester
- MSc in Music Therapy (Nordoff–Robbins)—Edinburgh.

All courses provide rigorous clinical, musical, and psychological training. Key areas of study are:
- Clinical context for music therapy
- Clinical improvisation
- Infant observation and child development
- Music therapy theory

- Psychoanalytic and psychodynamic theory
- Clinical case work and supervision
- Personal therapy
- Introduction to research
- Dissertation.

Students gain clinical experience with adults and children in a variety of settings, including:
- Psychiatry
- Special education
- Learning disability
- Communication disorders.

All music therapy students are required to have their own personal therapy during training.

Qualified music therapists are eligible to register as art therapists with the HCPC and as professional members of the BAMT.

Recommended reading

Ansdell G (1995). *Music for Life*. Jessica Kingsley Publishers: London.
Bruscia KE (ed) (1998). *The Dynamics of Music Psychotherapy*. Barcelona Publishers: Gilsum.
Bunt L and Hoskyns S (2002). *The Handbook of Music Therapy*. Brunner-Routledge: Hove and New York.
Wigram T and De Backer J (eds) (1999) *Clinical Applications of MT in Psychiatry*. Jessica Kingsley Publishers: London.
Wigram T, Pederson IN, and Ole Bonde L (2002). *A Comprehensive Guide to Music Therapy*. Jessica Kingsley Publishers: London.

Counselling

Key concepts

Counselling is a broad concept and will be considered here as a professional activity practised by skilled, trained practitioners accredited by the BACP or a similar regulatory organization. As with psychotherapy, there are many different models. The three primary counselling orientations are psychodynamic, humanistic, and cognitive behavioural (although, since the introduction of IAPT, CBT has become less associated with counselling). Context will also have an impact on the way that counselling is delivered. For example, a counsellor in private practice would be far more likely to offer a long-term or open-ended contract than would be the norm in an organization or agency with limited resources.

However, there are several key concepts that all counselling relationships will generally have in common, regardless of the practitioner orientation or context:
- The client needs to have engaged in the process voluntarily; counselling is not a prescribed treatment; it is a collaborative process and will not work, unless the client wishes to engage
- The client brings some element of distress that they wish to change or alleviate
- The counsellor is *there* for the client; there has to be a good therapeutic alliance which will be led by the client's agenda or needs, rather than those of the counsellor

- The counselling needs to be confidential; this is one of the guiding principles and extends to all aspects of the counselling contract, including the way notes and records are stored. Confidentiality can only be breached in certain specific circumstances, e.g. if there is a danger to self or others, and this is made explicit right from the start of the contract
- There are boundaries around the counselling relationship, including any contact outside the therapy room. Counsellors trained psychodynamically, however, may have stricter rules on boundaries than a humanistic, person-centred, or CBT-trained counsellor
- The counsellor receives regular clinical supervision

These tenets are covered in the BACP ethical framework and are there to protect the interests of the client and to give guidance on the ethical best practice for the counsellor.

So what happens in a counselling session? In many organizations, the client will be offered a brief intervention, usually between three and eight sessions. This means that every session, including a first assessment session, will need to count. This is where brief therapy starts to differ from longer-term where the process can unfold and the counsellor can adhere more easily to the purer principles of their training and chosen orientation. In brief therapy, a focus will need to be identified, and the practitioner will often take a more active or directive role, matching a range of interventions to suit the client and the client's situation. However, one of the key aspects of any counselling contract is that there should be a beginning, middle, and an end. In brief therapy especially, the end is always inherent, even in the beginning, and will need careful managing, especially if there are attachment issues involved. Often, the presenting problem is not what the real issue is, so the counsellor will need to be able to create the right environment for the client to feel safe enough to reveal relatively swiftly what the primary underlying problem may be. For this reason, one of the most important concepts of counselling is to be able to develop a strong therapeutic relationship or alliance. Whether this is understood in Rogerian terms of 'empathy, congruence, and unconditional positive regard' or a psychodynamic framing of transference and object relations, how the counsellor and client relate is vital to the success of the therapy.

Key contributors

- *Psychodynamic counselling*: although **Freud**, **Klein**, and other psychoanalysts (see ➜ Key contributors in Chapter 2, pp. 25–8) have been important in the evolution and understanding of the key ideas that underpin the psychodynamic model, the psychodynamic approach to counselling offers a broad perspective, drawing on many different schools of thought. The assumption that emotional problems have their roots in the past and that unconscious material will arise in the counselling through the client's transference reaction to the client and that the counsellor's countertransference in helping gain an understanding of the client and what they are feeling are key components of the model. In working with students and trainee doctors, other influential contributors are **Donald Winnicott** (see ➜ Key contributors in Chapter 2, pp. 25–8) and **John Bowlby** (see

➔ Key contributors in Chapter 2, pp. 25–8) in helping understand anxieties arising from early ruptured attachments. This becomes particularly pertinent during times of transition and also in the context of brief therapy.

- *Carl Rogers and the person-centred approach*: the use of the terms 'counsellor' and 'client' was introduced by **Carl Rogers** in the 1940s, when he developed the use of 'non-directive counselling', as opposed to psychoanalysis, in a non-medical setting. He believed that all people need to fulfil two primary needs—the need for self-actualization and the need to be loved and valued by others—and found that, given these conditions, people would find for themselves their own therapeutic pathway. The 'core conditions' of 'empathy, congruence, and acceptance' were deemed to be 'necessary and sufficient'. Many counsellor training courses now offer an integrative humanistic approach that combines Rogerian ideas with other humanistic models such as gestalt, transactional analysis (TA), and existential counselling. The humanistic approach differs from psychodynamic counselling in that it deals with the 'here and now', rather than looking back to how the past impacts the client today.
- *Cognitive behavioural and solution-focused therapy*: (see ➔ Cognitive behavioural therapy in Chapter 2, pp. 30–4, and in Chapter 5, pp. 172–84) most experienced counsellors, even if they are not specifically CBT-oriented, will usually have an understanding of the key techniques of CBT and often use these, especially in brief work. Solution-focused therapy (SFT) is also used by many counsellors. Developed by practitioners, such as **Steve De Shazer** and **Insoo Kim Berg**, from the work of **Milton Erickson** and initially used in family therapy, SFT is highly collaborative and looks to the solution or desired state, rather than the problem and is future-, rather than past-, oriented.
- *Integrative therapy*: many counsellors use an 'integrative' approach where they blend several different orientations. Some counsellors are 'eclectic' or 'pluralistic' (see ➔ Integration in Chapter 2, pp. 16–7), having a broad range of interventions and approaches at their disposal to use when appropriate. Another strategy for achieving integration has been to find a central theoretical concept or framework, in which all existing approaches can be subsumed. The central concept is 'problem management' and is broken down into three stages: 'exploration (present scenario)', 'understanding (and to articulate preferred scenario)', and 'action (strategies on how to get there)'. This is a very practical model, and many counsellors will use it as a framework, regardless of their orientation.

What is the evidence base?

There is much research which demonstrates the effectiveness of counselling. A number of systematic reviews have been conducted which provide evidence that counselling has greater clinical effectiveness, compared with usual care. Counselling has been demonstrated to be as effective as CBT, and a review for common mental health problems, such as anxiety or depression, found no significant differences between

CBT, non-directive counselling, and problem-solving therapy. There is also evidence that many people indicate a preference for counselling over antidepressant medication, and patients receiving counselling tend to be more satisfied with their treatment than those receiving CBT or usual care.

In terms of counselling students, a major BACP research project took place in 2011/12 looking at the impact of counselling (provided in-house) on academic outcomes in further and higher education. The research, based on responses from over 5000 students from 65 different institutions across the UK, demonstrated that counselling helped the student stay at university, improved their academic achievement, improved their overall experience of being a student, and helped them develop employability skills. An RCT is currently in progress to give further evidence for the efficacy of in-house counselling for students in further and higher education.

Counselling training

As counselling is currently unregulated, in theory, anyone can call themselves a counsellor. In order to ensure standards and protection for clients, the BACP have a registration and accreditation process, which most counsellors will need to engage with, in order to secure employment. The most conventional training pathway is a year-long part-time certificate in counselling, followed by a 2-year part-time postgraduate diploma, ideally on a BACP accredited course. Many will top this up with a Masters qualification (1 year full-time or 2 years part-time). Most training programmes, unless attached to a specific organization which provides its own training, either take place in or are validated by a Higher Education Institute. In recognition of the many ways counsellors can be trained, the BACP criteria for accreditation is that the applicant should have received a minimum of 450 tutor contact hours. In addition, all applicants for accreditation must have undertaken at least 450 hours of supervised practice accumulated within 3–6 years of training (150 hours after completion of practitioner training). Personal therapy is not essential for BACP accreditation (although, for many courses, particularly psychodynamic ones, it will be mandatory), but applicants must be able to demonstrate high levels of personal awareness. Once accredited, the counsellor needs to be reaccredited annually, having satisfied the criteria for ongoing CPD and supervision.

Recommended reading

British Association for Counselling and Psychotherapy (2012). *Evidence for Counselling Psychotherapy.* Available at: ℘www.bacp.co.uk.

Cooper M (2008). *Essential Research Findings in Counselling and Psychotherapy.* Sage Publications: London.

Cooper M and McLeod J (2011). *Pluralistic Counselling and Psychotherapy.* Sage Publications: London.

Egan G (1994). *The Skilled Helper: A Systematic Approach to Effective Helping,* fifth edition. Brooks/Cole: Belmont, CA.

Mcleod J (2009). *An Introduction to Counselling,* fourth edition. Open University Press: Maidenhead.

Rogers CR (1961). *On Becoming a Person.* Houghton Mifflin: Boston.

Chapter 3

General therapeutic competencies

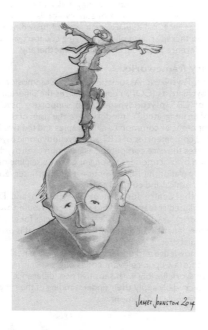

Competencies framework

Generic competencies

Generic competencies refer to the basic standards expected of any modality of therapy for it to be effective, and can be demonstrated in therapists working within any given therapeutic framework. Effective therapists demonstrate a sophisticated set of interpersonal skills and perceptiveness, and are able to bring warmth, empathy, openness, and acceptance to the work with a patient. The patient's acceptance and trust of the therapist stem from subtle verbal and non-verbal cues which signal empathy and expertise right from the start of the therapy. The therapist is then able to create a collaborative environment where: (1) there is a shared understanding of the patient's difficulties and (2) goals of therapy can be agreed upon together. This process paves the way for a robust *working alliance*.

A competent therapist is one who understands that a psychological explanation for an illness needs to be accepted by, and adapted to, the patient who can then go on to make sense of the treatment plan by linking it to his or her own lived experience.

When looked at in the context of the therapeutic process, generic competencies include the knowledge and ability to: apply appropriate competence frameworks; establish a good therapeutic alliance and thus engage the patient; manage effectively the journey of therapy, including responding appropriately to, and managing, risk and emotions; and finally manage endings. Appropriate use of supervision is included in generic competencies as well, particularly as a way of providing support and guidance to the therapist, as well as managing countertransference processes with reference to psychodynamic psychotherapy.

Competency frameworks

The American Psychiatric Association (APA) Commission on Psychotherapy by Psychiatrists (COPP) conceptualizes the different, but linked, approaches of CBT, psychodynamic, and supportive psychotherapies in the form of an integrated 'Y' model where the stem of the Y stands for the core competencies common to all therapies and the two branches as the specialized competencies of CBT and psychodynamic psychotherapy. Plakun delineates the core competencies common to all psychotherapies when practised by practitioners belonging to the discipline of psychiatry, which include: relationship, intervention planning, intervention implementation, and ethical and cultural sensitivity.

In the UK, the Centre for Outcomes Research and Effectiveness (CORE) has collated research findings which contribute towards identifying core (generic), as well as specific, competencies for all psychotherapies. Within the generic competency framework, what is expected of an effective therapist are:

• A working knowledge and understanding of mental health problems
• The ability to draw upon relevant codes of practice
• An ability to work flexibly with sensitivity to 'difference'
• An ability to credibly apply their understanding of their model of therapy to the individual patient.

Knowledge and understanding of mental health problems

(See ➲ Formulation in Chapter 4, pp. 122–4.)

Therapists are expected to have a good working knowledge of mental health problems, with reference to their antecedents, development, pattern of symptoms, impact on functioning, and the effects that poor functioning can have, in their turn, on mental health. The therapist also needs to acknowledge and manage the risk of escalation of interpersonal difficulties during therapy. This may be understood as linked to the underlying mental health problem and the ways by which long-standing unhelpful patterns of behaviour in relationships tend to come to the fore when they are examined in greater detail in therapy. In practical terms, a diagnostic label may be less useful to the medical psychotherapist than a biopsychosocial formulation with an emphasis on early experiences, which inform later patterns of functioning. It is probably important to know how certain symptoms and difficulties cluster together and form distinct clinical entities, e.g. an anxiety disorder with phobic avoidance or a depressive disorder triggered by loss/bereavement. Understanding the patterns of clinical presentation from a psychiatric perspective is often useful to take into consideration when planning the psychotherapeutic approach to the problem. Whilst a basic knowledge of classifiable mental disorders and symptom profiles is expected within medical psychotherapy, it is important to distinguish between a biologically driven diagnosis and a deeper psychological understanding of the patient's problems.

Knowledge of, and ability to operate within, professional and ethical guidelines

(See ➲ Chapter 9.)

All psychotherapists need to practice within the appropriate ethical and legal framework of their own professional body. For medical psychotherapists, therefore, the GMC guidelines regarding good practice will form the basis to a knowledge and understanding of other appropriate legal frameworks that apply to professional practice such as the Mental Capacity Act, Mental Health Act (MHA), Human Rights Act, and Data Protection Act. In the context of the therapist–patient relationship, this may relate to the ways in which the frame for therapy is set up and thought about. For example, for a patient who is in therapy and is also receiving care for an episode of acute illness, careful consideration needs to be given to the role of the therapist, whilst also being mindful of the involvement of other services. Such a discussion is only possible if the therapist is aware of, and able to take to supervision, the competing interests of various legal frameworks in patient care, and is thoughtful about their own position as the patient's therapist.

Therapists are expected to be conversant with the national and local codes of practice that apply to all health care professionals. Examples would be codes of practice relating to: obtaining informed consent, maintaining confidentiality and record-keeping standards, maintaining professional standards through CPD and training, and safeguarding the patient's interests both within the therapy, as well as in all interactions with the team. Every profession has a requirement to keep up with national and international standards of practice, as well as with the latest research evidence that may inform and improve current theory and practice. The task of examining and recognizing one's own limitations needs to be revisited time and again in a therapist's working life. It is the duty of the practitioner to take steps to ensure that they are fit to practise.

Ability to work with difference (cultural competence)
(See ➲ Ethnicity and culture in Chapter 6, pp. 297–8; Outcome research in psychotherapy in Chapter 11, pp. 518–19.)

Cultural competence has been a much examined term over the past few decades and is enormously relevant, not only given the increasingly multicultural nature of the patient population, but also with regard to differences between the therapist and patient in terms of their respective backgrounds and value systems. The therapist and patient are inevitably confronted with these differences in the consulting room. Cultural competence refers to an awareness of the significance of these differences and an understanding of the impact of these on therapeutic work. The domains that are often considered are religion, ethnicity, culture, class, gender, age, disability, and sexual orientation. Whilst earlier research suggested that 'ethnic match' and 'cognitive match' enhances positive therapy outcomes, it is now becoming clear that generic skills of a therapist include an ability to work across difference by: (1) understanding the social and cultural impact of a proposed intervention and (2) when accessibility is an issue, to tailor the therapy with the aim of providing maximum benefit to the patient within their cultural and social context. The other important point to acknowledge would be that the idea of a therapist–patient difference may well operate in the case of *all* patients, and not just in the case of self-identified or minority patients who actively bring a particular need for recognizing difference in the therapeutic context. A therapist's sensitivity to this quality of 'otherness' brought by the patient can significantly challenge, inform, and enhance treatment outcomes.

Knowledge of a model of therapy, and ability to understand and employ the model in practice
(See ➲ Chapter 2; Common factor research in Chapter 11, pp. 519–22.)

There are certain overarching factors inherent to understanding one's own model of therapy and applying it to an individual patient and to populations. These include knowledge of the underlying theory and principles of the model being used. All psychotherapies operate within a framework of being supportive, offering a reflective space in which new learning can occur. In being supportive, therapy fosters a trusting relationship within which the patient can actively explore their concerns with a professional who is compassionate, respectful, and encouraging. In this way, the therapist and the therapeutic relationship enhance the patient's personal effectiveness. Internal frames of reference are explored, in order to understand problematic experiences, both past and present, in new ways. Systems-based therapy modalities refer to this process as 'reframing the problem'. However, for all therapists working in all therapeutic modalities, applying theoretical constructs to the work with individual patients involves the therapist retaining some creativity and flexibility in this process. Experienced and effective therapists trained primarily in one therapeutic modality are able to adapt their core technique appropriately for the specific needs of the patient, which may involve 'borrowing' or incorporating techniques and skills from other modalities, whilst being mindful of the rationale behind such modifications and their effects on the therapeutic process.

Therapeutic alliance

(See ➲ Chapter 2; Research in psychotherapy in Chapter 11, pp. 508–26.)

The idea of the therapeutic alliance as a distinct entity, driving treatment outcomes independent of modality, technique, premise, and the nature of human dysfunction, finds its roots in psychoanalysis; in Freud's work and in the discovery of transference. Over the years, this has been viewed in the context of various therapeutic modalities, and it was in the mid-1970s that the notion of the *relationship variable* being a common one across all forms of therapy took root. In the present day understanding of this construct, the notion of *collaboration* is key. A collaborative relationship thus not only offers a safe environment within which to explore difficult experiences, but also enables a proper examination of relational problems: past, present, and future. By becoming a particular type of figure in the patient's life—one who is curious and interested in the patient, yet able to maintain professional boundaries—the therapist makes possible an integration of technical and relational elements of the theory underpinning the therapy. This, when taken together with the interactive nature of psychotherapy, fosters an atmosphere within which positive change is possible for the patient.

A good therapeutic alliance sits at the heart of any effective therapeutic encounter, independent of modality, and the ability to facilitate this with the patient is a necessary core competency in a therapist. However, in addition, a good therapeutic alliance means consensus between therapist and patient on shared goals, and the patient's acceptance of the techniques used in therapy. This involves trust; that which grows in a situation where the therapist is open, self-reflective, and honest with the patient. It stands to reason that an aloof, critical, or rigid therapist bent on imposing what may feel like an alien system of thinking on the patient will have little success by way of fostering a healthy working alliance.

Engaging the patient

(See ➲ Beginning the therapy in Chapter 5, pp. 158–9; Therapy in clinical practice in Chapter 5, pp. 154–63; What constitutes good therapy? in Chapter 11, pp. 523.)

A good therapeutic alliance goes a long way towards engaging a patient, once the therapy is firmly established. However, at the start, it requires an interested, concerned, and committed therapist who can convey a sense of optimism and confidence in themselves, in order to enable the process to begin. An ability to adapt personal style to the patient, as well as pragmatically meet change as it happens in the therapy, is a crucial skill that fosters positive engagement in a genuine process between therapist and patient. Being non-judgemental means that the therapist is open and curious, encourages the patient to speak openly, and is sensitive to a different world view. Thus, such a therapist is not threatened by the patient's curiosity, reluctance, or hostility, and will instead seek to understand the reasons behind such a stance. Any therapy runs the risk of alliance ruptures, and often it is the way in which the therapist addresses these—sensitively and in the interest of the patient—that can ultimately strengthen and deepen the therapeutic relationship. It is important for a therapist to be able to admit to their own contribution towards an alliance rupture, whilst seeking to understand it better. As is often the case, such threats mimic similar ruptures in relationships in the patient's external world, and a skilled therapist is able to point this out sensitively to their patients in a way that helps them to think about their experiences in a safe setting. An ability to create just such a dynamic process, of moulding an intervention to the here and now of the patient, could be thought of as a key engagement skill in the repertoire of an experienced therapist.

Dealing with emotions

Sitting with a patient who is in emotional distress is a challenging process. The desire to reach out, metaphorically and physically, to provide some comfort and the wish to help are often mobilized and, in other circumstances, can be acted on. However, working in a therapy setting changes the dynamics considerably. This can lead to junior therapists feeling that to want to help their patient will be frowned upon or seen as a breach of the often mentioned boundaries of the therapy. However, maintaining boundaries does not have to lead to a clinician becoming robotic, cold, or aloof. An emotional response is elicited from a therapist by the patient, because of the nature of their relationship and the transference.

Although some therapeutic modalities may more explicitly focus on the exploration of emotional states than others, the ability to deal with the emotional content of sessions is one of the generic therapeutic competencies that apply to all psychotherapies. This includes the ability to facilitate the processing of emotions by the patient—to acknowledge and contain emotional levels that are too high (e.g. anger, fear, despair) or too low (e.g. apathy, low motivation); the ability to deal effectively with emotional issues that interfere with effective change (e.g. hostility, anxiety, excessive anger, avoidance of strong affect); and the ability to help the patient access, differentiate, and experience his/her emotions in a way that facilitates change.

The processing of emotions is an active process for all human beings from the outset. An infant has needs that feel overwhelming, and there is a search for help to make sense of these. The ability of a mother (or other caregiver) to take in the projections of the infant and help them to process, or 'metabolize', them is crucial in helping the infant to develop a capacity to do that for themselves. In a similar way, the therapist's role is to help the patient process difficult emotions in order that they are less distressing.

Patients may present with differing emotional states, ranging from labile states to emotional detachment. The therapist will need not only to recognize the state of the patient, but also to notice how the patient perceives their own emotional state. For example, patients who have learnt to detach themselves as a defence against sadness or loss may describe traumatic memories with little emotion. The therapist will then need to observe, reflect, and discuss this with the patient, in order that they can then notice the pattern and manner by which they have learnt to manage. The process of observation of both the patient's and the therapist's affect forms a crucial part of the therapeutic work; the feeding back to the patient of these observations is in order to help them to recognize patterns of behaving and relating.

Therapists may encounter the more uncomfortable feelings of hostility, anger, or aggression directed towards them. The therapist's ability to manage their instinctive desire to react, and instead to think about why these feelings are being expressed now, is important in allowing the patient to develop a capacity to tolerate these types of feelings. The importance of knowing which feelings belong to the therapist and which belong to the patient is important and can be difficult to distinguish in the early stages of training (see ➡ Countertransference in Chapter 2, pp. 25; Balint groups in Chapter 10, pp. 484–96).

Vignette 1: less complex

A patient in her forties was in once-weekly CBT. She described long-standing difficulties of trust and intimacy. She was one of several siblings and had a strict upbringing. Her father was described as being a rather repressed individual who appeared to display little emotional reaction, whilst her mother was strict and keen to impress on her children the need to be 'good'. Her parents had clear expectations of how children should be 'seen and not heard'; she felt the weight of expectation to be a 'model child' and had learnt that displaying any 'negative' emotion was met with rebuke and punishment. She had invested heavily in portraying herself as good and unlike her siblings whom she perceived as angry and ill-behaved. As a result, she had developed a pattern of distancing herself from strong emotional states and found these difficult to put into words.

During the course of her sessions, she became able to speak more freely about her own emotional state and recognize the ways in which her own thinking style had led to particular ways of behaving. In one session, she spoke of her unhappiness with the way in which she had been raised and was more vocal in her own opinion. She then became distressed and demonstrated catastrophic thinking, believing that her negative comments carried more weight than any other statements. The result in her mind was that she was just like her siblings, bad and ill-behaved, and any sense that she was good was shattered momentarily.

During the course of CBT, the therapist helped her to identify and challenge her entrenched patterns of thinking. Not only did this give her great relief, but it also led to an increase in her self-confidence, as she had been able to test and challenge these thoughts with the therapist in a safe environment.

Vignette 2: more complex

A male patient in his twenties had sought help after repeatedly getting into relationship difficulties which ended in violent outbursts, with him causing damage to property. He was fearful that these incidents would continue, escalate, and end in him harming someone. He had a background of significant emotional deprivation. His father was unknown to him, and his mother had struggled to manage alone. His mother recounted to him a history of violence perpetrated by his biological father. Later she went on to have a series of relationships in which she was repeatedly subjected to domestic violence, often witnessed by the patient. The patient's behaviour was described as difficult to manage, and he had had multiple short-term placements in respite care to allow his mother to continue to care for him. He loved his mother but repeatedly described her as weak, easily overpowered by him, and fragile. He was able to find employment and form relationships, but these would repeatedly break down.

He saw a female therapist for a period of a year for psychodynamic psychotherapy within a forensic psychotherapy service. This therapy was characterized by frequent absences on his part, particularly after a break. He spoke of his difficulties in managing these breaks, but stayed in the therapy and continued to struggle. His therapist informed him after a year that her post was changing, and she would be leaving in six months. When informed, he became hostile, threatened the therapist, and moved his chair, appearing to block the therapist's exit. The therapist felt extremely vulnerable, fearful for her safety, and uncertain as to what was going to happen to her. She felt as if she was frozen, watching the patient, and found herself breathing in a shallow manner. She looked at the patient who was looking at her in an angry manner and watching her reaction. She realized that he had not commented on her leaving. Her thinking cleared a little, and she was able to recognize that some of the feelings she was experiencing were being projected by him; her absence had served to remind him how small and vulnerable he felt and how he may need her. The threat of her loss was enormously anxiety-provoking, and so he was trying to manage the situation, as he had always done—by trying to control her with threats and hostility, as he had with his mother. Gradually, the therapist was able to articulate this to him, at which point he broke down. He was able to acknowledge his feelings of hostility and anger towards her and how terrified he had felt when he heard her announce her leaving.

Over the course of the next few months in therapy, the patient continued to struggle with these feelings but did not act on them. There was a gradual recognition that his behaviour had echoes of the men he had seen abusing his mother in childhood and were his reference for a male identity. The therapist's ability to separate her feelings and those of the patient's was important in helping her to communicate with him. She was able to demonstrate a capacity to metabolize some difficult and strong emotions that the patient could not manage at that point. His experience of being understood proved difficult but helpful, and enabled him to move towards a change in this way of relating.

Dealing with breaks and endings

(See ➲ Transitions and disruptions in Chapter 6, pp. 298–311.)

Breaks and endings offer unique opportunities within therapy to explore ordinary feelings of loss, as well as a more permanent loss that lends itself to the mourning process. In psychodynamic psychotherapy, both breaks and endings are conceptualized as having immense significance, often evoking feelings associated with primitive, early responses to separation and loss. Managing both in a therapy appropriately and creatively, however, is a core skill in all modalities of psychotherapy.

For most patients, breaks bring up separation anxieties; for some, they can feel like endings. The patient's response, or the lack of it, must be picked up sensitively by the therapist; no two patients are alike, and perhaps the only universal truth is that breaks and endings bring up strong, sometimes unexpected, responses in both the therapist and the patient.

The therapist needs to be able to discuss the ending of therapy with the patient in a way that makes it possible to talk openly about the feelings associated with loss, as well as anxieties about how they are going to manage without the therapist. Being able to say goodbye in an ordinary and compassionate way, keeping in mind the patient's feelings, is a vital skill. Planning for this may include discussing the ending at the start and returning to it periodically in a way that helps to review the work done in therapy. Patients, as well as therapists, can get caught up in enactments around endings, and the work done in understanding this together is often crucial for the patient and goes a long way towards addressing earlier losses, both real and in fantasy. The following vignette illustrates this.

Vignette: ending

A man in his 50s was seen once weekly in psychodynamic psychotherapy over three years. He came to therapy with a long-standing difficulty with relationships, within which he struggled to trust others' motives towards him. The patient's problems were rooted in a difficult childhood in which he watched his beloved mother being undermined and dismissed constantly by his father. His mother went on to die of a sudden illness, whilst the patient, a young man, felt helpless. The patient himself felt held back and limited by his father, going on to feel that he had never achieved anything significant. The therapist noticed how the patient undermined his own family who were supportive and loving, and the work in therapy went some way towards exploring the identification the patient had with his father. The ending was planned over six months; however, the patient suddenly insisted on a premature ending, stating that he could not see the point in prolonging the therapy when a few months 'meant very little' in the grand scheme of things. The therapist felt thrown by this initially, and felt a bit useless and superfluous. However, on reflection, she was able to understand the patient's unconscious need to make her feel this way, in order to avoid his own feelings of humiliation and loss at the ending of a valued relationship. When this was brought up sensitively, the patient was able to admit to his fears about the future without therapy and feelings of anger towards the therapist, as well as mistrust of her motives at 'leaving' him. Thus a more realistic ending was possible in that the patient could experience some compassion and understanding from the therapist, whilst acknowledging that there was something he had gained from the experience of the ending.

Assessing and managing risk

Risk assessment

Risk assessment in mental health is traditionally divided into the *actuarial approach*, which measures static and historical factors associated with risk (such as age, gender, socio-economic status, and history of previous self-harm or risky behaviour), and the *clinical approach*, which measures dynamic factors (such as intimacy problems and chaotic lifestyle). Although psychotherapists may be more interested in the latter and may tend to assess risk on the basis of their individual clinical judgement measuring dynamic aspects of the patient, a psychotherapeutically based risk framework should take account of both clinical and actuarial evidence-based risk factors (e.g. knowing that, from an actuarial risk perspective, an older man living alone, with a previous history of a suicide attempt, poses a much higher risk of completed suicide than a younger woman with a history of self-harm). As well as elucidating the frequency, patterns, and precipitating circumstances of any identified risk factors, it is also important to consider their meaning for the individual as they occur in the therapeutic relationship and setting, as well as in the patient's external life. In recent years, the elucidation of *protective factors,* such as the presence of supportive relationships in the patient's life, has become more prominent in risk assessment.

The assessment of risk with psychotherapy falls into two defined areas. The first is an assessment in relation to the suitability for therapy, and the second is the ongoing dynamic risk assessment and management that take place in the context of an ongoing therapy. Risk assessment and management should be less concerned with prediction and more concerned with making a formulation about risk. This will assist clinical thinking about whether, and under what clinical conditions, a psychological intervention can take place safely for a particular individual.

Risk assessment begins when the referral is received by the clinician. At this point, attention is paid to the urgency of the referral and the nature of the case, and associated risk factors will be noted. These include the use of alcohol, illicit substances, forensic history (including acts of violence and aggression), active mental illness, acts of self-harm, and suicide attempts. The assessing psychotherapist may also request additional information from the referrer, e.g. previous psychiatric reports, probation or police records, court reports, etc., before deciding to assess the patient for psychotherapy.

The assessment process is usually comprised of one meeting or a short series of meetings which are aimed at identifying whether therapy is likely to be beneficial for the patient and, if so, what the most appropriate type of therapy is. The process should not be seen as the *patient* being suitable, but as what is likely to be the most helpful intervention at this point in time for the patient. The process looks at the presenting problem that the patient brings and how they hope to think about it.

Throughout the psychotherapy assessment process, information should be gathered regarding all relevant risk factors, so that the clinician becomes aware of the presence of mental illness, history of suicide in the patient or the family, use of drugs (prescribed and recreational) and alcohol, self-harming behaviours, or harm to others. For the latter, the circumstances in which the patient self-harms (or is violent towards others) are also explored, paying particular attention to the antecedents, feelings, and impulse to self-harm (or harm others) and the ability to withstand these or not. Attention is also paid to whether harm to self or others occurs in the context of disinhibiting substances such as alcohol or illicit drugs. Emotional deprivation is an important area to explore, as this will form the basis of the template of engagement with a therapist. If there have been experiences in the patient's life of good and reliable 'others' being present, whether primary caregivers or not, this gives some clues as to the emotional engagement of the patient and how they may withstand separation and loss. Conversely, those with complex, multiple attachments or abusive caregivers are likely to have more difficulty in not only establishing a trusting therapeutic relationship, but also managing loss, separation, and endings.

In psychodynamic terms, the clinician is identifying the ego strengths of the patient and their ability to withstand stressful or difficult internal feelings, and whether they are likely to act out in particular ways during therapy. Past behaviour, such as taking an overdose in response to difficulties in a relationship, may be re-enacted, e.g. during a break or ending.

If therapy is thought to be helpful, these risks can be addressed directly with the patient during a business meeting with the prospective therapist. This meeting is usually a brief appointment, which is not a therapy session, during which key issues, such as the timing and dates of future sessions, are agreed and support networks are identified. There should be mention of a crisis plan and an acknowledgement from the therapist that things may be difficult at periods during therapy and may lead to the patient feeling in a similar state to when they had experienced difficulties in the past. The adage of past risk predicting future risk should be borne in mind, as well as the concept that an individual may feel more disturbed at times during therapy.

Risk management

(See ➔ Dealing with breaks and endings in Chapter 3, pp. 103; Transitions and disruptions in Chapter 6, pp. 298–311.)

During therapy, the risk assessment should be reviewed regularly by the therapist. Identified periods of difficulty are likely to be around the breaks and ending. Again, the therapist will need to bear in mind the developmental history of the patient and their reaction to these scenarios in the past. If there are concerns that a patient is struggling to manage, such as becoming depressed or becoming suicidal, then an assessment of these states will need to become the focus, as safety is paramount. However, the context of the setting and the difficulties being encountered must be taken into account as well. Additional support in the form of contact with general psychiatric services, or additional social support, can be identified and pursued directly by the therapist. If there are indications for pharmacological treatment, then the therapist can liaise with the general practitioner or psychiatrist. Additionally, if the patient is known to be at higher risk in terms of self-harm and/or active mental disorder and is known to psychiatric services, it is helpful to communicate regularly from the outset of the therapy with other professionals involved in the patient's care, in order to appraise them of pertinent risk issues, within the limits of confidentiality of sessions.

Another matter which can often prove difficult for a therapist is the discussion of violent or sexual fantasies by a patient. If these are present, their disclosure by the patient is often after some time in therapy, after a level of trust has developed between the patient and therapist. The idea of a patient saying what is actually on their mind, and not providing a level of filter, can provide rich unconscious material to the therapist and help them to build a more accurate formulation. The anxiety that is raised in the therapist, however, is whether the patient will act on disclosed fantasies. For the most part, this is what is brought to the room, and the feelings stirred up in the therapist can be managed through careful clinical supervision of the case. Again the history of the patient will need re-evaluating; have they acted on their fantasies before? What are they trying to communicate, and why are they saying this now? Is this in relation to a break or ending, and what do they think the therapist will do?

Confidentiality and disclosure
(See ➋ Confidentiality and psychotherapy in Chapter 9, pp. 452–4.)

If there are concerns about identified serious risks of harm to the patient or to another person, particularly a child, the therapist may breach confidentiality, in order to share this information with other relevant parties. Any information sharing or disclosure should be considered within the framework of existing professional guidance on confidentiality from the Royal College of Psychiatrists, the GMC, and the Department of Health, which advise that it may be justifiable for a doctor to pass on patient information without consent or statutory authority if there is a risk of serious harm arising without disclosure.

Disclosure may, however, have potentially negative effects on a therapy, if it is not dealt with carefully, and the rationale behind disclosure not being clear in the therapist's own mind. Disclosure without the patient's consent may have a negative impact on the therapeutic alliance and on that of other patients, e.g. where the treatment is group therapy. Situations where disclosure is considered arise more commonly in the treatment of the offender patient population group where the risks are heightened during therapy if the patient is prone to resort to violence as a maladaptive response to dealing with emotional distress. In all cases, the respective risks of breaching confidentiality versus the risk of the patient causing harm to themselves and/or the public if disclosure does not occur should be carefully considered and balanced. Cases should be discussed within supervision and with other senior members of the team, including the Caldicott Guardian, where necessary, before any decision to disclose is made. All discussions and decisions should be carefully documented in the patient's record.

Vignette: managing self-harm
A 23-year-old female patient was attending once-weekly psychotherapy. She had been referred by her community psychiatric nurse (CPN), after speaking

about issues from her past that she was keen to address. In the assessment, she described being raised by parents who were self-absorbed and had difficulties in sustaining their own relationship. Her mother was described as needy and chaotic, and her father as charismatic but erratic. Her maternal grandparents had proved to be a consistent presence during childhood, and she frequently sought refuge with them. During adolescence, she struggled with intimacy and forming lasting relationships, and began to self-harm at times of distress. Following discussions with her CPN, she had agreed to a referral, as she was keen to 'sort out' her past.

Areas of risk identified during the assessment were the likelihood to self-harm at times of stress and breaks, alongside difficulties in sustaining the therapeutic relationship. She commenced therapy and appeared to be able to engage well, about which the therapist was pleased. During her eighth session, she spoke to the therapist about a situation in which she had managed to avoid her usual response and had felt positive about this. The therapist had also felt this was a positive step and felt the urge to comment on this. Afterwards, he noted how this had taken him by surprise, and he felt a little unsettled by this.

At the next week's session, the therapist was shocked to see that the patient's arm was bandaged. She went on to reveal that, following the last session, she had got drunk and harmed herself by cutting her wrists. She was unable to recall the previous session and was surprised by this, but in a manner that was not curious. The therapist felt anxious that he had missed something. He was able, during the course of the session, to manage his own feelings of anxiety and think about what had happened. He recalled the previous session as demonstrating a positive move, and this had been acknowledged. He wondered aloud with the patient whether the incident in the last week had been a response to this. He was able to note to himself a pattern in which the patient would punish both herself and the therapist, and there was a difficulty for her to stay in touch with difficult feelings, hence her forgetting the previous session. For her, more positive interactions were difficult, as was the sense of the therapist being interested in her as a person.

The patient denied this initially but then spoke during this and subsequent sessions about how having a therapist who was interested in helping her was difficult, because it was a painful reminder of the inadequacies in her own childhood. She was able, over the course of a longer therapy, to identify that this led her to act in destructive ways in an attempt to spoil the therapy to escape the painful feelings it stirred up.

Using supervision

Supervision is a vital part of clinical work. The rationale for this is to evaluate the material from the patient and to help the therapist recognize patterns in this material, as well as to differentiate which feelings are from the patient and which are from the therapist. For those undertaking long-term psychodynamically orientated work, regular supervision allows for the content of the session to be reviewed through this lens, allowing themes to evolve and be discussed, the development of the transference to be noted, and other material, such as dreams, to be thought about. It is good clinical practice to have regular supervision. To not participate in supervision, particularly when inexperienced, is not safe practice and leaves the therapist more vulnerable to shifting away from a therapeutic stance towards acting out. Even experienced therapists have regular and ongoing clinical supervision to ensure scrutiny and safety.

The ability to make use of supervision is one of the recommended generic therapeutic competencies for all psychotherapy modalities and includes the ability of the therapist to work collaboratively with the supervisor; the ability to develop capacities for self-appraisal and reflection, and for active learning; the ability to use supervision to reflect on the therapist's developing personal and professional role; and the capacity to reflect on the quality of supervision.

Trainee therapists will typically be part of a regular (usually weekly) supervision group, with an experienced therapist as their supervisor. This often involves the therapist making detailed process notes after a session in which the emotional affect of both the therapist and the patient is recalled and noted, alongside the content of the verbal and non-verbal communication of the patient and the therapist's response to this. These notes are then presented to the supervisor who may themselves make notes, will assess the themes within the session, and comment on the observations made by the therapist. Therapies, such as CBT or MBT in which sessions are directly recorded, may use supervision for the therapist and supervisor to listen to, or view, the recordings, which may provide a more accurate picture of the therapy than the therapist's recollected process notes.

The supervisee is encouraged to think further about the sessions being presented and to begin to develop a capacity to reflect on his or her own practice. For dynamic therapists, this will include the ability to recognize unconscious communications between patient and therapist, as well as the conscious communications. Areas identified for development of the therapist's clinical skills are kept under review, with regular discussion in relation to the expected competencies.

Recommended reading

Gabbard GO, Beck JS, and Holmes, J. (eds) (2005). *Oxford Textbook of Psychotherapy*. Oxford University Press: Oxford.

Horvath AO and Greenberg LS (eds) (1994). *The Working Alliance: Theory, Research, and practice*. John Wiley & Sons, Inc.: New York.

Plakun E (2008). A view from Riggs: treatment resistance and patient authority—introduction to paper IX: integrative psychodynamic treatment of psychotic disorders. *Journal of the American Academy of Psychoanalysis and Dynamic Psychiatry*, **36**, 737–8.

Assessment

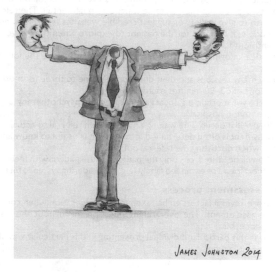

JAMES JOHNSTON 2014

Is my patient suitable for psychotherapy?

What does the word suitable mean? The dictionary definition is 'right or appropriate for a particular purpose'. Does this mean the patient will be unsuitable if refused therapy? As the medical psychotherapy referral process may take several months, and the referrer may naturally instill hope that 'psychotherapy is what you need', for the patient then to be told that they are 'unsuitable' at the end of the assessment could exacerbate feelings of rejection, failure, or worthlessness. Terms, such as 'useful', 'helpful', or 'available', may reduce the (possibly stigmatizing) impact this evokes in patients or professionals.

The purpose of assessment is to determine whether psychotherapy is helpful for an individual, and, if so, what modality might be the most appropriate. However, there is not any guarantee that a specific therapy will work for a particular patient. Moreover, there are many different ways of conducting assessments in psychotherapy, and to recommend a generic, prescriptive assessment process would not do justice to the practice of assessment in the many different modalities of therapy available today.

Practicalities of the assessment

The practicalities of the assessment process differ between modalities and local protocols. Local departments may use their own questionnaires as part of gathering background information in the assessment process. Before the assessment, when the referrer first discusses the possibility of therapy with the patient, it is often useful for the patient to be aware of what the assessment process might entail. The referrer may wish to give leaflets or suggest credible websites (specific to different models of therapy) for the patient to explore when they leave their appointment.

Practical information about the assessment may include the following details:

- How many sessions and their duration, e.g. one to three (or more) sessions of 60–90 minutes each?
- Where will it occur, e.g. local general practice, psychotherapy department, hospital?
- When will it occur? The waiting time between referral to actual assessment is often determined locally, but it is useful to know about this, when discussing the referral options.
- Who will be invited, e.g. only the patient, or the patient with their partner/friend or extended family (e.g. if considering systemic therapy).

The assessment process

There are several factors to be taken into consideration when conducting the assessment. The overarching question throughout the assessment process is:

- Why is this particular individual presenting in this particular way at this point in time?

Whichever modality of therapy, it is helpful to consider the following, when assessing patients:

- Does the patient have the capacity to be curious? Is the patient interested enough to want to work on the problem? Does the patient think that there is a psychological connection to their difficulties, or do they think that their difficulties are due to a mismatch in their neurochemistry or because of an external factor?
- Does the patient have the capacity to be reflective? Is the patient able to consider their difficulties in the context of themselves and to take some ownership of their problems?
- Is there evidence of motivation to attend the therapy? Although this question seems obvious, therapy without the patient is a non-starter. Has the patient attended the assessment session, or do they cancel repeatedly with poor, or even no, reasons? This can often signal how sessions may unfold.

Often a helpful measure of the triad of curiosity, reflection, and motivation can be whether the patient has had previous experience of therapy and their use of it.

There are certain aspects of the assessment that are modality-specific. For example:

- *CBT*: is the patient able to identify a current problem and clear goals for therapy? Are they aware of the importance of homework tasks and able to work collaboratively with a therapist? (See ➲Cognitive behavioural therapy in Chapters 2, pp. 30–4, and in Chapter 5, pp. 172–84.)
- *Psychodynamic therapy*: is there any evidence of psychological mindedness, i.e. a capacity to understand problems in terms of their psychological nature? How does the patient respond to trial interpretations? Do they have sufficient 'ego strength' to tolerate anxiety and bear frustration? Is there recognition of an unconscious mental life or a capacity to free-associate? (See ➲Psychoanalytic psychotherapy in Chapters 2, pp. 20–30, and in Chapter 5, pp. 163–72.)
- *Family therapy*: it is important to examine the family view(s) of the problem. Do the difficulties involve the whole system, and is a shared problem recognized? (See ➲Systemic family and couple therapy in Chapters 2, pp. 34–42, and in Chapter 5, pp. 184–8.)
- *Group therapy*: the effect the patient may have on a group and the group on the patient should be considered, as well as the ability to work in a group without too much anxiety. 'Special' (i.e. complexity or diagnosis-specific) groups need an assessment tailored to that particular group. A trial assessment within the group itself could be helpful (see ➲Group therapy and group analysis in Chapters 2, pp. 42–7, and in Chapter 5, pp. 188–94).
- *IPT*: the emotional difficulties are explored in the context of the individual's role with regard to life events and relationships. Areas of significance include grief, interpersonal disputes, change of roles, and interpersonal deficits (see ➲Interpersonal psychotherapy in Chapters 2, pp. 52–5, and in Chapter 5, pp. 203–7).

Patient and therapy acceptability

Is this therapy acceptable to the patient? Is the patient acceptable for this therapy? Before answering these questions, it is important to reflect upon *who* actually wants the therapy.

Prior to the assessment, the assessor needs to take into account why the patient has been referred and by whom. There may be numerous reasons. For example:

- Is the referrer wanting the assessment because *they* feel that the therapy will be helpful for the patient?
- Is the referrer being pushed into referring the patient by the patient's carer, family, or health-care team?
- Does the referrer want to discharge the patient and hope that psychotherapy will 'take the patient off their hands'?
- Is the referrer stuck and does not know what else to consider?
- Is the patient wanting to have therapy because of certain external conditions (e.g. probation, courts, benefits etc.)?
- Does the patient want therapy because of their impression of why it might be beneficial (e.g. due to NICE guidelines recommendations or the Internet states that this is what will help them)?
- Does the patient want therapy, because they are curious and want help?

Whatever the reason for referral, a discussion prior to a formal referral between the referrer and assessor can be immensely beneficial. The referrer can liaise with their local psychotherapy department to determine whether a referral is appropriate. This links to patient acceptability, because, although self-explanatory, if the patient does not actually want the therapy, then it is clearly not going to be acceptable for them.

- *Is this therapy acceptable to this particular patient?*
  - For this question to be answered, the patient must have an understanding of this type of therapy. There needs to be a degree of psycho-education during the assessment process regarding the therapy on offer.
- *Can the patient work within this particular model?*
  - The patient needs to have had an experience of the particular modality on offer during the assessment, e.g. a trial interpretation in psychodynamic psychotherapy or defining the problem and treatment goals within CBT. If there is clear evidence that they have not responded to such modality-specific interventions, then this may be a useful indicator that these particular therapies may not be helpful for this patient.
- *If the assessor concludes that a particular type of therapy will not be helpful, what are the alternatives?*
  - The following questions may be helpful to bear in mind:
    —Will any type of therapy be appropriate and helpful for this patient at this time?
    —What other options are available? This might not always be an option due to the local availability/resources/constraints.
    —The voluntary or private sectors may offer other types of assessments sooner, but is this a viable option for this patient?

—Does the patient wish to wait for an alternative assessment for a different type of therapy, bearing in mind often lengthy waiting lists?

All of the above questions need to be considered in a sensitive manner, as the patient may have pinned all hopes onto this one assessment.

Choice

Within the sphere of evidence-based medicine, patient choice has become paramount. With the advent of the ever expanding Internet, information is widely available at the click of a button. It is far easier nowadays for a patient to ask for, or even demand, a particular type of therapy, based on what 'NICE has said . . .' Patients may also ask to see a therapist of a particular gender, ethnicity, or sexuality. However, a patient's request for a particular therapy or therapist may not always be a realistic option, based on what is available. It is important to think about the risks in this context, as well as the potential benefits, and also about the supporting structures around the patient. For example, if there is only one form of therapy available, and it is not what the patients wants, it may be counterproductive, and even unethical, to shoehorn the patient into it.

Choice should be maintained within realistic parameters. The public sector is limited in terms of the different therapies available and the length of treatment that may be offered. A patient may sometimes be given the option of seeing a private psychotherapist, if this is available and appropriate. Low-fee schemes provided by psychotherapy training organizations and charities are also an option in some areas.

What about therapist choice? There may be occasions when a therapist feels they cannot work with the patient they have assessed. In certain modalities (e.g. psychoanalytic), this can be useful material within the assessment that may be taken up within the room with the patient. In other modalities, what happens if the therapist does not feel they can 'get on with' the patient? If, after the assessment, the therapist feels that a particular modality of therapy may be useful, then this needs to be explored further. It is always helpful to discuss the patient in a referral meeting or in supervision. If still deemed appropriate and resources are available, another therapist may be able to see the patient. It is well known that the therapist–patient relationship is crucial for the success of a therapeutic intervention. Whatever the outcome, it is vital to have an open, sensitive, and honest discussion with the patient.

Consent

(See ➔Consent and psychotherapy in Chapter 9, pp. 452–4.)

Consent is necessary to help ensure that a patient's decision to have therapy is informed, voluntary, and rational. The fact that the patient has attended the assessment does not necessarily mean that he or she has consented to treatment. The patient must be able to be given enough information pertaining to that specific therapy to make an informed decision.

Consent for therapy can be viewed as being akin to a surgical or medical procedure; you would not expect to have an operation without giving consent to do so. You would want to know the efficiency, efficacy, and safety of the surgery (therapy), along with the consequences if no surgery (therapy) or alternative was undertaken.

The benefits of a consent process within psychotherapy include:
• Helping to protect the patient, e.g. to ensure an awareness of the impact of the therapy such as feeling more emotionally disturbed at times during the therapy
• Helping to protect the therapist, e.g. ensuring the patient understands that the relationship with the therapist is a professional one only
• Allowing the patient to have ownership of their treatment decisions (autonomy)
• Allowing the patient to own their therapy (responsibility)
• Giving the patient an idea of the limitations of therapy
• Helping to dispel the myths or fears around therapy (through explanation of the therapy)
• Helping to encourage the working alliance between therapist and patient
• For psychoanalytic modalities, allowing the unconscious free rein with the knowledge that external reality has been acknowledged.

As with any consent process, it is vital that the language and cultural needs of the patient are taken into consideration when delivering the information.

The consent process may be implemented in clinical practice by taking the form of a discussion during the assessment session, which is then recorded by the therapist, or may be carried out formally during a separate business or care plan meeting between therapist and patient. A therapeutic contract is sometimes drawn up. A contract has the added advantage that the patient can go through a written document with the therapist before signing and both parties can have a copy to refer to.

The contract may incorporate the following components:
• Details of the patient (name, date of birth, address)
• Name of the therapist
• Type of therapy offered
• Time and date of appointments
• Duration of each session
• Frequency of sessions
• Confidentiality and any reasons for its breach during therapy
• Where information will be held/recorded
• Any known breaks (therapist and patient)
• Procedure for cancellations or missed sessions
• Patient's support network with specific names (if possible)
• Emergency contact numbers
• A brief description of the therapeutic modality
• Information about supervision of case material
• A statement that excessive use of drugs and alcohol will not be tolerated during the sessions and terminated if the patient arrives to the session under the influence of drugs or alcohol
• Information on the type of therapeutic relationship (professional, not social or personal)

- Possible benefits of therapy (generic and perceived)
- Possible risks of therapy (generic and perceived)
- Signed and dated by the therapist and patient, with a copy for both parties.

Risk–benefit equation

(See ➲Risk assessment in Chapter 3, pp. 104–5; Beneficence and non-maleficence in psychotherapy in Chapter 9, pp. 451–2.)

Primum non nocere—first do no harm

As with all treatments in medicine, it is important to remember the risk–benefit equation. Do the benefits of therapy outweigh the risks of not having therapy at this point in time for this patient? Furthermore, it is important that some form of risk assessment on the patient is completed at the assessment. This may take the form of specific risk assessment tools, based on local trust or organizational procedures.

The list of potential risks can be endless. However, whatever modality of therapy is being offered, it is crucial to note:

- Previous/current alcohol or drug misuse
- Previous/current self-harm
- Suicidal ideation and previous suicide attempts
- History of violence to others or other forensic/offending behaviour.

For some patients, and especially in relation to certain modalities such as psychodynamic therapy, therapy may be too destabilizing at that point in time, if risk factors are in the ascendant. On the other hand, in some instances, although therapy may be temporarily destabilizing, the overall benefits may outweigh the risks in the opinion of the assessor. These decisions can be difficult to make solely by the assessor, and it is often helpful to discuss the case with the referrer or psychotherapy colleagues, or within the departmental team meeting (if available locally).

Contraindications

It is often helpful to distinguish between an indication and a contraindication. In medicine, an indication is 'a condition that suggests a specific medical treatment is necessary', whilst a contraindication is 'a condition that suggests a particular treatment is inadvisable'.

In terms of contraindications and psychotherapy, it can become very difficult to delineate between contraindications and 'unsuitability'. Contraindications to psychotherapy can be viewed similarly to those when prescribing a particular medication; we can divide them into absolute and relative. In psychotherapy, however, there may not be absolute contraindications, but there will be relative contraindications specific to that modality of therapy. In addition, a contraindication for one therapy, such as psychoanalytic psychotherapy, may not necessarily be a contraindication for another, e.g. CBT.

Ultimately, whatever list of contraindications is produced, it is unlikely to be comprehensive and universally agreed upon. It will be up to the therapist and patient as to whether a particular contraindication will mean that psychotherapy will not be helpful for the patient at that time.

The following contraindications can potentially be relevant to all types of therapy modalities:
- Acute psychosis
- Acute suicidality
- Acute mania
- Organic brain disease
- Persistent use of illicit drugs or alcohol
- A patient without motivation to attend therapy
- A patient who is unable to commit to the possibility of change.

All of the above scenarios may suggest that the patient is not available for therapy at that particular point in time, and an alternative, more appropriate treatment (possibly biological) may need to be considered.

In terms of modality-specific contraindications, the following need to be thought about:
- *Psychoanalytic or psychodynamic psychotherapy:*
  - Poor impulse control either towards self or others
  - Poor ego strength
  - Severe paranoid personality traits
  - A lack of good object relationships in childhood (based on the patient's story and how the patient is with the assessor in the room)
  - Evidence of a complete lack of willingness to take responsibility for their actions
- *Family therapy:*
  - No shared motivation for change within the family
  - The chronicity and severity of the family disturbance is so great that therapy is unlikely to be able to make an impact
  - The psychopathology of a family member is too fragile to withstand the demands of family therapy and therefore therapy may lead to further destabilization
  - Families that are in the process of breaking up
  - Families that believe that the symptoms that need to alter are a result of organic disease in one family member, as opposed to a multifactorial problem within the family system
- *CBT:*
  - Patients who are unable to access their automatic thoughts
  - Patients who are unable to ascertain that there may be a connection between their negative thoughts and emotions
  - Patients who believe that their difficulties are purely due to a biological dysfunction
  - No evidence of a desire to work collaboratively with the therapist
  - No degree of personal responsibility for their work in therapy (e.g. no willingness to do homework or exercises outside the sessions), and a view of themselves as completely passive in the therapy
- *Group therapy:*
  - A lack of ability for self-disclosure
  - Problems with intimacy leading to severe distrust
  - Patients who use the defence of denial excessively

- Patients from very large families
- Patients with severe narcissistic or ASPD (although there may be a group tailored to such individuals in specialist centres)
- Patients with severe dependency issues
- Patients in an acute crisis.

With any type of long-term therapy, one clear contraindication is if the patient is simply wanting a 'quick fix'.

Outcomes of assessment

It is useful to have a discussion with the patient at the beginning of the first assessment session to give an idea of the possible outcomes of the assessment process. The patient may assume that an assessment will automatically lead to therapy; frequently, this may not be the case. The various outcomes could include:

- To commence the particular therapy offered (and a note that the assessor may not be the treating therapist)
- Therapy is not deemed to be helpful for the patient at this point in time and discharge back to the GP
- Refer to the GP (or psychiatrist if already involved) if there is an acute problem (severe depression, psychosis, suicidal intent) that requires an alternative medical management
- Referral for an assessment for a different form of therapy.

Recommended reading

Coltart N (1988). The assessment of psychological-mindedness in the diagnostic interview. *British Journal of Psychiatry*, 153, 819–20.

Cooper J and Alifille H (1998). *Assessment in Psychotherapy*. Karnac books: London.

Crown S (1983). Contraindications and dangers in psychotherapy. *British Journal of Psychiatry*, 143, 436–41.

Lemma A (2006). *Introduction to the Practice of Psychoanalytic Psychotherapy*. Wiley: Chichester.

Mace C (1995). *The Art and Science of Assessment in Psychotherapy*. Routledge: London.

Margison F and Brown P (2007). Assessment in psychotherapies. In: Naismith J and Grant S, eds. *Seminars in the Psychotherapies*. pp. 1–27. Gaskell: London.

What type of therapy?

Different forms of therapies

Although attempts have been made, with some success, to recommend specific therapies for specific disorders, a more complex picture must be considered in real-life situations. This includes patient characteristics (personality traits, interpersonal relationships, strengths and weaknesses, co-morbidities, and preferences), family and social context, and local service availabilities.

Selecting the right type of therapy, by the right therapist, at the right time, for the right patient is important. However, there is little evidence base to guide clinicians when choosing the type of therapy offered to a patient. Moreover, some evidence suggests that selection is more important for some therapies (psychodynamic) than others (CBT). Merely matching a modality to a particular disorder is inadequate. In general, clinicians consider the following:

- *Demographic factors*, e.g. patient's age group, cultural background, and command of the language in which therapy is conducted
- *Psychological capacity and ego strengths*, e.g. a weaker ego and higher risk of acting out would favour supportive over explorative therapy
- *Response to previous therapies*
- *Patient preference*, e.g. regarding theoretical inclination, willingness to travel, willingness to wait, willingness to pay for private therapy
- *Local availability*, e.g. waiting times, possibility for being taken on as a training patient, possibility of accessing therapy via the private sector or charities
- *Constraining factors*, e.g. physical illness or disability, timing of sessions relative to other commitments such as work, childcare, etc.
- *Problem to be addressed*: although specific illnesses cannot be strictly matched with particular modalities, some therapies have been established for the treatment of certain conditions:
  - Circumscribed clinical problems, e.g. depression (IPT, CBT, behavioural activation), specific phobias (behavioural therapy), BN (IPT), BPD (MBT, DBT)
  - Difficulties affecting global psychological functioning (psychoanalytic therapy, systemic therapy)
- *Goals*: are the outcomes predetermined (IPT, CBT, BT) or not (psychoanalytic therapy)?
- *Frequency*: once weekly, less than once weekly, more than once weekly
- *Open-ended or fixed-term*
- *Timescale*:
  - Short-term—up to 20 sessions (CBT, IPT, brief dynamic therapy)
  - Long-term—more than 20 sessions (psychoanalytic psychotherapy, group therapy, TC)
- *Format*:
  - Individual
  - Group—intolerance of groups (as in extreme social phobia) and the availability of a suitable group must be taken into account
  - Family or couple therapy for relational problems
  - TC.

Specific factors may favour a particular modality

- *Long-term psychoanalytic psychotherapy* (see ➜Psychoanalytic psychotherapy in Chapter 2, pp. 163–72, and in Chapter 5, pp. 163–72):
  - Diffuse personality difficulties stemming from early developmental problems
  - Difficulty identifying a discrete conflict
  - Problems with general interpersonal functioning and forming relationships (e.g. difficulties with dependency, control, or intimacy)
- *Short-term dynamic therapy*:
  - Clear treatment goals, which can be expressed as a specific conflict
  - The patient's capacity to formulate the problem with help from the therapist
  - Recently arising problems

- Problems with conflicted triangular relationships (Oedipal, rather than, pre-Oedipal)
- Ability to tolerate frustration in therapy
- Ability to work within a predetermined time limit
- *IPT* (see ➲Interpersonal therapy in Chapter 2, pp. 52–5, and in Chapter 5, pp. 203–7):
  - A particular issue (e.g. unresolved grief or change in roles) that needs working through
  - Evidence that interpersonal difficulties are associated with depressive symptoms
- *CAT* (see ➲Cognitive analytic therapy in Chapter 2, pp. 47–52, and in Chapter 5, pp. 194–202):
  - The presence of clearly identifiable relational patterns which need addressing
  - Complex and interlinking themes
- *CBT* (see ➲Cognitive behavioural therapy in Chapter 2, pp. 30–4, and in Chapter 5, pp. 172–84):
  - Ability to identify focal problems
  - Clear treatment goals, based on the patient's thoughts and behaviours
  - The patient's capacity for active collaboration within a focused approach
  - Ability to form a trusting and collaborative relationship with the therapist
  - Chronicity and some traits, such as perfectionism, have been shown to predict poorer outcome with CBT
  - Patients with avoidant personality disorder respond better to CBT than to IPT
- *Group therapy* (see ➲Group therapy and group analysis in Chapter 2, pp. 42–7, and in Chapter 5, pp. 188–94):
  - Problems in interpersonal settings
  - Tendency to avoid responsibility for change through reliance on others
  - Ability to work with confrontation and tolerate group settings without severe anxiety
  - The patient has limited capacity to initiate exploration
- *Family and marital therapy* (see ➲Systemic family and couple therapy in Chapter 2, pp. 34–42, and in Chapter 5, pp. 184–8):
  - Difficulties involving a couple or several family members
  - A family member is scapegoated (the identified patient)
  - Family members (or a couple) recognize a shared problem and wish to work collaboratively
  - Enmeshed family relationships
- *TCs* (see ➲Therapeutic communities in Chapter 2, pp. 75–80, and in Chapter 5, pp. 243–50):
  - A risk of extreme regression in a patient who would be generally suitable for psychodynamic therapy
  - The need for structured and stable boundaries
  - Severe and disabling problems
  - Living in the community is practicable.

Short-term versus long-term

There is no unanimous view regarding the cut-off point between a short-term and long-term therapy, but most would agree that a therapy longer than 25–30 sessions would be seen as long-term. Whilst 'short-term' or 'long-term' refers to the length of time over which therapy will be delivered, 'open-ended' and 'time-limited' signifies whether the number of sessions has been preset at the beginning of the therapy.

Short-term therapy is likely to have a predetermined number of sessions (e.g. CAT, IPT) which will be agreed at the start of therapy. However, the number of sessions can remain under ongoing review, dependent on progress (e.g. CBT).

Long-term therapy can be either open-ended (e.g. psychoanalytic psychotherapy) or time-limited (e.g. DBT typically lasts 1 year, and psychodynamic psychotherapy will involve between 30 and 40 sessions).

There is no definite agreement regarding the superiority of long-term over short-term therapies or on whether effectiveness is determined by length or modality. However, some evidence suggests that, whilst short-term dynamic and cognitive behavioural therapies are effective for acute and circumscribed problems, long-term dynamic psychotherapy is superior to less intensive forms of psychotherapy in complex mental disorders. Preliminary data suggest greater stability of positive outcomes with long-term therapies. Thus, therapy length should be matched to the individual patient (see ➲Outcome research in psychotherapy in Chapter 11, pp. 518–19).

A few questions should be borne in mind:
- *Can the problem be seen in focal terms?* If so, is a brief therapy feasible? Circumscribed problems can be addressed with short-term therapies (CAT, IPT, CBT) or medium-term therapies (brief dynamic therapy), but diffuse issues, such as personality disorders and difficulties, are more suitable for longer-term therapy (psychoanalytic, schema therapy, systemic, DBT, TC).
- *What can the patient tolerate?* There is marked variability amongst patients' abilities to tolerate different frameworks and settings. Whilst long and open-ended therapies may appear uncontained and stir up anxiety in some patients, time limits may evoke feelings of pressure in others.
- *What is available locally?*

Limitations in availability

It is widely known that psychotherapy is a limited resource, and waiting lists may be very long.

Availability is likely to be determined by:
- *Modality*: some modalities are more available (e.g. CBT)
- *Length*: short-term therapies are more available than longer-term ones
- *Therapist qualification*: a patient's readiness to see a trainee therapist will shorten the waiting time. This is especially true in training centres where training therapists are seeking training patients
- *Locality*: it is likely that therapist availability will be greater in larger urban centres, especially with developed training programmes, and scarcer in rural settings, although there are exceptions
- *Funding*: patients able to self-fund therapy, as opposed to being financed by public funds, are likely to have greater access and choice.

Thus, to maximize local availability, in addition to referrals for public-funded therapy (the NHS in the UK), it is important to think outside the box in considering:

• Private insurance schemes
• Private therapists will sometimes have fees on a sliding scale, dependent on patients' income
• Private psychotherapy training organizations usually offer reduced fee schemes
• Charities: national (e.g. MIND, Rethink, Cruse in the UK) or local. These organizations either provide therapy free of charge or have a sliding scheme according to patients' ability to pay. Some have a particular field of work (e.g. eating disorders, victims of sexual abuse).

In addition to referencing national registers of psychotherapists and listings of professional organizations, it can be useful developing a catalogue of local resources and distributing it to possible referrers in an area.

Patient preference

(See ➲ Common factor research in Chapter 11, pp. 519–22).

Patient preferences are determined by an interplay of numerous personal, cultural, and practical issues. There are three recognized components of preference:

• *Role preferences*, e.g. active and advice-giving therapist v. a listening role, being a member of a group v. an individual
• *Therapist preferences*, e.g. years of clinical experience, similar ethnic background, therapist's gender
• *Treatment preferences*: the type of intervention to be used, e.g. CBT v. psychodynamic.

Patients matched to their preferred therapy conditions are less likely to drop out of therapy prematurely and show greater improvements in treatment outcomes, although it is more important to consider patient preferences when treating anxiety, depression, or substance abuse, compared to serious mental illness.

Previous experience of therapies can contribute to specific preferences. However, this may be complicated by misconceptions based upon the portrayal of various therapies in the media and popular culture.

Superior treatment outcomes are noted when treatment is culturally adapted in terms of:

• *Language, race, and ethnicity*: clients may prefer therapists matched to their race, ethnicity, and native language, but equally may have no preference or prefer a therapist who is relatively different from them in these terms
• *Metaphors and cultural concepts*: metaphors, proverbs, and culture-specific references are useful for conveying meaning
• *Cultural content*, e.g. some cultures place more value on collective aspects of mental life, and individuation may not be a predominant desired outcome.

In patients for whom spiritual outcomes are highly valued, psychotherapy accommodating religious and spiritual components can be considered a treatment of choice.

Some commonly encountered practical issues are:
- *Timescale and frequency*: beside any anxieties that the duration and intensity might stir up in an individual, there are also practical considerations regarding how much time the patient is able and willing to set aside for therapy
- *Timing of sessions* in the context of other commitments—work, childcare, etc. The working population will struggle to attend more than one session per week within office hours
- *Distance to therapy sessions* and willingness to travel
- *Physical illness or disability*, including availability of appropriate accessible consultation rooms.

Recommended reading

Coleman HLK, Wampold BE, and Casali SL (1995). Ethnic minorities' ratings of ethnically similar and European American counselors: a meta-analysis. *Journal of Counseling Psychology*, **42**, 55–64.

Margison F and Brown P (2007). Assessment in psychotherapies. In: Naismith J and Grant S, eds. *Seminars in the Psychotherapies*. pp. 1–27. Gaskell: London.

Smith TB, Rodríguez MD, and Bernal G (2011). Culture. *Journal of Clinical Psychology*, **67**, 165–75.

Swift JK, Callahan JL, and Vollmer BM (2011). Preferences. *Journal of Clinical Psychology*, **67**, 155–65.

Watzke B, Rüddel H, Jürgensen R, *et al.* (2010). Effectiveness of systematic treatment selection for psychodynamic and cognitive-behavioural therapy: randomised controlled trial in routine mental healthcare. *British Journal of Psychiatry*, **197**, 96–105.

Worthington EL, Hook JN, Davis DE, and McDaniel MA (2011). Religion and spirituality. *Journal of Clinical Psychology*, **67**, 204–14.

Formulation

Formulation is recognized as a core competency for all psychiatrists. However, there is wide variation in how it is understood and constructed, depending on the underlying theoretical model used to inform it. A formulation is a process, or the end result of a process, that seeks to explain how a situation is developed, maintained, or resolved. A key feature of a formulation is that it is explanatory, rather than solely descriptive—in this way, it differs from a diagnosis.

Formulations vary in their degree of focus, explicitness, comprehensiveness, process, and degree of sharing. All formulations are hypotheses that are provisional and open to revision, especially in the light of new information. Moreover, there may be several ways in which to elucidate and organize the information available—no one way of understanding or theoretical model is definitive.

Using formulations in clinical practice may have several benefits, including bridging different models of understanding (e.g. biological, psychological, and social), providing a language and framework for dialogue, strengthening team working and therapeutic relationships with patients, encouraging awareness of areas of uncertainty, improving assessments, and guiding interventions.

There are many different models which include theorizing about how causal factors are linked and which may be used to inform the process of formulation. The most widely used explanatory models include those based on biopsychosocial, attachment, psychodynamic and psychoanalytic, systemic, cognitive behavioural, cognitive analytic, narrative, and dialogical theories, respectively. Other more 'atheoretical' models, such as the '3 Ps', may be helpful for organizing information but do not necessarily include a coherent explanatory narrative to link the different factors.

Biopsychosocial model

The biopsychosocial model groups aspects of a patient's difficulty into three categories: biological, psychological, and social. This can help understand the nature of the difficulty. Robert Money Kyrle's three 'facts of life' can be linked with these categories.

- *Biological factors*:
  - *Examples*: genetic predisposition, brain injury, drug use
  - *Fact of life*: we will all eventually die
  - Like death, biological factors are relatively fixed and unchangeable. How does the patient respond to factors over which they have little control such as a chronic physical illness or a disability?
- *Psychological factors*:
  - *Examples*: trauma, loss, impulsivity
  - *Fact of life*: we have no part in our own creation
  - We are separate to our parents, which opens up the possibility of psychological freedom and independence, but also aloneness and exclusion. How does the patient respond to evidence of their separateness?
- *Social factors*:
  - *Examples*: life events, socio-economic status, culture
  - *Fact of life*: we are born utterly dependent on our parents.
  - We remain dependent on, and inter-dependent with, others. How does the patient relate to those upon whom they depend (e.g. family or the state) and to those who depend upon them (such as their children)?

Fig. 4.1 shows the relationship between the biological, psychological, and social factors, and relates these to Money Kyrle's facts of life.

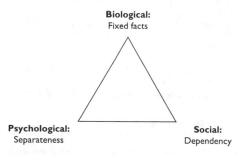

Biological:
Fixed facts

Psychological:
Separateness

Social:
Dependency

Fig. 4.1 One relationship between biological, psychological, and social factors (in bold) and Money Kyrle's facts of life.

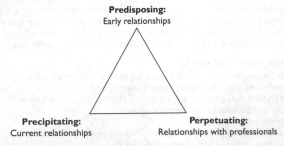

Fig. 4.2 One relationship between predisposing, precipitating, and perpetuating factors (in bold) and object relations.

3 Ps in formulation

The '3 Ps' (predisposing, precipitating, and perpetuating) can be one way of attempting to find a temporal order to factors relating to a patient's difficulty. They can also focus attention on how the patient relates to others, i.e. their object relations.

- Predisposing:
  - Which factors *in the past* predispose to this problem, e.g. previous illness, childhood neglect?
  - What *early relationships* with caregivers are described which may predispose to the problem?
  - How does the patient describe their early relationship with their parents? What is their first memory? What was growing up like?
- Precipitating:
  - Which factors *in the present* (or more recent past) may have precipitated the problem, e.g. bereavements, life events?
  - What *current relationships* are there in the patient's life, which may have precipitated the problem?
  - How does the patient describe their current relationships with significant others? Why did the patient seek help?
- Perpetuating:
  - Which factors *in the future* may perpetuate the problem, e.g. chaotic lifestyle, poor coping mechanisms?
  - What is the *relationship with professionals* (e.g. the transference) which may perpetuate the problem?
  - How does the patient relate to the professional? Are they able to seek and use any help that is offered?

Fig. 4.2 shows the relationship between the '3 Ps' and relates these to object relations.

Recommended reading

Johnstone L and Dallos R (2014). *Formulation in Psychology and Psychotherapy: Making Sense of People's Problems*. Routledge: Hove.

Money-Kyrle R (1971). The aim of psycho-analysis. *International Journal of Psychoanalysis*, 52, 103–6.

The British Psychological Society, Division of Clinical Psychology (2011). *Good Practice Guidelines on the Use of Psychological Formulation*. The British Psychological Society: Leicester.

Psychodynamic assessment and formulation

(See ➔Psychoanalytic psychotherapy in Chapter 2, pp. 20–30, and in Chapter 5, pp. 163–72.)

Assessment for psychodynamic psychotherapy is a skilled and mul-tilayered process comprising several functions, including the provision of a diagnosis; formulation of the patient's difficulties in psychodynamic terms; consideration of the patient's suitability and motivation for psy-chotherapy; assessment of risk, e.g. of depression, self-harm, or sub-stance misuse; and providing an opportunity for the patient to have an initial experience of the psychodynamic approach, so that he can make an informed decision about whether this type of treatment is suitable. Psychodynamic assessment puts most emphasis on the direct encounter with the patient, rather than other forms of assessment tools such as personality inventories or cognitive tests. The experience of both patient and assessor within the clinical interviews with the patient, particularly the nature of the relationship that emerges between patient and asses-sor, can yield the most meaningful information regarding the unconscious processes and interpersonal functioning of the patient.

The assessment process may be subdivided into the following stages:
• Initial referral
• Conducting the assessment
• Psychodynamic formulation
• Outcome.

Initial referral

The ways in which the patient is referred may reveal useful information about their motivation and predict subsequent engagement in therapy. Patients may be referred for psychotherapy by their GP or other mental health professionals, or are 'sent' by concerned spouses or relatives to address problematic behaviours (e.g. drinking, gambling), whereas the patient himself has little inclination to change. Even seemingly motivated patients who are actively seeking therapeutic help may have little idea of the different modalities of psychotherapy and how engaging in psycho-dynamic therapy may involve periods during which they will feel more disturbed, as defences are challenged and underlying anxieties explored. Some psychodynamic psychotherapy services request that the patient complete a written questionnaire in advance of the clinical interview, which asks details about the patient's presenting problems and personal and family history. Whilst this may enable the assessor to focus on the emotional experiences of the patient in the clinical interviews and trans-ference/countertransference dynamics, rather than historical informa-tion gathering from the patient, this may prove to be an obstacle for patients with difficulties in literacy.

Conducting the assessment

The assessment interview may be the first exposure the patient has to a psychoanalytic way of thinking, which, for some, may be a strange, or even threatening, experience. The manner in which the therapist conducts the first meetings with the patient is critical for future engagement in therapy.

The clinical interviews form the mainstay of the assessment process and provide an opportunity for the assessor to both collect the necessary information about the patient to make an informed decision about his suitability for psychodynamic psychotherapy, as well as create an experience for the patient that will give him some idea of the nature of the psychodynamic process. The assessor therefore alternates between the subjective and the objective—on the one hand, empathically eliciting the patient's difficulties by creating an atmosphere conducive to the emergence of unconscious material, and, on the other hand, objectively gathering sufficient factual information.

Ideally, the assessment should involve more than one meeting to allow sufficient space and freedom to address the various factors that should be examined during the assessment process and allow time for the careful introduction of different technical stances and observation of the patient's responses. An extended assessment allows time to consider the following aspects and questions about the patient:

• Appraisal of the patient's ego strength, defences, and modes of relating.
• Motivation for therapy: does the patient attend all the sessions offered? Is he on time?
• What does the patient make of the meetings? Is he capable of reflection between sessions and able to tolerate the anxiety associated with the open-ended process of psychotherapy?
• Can he tolerate exploration of the meaning of difficulties and 'not-knowing', or does he demand immediate solutions, advice, or symptom cure?
• How does he respond to silences?
• How does he relate to the assessor? Is he capable of forming a good rapport or working alliance?
• What is the patient's response to *trial interpretations*? These are interventions based upon a tentative psychodynamic hypothesis that is offered to the patient to see if he can think about himself in a different way.
• Does he have the capacity to respond affectively within the assessment sessions, e.g. allowing the expression of feelings of anxiety, sadness, or anger?

It is useful for the initial meeting to take the form of an unstructured interview to observe the patient's ability to free associate, and to assess the presence and quality of emotional contact within the session and the degree of access to his internal world. The assessor will listen very attentively to how the patient tells his story, his tone, pace, and affect in describing events and relationships, noting significant omissions and being attuned to the unconscious themes that emerge. This will also include carefully observing the relationship that the patient develops with the assessor which may represent the beginning of a transference, as well as the assessor's emotional reactions or countertransference, although the therapist may be tentative in interpreting these at this early stage. Some patients may find the unstructured nature of the interview anxiety-provoking or persecutory, and the assessor may need to intervene sooner than with a person whose ability to tolerate anxiety is greater. Patients with a limited capacity for reflection, or who have constructed lifelong defensive strategies to avoid thinking and feeling, may experience being invited to talk about their difficulties as threatening or associated with shame and stigma.

In subsequent interviews, the assessor can focus on more active history taking and obtaining essential information about the patient. This should include:

- Current difficulties, and why they have sought treatment at this particular point in time
- Family history, details of the patient's family, and relationships with key family members
- Developmental history, including history of major traumas, losses, separations from parents, and history of abuse
- Education and employment history
- Psychosexual development and relationships
- Dream life
- Interests and hobbies
- Current sources of both stress and support
- General health
- Past psychiatric history, including risk of self-harm, previous psychiatric or psychological treatment, alcohol or substance misuse, and any psychiatric diagnosis such as depression, psychosis, or personality disorder that the patient has received
- Forensic or offending history.

Psychodynamic formulation

The formulation brings together the information gathered in the assessment to generate a hypothesis that will inform the choice and goals of treatment. A psychodynamic formulation is based on an underlying theoretical framework which emphasizes the importance of:

- *Unconscious processes*
- *Intrapsychic and interpersonal mechanisms*, including internal conflicts, object relationships, and transference and countertransference
- *A developmental approach*, in which links and patterns are identified between past and present, and how significant events and relationships in the person's history have influenced their psychosocial and emotional development and current functioning.

Structuring the psychodynamic formulation

A variety of frameworks may be used to structure the formulation. As with any formulation, a psychodynamic formulation should be descriptive, explanatory, and predictive, and will include:

- *Description* or summary of the patient's background
- *Explanatory hypothesis* generated by systemic inferences about the dynamics of the clinical situation, focussing on the nature and timing of key developments in the person's history that have contributed to the current clinical picture

- *Prediction* about the person's prognosis or what is likely to happen in the future, based on the identification of recurring patterns of behaviour and relationships.

A psychodynamic formulation may follow the 3 Ps model in elucidating the main difficulties for the patient and their predisposing, precipitating, and perpetuating or maintaining factors, both external and internal.

However, a more specifically psychodynamic framework is to identify repeating themes or patterns in the patient's relationships. These occur because a person will bring to any relationship specific needs, expectations, and reactions based on earlier experiences, so that parallels will be seen in how the person reacts in different situations and relationships, past and present, including that with the assessor. The identification of recurring patterns of the patient's self-experience, behaviour and relationships with others may then be used to make inferences regarding the person's psychodynamic functioning, much of which may be unconscious, including their core conflicts; internal object relationships, including their experience of self and others, and capacity for attachment; and their psychological defence mechanisms, including ways of managing stressful situations and underlying threatening emotions and impulses.

The psychodynamic formulation may therefore usefully be seen in terms of a tripartite structure, bringing together common themes emerging from the three main areas covered in the assessment:
- The patient's current difficulties
- The patient's history of infantile or childhood conflicts or deficits
- The experience that emerges in the assessment, especially the transferential relationship with the assessor.

Mace has outlined the different levels involved in a phased method for structuring a psychodynamic formulation:
- *Recognizing the psychological dimension*: the patient is seen not solely as a diagnostic entity or someone whose difficulties are biologically determined, but as a person whose problems may be understood in relation to the psychological influence of previous experiences and characteristic patterns of reacting and relating.
- *Constructing an illness narrative*: significant events and experiences are identified in the patient's account of his history and links made between past and present.
- *Modelling a formulation*: here a more structured and dynamic understanding of how different pathogenic factors operate and interrelate with each other is formulated, which allows simple predictive hypotheses to be made about how patients are likely to react in future, including their relationships with professionals.
- *Naming the elements*: this stage leads to a theoretically sophisticated formulation of identified dynamics. The focus will depend on which specific theoretical orientation is used but is likely to incorporate specific dynamic understandings in terms of defence mechanisms, characteristic object relations, and attachment style.

Martindale and Summers emphasize three features of the psychodynamic approach that mitigate against subjective biases which may interfere in the process of formulation through the influence of theoretical orientation, social and cultural context, and transference and countertransference pressures:

- *A tentative attitude*, in which formulations are not seen as knowledge, but as hypotheses which may be reviewed and revised in the light of new information. This should include the capacity to tolerate ambivalence and not knowing, and awareness of one's own biases and selective interpretation of the facts.
- *A space for reflection*, in which there is protected and valued time to think about the case with the team, supervision group, or other involved professionals, that is free from practical and emotional demands. This should be supported by the management and leadership of the organization.
- *Different perspectives*. Different professionals involved may have different experiences of the same patient. Whilst this is often conceptualized as reflecting the patient projecting different aspects of themselves into different people or situations (splitting), it may also be the result of unrecognized countertransference responses in the clinicians that may distort the formulation. Discussion with others in supervision or team group discussions and considering the range of different perspectives of everyone involved can be helpful in clarifying countertransference patterns. It is also important to consider the patient's perspective of his difficulties and experience of care, and understand the reasons why this may differ from the views of others involved.

Clinical uses of psychodynamic formulation

A psychodynamic formulation has several uses in clinical practice. Its use is not confined to the psychotherapist but may help all psychiatrists and other professionals involved in clinical work in understanding what their patients are thinking and feeling, and understanding why. Exploring the patient's subjective experience is associated with strengthening the therapeutic alliance, increasing medication compliance and positive treatment outcomes. Formulation may be used to predict how patients will respond to therapy and guide future treatment and management. Psychodynamic principles may be used in formulation in everyday practice and complement other frameworks, including the biological, to deepen understanding and enhance the management of a variety of clinical situations occurring at different levels, from those concerned with the individual patient to those involving complex institutional dynamics.

Uses of psychodynamic formulation include:

- To understand and predict how a particular patient responds to being ill
- To understand and predict the patient's likely responses to treatment
- To summarize psychodynamic factors contributing to current difficulties
- To understand the interpersonal relationships that are central to the patient's recovery
- To provide a psychodynamic risk formulation

- To provide a map of treatment to guide the treating psychotherapist and supervisor
- To draw up recommendations for further treatment
- To evaluate the effectiveness of any subsequent psychotherapy
- To enhance the understanding of staff countertransference responses and reduce unhelpful responses and acting out
- To enhance the understanding of team or institutional dynamics
- To enhance other models of understanding, e.g. psychodynamic formulation in psychosis can complement a biological framework.

Outcome of assessment

The final stage of the assessment process is the outcome—first, reaching a decision regarding the patient's suitability and willingness to engage in psychodynamic psychotherapy; second, a carefully considered sharing of some of the details of the formulation with the patient, based on what seems most appropriate and helpful for him to hear at this stage; and third, a consideration of the treatment options available. This should involve a collaborative discussion with the patient about the availability and practicalities of treatment, including the setting, times and frequency of sessions, breaks in therapy, and the expected length of treatment, particularly if it is time-limited, as in the case of most NHS settings. Whilst psychodynamic psychotherapists do not usually set explicit goals or get the patient to sign contracts or treatment plans, it is good practice to gain the patient's informed consent by giving him sufficient explanation and opportunity to ask questions regarding the general nature of the therapy offered, as well as informing him about other psychological treatment modalities such as CBT. There should also be some discussion of the possible risks of therapy, such as feeling more depressed or anxious, or an increased risk of pathological behaviours such as self-harm, substance misuse, or becoming involved in risky relationships, which the patient may employ as maladaptive solutions to deal with disturbing feelings. If it is thought that there is a significant risk to self or others, other professionals may need to be actively involved in the patient's care such as their GP or general adult psychiatrist, particularly during breaks in treatment.

Vignette of psychodynamic assessment and formulation

Initial referral

Lucas was a 22-year-old man with chronic renal failure, referred for an assessment for psychodynamic psychotherapy by a liaison psychiatrist Dr X, who had been seeing him for the treatment of depressive symptoms related to his physical illness and difficult relationships with his family. In her referral letter, she noted that he presented as superior and cynical and experienced her as useless, often cancelling their appointments, only to ring in a state of semi-panic asking to see her urgently.

Assessment

The assessor, an experienced female consultant medical psychotherapist, saw him on three occasions as part of an extended assessment. He presented as a tall, good-looking young man, who was clearly intelligent and seemed keen to impress this on her from the start. In the first meeting, the assessor introduced herself, saying she knew a little bit about him from Dr X, but invited him to tell her about himself and why he thought he had been referred. Lucas said he had a rare renal condition diagnosed a few years ago, had recently been diagnosed with end-stage renal failure, and was awaiting a renal transplant, which would probably be from his mother. He complained bitterly about the doctors treating him, who had missed the diagnosis of renal failure until it was too late. However, it later emerged that he had put up with symptoms of lassitude and fatigue for a long time before seeking medical attention, and had missed several of his routine check-up appointments. He was now on renal dialysis, which made him feel terrible and at times suicidal. This was all related in a mechanical affectless way, as if he were a dialysis machine.

The therapist commented that he sounded quite depressed. Lucas looked annoyed and snapped, 'Yes, of course I am—that's why I've been referred! Didn't you read my notes?' He immediately went on to complain about his parents and how he had being unable to distance himself from his family, particularly his mother. He was just beginning to feel independent, having left home to go to university, when he became ill, and it was as if he had become a baby again, and she had to look after him. In the year before the referral, he felt that the only way he could survive was to break off contact with them altogether. He moved into a hall of residence and tried not to contact them, but this was impossible. However, when he saw them, he would get into horrible arguments with them, which made him feel guilty, but then felt angry about 'being made to feel guilty'.

At some point, he spotted a file on the assessor's desk and said, 'You have probably read my notes from Dr X and the other doctors. I'm sure they have said how difficult I am.' The therapist said that perhaps he was worried about what she would think of him and whether she could offer therapy that might be helpful. At this point, he became more animated and told her that all psychiatrists want to do is to prescribe antidepressants, but he refused to take them. He started to talk about his younger brother, whose behaviour and mental state had deteriorated recently, becoming paranoid, violent, uncooperative, and hallucinating. He said that their GP was useless, as he had failed to treat him in time, and his brother had ended up having to be sectioned. He was diagnosed with schizophrenia and 'incarcerated in a loony bin and drugged up to the eyeballs'. He was now living at home but was still psychotic. At this point, Lucas started asking the therapist her advice about what psychiatric care his brother could get. She said that she thought his anguish and concern about his brother reflected his own fears about what would happen to him and who would look after him, and drew a parallel with how his brother was now dependent on his parents and his fears that he would be as well. Lucas laughed somewhat menacingly and said that he would rather be dead than be in his brother's situation.

During this meeting, the therapist felt she had to tread carefully in how she worded her interventions, feeling rather sad and somewhat protective towards this vulnerable young man, yet at the same time found him somewhat intrusive and controlling in his interactions with her. At the end of this meeting, Lucas appeared to find it difficult to leave, asking questions about the therapist's experience and qualifications, which resulted in her being unable to end at the appointed time.

After this first appointment, Lucas phoned to cancel the next and requested another, which the therapist sent to him, but to which he failed to turn up. She wrote to him, asking if he wanted another, and immediately received a phone call saying that he did. When she saw him on this second occasion, he apologized for the missed sessions but then admitted that, when he had received her second appointment, he had already arranged to go for a long weekend away with his girlfriend and remembered thinking, 'Why should I arrange my life to suit her appointments?'

During the second assessment interview, the therapist took a more active stance in asking him more details of his history. He remembered an unpleasant atmosphere growing up, with constant arguments between his parents and his father being physically abusive towards him and his brother. He enjoyed primary school, but, when he became ill, he was bullied at school for being 'sickly', of which his parents were apparently unaware.

He did not do as well as he wanted in his final exams, due to his unhappiness at school, but persuaded his parents to send him to London to study where they had relatives with whom he could live. For the first year of university, he studied very hard and did well, but, in the second year, he was diagnosed with renal failure and failed his exams, and had to take a year off. He was now in his final year.

He had had one serious relationship with a female student on his course. He felt very attracted to her, but he was also worried that she was the more masculine one in the relationship and 'wore the trousers'.

There was another delay of a few weeks between the second and third assessment, Lucas cancelling again, saying that he had exams, and the therapist not being able to offer him an appointment shortly afterwards because of her summer holiday. In the third assessment interview, he appeared somewhat calmer and more available, reporting that no arguments had occurred between him and his family since he had last seen the therapist. He had passed his exams, about which he was pleased. However, he felt tormented by his girlfriend, who had broken up with him in a painful way. He said he was therefore talking to his mother several times a day, which he regretted, but there was no one else to talk to. However, he also wondered whether he could just do it all himself. The therapist linked his difficulties in separating from his girlfriend with his difficulties in separating from his parents, and also his experience of the help he had received from doctors, in that, on the one hand, he felt he desperately wanted it, but, when it was offered, he felt it was not good enough. She said that perhaps he felt a bit the same here, in that she was not able to see him as soon as he wanted after his exams. This time, Lucas did not get annoyed and appeared to accept the interpretation.

He then mentioned a distressing experience he had had with a nurse. The nurses were 'lovely but pretty stupid' and did not know anything about the science of haemodialysis, unlike him who had done a lot of

Internet research. He said that, with his own particular type of renal failure, he did not need much fluid removed. On this occasion, the nurse told him she was going to remove 1.5 litres of fluid. Lucas objected, saying it was not appropriate for him, and asked to see a doctor, but the nurse refused to call for one. He then said he was going to have to ask her to stop the dialysis, as he knew what she was doing was dangerous. Again she refused. He described feeling completely trapped and terrified, connected to machines with needles stuck in him.

Formulation

In her formulation, the therapist noted his personal and family history, and that Lucas was a young man presenting with depression and an antagonistic and conflictual relationship with his parents (*initial description of his problems*). Although there are possible biological factors contributing to his mental state (e.g. the first-degree family history of schizophrenia), the key factors may be understood in relation to the psychological influence of previous experiences, particularly his early relationships (*recognizing the psychological dimension*). She identified a prominent common pattern or *core conflict* in his object relationships, centred on anxieties around dependence and separation, which appeared to repeat itself in Lucas's relationships with others. This was evident in the three key sources of information in the assessment:

1. Lucas's account of his childhood experiences of being physically abused by his father and bullied at school, experiences over which he felt he had little control, and that people who should have been able to protect him—notably his mother and teachers—were unavailable (*this can be seen as identifying predisposing factors, as well as constructing an illness narrative*).

2. His current problems in him becoming physically ill and regressing to a more infantile state, in which he is again dependent on his parents and parental figures, including the doctors treating him (*precipitating factors*), but fights against this, in his wish to be independent. His description of his psychotic brother who could be forced to have medication depicted his own terrifying fears of a body out of control and at the mercy of others.

3. The transference–countertransference dynamics that emerged in the assessment: Lucas appeared to experience some of the therapist's comments in the assessment meetings as intrusive and persecutory, whilst the therapist's countertransference experience was similar in feeling intruded upon and controlled. This can be conceptualized as Lucas unconsciously manipulating the interaction with the therapist, so that his conflict is located in her via *projective identification*.

Perpetuating factors in maintaining Lucas's conflicts were not only his ongoing physical ill health, but also a vicious circle of arguments with parents and carers in which his aggression served to, on the one hand, distance himself from his fears of dependence, but, on the other hand, left him with a sense of guilt, which was quickly defended against by further anger and self-assertion which fuelled the conflict.

Lucas had some conscious awareness of this conflict in his expressed fears of dependence on his parents, but deeper understanding of his object relationships and their genesis, particularly in relation to women and his precarious sense of masculinity, remained less accessible to him. The therapist noted how the dynamic that was evident in the (female) referrer's description of him, on the one hand as being very dismissive of her efforts and on the other ringing her frantically for urgent appointments, was repeated in her experience of him cancelling and demanding appointments during this assessment. She also noted his anxieties about his girlfriend being the dominant one in their relationship. Lucas's vivid description of his experience with the nurse reveals some of his unconscious anxieties and fantasies of being overwhelmed and trapped by a female object, who professes to be caring but is experienced as dangerously intrusive, overwhelming, and obliterating of him, and from whom he needs to defend himself at all cost. The possibility that he might actually receive a piece of his mother's body in her donated kidney could only exacerbate his unconscious terror that he could never separate from her.

These links allowed the therapist to *model a formulation*, in which she predicted that the dynamics that she had observed in his object relations would most likely be repeated in the patient's relationship with the therapist, if he were offered therapy, and that resistances in the form of cancelled sessions, a demanding and dismissive attitude towards the therapist, and reactions to breaks were to be anticipated. However, there was also some evidence in the assessment that Lucas could reflect and make links in his more accepting response to the therapist's *trial transference interpretations* in the final meeting, which he did not reject but led instead to the association to the nurse.

In *naming the elements of the formulation*, the therapist hypothesized that Lucas's attachment style would be characterized as insecure avoidant. He used primitive defence mechanisms, such as omnipotence, denigration, projection, and projective identification, to defend a vulnerable self-identity against anxieties stemming from a core unconscious conflict centering on the fantasy of a powerful and dangerous maternal object, for which he desperately longed and yet by which he was terrified of being overwhelmed and controlled. These unconscious dynamics underpinned all his relationships in which he was unable to achieve any sense of security or genuine intimacy.

Outcome

The therapist thought that, despite the likely challenges, Lucas could benefit from a year of psychodynamic therapy, in which some of these anxieties might become more consciously available to be explored, if a stable and containing therapeutic relationship could be established. She did not share all of her formulation with Lucas but said that it was likely that he would find the therapy difficult at times and that he might feel more depressed and despondent. For this reason, she thought it was a good idea for both the liaison psychiatrist and GP to remain involved to monitor his mental state and review the need for antidepressant medication, as well as offer an overall containing therapeutic structure in which 'parental figures' could work constructively in Lucas's best interests.

Recommended reading

Cooper J and Alfille H (eds) (1998). *Assessment in Psychotherapy*. Karnac Books: London.

Garelick A (1994). Psychotherapy assessment: theory and practice. *Psychoanalytic Psychotherapy* **8**, 101–16.

Mace C and Binyon S (2005). Teaching psychodynamic formulation to psychiatric trainees: Part 1: basics of formulation. *Advances in Psychiatric Treatment* **11**, 416–23.

Summers A and Martindale B (2013). Using psychodynamic principles in formulation in everyday practice. *Advances in Psychiatric Treatment* **19**, 203–11.

Cognitive behavioural assessment and formulation

(See ➔ Cognitive behavioural therapy in Chapter 2, pp. 30–4, and in Chapter 5, pp. 172–81.)

Assessment: general criteria

Before offering any therapy, the key question is whether the potential patient is likely to benefit or not, and this must be determined at assessment. This is necessary, because:

- We need to prioritize the use of scarce resources
- The process of helping someone define their problem and explore appropriate treatment options is itself therapeutic
- It is unethical to offer treatment where success is unlikely, as this can lead to demoralization of both client and therapist
- Because CBT does not work for all.

Safran and Segal developed a *suitability scale* which defined nine criteria to determine suitability for cognitive therapy, which were:

1. *Accessibility of automatic thoughts*: is the patient able to recognize their negative automatic thoughts?
2. *Awareness and differentiation of emotion*: are they able to recognize and distinguish between different emotions?
3. *Acceptance of personal responsibility for change*: do they recognize the part they have to play in addressing the problem?
4. *Compatibility (of problem) with cognitive rationale*: can we make sense of the problem using the CBT model?
5. *Alliance potential—in-session evidence*: will you be able to work together?
6. *Alliance potential—out-of-session evidence*: will they put the necessary work in between sessions?
7. *Chronicity of problems*: the less chronic, the better!
8. *Security operations*: in what behaviours do they engage which keep the problem going, and are they prepared to address these?
9. *Focality*: is there a focus for the therapy, rather than a vague global issue?

In practice, assessment involves the juggling of several criteria and questions, which are essentially:

- Does the patient have a problem on which they want to work, and are they able to define this?
- Is this a problem for which CBT is indicated, or would a different approach have a greater evidence base or be more useful?

- Is it possible to begin to formulate this problem in a CBT way?
- What is the patient looking for in a therapy?
- What do they make of the CBT model?
- Do they want to work in a practical, structured, here-and-now way?
- Are they prepared to do homework and monitor their problems or carry out behavioural experiments?
- Are they looking for a more exploratory approach?

Patients with more straightforward problems may be able to score highly on the Safran and Segal scale, which indicates that they are likely to do well. However, with more complex patients, poorer scoring is the norm, or, at a one-off assessment, it is not possible to accurately score some of these criteria so, whilst this scale can be a guide, these latter questions may be more useful in determining whether to offer a course of therapy or a trial of therapy, e.g. six sessions, or to decline offering this type of therapy at all.

Assessment of information needed
- Getting an understanding of the problem the patient is experiencing
- Finding out what they want from therapy, i.e. initial goals
- Getting enough information about the problem to begin to formulate it, in terms of thoughts, feelings, behaviours, and physiology
- What triggers it?
- Who triggers it?
- Where does it happen?
- What helps?
- What makes it worse?
- History of the problem
- Any current treatment?
- Any previous treatment?
- Response to treatment/previous therapy?
- Previous psychiatric history
- Family, personal, and social history
- Drug and alcohol history
- Risk assessment
- A personalized discussion about how the CBT model might help address this problem and what therapy might involve
- Alternatives to CBT.

Formulation
Formulation is an umbrella term used to describe a way of understanding someone's difficulties and organizing information about them. In CBT, when we discuss formulation, we are talking about understanding someone's difficulties with reference to the CBT model, and, as such, it is a link between known CBT theory and the individual's particular presentation. It is central to CBT practice, and without one therapy cannot proceed. It helps us understand how someone's difficulties have developed and what is maintaining them, suggesting ways to intervene to turn the problem around. It is always constructed together with the client and is dynamic and tentative, something that can be added to or changed where new information emerges. In CBT, the formulation is usually diagrammatic,

and the development of this diagram can be likened to mapping out the patient's problems in terms of thoughts, feelings, behaviour, and physiology. This map can then be used to guide the appropriate intervention.

Why bother with formulation in cognitive behavioural therapy?

At beginning of therapy the formulation:
- Provides an alternative explanation for difficulties
- Helps build a therapeutic relationship
- Helps the patient feel understood and validated
- Helps the patient become aware of their individual thoughts, feelings, behaviours, and physiology
- Helps clarify the problem and makes it seem more manageable.

Throughout treatment the formulation:
- Acts as a tool for moving between specific issues and the bigger picture
- Suggests appropriate areas for intervention, e.g. changing particular patterns of thinking or behaviour
- Helps anticipate anything that might get in the way of treatment
- Helps address any problems that arise in the course of therapy or can be referred to, when expected change does not happen
- Useful in supervision.

At end of therapy the formulation:
- Helps identify areas on which to build for the future.

Types of formulation
- Can be an individualized version of a particular disorder-specific model or can be constructed from first principles, drawing on the therapist's knowledge of CBT theory and disorder-specific models
- Can focus on maintenance factors alone or include developmental factors.

How to construct a cognitive behavioural therapy formulation
- Begins before we have met the patient. What journey has led the patient to us? What information is available? What is the problem? What is keeping it going?
- Continues at first meeting. What is the problem the person is bringing to therapy? Get the history of the problem.
- Can they bring a particular example of that problem, so that we can begin to make sense of it, in terms of thoughts, feelings, behaviours, and physiology?
- Ask about this situation in micro detail.
- Do not be afraid to be gently curious. If you have not got a clear picture in your head, ask for clarification.
- Begin mapping this out on a whiteboard or shared piece of paper.
- Ask purposeful questions to try and understand in what sequence events occurred, rather than fill in random boxes of thoughts, feelings, behaviour, and physiology.

- Note relevant information regarding the background, self-criticism, obvious beliefs, or rules.
- Map out additional situations over the next few sessions.
- Look for the overall pattern.
- Add to the picture, as new information emerges.

Useful Socratic questions to help guide formulation

(See ⊃ Chapter 5, 'Socratic questioning and guided discovery' bullet point, pp. 173–4.)
- Can you tell me about a recent time when you have experienced this difficulty?
- When did this happen? At what time? Where were you? Who were you with? What were you doing?
- When this happened, what was going on in your head? What were you thinking?
- When you began thinking x, how did that make you feel? What emotions were you experiencing?
- Sometimes people get confused between thoughts and feelings. It can be useful to clarify that thoughts are strings of words, whereas emotions are single words to describe how you feel inside.
- When you thought x and felt y, did you experience any physical sensations in your body? What effect did that have on your body? What happened in your body?
- When you thought x and felt y, what did you do?
- How did doing that make you feel?
- What effect did that have on how you were thinking?
- Was it helpful?
- What happened next?

Often, particularly when working with specific mental illnesses, a maintenance formulation may be enough (see Fig. 4.3). The therapist should be aware that, for certain mental disorders, e.g. panic disorder, social anxiety, OCD, PTSD, and GAD, there are specific well-validated models

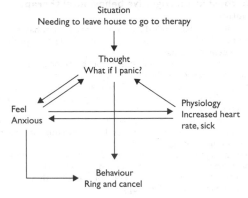

Fig. 4.3 Initial maintenance formulation.

which have identified common processes particular to that diagnosis, and the therapist, when working with such a diagnosis, should consider and base their formulation on these. However, it is important to stress that therapy is not about fitting someone into a box and rigidly following a protocol, but more about developing an individualized formulation, based on the validated model.

Longitudinal formulation

As you learn more about the patient, their history, and patterns of thinking and behaviour, you will learn pieces of information which help explain how a problem developed over time (see Fig. 4.4). This is particularly important with complex patients and with depression.

As relevant pieces of background history emerge, these can be noted. These can give us clues as to why a person thinks the way they do.

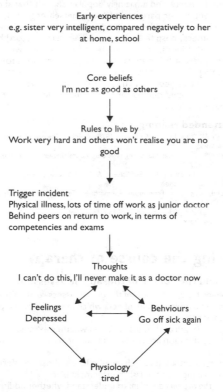

Fig. 4.4 Longitudinal formulation.

Similarly, patients' negative automatic thoughts reveal their beliefs about themselves, e.g. 'I'm useless', 'I'm worthless', 'Others are not trustworthy', or 'The world is a dangerous place'. These correspond to Beck's concept of *core beliefs*. How the person lives their life and what they do, as well as careful questioning, will help articulate strategies to which they adhere in life, perhaps learnt from key figures, such as parents, or developed over time to help cope with core beliefs. These correspond with Beck's idea of *dysfunctional assumptions* or Fennell's *rules for living*.

Observations can be shared with the patient, noted, and ultimately used to collaboratively map out a more detailed or longitudinal formulation.

Case example

Joanne described herself as having a reasonable childhood, other than growing up in her sister's shadow. She described her sister as beautiful, intelligent, sporty, and amazingly popular. She felt that she was a big disappointment to her parents and found herself negatively compared to her sister at school. Unsurprisingly, she developed a belief 'I'm not as good as others', despite having a good academic record herself and a good circle of friends, and was quite self-critical. She worked incredibly hard to prevent being found as lacking, and made it to vet school. She was doing alright, until she had to take time off due to physical illness, and then struggled to catch up with her course work, became very self-critical, developed depression, and went off sick. Fig. 4.4 shows her longitudinal formulation.

Recommended reading

Beck AT, Rush AJ, Shaw BF, and Emery G (1979). *Cognitive Therapy of Depression*. Guilford Press: New York.

Blenkiron P (1999). Who is suitable for cognitive behavioural therapy? *Journal of the Royal Society of Medicine*, **92**, 222–9.

Fennell M (1999). *Overcoming Low Self-Esteem: A Self-Help Guide Using Cognitive Behavioral Techniques*. Robinson: London.

Persons (2008). *The Case Formulation Approach to Cognitive-Behavior Therapy*. Guilford Press: New York.

Safran JD and Segal ZV (1990). *Interpersonal Process in Cognitive Therapy*. Rowman & Littlefield Publishers: New York.

Assessing the course of therapy

Why should the course of therapy be assessed?

- *Determining the effectiveness of therapy*: to assess relative benefits in relation to possible harmful effects which may have developed since commencing therapy
- *Planning the length of therapy*: to assess whether extensions to the therapy duration are needed, if that coheres with the model (e.g. CBT)
- *Risk management*: to assess changes in levels of risk to inform any necessary changes to the risk management plan
- *Updating the overall care plan*: to understand whether additional interventions (e.g. pharmacological or social) might be beneficial

- *Clinical governance*: to monitor and improve the level of care provided. Increasingly, NHS psychotherapy departments routinely use the Clinical Outcomes in Routine Evaluation–Outcome Measure (CORE-OM)
- *Research*: if the patient is participating in a research project.

Who should assess the course of therapy?

- *Therapist*: this is commonly the case, since the therapist will have the most intensive contact with the patient
- *Referrer*: GP, psychiatrist, or mental health nurse might independently, or in liaison with the therapist, assess the progress of therapy
- *Care coordinator/key worker*: who oversees the patient's overall care and coordinates various elements of the patient's care
- *The patient him/herself*: depending on the modality and personal preferences, the patient might keep a mood/thought diary, use a standardized self-monitoring form, or just form a general opinion. Patient-reported outcome measures (PROMs) or experience questionnaires are now commonplace in NHS services and often required by commissioners
- *Research assistant or assistant psychologist*: especially if the patient is in a research study.

How should the course of therapy be assessed?

- *Clinical assessment*: there are certain indicators which are useful for all psychotherapies, and others which are more specific to a particular modality. The patient's attendance is an obvious signpost to their ability to utilize the therapy appropriately, although this is a very general indicator and can be misleading—as when the therapy is used as a way of enacting a certain unconscious dynamic which might be ultimately destructive, rather than therapeutic. This will also depend on an appropriate match between patient and therapist. Depending on the modality and theoretical constructs, the ongoing assessment will vary. For example, in psychodynamic/psychoanalytic therapy, the therapist will observe and assess the development of transference in relation to the analytic framework and changes in the patient's reaction to breaks, response to interpretations, state of integration, use of defence mechanisms, dreams, external object relations, and reported symptoms. In CBT, the therapist will assess the patient's active engagement, commitment to task completion, and changes in cognition and behaviours.
- *Psychometric instruments*: quantitative (self-reported scales or semi-structured interviews) or qualitative (see ➲Assessing the outcome of therapy, pp. 142–5).

When and how frequently should reviews be held?

- *Regular planned reviews*: these can vary in frequency from weekly to yearly reviews. The frequency depends on the modality, local policies, and the patient's risk profile (i.e. patients with higher risks might need to be reviewed more frequently).
- *Ad hoc reviews*: in emergency situations involving a change in functioning or increased level of risk, significant acting out, or other unforeseen events.

In which setting should reviews be held?

- *Therapy sessions*: naturally, the therapist constantly, and consciously or unconsciously, makes judgements, assesses the patient's responses, and adjusts his/her interventions. However, this is not necessarily actively and explicitly communicated to the patient. Depending on the modality, at certain times, the therapist may provide the patient with feedback and plans regarding the future course of the therapy.
- *Supervision*: most therapists, whether fully trained or in training, will have a space to reflect on the progress of therapy. Here, they will benefit from a third person's perspective on therapeutic developments and the patient's progress.
- *Other health-care settings*, e.g. the outpatient clinic or GP consultation room where the therapy is not taking place. This process can either involve the patient or be at a professionals' meeting (e.g. a multidisciplinary team meeting where the patient's care is being reviewed).

Assessing the outcome of therapy

(See ➜ Outcome research in psychotherapy in Chapter 11, pp. 518–19.)

Contrary to Eysenck's proclamation in 1952 that patients in psychoanalysis improved no more than untreated controls, the overall conclusion from over 1000 studies is that psychotherapy is effective. Assessing psychotherapy outcome is important for clinical and research purposes. Measuring change is easier if problems are circumscribed and expressible in behavioural terms. Thus, clinical improvement in panic disorder or bulimia is measurable as a reduction in frequency of panic attacks or binge–purge behaviour. Measuring changes in subjective terms (e.g. mood, anhedonia) is more complex. Severity (e.g. for OCD) can be assessed using a Likert-type scale.

Crucial concepts in measuring therapeutic outcome

- *Validity*: is the outcome assessment method measuring what it sets out to measure?
- *Reliability*: is the outcome assessment method consistent, given the same conditions, over time and between different assessors?
- *Sensitivity*: is the outcome assessment method sensitive enough to pick up subtle changes? Different approaches differ in sensitivity to the same amount of change. Concepts of effect size and reliable change are introduced to quantitatively assess whether enough change has occurred (see ➜Chapter 11).

Who can assess the change?

- *Patients*: patients may consciously or unconsciously under- or overrate change for a number of reasons, e.g. it could be overrated in patients in whom substance misuse is a problem, due to a wish to deny the problem.

- *Professionals*, e.g. therapist, referrer, care coordinator, researcher. The therapist's personal investment in the outcome of therapy may limit reliability.
- *Significant others*, e.g. parents (child psychotherapy or family therapy), partners (marital therapy), educators (family therapy). A caveat is that reports from family or teachers can be affected by their own wishes in relation to the patient.

What can be the measured outcome?

- *Clinical indicators*:
  - Symptom reduction (e.g. depression, anxiety, obsessions, compulsions)
  - Increased functionality (better adjustment to life's demands and challenges, greater flexibility, less rigid behavioural patterns, improved motivation)
  - Reduction in problematic behaviours (e.g. substance use)
  - Acceptance (attitudinal change towards the problem)
  - Biographical self-understanding
- *Objective measures* can be used for characteristic problems and in cognitive and behavioural therapies. Examples include:
  - Clinical examination (e.g. body mass index in eating disorders, scars in self-harm)
  - Monitoring physiological reactions (e.g. to fearful stimuli)
  - Urine tests (e.g. for substance misuse)
  - Behavioural data monitoring (e.g. frequency of outings in agoraphobia)
  - Number of accident and emergency attendances
  - Inpatient admissions
  - Sickness absences
  - Medication use
  - Neuroimaging (in research)
- *Psychometric tools* can measure a number of variables, either used as self-reported scales and questionnaires or interviews conducted by professionals. Examples include:
  - Personality questionnaires, measuring personality traits or dimensions (e.g. Minnesota Multiphasic Personality Inventory, Freiburger Personality Inventory)
  - Symptom scales (e.g. Beck Depression Inventory, Symptom Check List-90, Hamilton Rating Scale for Depression, Yale Brown Obsessive Compulsive Scale)
  - Specifically theoretically defined constructs (e.g. Rosenberg Self-Esteem Scale)
  - Self-report scales assessing idiosyncratic problems. The therapist and patient may jointly formulate the client's target complaints and level of personal concern (e.g. Target Complaints)
  - Instruments focusing on the quality of interpersonal relationships (e.g. Inventory of Interpersonal Problems, Social Adjustment Scale)
  - Self-report questionnaires developed specifically as outcome measures. These measure areas of proven sensitivity to therapeutic change, such as well-being, psychopathological

symptoms, and life functioning (e.g. Outcome Questionnaire-45; CORE-OM)
- Satisfaction evaluation
- Qualitative assessor-conducted structured interviews (e.g. Client Change Interview).

Construct validity (the extent to which the chosen assessment method measures what is intended) is increased by employing a range of assessment methods (clinical, self-reported, structured interview), measuring different variables simultaneously (symptoms, functioning, and satisfaction, both objectively and subjectively), and combining perspectives (patient, therapist, other professionals, significant others).

Two different therapies for depression may be equally effective, although for different outcomes, e.g. symptomatic relief of core depressive symptoms (poor motivation, anhedonia, and anergia) versus improvement in interpersonal functioning.

Measuring change can depend on theoretical constructs specific to the different therapies:

- *Psychoanalysis*: structural reorganization of personality, resolution of unconscious conflicts, insight into intrapsychic events, superego modification, withdrawal of projections, integration. Symptom relief is an indirect result
- *Psychoanalytic psychotherapy*, partial reorganization of personality and defences, resolution of preconscious and conscious derivatives of conflicts, insight into current interpersonal events, improved object relations. Symptom relief is a goal or a prelude to further exploration
- *Supportive therapy*: reintegration and ability to cope, strengthening of defences, better adjustment or acceptance of pathology, symptom relief
- *CBT*: change in cognitive contents and/or observable behaviour which are more amenable to measurement (e.g. depressogenic cognitions can be measured using the Beck Hopelessness Scale, Dysfunctional Attitudes Scale, and Automatic Thoughts Questionnaire)
- *Family therapy*: change in family dynamics
- *CAT*: shift in roles and patterns of behaviour.

Lambert and Hill's (1994) conclusions about measuring therapeutic change, based on outcome research, are as follows:

- Measurements from therapists and non-blinded clinicians produce larger effect sizes than data from other assessors
- Gross measures (improved, not improved) produce a greater estimation of change than specific ones (symptom ratings)
- Measuring specific targets of therapy (e.g. self-harming) produces larger effect sizes than measuring generic psychotherapy outcomes (changes in personality)
- Data collected soon after therapy ends show larger effect sizes than data collected later (although this is not necessarily the case with psychoanalytically informed therapies)
- Physiological measures (e.g. heart rate) usually produce small effect sizes, compared to other measures, even when specifically targeted in psychotherapy.

Recommended reading

Eysenck HJ (1952). The effects of psychotherapy: an evaluation. *Journal of Consulting Psychology*, **16**, 319–24.

Lambert MJ and Hill CE (1994). Assessing psychotherapy outcomes and processes. In: Bergin AE and Garfield SL, eds. *Handbook of Psychotherapy and Behavior Change*, fourth edition. pp. 143–89. Wiley: New York.

Consultation

(See ➔Reflective practice groups in Chapter 10, pp. 497–505.)

Different forms of consultation

There are different forms of consultation involving the patient, the professionals, and the link between them:

A. *Consultation to professionals and teams*
- One-to-one consultation following referral with a colleague
- One-off staff meeting following a serious incident
- Reflective practice groups in wards, teams, or training
- Educational activity such as consultancy workshops

B. *Consultation to the patient (assessment)*
- Assessment to inform understanding and treatment
- Formulation to inform understanding for the patient
- Advice regarding alternatives to therapy for the patient
- Inform the ongoing management of the patient
- Liaison with the wider system of professionals

C. *Consultation to the patient and professional*
- Initial meeting with the professionals involved, only to decide whether assessment is in the patient's interests
- With or without assessment of the patient, gather countertransference data
- Formulation and recommendation
- Follow-up with professionals
- Review with the patient, if indicated
- Supervision.

Of the different forms of consultation above, it is category C, focusing on the patient and professional relationship in stuck clinical scenarios, that is the main subject of this section, with category B—consultation to the patient (assessment)—described earlier in this chapter (see ➔ Is my patient suitable for psychotherapy? pp. 110–17), and category A—consultation to professionals and teams—included in the reflective practice section in Chapter 10 (see ➔ Reflective practice groups, pp. 497–505).

Consultation as acute reflective practice

Consultation can be conceptualized as acute reflective practice, whereas reflective practice can be seen as chronic consultation. One patient is the subject of reflective practice in a single consultation, often with an acute sense of need for help with a risk-driven or stuck situation. Many patients are the subjects of the reflective practice group over a long period of time, with a chronic aspect in the length of time the space is offered and in the sustained and cumulative quality of revisiting patterns of problems again and again, with different patients.

The patient and professional link
The patient is usually seen as the centre of clinical activity, and the task of consultation is to shift this focus to a space *between* the patient and the professionals trying to help them. When it is recognized that it is the link and the breaks in these links, whether attacked or missing links, between the patient and professional that is the primary focus of interest, the process of consultation begins to make sense. However, the clinical culture of wanting a patient to be taken on (or taken away) for some other form of treatment means the intervention of not accepting the patient for another form of help itself subverts expectations that the problem will be relieved with the solution of another form of treatment equally susceptible to breaking down. The clinical tool of consultation is the offer of reflective space, an application of the therapeutic space and therapeutic attitude derived from it. It is not an offer of therapy to the patient, but it is an offer to the professionals to consider their relationship with the patient, without this becoming an offer of therapy to the professionals.

Distinction between consultation and assessment
(See ➔ Psychodynamic assessment and formulation in Chapter 4, pp. 125–35.)
The primary task in consultation is to meet the professionals, not the patient, though this is not what professionals commonly expect. The first task in the meeting with professionals is to think with them—is an assessment in the interests of your patient? Sometimes the terms consultation and assessment are confusingly used to describe the same thing: a meeting with the patient (see category B above). Consultation is being used here to describe meeting the professionals to think about the patient, whereas assessment is used to describe meeting a patient to think about their problems. As part of a consultation, the assessment of the patient serves the primary task of informing the consultation with the professionals about their work with the patient.

Consultation with assessment: consultation goldfish bowl
When a psychotherapist meets a patient for an assessment as part of a consultation, the goldfish bowl context is in the other professionals being observers of this assessment. The referring professionals who have requested an opinion from the psychotherapist are in the wings when the patient is seen and want information from the assessment. The dynamics of confidentiality and expectation are therefore different from an assessment where there is no expectation that the information gleaned will be communicated in detail to other professionals. Sensitivity about this experience of being observed, how far it might compromise the therapeutic relationship, and the discussion about the nature of the boundaries of the process make for a distinct experience which is further complicated by the potentially disappointing fact that the outcome of assessment of the patient is unlikely to be an offer of psychotherapy; this is a lot to ask of the patient.

Who can use therapeutic help?

If a consultation referral is appropriate, this will be of a patient who is struggling to benefit from, or use, the help they are being offered in the other parts of the service. The professionals who refer the patient commonly feel stuck, and, in part, they are consulting with the hope that psychotherapeutic understanding might help them think about this. The focus of consultation is therefore not solely on the patient, but on the patient and professional relationship, including the wider system. A question lies in the use of therapeutic help offered to the professionals, as this may not be entirely what is expected or hoped for.

Great expectations: patient and professional

However, great expectations come with great impasse. Harboured desires for psychotherapy to be the answer are often in the background for professionals understandably longing for a solution. The desire for psychotherapy may also be awakened in a patient offered assessment, and, if it is likely, on the basis of what is gleaned in a professionals' meeting, that they will not be able to make use of psychotherapy, it is maybe a cause of iatrogenic harm to offer an assessment.

Consultation without assessment

The psychotherapist who decides with the professionals that it is not in the patient's interest to be seen for assessment is then left only with the discussion with the professionals to inform their formulation. This inevitably limits the data they have to the countertransference of their colleagues without direct contact with the patient and limits what they can offer. The risk in offering a view of a patient without assessment is that it may be too remote or theoretical and prone to speculation not grounded in direct clinical observation. This is like clinical practice with one arm tied behind one's back; the examination of the patient is one-sided, missing the emotional experience of the therapist.

Learning from the experience of others

However, in practice, reflected in the experience of supervision or reflective practice or leading a Balint group, the skill in listening to the countertransference of colleagues and discerning the patterns of their feelings and the meaning in their dilemmas can be developed and focused in the task of articulating some therapeutic understanding.

Cure and curiosity

The leitmotif of this therapeutic understanding in consultation is with people who are, by definition, hard to help and centres on facing the painful limitations of what is possible without despair or retaliation. Consultation aims to help professionals to moderate their hopes and manage their therapeutic zeal or resentment towards patients who resist their best efforts to cure them. Given that interest can be lost when treatment fails, maintaining curiosity in the face of therapeutic impotence is a painful challenge. A central aim in consultation can therefore be seen to lie in replacing the desire to cure with curiosity.

Medical psychotherapy consultation

The affects of the consultation when it is emotionally effective include conflict, shame, and doubt for the professionals, both in and between them. The space between patient and professional is the focus of consultation, and the space between the consulting professional and the professionals seeking the help carries an emotional echo of the experiences of the stuck scenario that caused the need for outside help. The credibility of the consulting professional lies not so much in their knowledge or skill in psychotherapy, but in their tact and humility in recognizing the painful reality of facing limitations and the feeling of exposure in conveying therapeutic doubt and impotence to others. Although consultation described in this section has an evident psychoanalytic background, the feelings of being stuck, feeling fear about a patient, feeling hatred for a patient, or feeling hatred for the way a colleague is treating a patient can occur whichever therapeutic model is used.

The medical psychotherapist has a role in bridging the gap between psychiatry and other psychotherapeutic professions in consultation, as some psychiatrists may find it necessary to use the Trojan Horse of diagnosis to carry the enemy of empathy: their hidden feelings for their troublesome patient. Medical psychotherapists may hold the issue of diagnosis both lightly and with respect, and this can be an important link for psychiatrists who privilege this form of formulation as a primary means of talking about their relationship with a patient. This professional interface within a multidisciplinary team where there are different languages, and antagonism to the medical model defined as narrowly biological, can be common fault lines for splitting and unvoiced disagreement in a confusion of tongues which a medical psychotherapist can help to translate. The echoes of denigration and contempt are frequent emotional themes in the professional and patient impasse, and recognizing how this may play out between professionals, without making the understanding a form of therapy, requires confidence in psychiatry and psychotherapy, which medical psychotherapists can bring to the consultation process.

Dependency and destructiveness in consultation

The repeated psychological and physical themes for patients referred by professionals for medical psychotherapy consultation are problems of dependency and destructiveness. The problems the patient has with dependency are frequently a manifestation of early childhood deprivation and trauma, with the experience of obliviousness in the childhood environment becoming a disturbing companion to the patient's adolescent and adult relationships. Dependency problems in the psychological sphere are often shown in a profound split between longing and need, and suspicion and mistrust. Physical dependency with addiction to alcohol and/or drugs can take the place of relating and connection, complicating the clinical picture in which toxic relationships are replaced with toxic, but reliable, intoxicants used to numb contact with self, other, and reality.

Destructive patterns of relating to self and other in relationships permeate the patient and professional relationship, so that those who have experienced abuse soon find abuse echoed in other relationships, with professionals experienced as both abused and abuser. Anxieties associated with harm to self and other become the preoccupation of action or inaction, and cause doubt in professionals about the dependency needs of the patient. Destructiveness is often enacted in repetitive and relentless patterns of self-harm in a dependency on a sadomasochistic relationship, in which mental torment and suffering are evacuated into professionals. In this chaotic cycle of grievance, perverse distortions of pain replace loss, sadness, and grieving.

Doubt in the patient and professional relationship

The patient and professional relationship in stuck clinical situations can be understood in terms of doubt. There is doubt about the patient, their diagnosis, their legitimacy in seeking care, their motivations to receive help, and their intentions towards their caregivers. There is doubt in the minds of professionals about their capacity to help, their feelings for the patient, their feelings about carers and colleagues, and about their own intentions towards the patient. The destructive and abusive dynamic of the patient experience can find its counterpart in professional relationships with professionals coming to doubt the minds of colleagues, as they struggle with hostile, rejecting, or idealized rescuing impulses.

Doubt about dependency is frequently shown in a dilemma about viewing dependency in a split way, as either solely malignant or purely benign. The professional doubts about evading a malignant need and becoming stuck by reinforcing dependency tend to resonate with an economic organizational imperative to 'move the patient on', with a long-term need for help viewed with suspicion, as a toxic costly dependency. Professionals are unconsciously invited to hold doubt about the illness or life itself. Risk of death is a frequent companion to doubt in mental health practice.

Much of this doubt remains unconscious. Where a patient can hold doubt about their own mind, without being paralysed in the certainty of doubt, but mobilized in the uncertainty of self-reflective curiosity, there is psychological mindedness. Where there is psychological mindedness, the professionals and others in the dynamic field are unconsciously less pressured to hold doubt on behalf of the person who is more able to hold doubt about themselves.

Vignette of consultation without assessment

This medical psychotherapy consultation relates to a woman in her fifties in a CMHT, whom the psychiatrist had inherited from a colleague. Having had a diagnosis of bipolar disorder for many years, the psychiatrist had a different view—that she had an emotionally unstable personality disorder. However, he had continued to offer the medication she was used to receiving, and she had built up an idealized relationship with him. Every now and then, she presented in waves of suicidal despair. These tsunamis of pain had increased as the end of a counselling relationship loomed. The psychiatrist had hoped that the consultation would result in the patient being offered further psychotherapy to be seamless with the end of counselling.

The medical psychotherapist arranged a professionals' meeting, in which the care coordinator described how she felt the patient denigrated her and would not listen to her. In the meeting, the psychiatrist spoke over the care coordinator, not seeming to value what she had to offer. The psychiatrist spoke of the woman's history of sexual abuse and how he thought the counsellor was out of her depth and this counselling had been ill advised. In the meeting, he wondered whether she could be offered an assessment for further psychotherapy.

The consultant offering the consultation was reminded of the dynamic of the loss of identity in sexual abuse and the ways in which the loss of diagnosis could be experienced as a further loss of identity, as the patient was linked with a community of people suffering from bipolar disorder. The psychiatrist doubted the diagnosis and yet could not carry the courage of his conviction into withdrawing treatment, which was associated, in the patient's mind, with a legitimacy in being perceived to be ill and had incorporated an idealized transference of the potency of the prescriber. The care coordinator seemed to be placed in the position of holding the denigrated aspect of the patient, the silenced loss of identity in which she could not be heard. The patient apparently missed verbal cues when someone stopped speaking, coming in too soon in a way that was echoed in the psychiatrist speaking over the care coordinator and her seemingly being silenced.

At the end of the consultation, the psychiatrist asked the medical psychotherapist, 'All very interesting, but what are you going to do?'

The medical psychotherapist quoted the well-known frustrating psychotherapist's mantra, 'Don't just do something, sit there', advising that they wait until the end of counselling, and he would not offer assessment to the patient but would arrange a further professionals' meeting. He emphasized the split in which the care coordinator was the bad object holding the denigration and contempt from which the patient protected the idealized psychiatrist and the counsellor.

Psychoanalytic formulation: the ill legitimate or illegitimate patient? The vehicle of illness symbolizes potency both for psychiatrist and patient which cannot be mourned. There is privilege in retaining the illusion of illness and splitting of the devalued non-ill or illegitimate feelings which cannot be repaired and the patient cannot hear or cannot bear. The enactment of not being listened to in the consultation between professionals served as an echo of contempt. The attack on identity in illness being removed seemed to both repeat abuse and threaten the idealization of the psychiatrist.

Vignette of consultation with assessment

This consultation related to a woman in her thirties who was presenting a confused diagnostic picture of psychosis and borderline features, and the medical psychotherapist had seen her for assessment some years previously. The inpatient psychiatrist thought she presented a high and unpredictable risk, and the care coordinator described her as 'very hard to get hold of'. The patient led to the care coordinator feeling as belittled as the patient—in a measured, rather polite way saying she wanted other treatments, such as some form of therapy, which was better than the help made available now; referral, however, did not lead to her taking up assessments.

The consulting medical psychotherapist recalled in assessment that she had shown a dramatic split between, in the first assessment, presenting a worrying self-harming, reckless, drug-taking self, drawn to abusive partners, but, in the second assessment, presenting as if she was a different person, apparently considering a vocation to train as a doctor. Her rationale for this ambition and her accurate knowledge of the medical school application process made her seem to be a credible applicant, despite the prospect seeming remote. Following the 'doctor session', she then disappeared from assessment, leaving the psychotherapist with a doubt that she had killed herself.

The woman's presentation to inpatient services in the present had claustrophobic and agoraphobic elements, in which she sought to be in psychiatric intensive care units following psychosis and arson; she then absconded and, from a distance, would call professionals, begging for help. The professionals felt irritated with her and impotent.

The assessment some years before the consultation helped the medical psychotherapist to recognize that the woman's desire to train as a doctor also contained an unconscious motive of a desire not to allow herself to be a patient so that meaningful help could be offered to her; the ideal help is always remote, unrealistic, and impossible to reach.

Psychoanalytic formulation: the elusive patient

The professional and patient relationship of 'now you see me, now you don't' echoed her early object relations history of feeling she was hated by a mother who, to outward appearances, was competent. The psychiatric hospital or 'brick mother' is used by the patient for asylum from her mind, and, when she feels trapped, she takes flight, then panics at being bereft, leaving professionals with doubt and anxiety about her well-being. Her feelings of impotence and rage are projected into the professionals, as she searches for the idealized doctor to cure her elsewhere. In this consultation, the medical psychotherapist's direct experience of being confused by this split between a self-destructive and despairing patient and an idealized curative doctor helped him to process his assessment experience to inform the struggles of his colleagues which echoed his.

Recommended reading

Feldman M (2009). *Doubt, Conviction and the Analytic Process: Selected Papers of Michael Feldman (The New Library of Psychoanalysis)*. Routledge: Hove and New York.

Hinshelwood RD (2004). *Suffering Insanity: Psychoanalytic Essays on Psychosis*. Brunner-Routledge: Hove and New York.

Huffington C, Armstrong D, Halton W, Hoyle L, and Pooley J (eds) (2004). *Working Below the Surface: The Emotional Life of Contemporary Organizations (Tavistock Clinic Series)*. Karnac Books: London.

Menzies Lyth I (1989). *The Dynamics of the Social: Selected Essays, volumes I and II*. Free Association Books: London.

Obholzer A and Zagier Roberts V (1994). *The Unconscious at Work: Individual and Organizational Stress in the Human Services*. Brunner-Routledge: London.

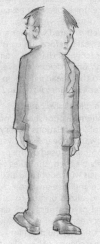

JAMES JOHNSTON 2014

Treatment

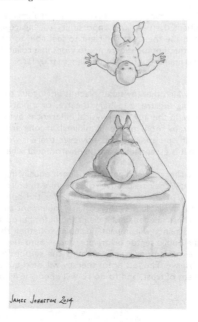

JAMES JOHNSTON 2014

Therapy in clinical practice

Psychotherapy, or therapy, is a carefully modulated encounter between a therapist and a patient, or a team of therapists and a group of patients, which requires sound foundations in order to work to best effect. Here the word 'therapy' or 'therapies' refer to a general therapeutic approach, unless otherwise stipulated. There are a range of therapeutic modalities described in this section of the Handbook which vary in many respects, in terms of the techniques used, the underlying philosophy, and the patients who are taken on. Alongside this, there are many common themes which form the building blocks of therapy and which require attentive management, in order to maximize the beneficial effects of therapy.

There are two central factors that are the responsibility of the therapist and which contribute directly to the development of a positive therapeutic relationship, sometimes referred to as the therapeutic alliance. The first of these is the environment in which the therapy takes place, which is here described as the setting. This includes the journey into and out of the therapy session, how the patient experiences this, and factors that can support a positive experience of therapy. The second is the functioning mindset of the therapist, that they are able to pay undivided attention to the patient and their difficulties, and to communicate and empathize with the patient in order to assist their improvement. This is not static, as the therapist will move in relation to the patient during the course of sessions, and at times moment-to-moment changes will take place.

When both the setting and the therapist are in a conducive place and space, the patient then has the opportunity to engage in therapy, to develop trust in the therapist sufficient to feel able to confide difficulties, and, using the therapeutic frame, to work in a collaborative way to understand and manage better the challenges they face.

Setting

The setting in which therapy takes place is analogous to a theatre, be that an operating theatre, a military theatre, or a place where actors construct a play. In therapy, the physical differences between a normal room and a therapy room may seem minimal, in comparison with a normal room and an operating theatre; however, there is work taking place in therapy, and it is essential to have an environment which is conducive to this function.

Although the therapist and patient are both equally important to the success of therapy, their respective roles require them to hold different responsibilities. The therapist is responsible for the operating theatre, for ensuring it is available, has the correct equipment and appropriate support staff where needed, and is clean and fit for purpose.

Real-life constraints will impact, including whether therapy is taking place in the public sector or private, and is outpatient or inpatient; however, some basic principles in creating the setting for therapy are essential to observe. The setting for therapy will be required to support the development of trust, and to do so will need a level of privacy and neutrality.

In public sector services, there will generally be a room which is multi-functional and used by a number of different staff. The therapist may have little say in how this is organized; however, it is important to ensure that the setting is fit for the purpose it fulfils. In private practice, the therapist may have more input to how the room is arranged, depending on whether they are working in a personal dedicated consulting room or a space which is rented. In either case, there are essential important aspects to the room and furnishings which will either support or detract from the therapy.

Prior to beginning therapy, it is good practice for the therapist to visit the setting where therapy will take place or, if this is impractical, to discuss this with a colleague who has worked there, or, in the case of a trainee, to ask their supervisor to confirm the setting is satisfactory. This can be a daunting task for the trainee starting out with their first patient; however, it can also be useful, as it provides a 'dress rehearsal'. Not only will the therapist check out the room, but they will also need to enter the building, go through a reception area, perhaps visit the toilet, find their way to the room, and sit in it for a while. This is helpful acclimatization, in preparation for therapy. It also gives an opportunity to begin to empathize with what the patient might experience, to understand how daunting the journey to that first therapy session can be, as well as gives an opportunity to get to know the reception staff and how they work.

In an ideal setting, such as a dedicated psychotherapy service, the receptionist will know therapists do not wish to be disturbed and will therefore not routinely pass on phone messages or communicate via urgent emails during therapy sessions. In other clinical settings, this may be usual practice, e.g. phoning through to let the doctor know their next patient is waiting, even when they are still with the previous patient. Therefore, it is an important part of setting the scene for the therapist to inform the reception staff they will be undertaking therapy and do not wish to be disturbed, unless, of course, there is an emergency such as the building being on fire. In line with this, mobile phones, on-call 'bleeps', and electronic devices (unless used in the sessions) should be turned off or on silent.

In public sector services, there are also often alarm systems which can be activated in case of emergency, and increasingly these are provided in therapy rooms as an essential part of health and safety regulations. Again these may have an impact on the therapy, so it is important to be familiar with these procedures and how to respond to both the alarm and curiosity of the patient about this.

The environment of the therapy room should be comfortable, with minimal distractions externally; for example, it should be relatively quiet, so that the intrusion that external noise can place on communication and thought is kept to a minimum. There should be a reasonable degree of sound proofing, so that the conversation taking place in an adjacent room is not audible, as this would indicate that the therapy taking place can be overheard and is therefore not confidential. The temperature should be reasonable and ideally controllable, though this can be difficult with modern clinical buildings. Blinds are preferable to curtains, as they provide a more clinical adjustment—drawing curtains across, even on a bright summer's day, may convey a message of potential sexual intimacy and is not recommended for working with vulnerable patients.

Furniture in a room which is multipurpose may include a desk with a computer, a desk chair, and a chair for the patient. The arrangement of the furniture is important, as is the need to ensure that equality is conveyed. Two people are meeting, in order to have a conversation; therefore, it is important not to place barriers in the way, e.g. as would be formed by the therapist sitting behind a desk, corporate style. It is better for the therapist and patient to sit on comfortable chairs of similar height where they can feel relaxed and are able to establish eye contact. Often it can be more comfortable to sit at an angle, rather than directly face to face, in order that the patient or therapist can easily look away at times, non-verbal communication being important in sessions. It may also be useful to position a clock where both the therapist and patient can discretely see it, but which does not intrude too forcefully into the session. This will enable the therapist to be able to end the session on time, without having to obviously check their watch, which may be experienced by the patient as the therapist being bored and impatient to end the session.

In some forms of therapy, there will be different arrangements, e.g. in psychoanalytic psychotherapy, the patient may lie on a couch, with the therapist behind them and out of eye line. In systemic therapy, there may be cameras in the room with a one-way screen, behind which the observing team are placed. Such variations will usually be discussed, and there may need to be consent, e.g. to record sessions, and a meeting with the observing team. Some specialist therapies take place in settings where the environment is changed to support materials and the space required, e.g. art therapy will usually take place in a room appropriately equipped, as will music therapy and group sessions.

In order to maintain neutrality, personal items, such as photos of family and religious symbols, are to be discouraged, as they may signal messages to the patient, which can inhibit their full and spontaneous participation in therapy.

The setting is one in which both the therapist and patient can feel safe and secure, so that they can relate as comfortably as is possible. Continuity is important for this, and the same room should be used for each and every session with the patient, as moving can be disruptive to the therapy. Ideally, the therapist would use the same room for all the patients they see in a particular area or clinic, as this ensures a better level of continuity for them. A consistent base from which to work also assists communication, e.g. if there is a need to cancel a session at short notice, the availability of a reliable person to take and pass on a message is invaluable. Without this level of support, the therapist may need to spend more time on keeping the setting working at optimum level.

Some patients may have disabilities and require special adaptations. This is often acknowledged during the process of referral to therapy and, if not anticipated, may lead to awkward rearrangements being required at short notice to accommodate limited mobility or other disabilities such as deafness.

Preparation for therapy involves the therapist arriving in time to check the room and make any required alterations. This may involve moving chairs, checking that no other patient notes are visible, and ensuring the therapist has available what they need for the session. It is often helpful, especially if working in a number of settings, to arrive with a few minutes to sit in the room and prepare the internal world of the therapist, which may include looking at notes of the previous session and possibly also supervision notes.

There may be an issue about whether or not a room and setting are suitable for therapy, and some level of compromise may be required, as not all settings are honed for this activity. However, it is important to remember that a surgeon would not perform in a place which does not provide the adequate hygiene, and the therapist similarly would need, as part of their role, to ensure that the room and setting in which it takes place is 'good enough' for the work to proceed.

The therapist
(See ➲Chapter 3.)

Ensuring the environment is conducive to therapy can be likened to laying the foundation stones for therapy. Next is needed a framework for the therapy to take place around. This is the work of starting the therapy, and the better footing it can have, the better it can proceed.

As in an operating theatre where there is an accepted process by which the surgeon 'scrubs up', so there is a process for the therapist to prepare for therapy. This involves personal preparation of their mindset and attention, so they can be open and receptive to the patient's material and active in processing and responding to this. As with donning the operating gown, the therapist will take on a mantel. Although this is an internal process taking place in the mind of the therapist, it is important to prepare a space, which can be thought of as the 'ready position'.

It is often said that the therapist should maintain a neutral stance. However, another way of thinking about this is that the therapist should always be able to pull themselves into a place in their mind where they are ready to engage with the patient. This can be described as the 'ready position', familiar to many who engage in sports. To illustrate this, the ready position on the tennis court is a stance adopted by the player preparing to receive a ball. The player will be positioned mid court, to give maximum reach, standing firmly but not rigidly, with both feet rooted symmetrically and soft knees, ready to spring into action. The racquet will be held centrally in front of the body in both hands, in order that it can be moved easily to either side, and, most importantly, the player is very attentive, watching carefully, as their opponent eyes up the court and decides how and where to place the ball.

Although therapy is not about competition, the 'ready position' is a helpful concept, as the therapist needs to develop a place where they feel grounded, balanced, and attentive. They are then ready to interact with the patient, able to reach out from a place of balance and, most importantly, able to return to the ready position on a regular basis. The therapy requires the therapist to move in and out of the ready position, and, when therapy is going well and smoothly, this will be happening, as a dialogue develops and deepens, each participant aware of the boundaries of the encounter. At times, there may be sharper movements, in response to which the therapist will move well out of their comfort zone and find themselves, to return to the tennis analogy, off balance and on the edge of the court, or even beyond the white lines. A strong outpouring of emotion from the patient may evoke this or the patient bringing in material that strikes a personal chord with the therapist. Whilst noting this and mentally flagging it up for later exploration or supervision, the therapist also needs to get back to the ready position as soon as possible, just as the tennis player would, in order to continue the therapy.

An example of this would be a therapist who has experienced a life event, such as losing a parent or sibling, or a miscarriage, hearing similar material from the patient in the therapy. This may block their capacity to think and respond to the patient, or skew their reaction. Generally, the therapist is not advised to work, if in severe distress; however, even when they may have worked through personal issues, there is a need to keep an eye on this and seek support and a place to think, such as in clinical supervision or their own personal therapy, in order to separate their own issues from that of the patient.

Beginning the therapy

(See ➜Therapeutic alliance in Chapter 3, p. 99; Engaging the patient in Chapter 3, pp. 99–100.)

Across all the therapies, it is important that the therapist and patient have an understanding of the therapy, including arrangements for meetings, the duration of a session, the expected overall number of sessions, especially in brief therapies, and how and who to contact in the event of a cancellation. Arrangements will differ, to some extent, with therapeutic modality, but, e.g. in psychodynamic therapy, a therapy session will usually be 50 minutes' duration, and will start and finish on time. The emphasis is based on the patient having uninterrupted space and time, in order that they can open up and explore issues which are troubling them and also consider how they are thinking and feeling whilst with the therapist. This discussion will be part of the therapeutic agreement, or contract, forming a base for the therapy.

Whilst setting the frame for therapy, there is also something very important taking place, as the therapist and patient are talking together and beginning to explore how the relationship is developing, beginning to get to know each other, and to form an attachment. Taken together, the therapy setting, frame, and relationship facilitate a secure base from which an attachment can form.

The therapist will also have a professional stance which again will differ, to some extent, according to the modality of therapy in terms of governing principles. The therapist is there to work with the patient, giving time and space to them to explore their issues, and, in order to maximize this, the therapist maintains privacy about personal matters such as their relationship status, family background, and more immediate pressures (see ➜ Knowledge of, and ability to operate within, professional and ethical guidelines in Chapter 3, pp. 97–8; Boundary setting and maintenance in Chapter 9, pp. 454–5).

It is the role of the therapist to follow closely what the patient says and does in the session, and to listen and be curious about the patient's life, experiences, relationships, and their internal world, including dreams.

It is not the role of the therapist to advise the patient, but rather to help them think about their situation and develop their own way forward in life. Focusing on the patient, the therapist may respond to material directly brought into the session and also will be trying to register under-currents, changes in mood, and emotional arousal.

Therapy has boundaries in the form of the setting and the therapeutic frame. It can be helpful to explain this, e.g. generally therapists do not hug or kiss patients, as this may be traumatic to a patient who has been abused. Similarly, they would not position chairs either very close together or too far apart, as this would convey untoward intimacy or distance (see ➔ Knowledge of, and ability to operate within, professional and ethical guidelines in Chapter 3, pp. 97–8; Boundary setting and maintenance in Chapter 9, pp. 454–5).

There should also be discussion about communication, e.g. to referrers and the GP, which is explored further in the sections below on public and private practice. Linked to this, the issue of confidentiality should be openly explored, along with the limits to this which may relate to risk factors. It is usual to ensure that therapy is confidential, especially when personal feelings and sensitivities are disclosed. However, if material emerges that presents new risk factors, such as self-harm or potential harm to others, or ongoing sexual abuse, there can be a need to inform and involve other agencies. In this situation, it is usual to discuss and revisit confidentiality with the patient and, as far as possible, ensure they are aware of the need for professional disclosure and are as involved in the process as is appropriate (see ➔ Confidentiality and psychotherapy in Chapter 9, pp. 452–4).

As therapy progresses through the middle working and ending phases, these early foundations are often revisited and reviewed.

Outpatient therapy

Most therapy will take place in outpatient settings where the patient attends on a regular basis, usually weekly, for their regular therapy session. The experienced therapist will usually see several patients in a single setting and generally will have 50 minutes with the patient, followed by a 10-minute break, in which to write notes and ensure they are comfortable, e.g. stretching their legs or opening a window to let air circulate to refresh their memory about the next patient.

The setting in which outpatient therapy takes place varies greatly, from a psychotherapy clinic or consulting room corridor, where a range of appointments are taking place, or a half-day session when a number of therapists are working side by side. Whatever the arrangement, it is helpful to the therapy to work in a place where this is understood and there is sufficient peace and quiet to allow the therapy to be undisturbed. It can also be helpful to therapists to have colleagues close at hand, to exchange thoughts over coffee during breaks. When trainees are taking on patients, especially for the first time, they can be reassured by the presence of other trainees, a supervisor, or secretary who knows how therapy is organized. This becomes then more of a routine activity and less anxiety-provoking for the trainee, which, in turn, assists the containment of the therapy and patient.

Outpatient therapy is voluntary; patients are expected to get them-selves to the sessions on time and be able to leave the sessions at the end. The therapist will usually go to a waiting area and greet the patient, inviting them to the therapy room and observing boundaries, e.g. not chatting to the patient, in that the therapy does not begin until both are in the room and the door is closed. Some patients will find this difficult at first but usually respond to the therapist's lead. During the outpatient session, the therapist will be mindful of the process of the encounter, that it has a beginning, a middle, and an end, following which the patient will leave and need to keep themselves safe for their onward journey and until they return for the next session. Outpatient therapy then requires a level of resourcefulness on the part of the patient. When arranging therapy sessions, the therapist will also remind the patient of dates of sessions and give advance notice of planned absences.

Inpatient therapy

Therapy in inpatient settings takes a number of different forms, from specialized residential treatment facilities to in-reach therapy on an acute psychiatric ward.

Inpatient therapies for patients detained under the MHA are provided in secure services. Such patients will usually be deemed to be a potential risk to others and require a specialist therapeutic approach to ensure relational containment, alongside the physical containment of the setting (see ➔ Psychological therapy in secure settings in Chapter 8, pp. 428–39; Forensic psychiatry: forensic psychotherapies, applications, and research in Chapter 12, pp. 550–6).

Specialized residential treatments, e.g. for personality disorder, are provided for small numbers of people who have been unable to engage in outpatient therapy and where there are high levels of risk through self-harm, and possibly some element of harm to others. These specialist treatment units require, for optimal functioning, a team approach, with excellent communication across the team of staff who work shift patterns around the clock. The care plan for each patient in specialized inpatient services will usually include group therapy, milieu therapy, individual therapy sessions, along with other treatment interventions such as medication and psycho-education. Residential therapy services usually offer intensive treatments and focus on patients with complex multifactorial needs (see ➔ Chapter 8).

Therapy also takes place in acute psychiatric wards and rehabilitation units where there will usually be group therapies involving activities, such as art therapy, psycho-educational groups, and individual work, often focusing on assessment, e.g. understanding self-harm or disclosure of abuse. Acute inpatient therapy services will include specific interventions such as CBT for psychosis and distraction techniques to assist with resistance to act on impulses (see ➔ Rehabilitation and social psychiatry: psychotherapies, applications, and research in Chapter 12, pp. 568–73).

Occasionally, a patient attending outpatient therapy will become unwell or decompensate, and need admitting to an acute psychiatric ward, in which case it may be possible and/or appropriate, in some circumstances, for the therapist to continue individual therapy throughout the admission, in consultation with the treating team. Conversely, therapy begun in acute inpatient settings would ideally continue beyond discharge to the community, though, with resources for inpatients and outpatients often being located in functional teams, it will usually be a different staff member from a community team providing the therapy, in which case the contract and purpose will need to be revisited, as part of the engagement process.

Public or private sector?

As noted earlier, therapy may take place in public sector services, such as NHS mental health trusts or primary care therapy services, or may be provided in the private sector. There are some differences that impact on the therapy, due to the background of the provider, which are considered further below.

Funding and its impact in public sector therapies

In the public sector, funding is arranged through contracts, which are usually for a specific block of services and will specify some constraints of therapy such as the population it is providing for, both in terms of geography and the nature of the disorder presenting, the type of intervention, and the duration. Increasingly, commissioners of services are also likely to require information not just about the numbers and demographic details of those patients engaging in therapy, but also about their outcomes. In practice, this transfers into some limitations in relation to the expressed wishes of the patient, e.g. they may not have access to long-term psychodynamic therapy or may have this as a second therapy having been stepped up from a lower intensity service (see ➲ Assessing the outcome in therapy in Chapter 4, pp. 142–5; Outcome research in psychotherapy in Chapter 11, pp. 518–19).

There are also attempts to provide very low-intensity non-face-to-face therapies in some primary care therapy services where the patient may be guided towards online learning or provided with telephone advice. Such approaches may be sufficient for a small cohort of people with transient difficulties; however, this can work against therapeutic engagement for patients with more severe and enduring difficulties, especially where trust and interpersonal frustrations are part of the problem; thus, the initial engagement with the patient referred into higher-intensity services can be made more problematic.

Funding in private therapy

In private settings, there can be contracts established to provide specific interventions such as employment assistance programmes; however, when private therapy is referred to, it is generally taken to mean that the patient pays directly for the treatment. There is then an additional transaction between the therapist and the patient, in which the therapist, or service in which they are working, sends a bill to the patient. In practice, it is usually the therapist who gives a monthly bill to the patient and requests payment. This can provide more choice to the patient, in that they are able to express a wish for longer-term therapy or attend more than one session per week. The usual convention is that patients are expected to pay for all sessions agreed with the therapist at the outset, even when the patient misses sessions, e.g. when they are ill or away on holiday or have other work commitments. Problems can arise if the circumstances of the patient change, e.g. if they lose their income through illness or loss of employment. Here it will be left to the discretion of the therapist to respond, either by terminating the sessions, continuing for a fixed period at a lower rate, or continuing without an income. Some therapists offer a sliding scale of fees, based on the income of the patient, whereas others operate with a fixed fee.

Referrals in public and private therapy

Referrals to therapy in the public sector will usually go direct from primary care to the locally commissioned service, though, in parts of the UK, this is changing, as there is an enhanced attention to patient choice developing. In the private sector, the patient will usually make a choice of therapist, based on their local availability, recommendation of friend or professional colleague, or information obtained through the Internet from a professional body such as UKCP, BACP, or BPC (see ➡ Appendix: Key UK-based psychotherapy organizations, pp. 581–6).

Teamwork and confidentiality

(See ➡ Confidentiality and psychotherapy in Chapter 9, pp. 452–4.)

In the public sector, there will be records kept describing the therapy, including letters and reports to referring doctors or other health professionals. Increasingly, these are being kept in an electronic format, and there are constraints put in place to ensure confidential material in therapy sessions is shared within carefully boundaried staff on a 'need to know' basis.

In the public sector, there are also often a number of people in different roles assisting the patient, and it is important that the work is joined up. This will usually include a senior clinician, often a consultant medical psychotherapist, providing clinical leadership for a service. For medical trainees, there will be a tutor assigned to support the trainee with aspects of training, which may include assistance in getting the setting organized and finding suitable patients. The tutor will also ensure there are supervision arrangements in place for the trainee, to support their learning and professional development.

Risk issues, especially access to crisis (urgent) services and sharing of risk information, are part of the team around the patient's function. In the public sector, it is argued that patients with higher levels of disturbance should be taken on for therapy, only if there is a wider network able to support them, e.g. between sessions. This might include the local crisis team, who would be able to be in touch with the therapist, and the GP bringing in additional support and services, as needed (see ➡ Assessing and managing risk in Chapter 3, pp. 104–7).

In the private sector, practices differ—some therapists will notify the patient's GP that they are in therapy, whereas others will not do so but may keep on record contact details of the GP, in order that, should the clinical presentation change, they could, if required, notify the GP.

Summary

Whatever modality of therapy is practised, the setting in which it takes place makes a crucial contribution to the quality of the encounter. Similarly, the therapist is required to look after their mind and ensure for each therapy session that they are in the 'ready position' and, when pulled out of balance, are able to return to this. The combination of the environmental setting and the internal workings of the therapist ensure that there is a sound frame for therapy and that the patient is able to engage constructively and creatively to pursue change across a range of clinical services.

Recommended reading

Casement P (2013). *On Learning From the Patient*, second edition. Routledge: Hove and New York.

Hobson RF (1985). *Forms of Feeling: the Heart of Psychotherapy*. Routledge: Hove and New York.

Holmes J (2013). *Storr's The Art of Psychotherapy*, third edition. CRC Press: Boca Raton.

Lemma A (2003). *Introduction to the Practice of Psychoanalytic Psychotherapy*. John Wiley: Chichester.

Weissman MM, Markowitz JC, and Klerman GL (2007). *Clinician's Quick Guide to Interpersonal Psychotherapy*. Oxford University Press: New York.

Psychoanalytic psychotherapy

(See ⟳Psychoanalytic psychotherapy in Chapter 2, pp. 20–30.)

Key techniques and competencies

Free association

The course of psychoanalytic psychotherapy is unstructured, in that the therapist does not direct the patient to talk about anything in particular or focus the sessions on specific topics or goals. This is based on the psychoanalytic technique of *free association*, in which the patient is encouraged to say whatever is in his mind, without censoring his thoughts, however trivial or disturbing. The psychotherapist's task, through a corresponding type of evenly suspended listening that Freud called *free-floating attention*, is to discover the unconscious themes that underlie the patient's discourse via the patient's slips of the tongue, associative links, and resistances to speaking about certain topics of which the patient himself may be unaware.

The setting

(See ⟳Setting in Chapter 5, pp. 154–7.)

In psychoanalytic treatment, patients are encouraged to lie on the *couch*, with the analyst sitting behind them. The relative sensory deprivation and inability to see the analyst's facial expressions facilitate the patient in free association and focusing on his inner world. In once-weekly psychotherapy, the patient may lie on the couch but is usually sitting up, and therapy is conducted face-to-face.

The creation of a protected psychic space in which the patient's unconscious material may safely emerge to be interpreted and understood is an essential component of the therapeutic relationship. This is achieved by maintaining the parameters or boundaries of the *analytic setting* or *frame*, which, in its external elements, includes consistency of the physical environment in which the therapy takes place, the reliability of sessions that begin and end on time, and, in its internal elements, includes the therapist's attitude of neutrality, anonymity, and abstinence. Here the therapist maintains clearly defined interpersonal boundaries, in which she is non-judgemental, minimizes self-disclosure, and maintains confidentiality.

Spectrum of interventions

The verbal interventions of the therapist can be categorized along a spectrum from the supportive to interpretive. The therapist may initially make more supportive or *empathic comments*; moving to *clarifications*— questioning or rephrasing what the patient means; to *confrontations*— pointing out inconsistencies in the patient's account or drawing his attention to subjects he may be avoiding; to *interpretations*. A contemporary Freudian therapist will usually work from surface to depth, analysing the patient's resistances and defences (e.g. his lateness to sessions or silences), before interpreting the content of underlying unconscious fantasies. This may differ from a Kleinian approach, in which the therapist may make 'deeper' interpretations of more primitive unconscious phantasies and anxieties earlier in the course of therapy.

Interpretations

Interpretations offer a new formulation of unconscious meaning and motivation for the patient and aim to promote insight and understanding. There are two main types of interpretation: *genetic* or *reconstructive*, and *transference* or *here-and-now interpretations*. A *reconstructive interpretation* links the patient's current thoughts or behaviour to their developmental or historical origins, making an explicit link with the past and aiming to help the patient understand how his current difficulties have been influenced by his history. In a *transference interpretation*, viewed by many contemporary psychoanalytic psychotherapists as the most mutative intervention, the therapist makes explicit reference to what appears to be happening in the 'here and now' of the patient–therapist relationship, focusing on the most emotionally charged moments, or *affective focus*, of the therapy session. Here the patient's feelings and behaviour towards the therapist point to conflicts from the past that are being re-enacted in the transference situation. These significant interchanges are not thought to solely represent repetitions of the patient's past experiences, but are new experiences created by the therapist being experienced as a *new object*, with whom the patient can identify in a healthier way than he may have with significant objects or relationships in the past (see ➲Transference in Chapter 2, pp. 25).

Use of countertransference

(See ➲Countertransference in Chapter 2, pp. 25.)

The therapist's countertransference has become an essential part of psychoanalytic psychotherapy technique in informing the therapist's therapeutic interventions and interpretations. The emotional feelings and responses of the therapist to the patient can be understood as reflecting, in part, the unconscious projection of the patient's unconscious mental states. Here the patient cannot bear to recognize their thoughts and feelings as internal to themselves and therefore projects and attributes them to others, including the therapist. The person who has been invested with these unwanted aspects may, via projective identification, unconsciously identify with what has been projected into them and may be unconsciously pressurized by the patient to act in certain ways. The therapist's evolving awareness of her countertransference feelings and their enactments may therefore act as possible clues to what has been unconscious and offer new access to the patient's internal world.

Working through

Understanding the meaning of unconscious conflicts, defences, and resistances, giving up old patterns of thinking and behaviour, and tolerating new ways of psychic functioning and relating to others all take time and emotional work. The therapist must be prepared to interpret the same difficulties with the patient over and over again, as they manifest themselves both within the transference and in the patient's external life, before the patient feels that he has sufficient insight and control over his life to effect lasting changes. This, at times painful, 'working-through' process is one of the reasons why psychoanalytic psychotherapists advocate that therapy should be longer-term and open-ended, as well as more intensive where sessions are offered more frequently than once a week.

What changes?

Psychoanalytic psychotherapy is not primarily aimed at symptomatic alleviation, but at the underlying unconscious conflicts, beliefs, fantasies, and personality traits that give rise to distressing symptoms and problematic patterns of behaviour. However, few psychoanalytic psychotherapists today adhere to a notion of analytic cure or fundamental restructuring of a patient's personality but would more modestly aim for the patient to have a greater understanding of himself, so that he may exert more control over his life choices.

Most contemporary psychoanalytic theorists acknowledge that there is no one view of psychic change and that it is likely to be a complex process involving multiple modes of therapeutic action. Interventions facilitating change may be categorized into three categories:

- *Those that foster insight, e.g. interpretation, free association*: these techniques prioritize interpretation of the patient's defences and resistance to allow insight into the origin of unconscious conflicts and strengthening of the ego. Change involves understanding and resolving the conflicts of the past, so as to lessen the hold that they exert on present functioning, and enables actions to be less unconsciously dominated by the repetition compulsion. Unhelpful defences and character traits, which may have defended against real anxieties and may have been essential to psychic survival early in development, are now recognized as disproportionate to current reality and actively impeding healthy functioning and relationships. Change also involves the relinquishment of omnipotent and idealistic fantasies and a more realistic acceptance of life's compromises and uncertainties, to which more adaptive solutions may be found. Interpretation of the transference and the way in which the patients' difficulties unconsciously manifest themselves within the relationship with the therapist is crucial in effecting therapeutic change.
- *Those that make use of aspects of the therapeutic relationship*: the non-verbal relational affective experience that develops between the

patient and therapist is also an important mutative factor. Change involves the internalization of a new relationship or more 'benign superego' with the therapist, who is reliable and not retaliatory, which may be very different from the relationships the patient has previously experienced with parental figures. Here, the identification of prominent transference–countertransference paradigms within the therapeutic relationship is important.

- *Non-interpretative strategies, e.g. confrontation and suggestion, exposure, problem-solving, affirmation, and empathic validation*: since Freud, there has been a gradual shift in emphasis on psychoanalytic technique from reconstruction of childhood experience and the recovery of 'repressed memories' to a focus on more current and immediate 'here-and-now' interactions between patient and therapist within the transference. Contemporary technique is aimed more at helping patients construe narratives and ascribe meaning to their early experiences than trying to accurately reconstruct historical events or facts. Change occurs through identifying and making explicit the patient's unconscious or implicitly coded relational patterns via their emergence in the relationship formed with the therapist. This involves an increased capacity for mentalization, self-reflection, and processing of emotional experiences. Such a capacity, which is disrupted in many individuals who have experienced early attachment difficulties and environmental adversity, may develop within the safe attachment relationship to the therapist (see ➔Mentalization-based treatment in Chapter 2, pp. 66–70; Theories of personality development: attachment theory in Chapter 8, pp. 380–1.)

Clinical population and contexts

Contraindications for psychoanalytic psychotherapy

Freud believed that psychoanalysis was a treatment for neurosis and that it was not suitable for patients with psychotic illnesses, addictions, or serious character pathology, whom he thought lacked sufficient 'ego strength' to withstand the psychoanalytic method. For these patients, exploration of underlying unconscious conflicts and analysis of their defences could release intense anxieties and could make their symptoms or pathological behaviours worse. However, from the 1950s onwards, there was a 'widening scope' of psychoanalysis and its application to the treatment of psychological conditions other than neurosis, including delinquency, perversions, personality disorders, and psychoses, as well as for children and adolescents. Nevertheless, many psychoanalytic psychotherapists today would advocate a cautious and modified approach for patients with severe mental illnesses or personality disorders, often in a more supportive, rather than interpretative, direction. People with violent or suicidal tendencies, or those with drug and alcohol addictions, may not be suitable, as their problematic behaviours may worsen, at least in the short term, with psychotherapeutic treatment (see ➔Violence and aggression in Chapter 6, pp. 304–8; Suicide and self-harm in Chapter 6, pp. 308–11; Substance misuse in Chapter 7, pp. 338–45; Personality disorders in Chapter 8, pp. 384–422; Forensic psychiatry: forensic psychotherapies, applications, and research in Chapter 12, pp. 550–6).

Other exclusion criteria include patients with organic brain damage, such as dementia, who are unlikely to be able to make use of psychotherapy. Individuals with very low intelligence will preclude effective treatment with a verbally based therapy. However, patients with mild learning difficulties may be able to benefit with a modified approach but may require referral to a specialist psychotherapy service (see ➜Intellectual disability in Chapter 7, pp. 368–71).

Indications for psychoanalytic psychotherapy

Patients with less severe mental disorders, such as mild to moderate anxiety and depression, or personality difficulties, particularly in the interpersonal realm, are most likely to benefit from psychoanalytic psychotherapy. However, a formal psychiatric diagnosis is less helpful as a suitability indicator than an ability to engage in the therapeutic process and to be able to form and sustain a psychotherapeutic relationship. When assessing a patient's suitability for psychoanalytic psychotherapy, it is important to consider:

• Whether the person's difficulties are understandable in psychological terms
• Psychological mindedness (see Coltart below)
• Motivation for treatment
• Ego strength
• Capacity to form and sustain relationships
• External factors, including:
  • Time
  • Money if therapy is fee-paying
  • Distance and mobility
  • Presence of other supportive relationships in the patient's life which may sustain him between sessions.

Coltart (1988) identified the following features of *psychological mindedness*:

• Acknowledgement of unconscious mental life affecting the patient's thoughts and behaviour
• Capacity to give a self-aware history and to have some awareness of the emotional significance and meaning of past events
• Capacity to recall memories with appropriate affects
• Capacity to step back from one's story and reflect
• Willingness to take some responsibility for one's difficulties
• Use of imagination, e.g. metaphors or dreams
• Some signs of hope and self-esteem
• Capacity to recognize and tolerate internal anxiety with wishes and conflicts, and distinguish from external reality
• Curiosity and concern about internal reality
• Ability to make links between past and present.

Service provision

Psychoanalytic psychotherapy within the NHS was traditionally offered by specialized psychotherapy departments located within secondary mental health services. However, because of long-standing difficulties in convincingly demonstrating the efficacy and cost-effectiveness of this form of treatment, psychoanalytic psychotherapy has arguably been more vulnerable than other therapeutic modalities to its services being reduced within the public sector in the current era of economic constraints and reorganization of mental health services. Psychoanalytic psychotherapy services continue to be available in the NHS but are increasingly reserved for patients with chronic and entrenched psychological difficulties, particularly those with personality disorders. Intensive psychoanalytic psychotherapy continues to be offered in the NHS; in the midst of dramatic reduction in the length of therapies, this is in the context of psychoanalytic work applied in consultation for teams working with complex cases in acute and community psychiatry. The intensive work informs the applied work. Much longer-term psychotherapy is carried out by trainees who are supervised by more senior analyst therapists.

Case vignettes

Case one

Gemma was a 22-year-old design student referred for psychoanalytic psychotherapy, following completing eight sessions of CBT in IAPT services. Although her presenting symptoms of anxiety, depression, and obsessional thoughts that she was worthless had improved with this therapy, it was felt that she could benefit from longer-term therapy to explore the historical roots of her difficulties. She was assessed by an experienced psychoanalytic psychotherapist who noted her to have a harsh superego which constantly criticized and undermined her, making her feel stupid and not good enough. Attempts to cope with these unmanageable feelings led to episodes of binge drinking at least once a week.

Gemma was the youngest of three children, with two brothers who were much older than her. Her father left the family, when she was 5 years old, to live in another country, and she had little contact with him until recently. Her mother recently told her that he had left her for another woman, with whom he lived for 10 years. Gemma felt shocked and devastated by this revelation, feeling betrayed that everyone else in the family, including her older brothers, knew about it, except her, and she had been unable to speak about it with her family since.

Gemma always felt shy and unattractive, and had not had any relationships until 18 months prior to the referral, when she had started a relationship with a fellow student of the same age. However, when this progressed to sexual intercourse, her feelings of sexual arousal gave rise to feelings of guilt and the onset of her anxiety and obsessive–compulsive symptoms, and she ended the relationship abruptly. Since this time, she had formed several brief relationships with other young men but reported a pattern in which she would become quickly convinced that the boyfriend would not be interested in her; she would then reject his sexual advances and break up the relationship, before he rejected her.

Gemma was offered 1 year of weekly psychodynamic psychotherapy with a male core psychiatry trainee who was supervised by the original assessor. Gemma initially appeared to engage well in the therapy. A prominent theme that emerged fairly early was about her feeling left out of 'family secrets' and that she was always the last to know about significant events. She initially claimed that she remembered very little from her childhood, except that she was a sensitive child who often fell out with people. Although she claimed to have always had a good relationship with her mother and stepfather, whom her mother married when she was five, a picture emerged of parents who were relatively unaware of their timid child's needs, instead being more preoccupied with their own problems. Gemma's sense that her parents were not that interested in her contributed to her feelings of poor self-worth and lack of confidence.

It also emerged that Gemma's first sexual experience and the subsequent onset of her symptoms had coincided with discovering the real reason as to why her father had left the family in her early childhood. The therapist linked her discovery of her father's sexual betrayal of her mother to Gemma's feelings of guilt and anxiety in relation to her own sexual feelings towards her boyfriend. The therapist suggested that, perhaps at an unconscious level, Gemma had identified sex as something that was destructive and wrong, and gave rise to her symptoms of anxiety and checking.

Gemma appeared to understand and accept this (Oedipal) formulation (see ➲The Oedipus complex in Chapter 2, p. 22) at an intellectual level. However, her attendance subsequently became more erratic, and, when she did attend, she reported drinking more. She then missed three sessions, following the therapist's planned annual leave of 2 weeks. When she finally re-attended, after the therapist had written to her encouraging her to return to therapy, she said that she had been depressed with the conviction that she was too unattractive for anyone to be really interested in her.

The therapist suggested that Gemma had perhaps felt that he also sometimes was not very interested in her, and that his 2-week absence might have exacerbated these feelings, which she blocked out by drinking too much. Whilst Gemma initially rejected this transference interpretation by insisting that she knew that he had to go on holiday, she was able to acknowledge that perhaps she did sometimes feel that he must find her boring.

Three weeks later, the therapist had to cancel a session at short notice due to a family bereavement. Again, Gemma did not attend the subsequent session but did attend the one after. She expressed irritation at the therapist having to cancel a session so soon after his break, saying that it was clear that he had better things to do than to see her. This time, the therapist was able to more directly interpret Gemma's feelings of anger at feeling left and rejected by him. He suggested that she was experiencing him in a similar way not only to her boyfriends, whom she became convinced were not interested in her, but also to how she may have experienced her father when he originally left the family. He added that perhaps she was afraid that, if she remembered what had happened, she might become overwhelmed by unbearable feelings of rage and abandonment. He suggested that she avoided these feelings in her relationships by pre-empting the feared rejections by rejecting her boyfriends first. However, she did not have any control over him cancelling the sessions, which made her feel furious, rejected, and desperate.

Following this interpretation, Gemma cried for the first time in therapy, saying that she had always secretly blamed herself for her father leaving and believing that she must have been worthless for him to lose contact with her. Over the next few months, Gemma was able to gradually explore in more depth the links between her feelings of self-hatred and fears of rejection, and her experiences in childhood. She was also able to acknowledge that she sometimes had similar feelings towards her therapist and to better tolerate the painful and humiliating feelings that this engendered. They explored how she had protected her family (and her therapist by missing sessions) from her anger by avoiding conflict and directing her aggression towards herself in self-destructive behaviour, which included drinking and repeatedly sabotaging her relationships. She formed a relationship with another young man but this time did allow it to progress to full sexual intercourse, and was surprised when she did not feel as self-disgusted and anxious as she had anticipated.

Gemma was able to end therapy in a planned way and attend the final session, facilitated by the therapist actively interpreting, in the weeks leading up to this, her feelings of being rejected yet again and her wish to end prematurely to avoid these.

Case two

Carlo was a 33-year-old man who initially presented to his GP with low mood, anxiety, and panic attacks that had started after being fired from his job following a work-related injury to his back. He was screened by the local IAPT services, but his presentation was felt to be too complex, and so he was referred to the psychology therapies service where he received 16 sessions of CBT from an experienced male psychologist. He engaged well, and his symptoms improved, but he requested further therapy. He was referred for longer-term psychoanalytic psychotherapy and offered 12 months of individual weekly therapy with a female higher trainee in medical psychotherapy.

Carlo came from a large family in Southern Spain and was exposed to violence and deprivation throughout his childhood. He reported a difficult relationship with his mother who showed little affection towards him and would also beat him for minor misdemeanours. His father was involved in criminal activities and rarely at home, but Carlo had always admired him and sought his approval. Carlo was made to work since the age of 13 to help support his family, which prevented him from continuing his education.

When he was 18, and about to begin his mandatory military service, he was involved in a violent incident in which he assaulted a soldier with a broken bottle. This occurred just after discovering that his father was not his biological father. He spent 2 months in a military prison and was fined £30000, which took him several years to pay off. Since then, although he frequently got into verbal arguments with others, he had not committed any further violent acts.

He moved to London to escape his home environment where he quickly learned English and worked in a pub, initially as a bartender and later as shift manager. He worked for the same company for 8 years and took his job very seriously. He believed that there was no reason for him being fired and was furious with his employer for not rewarding him with any compensation. He had violent fantasies of skinning his former manager and expressed his intentions in great detail in the first few sessions of therapy.

At the start of therapy, Carlo was threatened with eviction from his flat in which he had been living for 5 years. He was not aware that the flat was sublet to him, and the original owner unexpectedly returned to claim the property. Carlo managed to get a temporary injunction against his eviction, but the case was still unresolved and awaiting court proceedings at the time of his initial presentation.

Carlo attended his sessions regularly, although he was repeatedly 10 minutes late. He often appeared angry and agitated, talking at length in a concrete fashion about his current unemployment and threatened eviction, and painting a picture in which he was the victim of an unjust society. He complained that his Spanish background influenced the way people saw him, and believed that people thought he came across as aggressive and bossy and that no one could appreciate that he actually felt very vulnerable and might 'flip' and become violent or suicidal. He also expressed feelings of shame and worthlessness regarding his lack of education and that he had nothing to contribute. He frequently ignored the therapist's comments or interpretations and she often felt intimidated, silenced or viewed with contempt by him during the sessions. He complained that the sessions were not helping, unlike his previous sessions with his (male) therapist, or even his physiotherapist (who was also male).

A few months into therapy, Carlo was evicted from his property following the court hearing, but reported that this had been an empowering experience, as the (male) judge had been sympathetic and he felt listened to. He found temporary accommodation, which allowed him to continue to come to sessions regularly, and now on time. Having, until that point, appeared reluctant to discuss his past, saying that he was 'over it' and that it had nothing to do with his current situation, following his eviction, he began to discuss his family and childhood experiences more openly. He related much admiration for his stepfather but, when talking about his mother, would become angry and agitated. He described her as 'manipulative, ignorant, and evil' and attributed his move to London as an attempt to shake off any association with her.

He expressed how difficult it was for him to open up and show his weaknesses, particularly to a woman. He then asked whether he could attend the sessions once every 2 weeks for a period of 2 years, instead of weekly for 1 year, and expressed irritation when the therapist said this was not possible and suggested that it might be a way of prolonging the therapy without feeling too dependent on her. Nevertheless, the therapist felt that Carlo was gradually becoming more reflective in sessions and able to consider her interpretations, and he also reported feeling more positive in his external life.

However, Carlo did not return to sessions, following the therapist's 3-week planned summer break, and did not respond to letters. The therapist contacted his GP who reported that Carlo had moved out of the area. A few months later, the therapist was contacted by solicitors acting for Carlo to request a report on his therapy for his tribunal against his employers for unfair dismissal. When she declined to do this on the basis that this was not in the patient's best interests, she received a formal complaint from Carlo saying that the therapy had been useless and had made him more depressed.

The complaint was not upheld by the Trust, but, on discussion with her supervisor, the therapist reflected on the dynamics of the therapy and concluded that several factors appeared to have contributed towards Carlo's difficulties in engaging in psychoanalytic psychotherapy and in his premature termination of the treatment. At the time of referral, Carlo had been recently sacked from his job and threatened with eviction. This lack of external support and stability undermined an already fragile capacity for reflection or mentalization, and his initial presentation in sessions was very concrete. He appeared to have experienced his female therapist in the transference as a threatening maternal object on whom he was terrified of becoming too dependent. To defend against these anxieties, he employed primitive defence mechanisms of splitting, idealization, and denigration in comparing her unfavourably to his male therapists and the judge, defences that were also evident in his attitude towards his stepfather and mother. Although not overtly violent, his aggression was enacted implicitly in the sessions in his bullying and contemptuous attitude towards his therapist. However, after feeling 'heard' by the judge, representing a helpful paternal figure, he began to feel more 'heard' by his therapist, which seemed to open up a therapeutic space in which a more mutual and meaningful interchange could occur. However, he appears to have experienced her break as an abrupt rejection and betrayal, precipitating a regression into a more primitive and paranoid frame of mind, and re-enacting not only his initial presentation—the therapist is dismissed, as he was from his job—but also the original rejection by both his parents, which perpetuates his sense of victimization.

Recommended reading

Coltart N (1992). Diagnosis and assessment of suitability for psychoanalytic psychotherapy. In: *Slouching Towards Bethlehem and Further Psychoanalytic Explorations*. Free Association Books: London.

Gabbard GO (2010). *Long-Term Psychodynamic Psychotherapy: A Basic Text*, second edition. American Psychiatric Publishing: Arlington.

Gabbard GO and Westen D (2003). Rethinking therapeutic action. *International Journal of Psychoanalysis*, **84**, 823–41.

Greenson R (1967). *The Technique and Practice of Psychoanalysis*, volume 1. Hogarth Press: London.

Sandler J and Dreher AU (1996). *What Do Psychoanalysts Want? The Problems of Aims in Psychoanalytic Therapy*. Routledge: London.

Cognitive behavioural therapy

(See ➜Cognitive behavioural therapy in Chapter 2, pp. 30–4.)

Key techniques and competencies

CBT is not a series of techniques to be performed in a mechanistic way; on the contrary, CBT is an art, each therapy tailored to the individual via the formulation, with room for creativity in how the problematic areas are addressed. The range of CBT techniques available is huge, and the choice of technique will depend on the problem or diagnosis. What follows are some general principles to help the reader get started.

CBT treatment can be divided into three phases:

• *Assessment and formulation*: problems and goals are defined, and the formulation mapped out, detailing what is keeping the problem going and laying the foundations for interventions.

• *Intervention stage*: appropriate interventions, e.g. activity scheduling, behavioural experiments, thought monitoring, and restructuring are considered and carried out to bring about overall change in the problem.

• *Consolidation and relapse prevention stage*: key things that have been learnt in therapy are carefully detailed and noted, so that they can be generalized and referred to, should the problem recur in the future.

Underpinning competencies

The whole of the therapy will be underpinned by certain principles and techniques.

• *Structure and agenda setting*: the therapy is highly structured. At the beginning of each session, the therapist asks the patient the question 'What would you like to put on the agenda?' but also has an idea of what they would like to cover in the session. Standard items will include homework review, mood check (0–10), feedback from previous session, homework setting, and generally one to two items only on which to work in that particular session, relevant to the stage in therapy and preferably generated by the patient. At the beginning, the agenda is more likely to be therapist-led, whilst more patient-led as the therapy progresses. The rationale is that this keeps the therapy more focused and avoids the situation at the end of the session where the patient says that they need to talk about something very important, but there is no time left. It necessitates both patient and therapist doing some advance thinking and preparation regarding the oncoming session.

• *Collaborative nature*: the therapy is collaborative in nature, meaning that, whilst the therapist may be an expert in psychiatry and CBT, the patient is an expert in the nature of their difficulties, and both areas of expertise are equally important. The therapist does not assume superiority but relates to the patient with respect, as an equal. The idea is that the pair work together to solve the problem being brought to therapy. Both patient and therapist need to be equally active.

• *Feedback and summaries*: the therapist does not make interpretations. Instead they are careful to only use and summarize the words the patient has used. Indeed, they make frequent summaries and encourage the patient to do the same. Feedback is frequently requested both at the beginning and end of the session, but also throughout the session.

• *Socratic questioning and guided discovery*: the therapist uses a form of questioning called 'Socratic questioning', described as 'the cornerstone of cognitive therapy' (Padesky, 1993). This involves using questions to help guide the patient to think differently or come up with solutions to their own problems, rather than making suggestions for them to follow. The therapist adopts an attitude of genuine curiosity and is often unclear as to what the end result of the conversation will be. Poor Socratic questioning, however, can feel interrogative in nature, e.g. when the therapist asks questions in such a way that the patient believes they need to find the right answer, 'Dr Cooper, whatever is it you want me to tell you? Just let me know, and I'll tell you!'.

- *Formulation-driven*: therapy is not a mechanistic cook book procedure but is something unique to each patient, and treatment is based on an individual formulation of each patient (see ➜Cognitive behavioural assessment and formulation in Chapter 4, pp. 135–40). This is begun at the first meeting but is dynamic in nature, being constantly updated if new information arises, and is referred to throughout therapy to help guide interventions and explain any ruptures.
- *Therapeutic relationship*: engagement is crucial; unless the therapist builds some rapport with the patient in the early sessions, they are unlikely to return. In CBT, this is as important as in any other therapy, particularly with patients with complex disorders where the interactions between patient and therapist are prominent, and the formulation can be used to understand this better. However, unlike in some other therapies, whilst the relationship is important and necessary, it is not considered sufficient to bring about change.
- *Empirical nature*: CBT has held on to its behavioural traditions, and therapists are expected to keep up-to-date with the latest evidence base and use a standard treatment approach, if this has been shown to work. Various models and protocols for the treatment of specific disorders, including panic disorder, social anxiety disorder, PTSD, and OCD, have been developed and well validated, with which the therapist should be familiar and follow where this is the presenting problem. However, it is important to emphasize that therapy is never about fitting a patient into a box or model, and, even when using models, these are individualized for the particular patient. In addition, therapy itself adopts a scientific enquiry approach, with the carrying out of behavioural experiments to provide new information and test hypotheses (see ➜Cognitive behavioural therapy in Chapter 2, pp. 30–4; Outcome research in psychotherapy in Chapter 11, pp. 518–19).
- *Homework*: the majority of work takes place in the hours between sessions, with the patient first monitoring their problematic behaviours or thoughts and then practising new ways of thinking or behaving.

Key techniques

The choice of individual techniques will depend on the stage of therapy:

1. *Assessment stage*

By the end of this stage, the therapist should have:
- Socialized the patient to the format of a CBT session, e.g. agenda setting

- A written problem definition
- Goals for therapy
- An initial diagrammatic formulation of the problem (see ➲ Cognitive behavioural assessment and formulation in Chapter 4, pp. 135–40)
- A reasonable rapport with the patient.

A typical agenda for session 1 includes:
- Introduction
- Practicalities of therapy, e.g. how long the sessions last for, who will you contact if you cannot come, where the sessions will take place
- Current difficulties (aim for problem definition/beginnings of formulation
- Goals for therapy
- Feedback
- Homework.

Useful techniques include:
- *Problem definition:* aim for written definition of the patient's problem in terms of thoughts, feelings, behaviour, and physiology, e.g. 'I have a problem going out, because, every time I try to go out, I think that I am going to have a panic attack; this makes me feel very anxious, and I get lots of physical symptoms, and the only way to get rid of them is not to go out.'
- *Goal setting,* e.g. 'By the end of therapy, what will you be doing that you are not doing now? You say you want to feel better. If you are feeling better, what will be different, what will you be doing that is different? How will you know that you are feeling better?'
- *Socratic questioning* to develop formulation (see ➲ 'Socratic questioning and guided discovery' bullet point in Chapter 5, Underpinning competencies, pp. 173–4).
- *Monitoring techniques* to gain information for the formulation or about the problem, e.g. diaries to provide examples of problematic situations. This involves getting the patient to write down examples of the problematic behaviour or situation, and maybe looking at frequency or associated thoughts and feelings.
- *Behavioural experiments* to help patients gather information for the formulation or decide whether therapy is for them.

2. Intervention stage
In this stage, the therapist builds on the work done already, but particularly helps the patient make changes in some of the areas which are keeping the problem going. The formulation is used to identify these areas, which will tend to be in the cognitive or behavioural domain. The formulation, particular problem or diagnosis, and patient preference will dictate whether cognitive or behavioural techniques will be used first.

Behavioural activation
This is usually the first treatment of choice in depression, particularly in ruminators or where the person is too depressed to concentrate on their thinking. It involves helping a person first monitor their activities and corresponding mood, thus helping the patient and therapist get an overall picture of the activity level. It also helps the patient identify any activities which are associated with low mood or which improve it (see Table 5.1).

Table 5.1 Sample activity diary

	Mon	Tues	Wed	Thurs	Fri	Sat	Sun
7–8	Woke up 80						
8–9	Shower 75						
9–10	Sat on sofa, avoiding paperwork 90						
10–11	Did paperwork 70						
11–12	Sister came round 50						
12–1	Sister 50						
1–2	Sister 50						
2–3	On own, on sofa, surfing web 75						
3–4	Ruminating 80						
4–5	Avoid meeting 90						
5–6	Went to bed 90						
6–7	Bed 90						
7–8	Bed 90						
8–9	Bed 90						
9–10	Bed 90						

Fill in at least every 2 hours, recording very briefly what you did and the corresponding mood rating, e.g. depression on a scale of 0–100 where 0 = not depressed at all and 100 = the most depressed you could possibly be.

Once a baseline is established, and the patient buys the idea that activating is good, a plan can be developed to build on helpful activities, even if the person does not feel like doing so.

Values identification helps the patient identify areas in life that are important and meaningful to them, and thus they can work towards activities and goals that are meaningful to them and consistent with their values.

Cognitive techniques
Given Beck's original model suggests that it is not the situation that causes the problem but how we appraise it, then it is not surprising that a good part of the therapy may be directed at helping people make changes in their thinking styles. This may have to wait, until after mood has improved via behavioural activation, or may even be unnecessary. Different levels of cognition may be considered (see ➲ Cognitive behavioural therapy in Chapter 2, pp. 30–4).

Unhelpful thinking patterns: what are they, and what do we do with them?
Beck described typical thinking patterns that occur in depression, which have been variously called cognitive biases, dysfunctional thoughts, and

thinking errors, but may be more clinically acceptable and less pejorative if simply called unhelpful thinking styles. These are:

• Not unique to patients
• Habitual ways of processing information
• Can be unhelpful
• More prevalent/extreme in, e.g. depression/anxiety.

We tend to think that our thoughts are facts, but just because we think something does not make it true, e.g. 'The world is flat' was a prevalent thought for many years!'

Beck's original list comprised:

• *Arbitrary inference*: jumping to conclusions, fortune telling, mind reading, making judgements in the absence of supporting evidence, e.g. 'They are laughing. Therefore, they must be laughing at me.'
• *Selective abstraction* (mental filter): focusing on whatever went badly and ignoring anything else that may have happened, e.g. 'The IT failed, so the lecture was ruined.'
• *Overgeneralization*: one thing going badly means it is all bad, e.g. 'I've been turned down at one interview; therefore, I'll never get a job.'
• *Magnification and minimization*: when things go well, this is not important, but, when they go badly, this is given a disproportionately large level of significance.
• *Personalization*: taking things personally, e.g. 'I'm responsible for things going wrong.'
• *Absolutist, dichotomous thinking*: black-and-white/all-or-nothing thinking, e.g. 'I'm great or I'm hopeless. There are no shades of grey.'

Over the years, these have been modified and added to and adapted. Other useful categories include:

• *Unrealistic expectations/high standards*, e.g. 'I ought to be the best; I should always work hard; I must do everything perfectly.'
• *Catastrophization*, e.g. 'My husband is late home. He must have had a car crash.'
• *Disqualifying the positive*: rejecting anything positive such as compliments, e.g. 'He's only saying that to be nice.'
• *Emotional reasoning*, e.g. 'I feel awful. Therefore, it is awful.'
• *Self-criticism and name calling*, e.g. 'You idiot!'

How is this used in therapy?

Having identified problems to work on, the patient is asked to bring examples of these to sessions, and these are used to identify and explore the typical thinking patterns further, and the patient is helped to develop more helpful perspectives, initially in therapy and then on their own.

The following steps may be a useful guide:

• Introduce the idea of thought as an area which can be addressed to help improve mood
• Get the patient to monitor thoughts at times of low mood or problematic behaviour, using a thought record form with columns for situation, thoughts, and feelings (0–100%) (see Table 5.2).
• Educate, if necessary, regarding the difference between thoughts and feelings

Table 5.2 Sample thought record

Date/time	Situation	Thoughts (rate belief in thought, 0–100%)	Feelings (rate, 0–100%)	Alternative perspective

- Introduce the idea regarding 'hot cognitions', i.e. those thoughts which are particularly causing distress
- Introduce the idea of unhelpful thinking patterns: give handout, and see if any applies
- Look for any themes through monitoring
- Learn to 'decentre' from thoughts by noticing what the patient is doing and stating to self what they are doing, e.g. this is a catastrophic thought
- Understand where these thoughts come from, through joint exploration of history
- Look at pros and cons of thinking like this
- Learn to question these thoughts and hence develop new perspectives.

Questions to ask to help develop new perspectives
The therapist will use questions similar to these in sessions to help the patient begin developing new perspectives and to use time between sessions to question their thoughts independently, so learning to be their own therapist. Choice of question will depend on the problem and particular thinking style.

- What are the advantages and disadvantages of thinking like this?
- What is the worst thing that could happen? Would you cope?
- What has led you to come to this conclusion? What would you cite as evidence to support this viewpoint?
- What does not fit with this idea? What does not support this viewpoint?
- Can you think of other explanations? Other possibilities?
- What would you say to a friend or loved one who had this thought?
- What would a friend say to you regarding this?
- How would your friend cope with this situation?
- Are there things that you are overlooking, because you are distressed?
- Have you been in this situation before and felt differently?
- Have you coped when you felt like this before? What did you do? If you could remove yourself from this situation, what would you think?
- How would you view it in 5 years' time?
- Are there other ways of looking at this situation?
- What are you missing?
- Is it really so bad?
- Are you giving myself too hard a time? Are other factors or people involved?
- Regarding name calling, is this helpful?
- Would you say this to someone else?

Rumination/worry or obsessional thinking

In depression, when challenging seems to make things worse, it is likely that the patient is ruminating, and just encouraging further introspection is not helpful. In this case, taking a process-driven approach may be more useful:

- Am I ruminating?
- Is there anything I can do about this situation? If yes, do it!
- If no, distract, do, and act according to plan, rather than how you feel, e.g. behavioural activation! Notice the surroundings! Be in the here and now! Physical exercise.

Working with worry or obsessions will require a similar approach, and well-validated protocols have been developed to address these areas.

Summarizing

It is useful to draw things together, using Socratic questions such as:

- Bearing in mind what we have just discussed, do you still have the same conclusion, or have you come to any alternative conclusion?
- What is it?

Behavioural experiments (based on Bennett-Levy et al.)

Frequently, and particularly when working with anxiety, just discussing thoughts is not enough. Anxiety formulations usually demonstrate that, when confronted with a feared situation, patients have thoughts about the likelihood and perceived awfulness of the feared outcome, which make them anxious, and they behave in ways to prevent this feared outcome, known as safety behaviours, to reduce their anxiety. Unfortunately, behaving in this way only serves to reinforce the idea that the bad thing would have happened, if the person had not, for example, left the situation. But how do they know this is true, if they never stayed in the situation?

Clearly, therapy will involve them needing to learn to behave differently, getting rid of their safety behaviours, and allowing themselves to feel anxious. Behavioural experiments are used in such circumstances and are particularly powerful in helping patients make changes. Their use, of course, is not restricted to anxiety disorders and may be particularly helpful also in testing out rules for living.

These might be carried out to:

- Further develop the case formulation
- Evaluate the accuracy of problematic thoughts, or
- Help develop and test out more helpful ways of appraising things.

Experiments can further be divided into those that are principally about testing a hypothesis, e.g. 'When I walk down the street, everyone is going to laugh at me', versus those that are more about discovering information, e.g. someone with panic disorder may be unable to articulate or remember their exact cognitions when they are anxious, but an experiment to induce anxiety in session may help provide this information. Other discovery experiments might help the patient find out what happens, if they behave in a different way than usual.

Finally, they can additionally be divided into active experiments where the patient and therapist together design new ways to address problematic patterns and actively set up situations to test this out. By contrast, observational experiments involve the patient in a more passive role, gathering data, e.g. watching their therapist role playing or collecting information via a survey.

How to design a behavioural experiment
- *Planning*:
  - Is there a clear and explicit reason for the experiment, and is this shared by both therapist and patient, e.g. 'to find out whether my belief that everyone talks about me and laughs at me is true or not'?
  - What target thought are you testing out? Explicitly identify what thought you are testing out, e.g. 'When I walk down the road, people point at me and laugh.' How much do you believe this on a scale of 0–100? Is there a different way of looking at things?
  - Assess the intensity of emotions (0–100).
  - Are there any unhelpful safety behaviours which might get in the way? Do these need to be addressed first?
  - What is the best way to test this out?
  - Where and when?
  - What might go wrong? How will you cope if x happens?
  - Can we make it a win–win situation, no matter what happens?
  - How are you going to measure outcome? How will you record this?
  - Is it doable?
- *Do it!*
- *Reflect on what happened*:
  - What happened? What did you notice?
  - What sense do you make of this?
  - What have you learnt from this?
  - How does this fit with your beliefs?
  - What can you do next to build on this?

Learning to accept
Sometimes therapy is less about change and more about helping the individual realize that unpleasant thoughts and/or feelings are going to occur. For example, fighting intrusive thoughts in OCD only makes them worse, and having a target of getting rid of all such thoughts will not be achievable. Instead therapy helps one develop a different relationship with their thoughts, learning to cope with them, and carry on regardless. Similarly, many people struggle to tolerate distress or anxiety, and often therapy may be about helping people address this. For example, someone with social anxiety may need to learn that certain situations are always going to produce anxiety. However, just because they are anxious does not mean they cannot carry on functioning perfectly adequately. Learning that this anxiety will not go away but can be lived with is an important learning point.

Working with rules and beliefs
This should never be the first target for change. For many problems, it is not necessary to address these, but, in complex cases, they may need addressing. Possible approaches may be:
- Validating the development and holding of the rule or belief through careful exploration of history and origins of the rule

- Historical record to look in detail at life to explore history that does and does not fit with belief
- Introducing the idea that they are beliefs, not facts
- Exploring Padesky's idea of seeing negative beliefs as prejudice against the self
- Looking at the pros and cons for continuing to hold these beliefs
- Using imagery techniques to reconstruct traumatic incidents in childhood, introducing a kind figure to alter the situation
- Developing alternative rules
- Using behavioural experiments to find out what happens when a rule is not kept to
- Using continuums to help patients find shades of grey and be more flexible
- Developing positive data logs to identify information that supports a newer, more adaptive belief
- Constructing flashcards to remind them of their new beliefs.

3. Consolidation stage: summary of therapy

Ideally, therapy ending should be planned and worked towards. Rather than a sad affair, the ending can be likened to a graduation where the patient now has learnt skills that they can begin to use on their own in the world, and, although it may be a little scary, it is also exciting!

Around three sessions before the end, a useful task is to give the patient a homework task of writing a summary of what they have learnt in sessions, a written document to which they can then refer if things become problematic in the future. A handout with questions to guide the process is best such as:

- What was the original problem?
- What kept it going?
- What ideas have you learnt in therapy to help you deal with the problem?
- Write about these in detail.
- What effect have these had on the problem?
- How are you going to build on these ideas for the future?
- What are you going to do, if things go wrong in the future?
- Can you write a step-by-step plan to guide you for this possibility?

Remaining sessions provide an opportunity to review this, but it should primarily be the patient's own work, not written by the therapist.

What changes?

Beck's cognitive theory suggests that problems arise because of problems in the way we think, i.e. the negative automatic thoughts and underlying beliefs. Therefore, therapy is directed at helping patients change these thought patterns, thus leading to a shift for the better in the underlying problematic mood. Changing behaviour can also have this effect, either directly or through its effect on altering the underlying belief. The overall drive is towards symptom change.

However, particularly when working with worriers, ruminators, or obsessive thinkers, it is clear that focusing on trying to change these thinking styles is unhelpful and that therapy is more usefully directed at helping people learn to accept, change their relationship with their thoughts, or distance themselves from such thoughts, rather than trying to change or get rid of them. Indeed, the research shows that the challenging of traditional CBT itself works by helping people label and distance themselves from their thoughts.

Clinical populations and contexts

CBT is now used in most clinical settings. The IAPT programme (see ➔ Improving Access to Psychological Therapies services in Chapter 10, pp. 463–4) has led to the widespread availability of CBT in primary care settings across England, mainly for anxiety disorders and mild depression. More complex presentations, or those with additional risk issues, tend to be seen in secondary care settings where, dependent on resources, CBT is likely to be available and offered. NICE recommendations for all patients with schizophrenia to be offered CBT has led to some mismatch between assumed need and availability, although this has led to some initiatives to train community mental health staff in CBT. Within specialist services, such as eating disorder services, trauma services, personality disorder services, and CAMHS, CBT may be offered as a treatment of choice. In addition, there are examples of it being used within intermediary care settings and with inpatient populations.

Case vignettes

Case one

Bill was a 28-year-old man who worked as a teacher and was referred for therapy by his GP. He had been feeling increasingly low for the last 12 months, following the death of his mother, but had felt particularly worse over the last month. This recent deterioration had been precipitated by a row at work with a colleague, following which he had gone off sick, but there was also a pending disciplinary hearing about this.

Since stopping working, he had ceased to go out of the house. Although he had a wide circle of friends, he had stopped socializing and had not been answering the phone to them. He struggled to care for himself, no longer enjoyed anything, and spent most of his day on the sofa. He felt very tired, although he was not doing anything. Whilst on the sofa, he thought, 'How have I got myself into this mess? I'm going to get sacked and never find another job. It's all my fault—I really am useless. There is no point speaking to anyone, as everyone will think I'm a waste of space.' He had started to think that he might be better off dead, and, although he did not like this thought, as it made him feel even more useless, it kept niggling away at him.

Initial formulation helped him to identify that his constant barrage of negative thoughts only served to reduce his mood further, which made him very lethargic and led to the behaviour of isolating himself and doing nothing, which made him more tired and led to a further barrage of critical thoughts and compounded his low mood. Seeing this drawn out visually helped him recognize the vicious circle in which he was trapped and realize that the only areas amenable to change were his thoughts and behaviour. It was decided to focus on his behaviour first, which was his choice and also wise in this circumstance. Although Bill did not feel like being active, he accepted that he needed to act according to a plan to improve his mood by building activity. Indeed, he began speaking to his sister again, as well as contacting friends he was rather embarrassed to have dropped, and got a good reception. He began to notice that this made his mood lift slightly. He then contacted work and organized to meet with his managers, which he had been putting off. He also started playing his guitar again. With his mood lifting, he was then able to learn to notice the thoughts that led him to avoid situations, e.g. when the phone rang, he would think, 'It's work ringing to have a go at me. Everyone hates me' and not answer, and he was able to learn to question himself and also test out whether these thoughts were true. This allowed him to realize that most calls were concerned friends, and even work were more concerned about him, rather than wanting to have a go at him. He did eventually have a reconciliation meeting with the colleague which went well, and he was able to go back to work.

Case two

George presented with anxiety in public and subsequent difficulty going out. He lived with his elderly parents, and motivation for therapy was concern for how he would survive when they died. He had had a sexual relationship with his karate teacher when he was 18 years old and had since believed that this man spied on him, followed him, and generally kept tabs on him. As a result, he had been unable to get on with his life and now, at age 40, lived with his parents, unable to hold down a job or be in a relationship.

On going out of the house, he believed that people knew all about him, and this made him anxious. He tended to avoid eye contact, hurried in and out of shops, and spent a lot of time caught up in his head, worrying about others' views of him. From therapy, he wanted to be able to go shopping without scuttling out after 3 minutes, and attend some social groups and possibly educational courses.

Therapy involved mapping out the pattern of thoughts, feelings, and behaviours whenever he entered social or other situations outside his house. It also involved exploring the history that had led up to this and identifying that, because of his beliefs, he overestimated the likelihood that he was being followed and that there might be a more innocent explanation for why he bumped into people.

George gradually widened his social repertoire and became more comfortable outside his house through a series of behavioural experiments, checking out if anything terrible happened if he made eye contact. Whilst his underlying beliefs did not change, by the end of therapy, George was more active, had made a number of acquaintances, and had commenced on an art course at a local centre.

Recommended reading

Bennett-Levy J, Butler G, Fennell M, Hackmann A, Mueller M, and Westbrook D (2004). *Oxford Guide to Behavioural Experiments in Cognitive Therapy.* Oxford University Press: Oxford.

Moore R and Garland A (2003). *Cognitive Therapy for Chronic and Persistent Depression.* Wiley: Chichester.

Padesky CA (1993). *Socratic Questioning: Changing Minds or Guided Discovery?* Congress of the European Association of Behavioural and Cognitive Therapies: London. Available at: www.padesky.com

Teasdale JD, Moore RG, Hayhurst H, Pope M, Williams S, and Segal ZV (2002). Metacognitive awareness and prevention of relapse in depression: empirical evidence. *Journal of Consulting and Clinical Psychology*, **70**, 275–87.

Waddington L (2002). The therapy relationship in cognitive therapy: a review. *Behavioural and Cognitive Psychotherapy*, **30**, 179–91.

Wells A (1997). *Cognitive Therapy of Anxiety Disorders: A Practice Manual and Conceptual Guide*. Wiley: Chichester.

Westbrook D, Kennerley H, and Kirk J (2007). *An Introduction to Cognitive Behaviour Therapy: Skills and Applications*. Sage: London.

Systemic family and couple therapy

(See ➔ Systemic family and couple therapy in Chapter 2, pp. 34–42.)

Key techniques and competencies

Systemic family therapists employ a wide range of therapeutic skills and techniques, some more generic in nature, and others more specific to the particular theoretical orientation of the therapist.

General competencies

- Working with a team and accepting live supervision via a screen/ reflecting team
- Stance of neutrality, curiosity, and not knowing: the therapist uses their knowledge in a tentative and provisional manner as food for dialogue, rather than being authoritative
- Engaging with the family on their own terms, using their language, i.e. joining
- Assuming cultural relativity and a capacity to talk openly about culture, race, religion, class, sex, and power in a respectful manner
- Awareness of attachment patterns and trans-generational transmission (see ➔ Theories of personality development: attachment theory in Chapter 8, pp. 380–1)
- Awareness of family life cycle (see ➔ Life: cradle to grave in Chapter 6, pp. 284–93)
- Containment of emotionally intense interactions, facilitating the disclosure of feelings or divulging of family secrets (see ➔ Dealing with emotions in Chapter 3, pp. 100–2)
- Working/liaising with the wider system.

Specific techniques

- Questioning, e.g. who defines the problem? How does the family maintain the problem? How does the problem constrain relationships? What change in understanding, communication, or behaviour would shift the problem? What are the resources for change?
- Circular questioning such as:
  - Questions with an embedded suggestion, e.g. 'What would it be like, if *x* didn't come round every day?'
  - Triadic questions, e.g. 'What does *z* think when *x* and *y* are quarrelling?'
  - Future hypothetical questions, e.g. 'Where would you like to be in 5 years?'

- Connecting behaviour and emotion, e.g. 'Does x behave better or worse when you feel sad?'
- Process interrupting, e.g. 'So when you get angry at home, does x go quiet like she is now?'
- Normative comparisons, e.g. 'Do you think that x is typical of someone at that age/with a chronic illness, etc.?'
- Miracle questions, e.g. 'If you woke up and the problem had gone, what would it be like at home?'
- Reframing, positive connotation, inspiring hope.
- Hypothesizing, e.g. 'I wonder if what has happened in the family is that you have divorced your husband and married your son?'
- Self-reflexivity, e.g. 'It must be hard to imagine that a middle-class, middle-aged woman therapist can have much clue about the reality of your life as a young black man living in Brixton.'
- Externalization, e.g. 'How can anorexia have a less powerful influence in your life?'
- Scaling: 'Who gets most/least upset when mum gets drunk?'
- Modelling, e.g. of tolerance of difference
- Contracting, e.g. 'Take 5 minutes each to listen to the other's day.'
- Role play or 'interviewing the internalized other'. This powerful technique is when a couple role play each other in a discussion, thereby gaining experience of each other's attitude. They then come out of the role and reflect on what they have learnt.
- Use of genograms and mapping the wider system, e.g. social services, school, etc.
- Play techniques and use of drawing with younger children.
- Working with multifamily groups.

What changes?

Outcome studies have shown the general therapeutic effectiveness of family therapy, without analysing particular areas of improvement.

Specific areas which are clinically salient and merit further research include:

- Optimism regarding possibility of change and improvement
- Realism regarding the extent of possible change and acceptance of intractability of some situations
- Recognition of losses and regrets
- Diminution of blame and guilt
- Increased mentalization, awareness of the perception of the others in the family
- Improved direct communication with reduced mindreading and assumptions regarding the other
- Safer expression of negative feelings
- Enhanced self-respect of the family members
- Sense of empowerment to make changes and continue to develop after the end of therapy.

Clinical populations and contexts

Systemic family therapists are employed in primary care, CMHTs, inpatient settings, schools, social services, and third sector agencies.

However, given the extensive evidence base for the effectiveness and wide applicability of the model, it is striking how patchy and unsatisfactory the delivery of family therapy and family intervention has been across the UK, with notable exceptions.

Systemic family therapy has shown to be effective in the treatment and management of a wide range of mental disorders, illnesses, and problematic behaviours, including:

- Psychosis, including early-onset psychosis and puerperal psychosis (see ➔ Psychoses in Chapter 7, pp. 331–4)
- Personality disorder (see ➔ Personality disorder in Chapter 8, pp. 384–422)
- Mood disorders, including bipolar disorder (see ➔ Affective disorders in Chapter 7, pp. 326–31)
- Anxiety disorders, including agoraphobia (see ➔ Anxiety and anxiety disorders in Chapter 7, pp. 324–6)
- Conversion disorders
- Addictions, including dual diagnosis addiction and SMI (see ➔ Substance misuse in Chapter 7, pp. 338–45)
- Learning difficulties, including chronic severe problems, autistic features, challenging behaviours, with or without psychotic features (see ➔ Intellectual disability in Chapter 7, pp. 368–71)
- OCD
- Eating disorders (see ➔ Eating disorders in Chapter 7, pp. 334–8)
- MUS (see ➔ Medically unexplained symptoms in Chapter 7, pp. 359–63)
- Chronic physical illness
- Deliberate self-harm (see ➔ Suicide and self-harm in Chapter 6, pp. 308–11).

Systemic family therapy may be applied in a range of settings and services, including:

- Psychosis and rehabilitation services, e.g. Care Programme Approach (CPA) meetings may be used as family sessions, in which there is the opportunity to enhance communication, show respect for different family members' perspectives, and decrease mutual blame and negative expressed emotion (see ➔ Psychoses in Chapter 7, pp. 331–4; Rehabilitation and social psychiatry: psychotherapies, applications, and research in Chapter 12, pp. 568–73)
- Forensic services, e.g. family sessions with parents may be used to support the patient's move from inpatient to the community (see ➔ Forensic psychiatry: forensic psychotherapies, applications, and research in Chapter 12, pp. 550–6)
- Services for learning difficulties, e.g. family therapy may be indicated where families are disillusioned and cynical regarding services; to support the involvement of the family in decision-making; and addressing issues of over-involvement versus detachment (see ➔ Intellectual disability in Chapter 7, pp. 368–71; Psychiatry of intellectual disability: psychotherapies, applications, and research in Chapter 12, pp. 562–4)
- Services for older adults, e.g. addressing long-standing relationship problems exacerbated by dementia, disinhibition, challenging behaviour including domestic violence, living with physical

co-morbidity, or hoarding. Flexibility of model, offering therapy at home or in the clinic (see → Dementia in Chapter 7, pp. 372–6; Psychiatry of old age: psychotherapies, applications, and research in Chapter 12, pp. 565–7)

• Perinatal services, e.g. working in the mother and baby unit, with the wider system, alongside mother–infant psychotherapy and pharmacotherapy, multidisciplinary work (see → Parent–infant psychotherapy in Chapter 12, p. 559);

• CAMHS: 48% of children attending CAMHS have a parent with a mental health problem. Family therapy may be useful for behavioural problems, eating disorders, school refusal, encopresis, school disruption, adoption, and fostering (see → Child and adolescent psychiatry: child and adolescent psychotherapies, applications, and research in Chapter 12, pp. 556–61)

• Liaison with social services regarding child protection, across CAMHS/ adults services divide, support of parenting in mentally ill parents.

Systemic family therapy may also be used to address:

• Chaotic families with health and social service involvement, including child physical, sexual, or emotional abuse
• Couple relationship problems, including gay, lesbian, bisexual, transgender couples
• Family crises, e.g. adolescent suicidal behaviour, bereavement, new serious diagnosis.

Case vignettes

Case one

A married couple Jeff and Jenny presented with relationship difficulties linked to Jeff's bipolar illness.

Jeff had had several admissions over the previous 5 years and was in a job that he felt did not reflect his ability. He was depressed about his diagnosis and his career, and was significantly overweight. Jenny felt angry that Jeff used his low mood to avoid the hard work of bringing up their two young children. She found him self-absorbed and apathetic, and she felt lonely within the relationship and was considering separation. They argued but were also both worried about the effect on the children, particularly as they knew about the genetics of bipolar disorder.

Systemic couple therapy allowed for mutual ventilation of feelings of disappointment and resentment, but also positive descriptions of how the relationship had begun and what they would each like to change. A family tree allowed discussion of the different assumptions about family and marriage they had each absorbed in their own family of origin.

The distinction and overlap between the mental illness and the personality of Jeff could be thought about by both of them. How could he be excited about his new job, when she was anxious he was becoming hypomanic again?

Gradually, greater mutual sympathy developed towards the complexity of the other's position for both of them—they were discharged, realistic, but hopeful, about their future together.

Case two

A young woman Sarah was referred, housebound by severe OCD and agoraphobia. Unable to attend the outpatient clinic, she had not left the house for 5 years.

Sarah's mother, sister, and the clinical psychologist, who was working with Sarah individually, were seen for systemic family therapy. Videos were taken home for Sarah to watch. At a later stage, sessions moved to her home to include her.

Sarah's anxiety symptoms were entrenched, and her mother was entirely controlled by them, becoming tearful at any prospect of challenging the daughter. Sarah's sister was more robust, so a range of different opinions were discussed, balancing understanding but insisting on progress. A behavioural plan of increasing movement, out of the house (into the garden, the front doorstep), was implemented by the clinical psychologist.

The adhesive attachment between mother and daughter was challenged with future hypothetical questions about 'what will happen as mother gets old?'. The therapists needed to be aware of their own frustration and potential sadism or despair in this entrenched situation.

A degree of progress was achieved, with Sarah finally managing to leave the house occasionally, but her quality of life remained significantly impaired.

Group therapy and group analysis

(See ➲ Group therapy and group analysis in Chapter 2, pp. 42–7.)

Key techniques and competencies

All would-be therapists, especially those working in NHS services, should try and equip themselves with group skills. This includes competencies in the assessment of psychological distress, knowledge of group dynamics, and basic psychological communication and reflective skills.

A key technique for group therapists is the ability to monitor the experience of individuals in a group, whilst, at the same time, keeping the group on task and paying attention to group dynamics. Being a group therapist entails good communication skills, a sense of humour, and the capacity to manage one's own emotions, especially in those situations when group members are becoming distressed and angry.

Selection for groups

Before each member joins a group, there must be the usual psychotherapy assessment: of the would-be member's problems, what they want out of therapy and their usual defences against stress (see ➲ Assessing the course of therapy and Assessing the outcome of therapy in Chapter 4, pp. 140–2 and pp. 142–5, respectively). People who are acutely distressed or disturbed, and/or very paranoid, are unlikely to be able to use group therapy and may be disruptive to established groups. As for all therapies, it is important to have a good understanding of the patient's attachment style or representation, as this may influence how they relate to the therapist and to group members (see ➲ Theories of personality development: attachment theory in Chapter 8, pp. 380–1). It is also important to spend some time developing a therapeutic alliance with the patient and preparing them for what it may be like to explore their particular problem with others.

Patients who are referred for group therapy need to be able to come regularly, sit reasonably still, and be able to speak (again, not dissimilar to individual work). Very socially phobic people and those with avoidant attachment styles may find it hard to engage at the beginning. Some group therapists assert that patients who come from large families may find groups difficult, although this is not empirically tested and may reflect insecure attachment processes and/or childhood adversity, not family size per se. It also used to be thought that people with severe personality disorder (especially BPD) could not use group therapy. This has been shown not to be the case; however, it may still be true that people with severe narcissistic and/or paranoid personality dysfunction will struggle to engage with groups. There is evidence that people who score highly on measures of psychopathy do not benefit from groups, and may try and exploit fellow group members or therapists.

Group selection then depends on what type of group is being set up— whether themed or not, whether supportive or encouraging of change, whether it is therapist-led and directed, or led by the group membership. Supportive groups are widespread in the voluntary sector and in mental health services; their primary task is to help people manage a difficult life task and perhaps relate to it differently. The focus of the rest of this chapter is the process of group therapy that actively promotes psychological change in terms of increased reflective function and enhanced agency. It is sometimes useful to encourage people who have no prior experience of therapy to join a time-limited psycho-educational group that encourages curiosity and thought about a problem they face and, if this goes well, to then offer a long-term group that is led by group members' discussion and narratives.

Groups typically go through stages of interaction, although this is not a rigid or inevitable process. It is common for a new group of people to focus on how much they have in common and to take up a rather idealistic stance towards the group and the therapist(s). This stage then gives way to something more real and more conflicted, as people allow themselves to explore their differences from each other and the associated anxieties that this raises. Group members also experience disappointment, as they realize (as in individual therapy) that the therapist will not magically remove all their problems or distress, but that the problems are likely to be in the room and in the group, and they must work the issues out in the here-and-now. Like any therapy, the group process stimulates the attachment system, and some people with highly insecure attachments may experience high levels of anxiety and fear, and express this as anger or flight (see ➲ Theories of personality development: attachment theory in Chapter 8, pp. 380–1).

Defences in groups
(See ➜ Defence mechanisms in Chapter 2, pp. 22–4.)

Therapists need to understand, and be aware of, typical dynamics in groups. Group members will bring their own 'hand' of immature defences to the group, as part of their original complaint or problem. However, the group itself may function immaturely, using defences that reflect anxieties and dysfunctional ways of dealing with them.

These include:
- Pairing, i.e. when two group members make a bond in the group that undermines the group process—in terms of making others feel excluded and jealous, challenging the facilitator, and preventing the pair from engaging
- Domination of the conversation or withdrawal from the group, including absence, sleepiness, and toxic silences
- Excessive helpfulness to others
- Passive aggression (often linked with pairing)
- Idealization or denigration of the therapist/group
- Scapegoating (often of absent or silent members, or the therapist)
- Attempts to take the group off-task—usually setting up another task with an alternative leader
- Anti-groups, in which the group as a whole gets together to stop the process of thought or the task of the group. This may involve attacks on the therapist.

This list is not exhaustive. Group therapists need to be comfortable in managing the anxieties that generate these defensive behaviours, compassionate, even when being attacked, and understanding that people change defences slowly because psychological change is painful. They especially need to be able to manage their own responses to people in a group.

The group process
Co-therapy is a useful technique for running groups. Clearly, there need to be excellent relationships between group therapists, as well as a common understanding of what is being delivered. Supervision is essential for all groups, including psycho-educational ones—the dynamics described above occur in ALL groups that meet regularly, not just therapeutic ones.

Typically, people are advised to stay in a group for at least a year, because it takes this long for people to get used to the process, and 12 to 18 months of therapy is associated with better outcomes. Like individual therapy, group members are asked to make a commitment to come to therapy, even when they do not feel like it, and to speak honestly about their thoughts and feelings, both about their personal past and the here-and-now in the group. Groups typically last between 60 and 90 minutes; to some extent, this is a function of the size of the group. Smaller groups can run for an hour, but, if there are more than five or six people, then 75- or 90-minute groups are preferable to allow space for all to speak and for conversation to develop.

A group session often begins with some feedback from each member about where they are psychologically and what concerns them. A topic for discussion will then emerge; either it will be agreed explicitly or an implicit agreement to discuss this issue will follow. The group may stay with a topic or change. If the group is a themed one, the group therapist may need to help the group to stay on task. The therapist may need to help more silent members to speak, and more dominant members to help others to speak. Throughout, the therapist's main task is to help group members become a little more self-reflective and curious about their minds and the minds of others.

What changes?

The psychotherapeutic aims of group therapy resemble those of other therapies:

- Reduction in symptomatic distress and problem behaviours
- Improved social functioning and social mind-mindedness
- Improvement in self-reflective functioning about the nature of one's problems, especially with other people
- Enhanced sense of agency and engagement in one's own life.

It is unusual for people to seek out group therapy; in general, people seek psychological therapy and then are referred for group therapy, often somewhat reluctantly. This is partly because people in pain or distress apply the same medical model of individual treatment to their mental suffering, as they do to their physical suffering, and partly because people who feel anxious or vulnerable may feel particularly anxious in a group. However, groups may be especially helpful for people who have problems interacting with others, precisely because it is a form of therapy that engages and develops the social mind.

Yalom, in his seminal work on group therapy (now updated with Lesczc, 2005), described a number of factors that he believed were therapeutic in groups and brought about positive change. These are:

- *Universality*: the sense of being connected to others and reduction in social isolation
- *Altruism*: the experience of contributing to others' benefit, as well as one's own
- *Instillation of hope*: being with others who are struggling enables group members to see that change is possible, if hard or slow
- *Information giving and interpersonal learning*: the provision of information facilitates psychological change
- *Social experience in the group and cohesion*: undermines social isolation and shame
- *Imitation*: modelling oneself on others (including the conductor)
- *The experience of a different social experience in the here and now*: what is called 'a corrective experience'. This allows people to learn that they can experience others differently and be seen differently
- *Catharsis*: the expression and articulation of negative affects can facilitate emotional shift
- *Self-understanding*: this is closely linked to the process of reflective function that changes in MBT (see ➲ Mentalization-based therapy in Chapter 2, pp. 66–70, and in Chapter 5, pp. 229–34) and is, to some extent, common to all therapies.

Other therapeutic factors in groups include the process of mirroring, in which people see aspects of themselves in others (both good and bad), and the experience of transference in the group, both towards the conductor and between group members. Although therapeutic experiences, they are not always comfortable, and, for this reason, some group therapists offer additional individual therapy sessions, either with the same therapist or a different therapist who works closely with the group therapist. This model is the basis of the MBT programme of therapy for BPD (see ➲ Mentalization-based therapy in Chapter 2, pp. 66–70, and in Chapter 5, pp. 229–34).

For people who can make an attachment to a group and remain in therapy, group therapy is a helpful intervention, especially for those who are struggling with their social mind and identity. It may be especially helpful for those who have had very difficult interactions with parents or carers when they were children, especially those who had incestuous experiences with authority figures or who experienced extensive and persistent abuse from someone with whom they were dependent or intimate. For such people, being alone in a room with another adult, who is a comparative stranger and who has some authority or apparent power, may be highly anxiety-provoking and lead to early ruptures and dropout in therapy. This group of people may find it easier to be in small groups (of three to four people only) to get used to the idea of being in therapy at all.

Clinical populations and contexts

Group therapy is offered both as an inpatient and an outpatient intervention. It may be offered as part of a programme for a clinical problem (such as substance misuse or depression), or it can be a stand-alone intervention for psychological development and those with social and interpersonal difficulties. Groups are offered at every level of mental health care and in the voluntary sector, especially in relation to substance misuse (e.g. Alcoholics and/or Narcotics Anonymous).

The commonest form of group therapy is a psycho-educational group that provides information about therapy and helps prepare people for a more in-depth experience of group therapy. Such groups are used to good effect in psychotherapy services, as part of the assessment and preparation of potential group members for therapy.

Group therapy may be offered to a heterogeneous group of people who all (superficially at least) have different problems, or it can be offered to people who all have the same problem. The advantage of heterogeneous groups is that they enhance perspective taking and decrease social isolation by letting people see how much they have in common with people who, at first sight, are different to them. Thus, issues of assumptions and differences can be well explored in heterogeneous groups.

Focused or themed groups where everyone (apparently) has the same problem (e.g. trauma, bereavement, violence perpetration, eating disorders) offer alternative benefits—a reduction in sense of shame and social isolation, combined with an enhanced understanding that people can have very different responses to experience. This can be helpful for those who feel 'stuck' in their identity as a patient or trauma survivor, and for those who feel that no one else can understand their difficulties. Focused or themed groups include group therapy for:
• People with clinical depression
• People who have experienced childhood sexual abuse

- People with eating disorders
- People who have suffered bereavement
- Men's groups
- Mothers' groups
- People with personality disorders
- People who have suffered trauma in adulthood and chronic PTSD
- People who have been violent to others (including domestic violence, sexual assaults, and murder).

TCs are a particular form of social therapy, which usually are structured around a programme of small and large groups (see ➔ Therapeutic communities in Chapter 2, pp. 75–80, and in Chapter 5, pp. 243–50).

Case vignettes

A psycho-education group

Sarah has recently been seen by the crisis team, because she took an overdose. She is referred to the Complex Needs service. At assessment, it seems likely that Sarah might benefit from therapy, but she is ambivalent about starting with the Complex Needs programme. She is offered a place in her local Link Group: a 12-session psycho-educational group attached to her local CMHT. This group takes a theme or topic each week, which relates to the issue of mood disorder and negative affect management. The facilitators encourage discussion, question, and answer, and provide educational materials. Sarah is initially dubious, but she finds the topics relevant to her. She gets used to the idea of coming and sitting in a group each week, and to the experience of talking aloud about her feelings to others. By the end of the link group course, Sarah says she has a better idea of what the Complex Needs programme might be like to be part of, and she says she is willing to try it.

A heterogeneous psychoanalytic group for men and women with a variety of psychological problems

Karen (34) is a health-care professional who joins an established evening analytic group run by a consultant psychotherapist. The group is composed at the time of three men and three women, most of whom have been in the group for some time. They initially welcome Karen, who seems to fit right in very easily. She is helpful to others in the group and seems to present as empathetic and sympathetic. She also supports the group conductor, who notes to herself that Karen is almost like a co-therapist.

Karen describes herself as having chronic depression and sees her problems as stemming from an abusive relationship with her mother. She tearfully tells the group about her mother's cruelty towards her, whilst at the same time appearing to be understanding of her mother's problems. She denies any other problem, apart from at work where she accuses her (female) boss of being 'mean' to her, and at home where she jokingly describes her partner as a 'typical useless male'.

Gradually, the group therapist becomes aware that Karen's main self-narrative emphasizes how other people are mean and useless. Her account of herself is as competent and helpful, and that is the way she acts in the group. When the group therapist tries to gently suggest to

Karen that she herself might struggle with being mean or incompetent, Karen is hurt and offended. She feels criticized by the therapist and accuses her of being 'mean'. The rest of the group try to help Karen, but she is clearly uncomfortable with being a person in need of help.

The situation changes dramatically when a new group member starts, called Gloria. Gloria is larger than life and dramatic in the group; she also takes an instant (irrational) dislike to Karen and tells her so. Karen is devastated and becomes very distressed in the group. She manages to say that she has never felt disliked by anyone before, and it emerges that her helpfulness in the group (and at work) enables her to ensure that she never does or says anything that would lead to conflict or tension with others. She is helped to say how much she dislikes Gloria, even though this is a tense and difficult group discussion, with some people joining in to support either woman, and some furious with the group therapist for letting this type of conflict arise.

It becomes clear that Karen is actually struggling not so much with sadness, but anger—chronic, unexpressed rage towards her family of origin, herself, and the people she has looked after. The process of exploring being disliked by Gloria allows her to reflect on her mother's dislike of her and why that might be her mother's problem, and not hers. The rest of the group can now reflect on their expectations or wishes that the group be a 'nice' place where people are always 'nice' to each other, and how this might relate to their childhood experience in their own families. Gloria leaves the group before the expected year's attendance but is able to say that she learned something about her tendency to dismiss people.

Recommended reading

Bateman A (2008). 8-year follow-up of patients treated for borderline personality disorder. *American Journal of Psychiatry*, **165**, 631–8.

Callahan K (2004). A review of interpersonal-psychodynamic group psychotherapy outcomes for adult survivors of childhood sexual abuse. *International Journal of Group Psychotherapy*, **54**, 491–519.

Kanas N (2006). Long-term psychodynamic group therapy for patients with personality disorders. *International Journal of Group Psychotherapy*, **56**, 245–51.

Lorentzen S, Bogwald K, and Hoglend P (2002). Change during and after long-term analytic group psychotherapy. *International Journal of Group Psychotherapy*, **52**, 419–30.

McDermut W, Miller IW, Brown RA, et al. (2001). The efficacy of group psychotherapy for depression: a meta-analysis and review of the empirical research. *Clinical Psychology: Science and Practice*, **8**, 98–116.

Cognitive analytic therapy

(See ➔ Cognitive analytic therapy in Chapter 2, pp. 47–52.)

Key techniques and competencies

The practice of CAT assumes a range of fundamental therapeutic skills and competencies common to most effective therapies, especially those more relationally based (see ➔ Chapter 3). Acquisition of many of these skills would represent the aims and outcomes of an intensive training course, although certain underlying self-reflective and compassionate attitudes would be regarded as mandatory for such work.

General skills and competencies
These skills and competencies would include the ability to engage respectfully and work with a diversity of clients and presentations in a range of settings, from possibly dynamically complex institutional settings to individual independent practice. General skills would include the ability to conduct an initial assessment and make appropriate treatment recommendations, and to negotiate and set up a realistic and boundaried therapy framework, whilst also maintaining appropriate communication, as desired and required, with other professionals or services. Skills and competencies would include the ability to make a healing-containing and insight-generating use of the therapeutic relationship from the beginning and the ability to use the approach to notice, name, and repair threats to, and ruptures of, the alliance, and so to strengthen and sustain this key aspect of therapy. Key CAT skills include the ability to create joint writ ten and diagrammatic reformulations to aid therapy and to help make sense of problems and difficulties, and so to better negotiate possibly challenging interpersonal and systemic dynamics within and outside of therapy, as well as 'self-management' procedures (RRPs) and the development of self-reflection.

The CAT therapist should be able to:

- Judge how best to work in the so-called 'zone of proximal development' (ZPD) in a way that enables the client to engage with, and make use of, therapy without being demotivated or demoralized by a style of therapy which is confusing or beyond their current psychological and/or emotional capacities
- Set up aims and, where appropriate, formal tasks or '*behavioural experiments*' (see ➔ Cognitive behavioural therapy in Chapter 5, pp. 172–84) for the work of therapy, including in relation to interpersonal challenges and enactments within therapy
- Maintain or recover a compassionate and non-judgemental stance, even when experiencing frustration or hostile enactments from the client and possibly others. CAT skills include the negotiation and management of a clearly anticipated ending and placing 'ending well' as a fundamental aim of therapy in itself, and recognizing the dangers of not doing so and of engaging in collusive and unhelpful protracted therapies (see ➔ Dealing with breaks and endings in Chapter 3, pp. 103)
- Recognize the limitations of therapy both in dealing with aims negotiated with the client, but also in terms of the self-imposition of unrealistic and stressful aims upon themselves as therapist
- Recognize the need for, and make use of, ongoing supervision and reflective practice and be open at all times to this. This provides the necessary opportunity to check out potentially difficult interactions with the client and to seek support, feedback, and advice from colleagues (see ➔ Using supervision in Chapter 3, pp. 107–8)
- Recognize the need to look after one's self and seek help appropriately in often stressful (e.g. public health service) settings, particularly in working relationally and given the dangers of, for example, 'vicarious traumatization' and 'burn out'

- Recognize the social dimension of mental health and of therapy and be able to incorporate this within their work, as appropriate, and to recognize this and communicate with regard to the limitations that this may impose
- Conceptualize, describe, and evaluate the process of change in therapy from a CAT perspective (see ➔ What changes? in Chapter 5, pp. 197–8)
- Recognize the need for, and be able to implement, other interventions or other modalities, as appropriate, such as formal trauma processing work, group therapy, creative therapies, medication, or social rehabilitation.

Specific activities and techniques

CAT therapists would be expected to be able to participate effectively in a time-limited and structured form of relational therapy. Individual CAT therapy is most often conducted as an outpatient model of weekly 1-hour sessions lasting for either 8, 16, or 24 weeks, with one or more follow-up appointments. CAT therapists should be able to offer and manage therapy overall in a flexible, but structured, sequence of stages, maintaining throughout a responsive, reflective, and compassionate stance.

These stages include firstly undertaking an initial assessment for therapy. In CAT, this would normally be directed towards obtaining some general overview of the client's current difficulties and of their background, especially their early formative experiences. *The early sessions* in CAT (which could form part of the assessment process) would be somewhat more proactive and directed towards information gathering and understanding of the key issues. However, even in these early sessions, the style of the approach, in terms of understanding problems in terms of RRs and RRPs (see ➔ Cognitive analytic therapy in Chapter 2, pp. 47–52), would be commencing along with a recognition and exploration of how these might already be enacted within the therapy relationship. After a few sessions, the therapist would aim to draw together both a written ('narrative') and diagrammatic (map) reformulation. The letter written to the client aims to outline in a sympathetic and non-judgemental fashion a tentative understanding of the key issues (RRs and RRPs) and background to them in terms of formative relational experience. It aims to tell a client's story back to them, with the aim of validating this and 'bearing witness' to it.

The diagram or map would ideally be jointly constructed in the session through initial rough drafts and would aim to depict background formative relational experiences (RRs) and subsequent general coping patterns (RRPs). The reformulations act as a kind of 'route map' for the course of therapy, which is helpful for both client and also the therapist. They also act as a framework within which many other activities or interventions may be undertaken, depending on needs and wishes—although always seen in relation to the reformulations.

The *middle phase* of therapy is more open and may depend on issues arising both day to day in the life of the client, and also in terms of the need to work through and process past experiences, often of trauma or loss. No-send 'therapy letters' are commonly invited from the client, as a means of finding 'the words that need to be said.' Events, particularly conflicts and examples of self-sabotage from the preceding week, are broken down, discussed, and mapped out in the session. Alternative ways of dealing with these situations are discussed, and 'exits' are formulated and tried out before the next session. Threats to the therapeutic alliance, especially with the end approaching, are anticipated, brought into the dialogue, and added to the maps. Self-reflection is encouraged, using the metaphor of the 'observing eye'.

CAT stresses the importance of *ending well*, and focus on this is always maintained from the very beginning of therapy. In the *termination phase* of therapy, this is formally acknowledged by means of 'goodbye' letters written by the client and therapist to each other and read out in the last session. The letters reflect on the journey shared, the progress made, and the obstacles overcome, with anticipation of threats to progress that may be encountered after the therapy is over. Often there are one or more follow-up appointments to check progress and to offer 'top-up' reformulation and reflection. Some clients may subsequently need further help in the shape of more CAT, or a different individual approach, or joining an analytic therapy group. A group CAT approach is often suitable for clients who have overcome the initial disclosure of abuse and trauma in individual work but who are still held back in relationships and in their ability to negotiate intimacy and work environments.

What changes?

CAT aims at change of deep psychological structures and processes through therapy, in addition to the important roles of support, ventilation, and validation. Therapeutic change in CAT is seen in terms of changes and modifications to underlying RRs (and their associated feelings, cognitions, and behaviours) and in the repertoire of often unhelpful RRPs. These would include patterns of relating to others and also to self, as well as various symptoms and behaviours. An important aspect of change is seen as that brought about through the therapeutic relationship. This is achieved both through work on threats to, and rupture of, the therapy relationship, but also through the experience of the relationship itself.

In more serious 'borderline'-type problems, an additional therapeutic aim would be promoting integration of a self that is liable to fracture or split into different self-states and correspondingly to promote self-reflective capacity, insight, and executive function. In association with, and consequent to, these changes, it is anticipated and expected that improvements in mood, self-esteem, reduction in various symptoms, such as anxiety, depression, anger, irritability, substance abuse, insomnia, anorexia, self-harm, and so forth, would occur. Such changes have been evidenced in formal outcome studies.

Within therapy, change may be monitored by use of rating charts to evaluate recognition and change (revision) of target problem procedures (TPPs), and may be helpful to maintain focus. Likewise, keeping a notebook or diary can be helpful. In addition, CAT therapists would normally use some general outcome measure (e.g. CORE-OM) or the IAPT Minimum Data Set to formally evaluate progress. For more complex disorders, the Personality Structure Questionnaire (PSQ) may be used as a measure of fragmentation of the self. The C-CAT adherence tool may be useful in research studies and for training purposes.

Clinical population and contexts
Suitability
CAT adopts an essentially inclusive position towards suitability of clients for both individual and group therapy, and therapists would normally be prepared to offer a trial of therapy to most clients who request help. CAT regards 'motivation' or 'psychological mindedness' (see ➔ Psychoanalytic psychotherapy in Chapter 5, p. 167) as an aim of therapy, rather than as being a prerequisite. The only serious reasons not to consider a client for therapy would be serious and incapacitating substance abuse (or excess medication), acute psychotic disorder, or serious current risk of violent behaviours. High intellectual capacity is not required, and CAT is being increasingly used with appropriate modifications (e.g. use of colour coding, or pictures and cartoons on diagrams) in learning disability and forensic settings. Thus, CAT as a model is very open to working with a wide range of clients and problems, given that formative relational issues demonstrably underpin the vast majority of mental health problems and given its whole-person 'transdiagnostic' approach. Such presentations may cover a range of specific problems and difficulties or formal diagnoses.

Range of presentations and contexts
A major strength of CAT is its ability to engage 'difficult' or 'hard-to-help' clients and to create a strong therapeutic alliance and higher levels of engagement. CAT in the NHS is typically offered to more complex clients or as a second-line approach for clients with 'personality'-type disorders related to childhood abuse and trauma, eating disorders, bipolar disorder, substance abuse, medical illness and MUS, OCD, and gender identity issues, and in forensic and learning disability settings. CAT is also being offered and evaluated in a number of IAPT services for anxiety and depression (see ➔ Improving Access to Psychological Therapies services in Chapter 10, pp. 463–4).

CAT, being a relational and dialogic approach, is well suited to application in a group therapy setting. CAT groups have ranged from eight to 18 sessions for less complex problems or for groups of clients with similar presenting problems (e.g. anxiety, eating disorders, post-bariatric surgery) to closed and open groups running for a year or 18 months where abuse and trauma are common themes, single-sex groups, or for clients who have had extended spells in secondary care services (see ➔ Group therapy and group analysis in Chapter 5, pp. 188–94). CAT is also being increasingly used and evaluated as a consultancy tool for teams and services working with 'difficult' clients (e.g. assertive outreach teams), making use of extended 'contextual' reformulations.

Case vignettes

Case one

Steve was a young man in his early twenties who presented with a long history of low mood, poor sleep and anxious dreams, and general feelings of hopelessness about life. This had led recently to an overdose attempt and to a brief hospital admission. Subsequently, he had had interventions from a community team, which he felt had not helped and from which he had been referred for an assessment. At presentation, he appeared downcast and saw little point in trying therapy, and repeatedly blamed himself for his difficulties and failures, as he saw them, in life. He felt he would be wasting our time. However, he reluctantly agreed to fill in questionnaires (including the CORE in which he scored as 'moderately severe') and to 'give it a go'.

His background included upbringing as a middle child by parents who struggled financially. His father was in and out of work as a lorry driver, drank heavily, and was experienced as harsh and critical and who frequently argued with his wife who struggled to cope and probably had periods of depression herself. Steve did not do well at school, struggled to achieve any exams, and felt constantly that he was not good enough. He was often teased by pupils, partly because he tended to be overweight. He agreed that he had subsequently developed a tendency to try to entertain and please others to get by and to keep his real feelings to himself, including at home. After school, he did various odd jobs but could not afford to move out from home. He had one or two brief relationships which never worked out longer term.

In therapy, he initially struggled to see any point in coming but gradually began to open up and discuss his story and his formative experiences which were sketched out on maps (see Fig. 5.1). These he found 'interesting' and appeared to help him engage in therapy and to begin to understand how he tended to actually put himself down as a result of his 'critical' voice. Likewise, the reformulation letter appeared to have a powerful effect, provoking tears and acknowledgement of his struggle and hurt feelings. This was also helpful in flagging up how he might be naturally finding it hard to trust his therapist and tend to placate her also and 'put up a front'. A major turning point in therapy seemed to occur, when he came back to report one week that (as expressed in his 'aims'), instead of always offering to drive some friends to the pub at the weekend, as he always felt he should, he communicated that he did not feel great, and he had asked someone else to do it. To his astonishment, his friends had been sympathetic and offered to help out. This also appeared to improve his ability to trust his therapist and make use of therapy to reflect further, ventilate feelings, and work on further change, including noting and challenging the validity of his self-critical 'voice'. He appeared ready, although anxious, to end after 16 sessions and wrote a short, but touching, goodbye letter, in which he expressed his surprise and gratitude, but also his worries about the future. His end-of-therapy CORE score had improved to the high normal range, which only deteriorated slightly on 3-month follow-up.

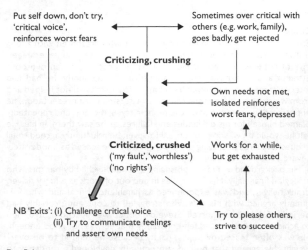

Put self down, don't try, 'critical voice', reinforces worst fears

Sometimes over critical with others (e.g. work, family), goes badly, get rejected

Criticizing, crushing

Own needs not met, isolated reinforces worst fears, depressed

Criticized, crushed ('my fault', 'worthless') ('no rights')

Works for a while, but get exhausted

NB 'Exits': (i) Challenge critical voice
(ii) Try to communicate feelings and assert own needs

Try to please others, strive to succeed

Fig. 5.1 Jointly constructed sequential diagrammatic reformulation ('SDR' or 'map') for Steve, showing key formative reciprocal role and subsequent reciprocal role procedures ('coping patterns') and how these reinforce the formative reciprocal role. Initial therapeutic aims or 'exits' are also noted on this map.

Case two

Chloe was a 22-year-old woman with a differential diagnosis of schizo-affective disorder and BPD. The consultant psychiatrist in charge of her care referred her for CAT and admitted to feeling in a 'catch-22' situation with her. There were times when she presented with self-harm by cutting and times when she presented in a psychotic state with paranoid features. When the community team attempted to help her, they usually found her hard to engage and wary of them. The harder they tried, by phoning her or attempting home visits, the more this tended to intensify her paranoia and trigger psychosis, for which she resisted medication. If the team held back and waited for her to contact them, they found that this was followed by periods of silence on both sides, usually culminating in Chloe turning up in accident and emergency (A&E) after a severe cutting episode. One of the liaison nurses in A&E happened to be CAT-trained and, on one such visit to A&E, had assessed Chloe and, during that discussion, had sketched out some reciprocal roles with her. Chloe turned up at her next outpatient appointment with her consultant psychiatrist and asked if she could be referred for CAT.

Chloe was seen for a 24-session CAT by a therapist who was aware of the background situation regarding her relationship with services. The therapist used Chloe's positive response to the rapidly sketched RRs in A&E to take a similar approach and diagrammed quickly with her in the first few sessions (see Fig. 5.2). It turned out that Chloe was as frustrated

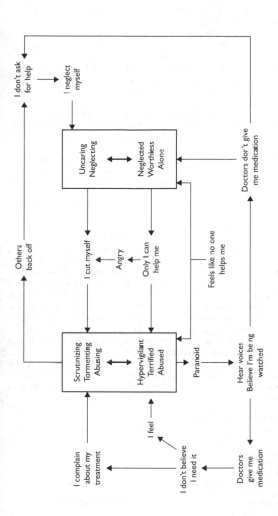

Fig. 5.2 Jointly constructed sequential diagrammatic reformulation ('SDR' or 'map') for Chloe showing formative reciprocal roles and subsequent reciprocal role procedures ('coping patterns') and how these reinforce formative reciprocal roles. The depiction of two key reciprocal roles and subsequent role procedures indicates a tendency to dissociate into different 'self-states' characteristic of 'borderline'-type disorders.

regarding her care as the consultant psychiatrist was, and the diagram naturally came to describe her relationship with services as they talked, moving in conversation back and forth between her childhood experiences and the present day.

Chloe's father had tormented her as a child by not only sexually abusing her, but also by spying on her at home and when she was out with friends or travelling to and from school. She would notice him behind trees or bushes looking at her and would often open her bedroom door at home to find him standing there, listening. He would sometimes creep up behind her and grab her. He often said to her, 'I am watching you' and 'you can't get away'. When she had a psychotic episode, these were frequently the voices she heard, and the feeling of being watched by someone somewhere was something she readily identified as belonging both to her childhood and to the present when psychotic or when 'hounded' by the community team.

Chloe's mother had been uncaring towards her as a child and had never protected Chloe from her father. She had provided food and clothes, but nothing else. Chloe had grown up feeling there must be something wrong with her to be so unlovable and had taken the anger out on herself.

The diagram and the reformulation letter that followed helped Chloe see the patterns that she and the community team were unwittingly acting out between them and how they replayed the patterns from Chloe's childhood. With Chloe's permission, the reformulation and diagram were shared with the consultant psychiatrist and the care coordinator. The second half of the therapy included useful negotiations with the community team that Chloe conducted herself, and together they designed exits to the diagram. The care coordinator agreed to give Chloe an appointment within a few days of any request, and it was agreed that it was appropriate for Chloe to ask when she was feeling alone and neglected. If the team felt concerned about Chloe at any time, then they agreed to make initial 'are you ok?' contact via Chloe's close friend who also agreed to that arrangement. Both Chloe and the team used these agreements well, and, within a few months, the relationship had become more mutually trusting and less mutually suspicious. By the end of therapy, there had been minor spells of paranoia and some thoughts of self-cutting, but no significant incidence of either kind.

Recommended reading

Bennett D and Parry G (2004). A measure of psychotherapeutic competence derived from cognitive analytic therapy (CCAT). *Psychotherapy Research*, **14**, 176–92.

Application in different settings

Hepple J (2012). Cognitive analytic therapy in a group. Reflections on a dialogic approach. *British Journal of Psychotherapy*, **28**, 474–95.

Hepple J and Sutton L (eds) (2004). *Cognitive Analytic Therapy and Later Life. A New Perspective on Old Age*. Brünner-Routledge: Hove and New York.

Kerr I, Dent-Brown K, and Parry G (2007). Psychotherapy and mental health teams. *International Review of Psychiatry*, **19**, 63–80.

Lloyd J and Clayton P (eds) (2014). *Cognitive Analytic Therapy for People with Intellectual Disabilities and Their Carers*. Jessica Kingsley: London and Philadelphia.

Interpersonal psychotherapy

(See ➔ Interpersonal psychotherapy in Chapter 2, pp. 52–5.)

Key techniques and competencies

The IPT process is collaborative and educative, and aims to foster a sense of interpersonal competence and expertise in the patient.

Early in the assessment process, the patient and therapist review the significant current relationships in the person's life, examining their quality, availability, reciprocity, and influence on current depressive symptoms. This is called the interpersonal inventory and is often represented in a simple diagram, which helps the patient to hold the broad network of people in their life in mind and to learn to tolerate thinking about the positive and negative relationships in their life as part of an integrated picture.

A collaborative formulation is developed with the person, and this focuses on one of the four focal areas: role transition, role dispute, grief, and interpersonal sensitivity. This is used to guide and contain subsequent work, and goals are agreed in relation to the chosen focal area.

Symptoms of depression are monitored during every IPT session, and changes are related to the immediate interpersonal environment. Interpersonal incidents related to the target problem area are preferentially discussed, with a view to resolving the recurrent problem and to break down the connection to depression. Discussion balances detailed attention to specific aspects of the problem area and engaging support in the person's current relationships. IPT attention is primarily focused on current relationships, rather than on the therapeutic relationship, which is carefully monitored but rarely explicitly discussed in IPT.

IPT pays close attention to the patient's affect, with the intention of enhancing self-awareness, emotional regulation, and the capacity to communicate clearly and effectively about significant feelings. This is integrated with repeated attention to the quality and character of the person's communication, and significant exchanges associated with a change in depressive symptoms are examined in fine detail, and more adaptive communication skills are developed.

What changes?

Research has repeatedly demonstrated change, in line with the two principal objectives of IPT:
- Reduction in symptomatic distress
- Improved social functioning.

IPT has repeatedly been shown to effect symptom reduction and recovery in a majority of patients with depression by the end of treatment, but a single package of IPT has not been shown to be sufficient to prevent further episodes of depression. Maintenance IPT, which is delivered monthly, following successful treatment, has been shown to significantly reduce the rate of recurrence and to prolong the period of wellness for people with recurrent depression. Improvement in social function and global functioning has been shown to continue in the period following treatment in a number of studies, often revealing a significant advantage over comparison treatments at follow-up assessment (see ➔ What is the evidence base under Interpersonal psychotherapy in Chapter 2, pp. 54–5; Affective disorders in Chapter 7, pp. 326–31).

When IPT has been used with non-depressed clinical populations, a reduction in relevant target symptoms have also been demonstrated, e.g. a reduction in binging and vomiting in BN and overeating in BED, a reduction in avoidance, hyperarousal, and re-experiencing in PTSD, alongside improvements in social functioning. When patients with depression and co-morbid anxiety symptoms are treated with IPT, those who respond demonstrate a reduction in anxiety symptoms, as well as depressive symptoms. Where anxiety and depression are both prominent in the clinical presentation, the speed of response is slower, and general outcome is poorer than when depression is the sole clinical complaint.

Each of the IPT focal areas has specific goals, which are tailored to the individual and targeted during treatment. Outcomes have been shown to be equivalent across the focal areas. These are as follows:

Role transition
- Facilitate mourning and acceptance of the loss of the old role
- Help the patient to regard the new role as more positive
- Help the patient to restore self-esteem by developing mastery of the demands of the new role.

Role disputes
- Modify non-reciprocal role expectations and faulty communication patterns to bring about a satisfactory resolution in the dispute.

Grief
- Facilitate the mourning process
- Help the patient to re-establish interest and relationships with the current network to substitute for what has been lost.

Interpersonal sensitivity
- Reduce the patient's isolation
- Encourage formation of new relationships.

Clinical populations and contexts

IPT was designed as an outpatient treatment for depression and is mainly provided in primary care. The inclusion of IPT in IAPT services has significantly increased the provision of IPT in primary care settings in England, with similar expansions of evidence-based practice across the UK (see ➔ Improving Access to Psychological Therapies services in Chapter 10, pp. 463–4). There is a much smaller provision in secondary care, often with liaison with local primary care services. Specialist eating disorder services and CAMHS often provide IPT. CAMHS and older adult services provision will increase with the inclusion of these services in IAPT. IPT is infrequently provided in trauma services, forensic settings, and inpatient settings in the UK.

Case vignettes

Case one

Louise is in her mid 50s and had worked in a large government agency for over 30 years, having been promoted through the ranks from a junior administrator to a senior management position. Following a change in management, Louise's long-term manager was replaced, and she felt bullied and undermined by his replacement. Over the course of a year, she was transformed from a confident successful woman to a timid and tearful shadow of her former self. She was medically retired, for which she felt unprepared.

Louise had no previous episodes of depression. She accepted the diagnosis, and her responsibility to learn about depression and talk to the people who were close to her about her diagnosis. Louise's husband was very supportive, and they agreed that he would temporarily take over some of the domestic responsibilities that she found difficult to manage, whilst Louise focused on reintroducing routines and activities that she found enjoyable and stimulating.

Louise's inventory revealed that, whilst her life had been well populated, the majority of people had been related to work, and she and her husband had led a private life. Louise was encouraged to maintain friendships with former colleagues, some of whom she had known for more than 20 years. She took this up and found that they welcomed her company and envied her escape from a stressful work environment.

Louise was helped to reconstruct the story of her working career, actively balancing the positive memories and achievements with realistic recollections of more stressful and difficult times. The final period of her working life was examined in detail, and the painful experience of being forced out by a new manager who did not respect or value the experience built up over many years by long-standing members of staff. Louise was able to chart out a timeline of her working life through the many highs and difficult lows of her career. This helped her to recognize that it had been some time since she had last enjoyed her working life, and there was little scope to engage in the aspects of her job she had most enjoyed, as the system changed and modernized around her.

With her re-established confidence in talking about her feelings and recognition of her administrative and planning skills, Louise put her time to good use by volunteering with a local charity. Louise soon became a valued and well-used member of the organization. This significantly bolstered her self-esteem and confidence, and introduced a new network of relationships that she enjoyed and used to fill her day. Louise increasingly valued the role other people played in her life and, through her active attention, developed a number of close and rewarding friendships.

Over the course of therapy, Louise's symptoms of depression reduced from the severe range to non-clinical. Her struggle to come to terms with the loss of her much valued career was fully resolved, and she no longer missed her job. She was fully and enjoyably occupied by her voluntary work and time with her husband and close friends, and was able to appreciate and enjoy the opportunity to slow down and appreciate her day-to-day experience that retirement allowed.

Case two

James was 24 years old and came for treatment one year after a friend's violent death. James had lived and worked with his friend, and, on the night of his friend's death, a local drug dealer, known to them both, called at their flat. James had been afraid of this man and left the flat as soon as he arrived. On returning home, he discovered that his friend had been violently murdered.

A number of friends were critical of his decision to leave his friend alone, and he thought they believed he had contributed to his friend's death. James became very isolated in the months that followed. He was unable to mourn, and his grief turned into depression, with significant self-blame, suicidal ideation, and hopelessness. His daily routine became unrecognizable, as he moved out of the shared accommodation to live in a small studio flat, was on long-term sick leave from work, and saw few of his former friends.

James was initially very reluctant to accept a diagnosis of depression and said he could not imagine feeling any other way in the circumstances. Despite having used drugs recreationally, James refused to consider using antidepressant medication. The similarities and differences between grief and depression were discussed at length, and comparison was made with the progress he knew other people who had known his friend had made in living with loss.

The IPT formulation highlighted two major difficulties—he was overwhelmed by the depth of his grief and loss, and was almost entirely isolated in his remaining relationships. Again James saw both as the inevitable consequence of his situation, but he was helped to appreciate how one contributed to the other by carefully reconstructing memories of his life when he and his friend had been at the heart of their social group and comparing it with the almost entire lack of support he faced now.

In order to stay close to the parts of his story that most directly fed into his depression, James was supported in talking about the events around the death. This focused particularly on his irrational guilt and the impact of most of his support disappearing in the immediate aftermath of the death. This was very painful for him, and the work had to be carefully paced to ensure he could tolerate the distress when he had so little support. In order to reduce this vulnerability, active attention was given to maximizing the interpersonal contact he had. This focused mainly on his girlfriend, who had been with him since before the death, and actively planning for his gradual return to work. The work progressed very slowly, because James had so few resources available to him at the time of starting therapy and had to build many routines from almost nothing.

James's phased return to work proved very beneficial. Some of his colleagues had known his friend, and they offered a sympathetic response, which slowly helped him to think in a more balanced way about his own self-blame and the angry and blaming response of other people in his life. After some weeks of planning, he also visited his friend's parents who welcomed him and made it clear that they did not blame him for their son's death. This marked a turning point for James, when he became more open to remembering his friend and reconstructing a fuller picture of the time they had known each other. In doing this, he found that intrusive memories of his friend's death started to lessen and were replaced with a more varied selection of memories, which he discussed in therapy and with his girlfriend.

James believed that some of the friendships he had had before the death were damaged beyond repair, and he began to build more of a routine with work colleagues and his girlfriend's friends, with whom he had previously had little to do. This created opportunities for enjoyable social contact that was not filled with memories of the past.

James's progress remained slow, but, after several weeks, he had improved sufficiently to be able to think again about using antidepressant medication, and this was added to his treatment. This helped with his sleep and appetite, both of which had been suppressed, and this, in turn, improved his mood and interest.

James continued to experience mild symptoms of depression at the end of treatment but was continuing to improve and planned to continue his antidepressant medication in the months ahead. He was gradually building up his social routine and was talking with his girlfriend about moving in together.

Recommended reading

Law R (2013). *Defeating Depression: How to Use the People in Your Life to Open the Door to Recovery*. Constable and Robinson: London.

Lemma A, Roth A, and Pilling A (2010). *The Competences Required to Deliver Effective Interpersonal Psychotherapy (IPT)*. Available at: http://www.ucl.ac.uk/CORE.

Ravitz P and Maunders R (eds) (2013). *Psychotherapy Essential To Go. Interpersonal Psychotherapy*. WW Norton and Company: New York.

Stuart S and Robertson M (2012). *Interpersonal Psychotherapy: A Clinician's Guide*, second edition. Hodder Arnold: London.

Weissman MM, Markowitz JC, and Klerman GL (2007). *Clinician's Quick Guide to Interpersonal Psychotherapy*. Oxford University Press: Oxford.

Psychodynamic interpersonal therapy

(See ➜ Psychodynamic interpersonal therapy in Chapter 2, pp. 56–61.)

Key techniques and competencies

In short-term work, PIT shares many non-specific competencies with other therapeutic models, including the provision of a safe, structured therapeutic environment (see ➜ Chapter 3).

There are key therapist behaviours which help promote the development of a collaborative 'personal conversation' between the client and therapist and the emergence of a 'feeling language'. These specific competencies include:

- An ability to listen and respond in such a way to convey an emerging understanding of the client's problems and perceptions by paying careful attention to the client's verbal, vocal, and bodily cues, such that the practitioner's responses match and complement the client's feeling state, and encourage further exploration
- An ability to phrase the majority of interventions in the form of a statement, as opposed to a question
- An ability to work collaboratively with the client to develop 'shared meaning' by using direct and collaborative language (e.g. 'I' and 'we') that facilitates the development of an active, mutual dialogue with the client

- An ability to help the client to stay with immediate bodily experiencing, to try to share something of that experience, and to wait for natural associations of images, prior experiences, and feelings to emerge
- An ability to use tentative statements (understanding hypotheses) which refer to how the client is feeling, based upon subtle non-verbal cues or other meaningful exchanges, which are not mere reflections of the client's feelings, but an attempt on the part of the therapist to take the exploration of the client's feelings a little further
- An ability to use statements that tentatively link feelings that have emerged in the therapy sessions to other feelings both inside and outside the therapy (linking hypotheses)
- An ability to use tentative statements (explanatory hypotheses) which introduce the possibility of underlying reasons for problems and difficulties in relationships, and refer to either a repeated pattern of behaviour or a warded-off unbearable feeling.

What changes?

Research has demonstrated change in both psychological and physical symptom distress, and improved functioning, including improved health status and quality of life. Improved outcomes appear to be maintained for at least 12 months post-therapy. For people with pain, tolerance to painful stimuli increases, following treatment. For people who self-harm, there is a reduction in self-harming behaviour post-treatment.

People who receive PIT have also been shown in several separate studies to use less health care post-treatment and to require less medication for their health problems.

As is consistent with the theoretical model, change in interpersonal functioning also occurs, following treatment. Qualitative work has shown that clients go on to make positive changes in their lives in the months following the ending of therapy, which they directly attribute to the therapeutic process. On an interpersonal level, this includes becoming more open with their partners and families about their problems and difficulties, ending problematic relationships, and forming new more stable and supportive relationships, and recognizing and solving interpersonal disputes at an earlier stage than previously and more effectively. People who report a past history of childhood sexual abuse have a preferentially good outcome with this model of therapy.

Clinical population and contexts

PIT is suitable for a broad range of people with a wide variety of presenting problems. It has a transdiagnostic approach to treatment, so can be used for clients who have multiple or co-morbid symptoms.

The evidence base suggests that it may be particularly useful for engaging clients who have 'treatment resistant' symptoms or who have not gained benefit from other treatment approaches. Clinical and research experience suggests the following kinds of problems areas may benefit from either brief or longer term PIT: depression and anxiety states, mixed depression and anxiety, treatment resistant depression/anxiety states, phobic disorders, eating disorders, self-harm, medically unexplained symptoms, people who have been hard to engage in psychological treatment, high users of health care, and clients with borderline personality disorder.

PIT can be used in a group format, and it has also been used in a couple therapy format. A condensed version of PIT (PIT-C) is also available which can be used to enhance other therapeutic approaches, such as behavioural activation or brief cognitive behavioural therapy.

Case vignettes

In PIT, there is a strong focus on the conversation between the client and therapist, and the therapist responds in a very particular way to the client. The therapist avoids asking questions, whenever possible, and uses tentative statements which are couched in a way so that the client can amend or reject them. The statements are based upon, and tailored to, the client's cues and should subtly and gently deepen the conversation. The therapist tries to help the client stay with and experience feelings, rather than talk about them in an abstract way.

It is within this conversation that the client's 'problem' is revealed. Rather than describe a full therapy, the next section describes the first 5 minutes of two PIT therapies. In this way of working, the key problem areas for the client are very quickly revealed, without having to know a lot of information about the client or ask a lot of questions. All the therapist's actions are determined by, and follow on from, cues from the client, so the sessions are very carefully paced. Exploration therefore only occurs in a collaborative and consensual way.

In the following clinical examples, the therapist is referred to by her first name, which is in keeping with the conversational model in which the therapist and client are on first name terms, as part of fostering a collaborative and supportive therapeutic alliance.

Case one

Adam was a man in his late forties who had been treated for mental health problems and pain for 6 years prior to therapy. He had been intermittently suicidal during this period and had had two admissions to an inpatient psychiatric bed for treatment for depression. He had been tried on several different antidepressants but suffered with severe side effects and had not been able to complete a course of treatment. He had found it difficult to engage with services and had an erratic pattern of attendance. His contacts with services were often challenging, and, on occasions, he had threatened to smash up waiting rooms, because of frustration at having to wait to be seen. He was never actually physically violent towards any member of staff. He had had several referrals for brief CBT-based treatments but had always dropped out of treatment and had never completed a course.

The first 5 minutes of the first session

Liz went down to meet Adam in the reception area. She spotted a tall man, with greying thick hair, who was pacing up and down outside the reception area, smoking a cigarette. A woman was with him, and they were deep in conversation. She appeared to be trying to persuade him to stay, and he appeared to be wanting to walk away. Liz checked with the reception staff that this was Adam and then went outside and approached the couple, introducing herself to both and offering her hand. Adam looked surprised but offered his hand back. Liz looked him firmly in the eye and smiled warmly, but he glanced away, and his handshake was limp. His hand was actually clammy and tremulous. Adam said, 'Oh . . . at least it's a woman.' The woman with him said, 'Look, you'll be ok with her . . . at least give it a try . . . I'll wait for you.' She smiled at Liz and said that she was Adam's wife Pat. 'His bark is worse than his bite . . . He's actually been up all night, worrying about coming this morning.'

Liz acknowledged Pat and calmly and clearly turned to Adam and said, 'I can see that this is very stressful for you, and it must be really difficult coming to see a stranger like me.'

(Pause)

'I can see you are in two minds and are not sure really about coming up to see me?'

Adam suddenly changed, and he smiled and said to Pat, 'I'll give it a go . . . Can't be worse than the last one.' His whole demeanour transformed into a 'cheerful, cheeky chappy'. 'Let's get on with it.'

Liz showed Adam up to her room. He jauntily followed her up the stairs, commenting on the pictures on the wall. Liz chatted back but was also reassessing in her mind what had happened downstairs.

Adam was clearly very ambivalent about staying for therapy. There was possibly an issue in relation to men, as he had commented that 'at least it's a woman'. Adam appeared to be expecting a negative experience and was near to avoiding even talking to Liz. She also thought about what his wife had said, 'His bark is worse than his bite'. She noted that there had been a dramatic change in his persona from a reluctant, wary, frightened person to a seemingly cheerful, light-hearted bloke.

It was the light-hearted bloke who sat down in her room.

Liz: Well you made it! (cue: picking up his jokey demeanour)

Adam: Yes . . . I thought I would be off. But here we are *AGAIN* (heavily accents this word). No offence.

Liz: No, of course not. But what you say sounds important. Like . . . you've been in this situation before . . . (*understanding hypothesis*)

Adam: Doesn't matter. Nothing matters. (He is smiling cheerfully, but not making eye contact and looking round the room.)

Liz: Look . . . It's been a struggle for you to come and see me today . . . We've not met before . . . It's often difficult meeting someone new for the first time, but it feels like there's a bit more than that going on . . . (*understanding hypothesis which focuses on the current 'problem'*)

Adam stops looking round the room and looks at her . . . then shrugs.

Liz: I'd like to try to get a sense of what you are feeling right now . . . here now . . . (pointing with hands) . . . (*focus on here and now*)

Adam: er . . . I've got to talk to yet another new person . . .

Liz: A sense of frustration . . . (*focus on here and now*)

Adam: Pat's made me come . . . I wouldn't be here otherwise . . . Nothing has ever helped.

Liz: So you are kinda seeing me, because Pat has asked you to?

Adam: Correct . . . That's the only reason I'm here (smile) . . . (longish pause) I drive her mad. She worries (his expression changes slightly, and the therapist senses some of Adam's anxiety coming back).

Liz: Sounds as if she feels you need some help, and you worry about the effect your problems have on her (*statement*).

Adam: She worries when I get suicidal.

Liz: Umh . . . (Pause) . . . I wonder if we could look at that . . . Perhaps you could tell me a bit more about that (*focus on feelings*).

Adam. What's the point? (*Client cues that he does not want to look at his suicidal feelings.*)

Liz: (*Picks up this cue and refocuses on Adam's ambivalence about the therapy.*) I may be wrong . . . But I'm wondering if you've really felt let down by people, whether you feel you've been left high and dry . . . (*understanding hypothesis*)

Adam: It's all . . . see you for 6 weeks, then bye bye . . . You feel like a parcel . . . passed from pillar to post . . . (*Adam responds to this hypothesis.*)

Liz: As if you are of no value? . . . No one cares? (*understanding hypothesis*)

Adam: (relaxing somewhat, beginning to make eye contact) . . . Yes . . . Just a number . . .

Liz: Well, the system can, I think, understandably make some people feel like you do . . . Passed on from one person to another . . . It feels to me as if you feel that no one has been listening to you . . . has really appreciated or heard how distressed at times you get? . . . And it's made you wary of embarking on something here with me . . . in case something similar happens . . . (*understanding hypothesis/use of 'I' and 'we'*)

Adam: Yeah . . . I mean I don't know you . . . Yet I'm expected to talk about how I feel . . .

Liz: Well in this therapy . . . we like to try . . . And try is a big word . . . We like to try to get to know the person . . . if we can. Try to understand what gets to them . . . the things that are important for them . . . and I think . . . and I'm not sure . . . but I am wondering . . . if for you . . . it really hurts . . . this feeling of being passed on from one person to another . . . (*understanding hypothesis/negotiation/exploratory rationale*)

Adam: . . . It takes a lot for me to trust anyone . . . Pat's the only person who I really trust . . . She's the only person who has stood by me . . . Why she does that . . . I don't know . . . I keep expecting she won't come back one day . . . She'll have given up like everyone else . . .

Liz: That's a big worry for you . . . (*understanding hypothesis*)

Adam: Yes . . . it is . . .

Liz: OK . . . well . . . I am aware there are some really big things going on for you . . . I'm also aware . . . that, in this therapy, we have 20 sessions . . . That works out at about 6 months of help . . . and that . . . having spoken to you for just a few minutes . . . you may feel . . . that once again . . . someone . . . me . . . is going to see you and then . . . there will be an ending . . .

Adam: No . . . I know . . . I mean the other lady told me . . . but I don't know . . . what's the point?

Liz: Well . . . I wonder if your problems feel so huge at the moment, so overwhelming that it feels that nothing will help . . . (*understanding hypothesis*)

Adam: Well . . . yes . . . I know you are doing your best . . . (beginning to make more eye contact)

Liz: Well . . . suppose . . . we . . . let's see . . . we've got about 40 minutes or so . . . today . . . I am very aware . . . you will not want to get into anything . . . and be left high and dry . . . but I am wondering if you would like to spend that time with me . . . and just see where we get to . . .

Adam: Pat would kill me if I walk out now . . . but I will give it a go . . .

Liz: Well perhaps we could start . . . with just if we could try and stay a bit with how you are feeling . . . feeling right now (*focus on here and now*)

Adam: Now?

Liz: Yes here . . . right now . . . (*here and now*)

Adam: I'm not sure . . . sickly . . . pit in my stomach . . . a bit dry

Liz: Well if you could just stay with that sickly feeling . . . in that hole inside? (*staying with feelings*)

Adam: I get like this ... when Pat's about to go out ... this awful sickness ...

Liz: Dread? I'm not sure (*amplification*)

Adam: Yes a dread ...

Liz: With that comes a fear ... (*amplification*)

Adam: Fear yes ... fear she won't come back ...

The session after this point continued for a further 40 minutes, and Adam was able to begin to talk about his feelings. Liz had noted that he had referred to suicidal ideas, so, at the mid-point of the session, she explored these with him and evaluated the risk. Adam returned the following week and completed the full course of therapy, which he found very helpful. The main focus revolved around his fears of being abandoned and being left all alone. Such was the strength of these fears that he began to realize that he pushed people away, both physically and psychologically, and he had even done this with Pat. This intellectual understanding of his problem, how-ever, was secondary to the experiencing of similar feelings in the session with Liz. Instead of automatically warding off all feelings of vulnerability, he was slowly able to stay with these feelings, and this generalized to his relationship with Pat. Adam's 'problem' was apparent in the first 5 minutes of the therapy and enacted in the here and now with the therapist.

Case two

Edith was a woman in her late sixties. She had presented to her GP with severe anxiety and sleep problems. She had been referred to IAPT and had received a low intensity intervention, consisting of behavioural acti-vation and also sleep hygiene. Neither had been helpful.

The first 5 minutes

Edith had arrived punctually for her appointment with her therapist Sarah. Sarah noticed, as she approached Edith in the waiting area, that Edith was sitting forward on the edge of her seat, with her hands clenched in a ball on her lap. She was smartly and neatly dressed, but appeared very tense and closed in on herself. Sarah greeted her warmly, and Edith responded with a smile and good eye contact. They talked about the traffic around the clinic, as they went upstairs, and Edith com-mented that she hated being late so had ordered a taxi that morning to ensure she got to the appointment on time.

Sarah could sense Edith's nervousness, as they sat down in her room.

Sarah: Just take a few moments to settle yourself down, get comfy. There's a clock over there, so you can keep track of the time if you wish, and we've got about 50 minutes this morning to talk about things ... It's a bit strange meeting someone like me for the first time ... (*focus on here and now*)

Edith: I don't know if I will be able to answer all your questions.

Sarah: Umh ... well ... that's ok ... I'm not actually going to ask you many questions ... in that, in this therapy, we try to get to know some-one, rather than know a lot about them ... but I understand it's a worry not knowing what to do or expect when you see someone like me (*under-standing hypothesis*)

Edith: Oh ... well ... I've written down some things, some notes, I thought that might be helpful. I sometimes forget what I mean to say ... and then remember later.

Sarah: I'd certainly like to see what you've written.

Edith passed the therapist a piece of paper with some notes, neatly written in the form of a list. The notes had been written in the early hours of the morning, and there were several entries on different nights in the last week.

Sarah read them carefully and then said, 'It sounds as if night-time is a very bad time for you' (*understanding hypothesis*).

Edith: Yes, terrible ... I can't sleep, you see ... I panic in the night ... every little noise ... I just can't settle.

Sarah: Umh ... that sounds really difficult ... Could we perhaps go back to one of these times you've written about ... maybe last night?

Edith: I was bad last night, I was worried about coming here ... I just couldn't settle ... It's a terrible feeling ... terrible ... (Edith clasped her hands and shook her head).

Sarah: And it feels as if you've felt a bit of that feeling just now ... I wonder if you could stay with that feeling ... I'd like to try to really understand what it's like ... (*focus on feelings/here and now*)

Edith: Oh ... it's a terrible fear ...

Sarah: Very distressing for you ... You feel it in your body too ... (*amplification*)

Edith: It's like a pressure ... I can't swallow ... Tightness here ... (pointing to her chest), I feel so scared ...

Sarah: (Also holding her chest) Scared ... as if something bad is going to happen (*understanding hypothesis*)

Edith: Yes ... I imagine ... someone's in the house ... someone's hiding in the house ... I know there isn't, but ...

Sarah: You don't feel safe ... (*understanding hypothesis*)

Edith: No ... that's it ... I don't feel safe ... I don't feel at all safe ... The lady I saw before ... told me when I couldn't sleep to get out of bed and do something else ... but I'm scared to get out of bed ... I put the covers over my head ... It's the only thing which helps ...

Sarah: I'd like to try to get you to stay with what it's like when you are in your bed and you are scared at night-time ... and you are alone? (*focus on feelings*)

Edith: Yes ...

Sarah: It must be very frightening (*focus on feelings*)

Edith: Yes ... it is ...

Sarah: And that fear's here now ... I wonder if any pictures or images come to mind ... (*staying with feelings*)

Edith: I can't bear this life ... I hate being alone ... It's so hard ... If I think about Frank (my husband), I feel worse the next day ... so I try and block him out ...

Sarah: He comes to mind?

Edith: Yes ... I lost him ... He died 5 years ago ... and since then, it's been hell. I struggle on ... but it's the nights that are the worst. He did everything for me. He sorted out everything in the house. Now ... I have to do everything ... everything by myself ...

Sarah: I'm very sorry for your loss ... You must feel very alone ... (*understanding hypothesis*)

Edith: I am ... It's unbearable ... Why am I still here? I had breast cancer 15 years ago ... We thought that I would be the one to go first ... not Frank ...

Sarah: Sounds like you really depended on him (*understanding hypothesis*)

Edith: He was my rock ... He really was ... I had a troubled upbringing ... I was always nervous ... but then I met him when I was 19, and he made me feel safe. I never felt nervous again ... until the last few years.

Sarah: Well it sounds to me as if all these things we have been talking about may be connected up with each other. The anxiety and fear at night-time, feeling alone, and the loss of Frank ... and it's a very big loss for you ... (*explanatory hypothesis*)

Edith: Yes ... it is ... It's like I've lost half of myself ... I don't feel a whole person ...

In this therapy, the focus centred on Edith's loss of her husband Frank, and her inability to function properly since his death. His loss had revealed an inner sense of frailty which had been present since her early adulthood but had been masked by her reliance upon him and the support he gave her. Edith felt angry and abandoned by his death, but had shut out these distressing feelings. Her fears had become large. The first stages of therapy helped Edith to tolerate and contain her anxiety in the sessions and also at home. Her fears at night-time became manageable.

The image of not feeling a whole person recurred as a theme throughout the therapy. Edith was able to stay with her fears in the sessions with her therapist, and, as she did so, she began to feel less frail and stronger as a person. She was able to consider the possibility of developing new friends and reconnecting with old friends, which previously had seemed impossible for her, as she felt, in some way, that she would be letting down Frank. She got back in touch with her sister, who Frank had never liked and who she had not seen for 20 years. She began to feel that, although Frank had been very protective of her, he had also been very dominant, and she had not been able to see friends and family as she would have liked. Her sister helped her have a burglar alarm fitted, security locks put on the windows, and security lighting. She began to speak to her sister every evening, and her anxiety gradually faded, and her sleep returned to normal.

She and her sister spent a lot of time discussing their childhood. Their parents had both died in a car crash when she was 12 years old, and they had both been placed in care. Edith made some links between how she felt during this period of time and her anxieties following Frank's death.

In the last phase of therapy, Edith joined an art group and a choir, both things Frank would not have allowed, if he had been alive.

Recommended reading

Hobson RF (1971). Imagination and amplification in psychotherapy. *Journal of Analytical Psychology* **16**, 79–105.

Hobson RF (1985). *Forms of Feeling: The Heart of Psychotherapy*. Tavistock Publications: London.

Meares R (2012). *Borderline Personality Disorder and The Conversational Model: A Clinician's Manual*. Norton series on interpersonal neurobiology. WW Norton: New York.

Meares R (2012). *A Dissociation Model of Borderline Personality Disorder*. Norton series on interpersonal neurobiology. WW Norton: New York.

Moorey J and Guthrie E (2003). Persons and experience: essential aspects of psychodynamic interpersonal therapy. *Psychodynamic Practice* **9**, 547–64.

Dynamic interpersonal therapy

(See ➲ Dynamic interpersonal therapy in Chapter 2, pp. 61–63.)

Key techniques and competencies

Phases of treatment

The DIT model can be conceptualized as consisting of three phases, each one with its own distinctive strategies:

- An engagement/assessment phase (sessions 1–4)
- A middle phase (sessions 5–12)
- An ending phase (sessions 13–16).

Initial phase

The primary task of the *initial phase* (sessions 1–4) is to identify one dominant and recurring unconscious interpersonal affective pattern (IPAF) (see ➲ Dynamic interpersonal therapy in Chapter 2, pp. 61–63) that is connected with the onset and/or maintenance of the depressive symptoms. This pattern is underpinned by a particular representation of self-in-relation-to-an-other that characterizes the patient's interpersonal style and that leads to difficulties in his relationships because of the way in which it organizes his behaviour. These representations are typically linked to a particular affect(s) and defensive manoeuvres. Affects are understood to be responses to the activation of a specific self-other representation.

Past experiences are not the major focus of DIT. They are included in the formulation shared with the patient, so as to frame his current difficulties in the context of his lived experience, but they are not a central component of the therapeutic process. Rather, given the brief nature of the therapy, the focus is on a core segment of the patient's interpersonal functioning closely connected with the presenting symptom(s). The therapist identifies the most important current and past relationships but does so with emphasis on present relationships. The therapist strives to establish the form of a relationship, the key processes employed in maintaining it, if it has changed over time, and how it relates to problems.

Middle phase

The IPAF guides the therapist's interventions during the *middle phase* of the therapy (sessions 5–12). During this phase, the therapist helps the patient stay focused on the IPAF and think about new ways of resolving their interpersonal difficulties. A consistent effort is made to encourage and support the patient to make psychological sense of what is happening in his own mind and others' minds, and in important interactions.

Ending phase

The last four sessions constitute the *ending phase* (sessions 13–16) and are devoted to helping the patient explore the affective experience and unconscious meaning of ending the therapy, to reviewing progress, and to helping him to anticipate future difficulties/vulnerabilities.

Techniques

In DIT, the therapist intervenes to generate, clarify, and elaborate interpersonally relevant information. A key intervention is to help the patient stay focused on the agreed IPAF. All the techniques used support this core aim of helping the patient understand what is happening for him in his mind when things go wrong in his relationships, including how the IPAF is enacted in the therapeutic relationship. To this end, DIT draws liberally on supportive and expressive techniques, whilst also making judicious use of directive techniques to support change. Confrontation or challenge is an equally important aspect of DIT (see ➔ Spectrum of interventions in Chapter 5, p. 164).

Because DIT is used with patients whose depression ranges from mild to severe, the therapist needs to titrate the level of supportive interventions. The less impaired patient, with a higher level of interpersonal functioning, is more likely to make greater use of expressive techniques, without requiring more supportive interventions. The ability to apply the model flexibly and to balance supportive and expressive techniques is therefore essential.

The DIT therapist's greater activity does not usually involve giving advice, but it requires that the therapist is alert to any deviations from the agreed focus so as to redirect the patient. It also requires that the therapist explicitly supports the patient's attempts to change. To this extent, some *directive* techniques are used during the middle part of treatment, which may well be less familiar to analytically trained therapists. Such interventions include more freely asking questions to clarify the patient's experience, and active encouragement to try out different ways of approaching a conflict with another person. They are considered to have a subtle structuring impact on the patient's perspective on his experience.

The way directive techniques are deployed in DIT is nevertheless framed in the context of a good understanding of the meaning that the therapist's more directive stance may acquire for the patient in light of the IPAF. For example, an anxious patient for whom separation is felt to be terrifying may well be very compliant with the therapist's direction, because non-compliance is felt to be a threat to the relationship. In such an instance, the DIT therapist would be attuned to the unconscious meaning that may be latent in the patient's wish to please the therapist and would actively address this, linking it to the identified IPAF.

What changes?

The DIT therapist has two aims:

• To help the patient understand the connection between his presenting symptoms and what is happening in his relationships by identifying a core, unconscious, repetitive pattern of relating

• To encourage the patient's capacity to reflect on his own states of mind and enhance his ability to manage interpersonal difficulties.

A distinguishing feature of DIT is that it approaches the exploration of problematic interpersonal patterns not by addressing the patient's behaviour, but through its consistent focus on the patient's mental states (beliefs, feelings, wishes, and thoughts) in themselves and in others. A primary aim is to provide the patient with an experience of being with another person who is interested in *thinking with* the patient about what distresses him, so as to stimulate the patient's own capacity for reflecting on his own experience.

This is what we call the *collaborative stance*. The goal is not simply to work on an unconscious conflict, but to use the patient's reports of his interpersonal experiences as a way of helping him develop his own capacity for thinking and feeling his experience. This focus is fundamental to DIT, and it informs technique in so far as the helpfulness of the therapist's interventions (e.g. the interpretation of transference) (see ➡ Psychoanalytic psychotherapy in Chapter 2, pp. 20–30) is evaluated against the criterion of whether they help stimulate the patient's capacity to reflect on their own subjective experience. The DIT therapist is particularly interested in making explicit what has effectively become procedural, so that the patient is better able to effect change in how he manages his relationships.

Clinical populations and contexts

The protocol was originally developed for use within primary care services in the UK with depressed patients referred to IAPT services (see ➡ Improving Access to Psychological in Chapter 10, pp. 463–4). At the time of writing, we have observed a trend towards a growing interest in its applicability in secondary care generally and more specifically with somatizing patients, as well as with adolescents who are depressed.

Case vignettes

Case one

Sam was in her late twenties, when she first became depressed following a termination of pregnancy. She had separated from her boyfriend some months after the termination. Her boyfriend said he felt too young to commit to starting a family, and, at the time, Sam had been of like mind—at least consciously.

By the time she started DIT—over a year after the termination—Sam struggled to go into work and had withdrawn from her social circle. She said she could not feel happy, and she harboured suicidal thoughts. When her therapist examined her relationships, past and present, more closely, a pattern emerged—Sam typically experienced others as 'pushy', and she experienced herself as 'insignificant'. This experience was associated with feelings of helplessness, which she managed by typically complying, appeasing, and pleasing the other, whom she feared would otherwise punish her in some way and who emerged as very powerful, relative to her own experience of herself (this became the IPAF). It became clear that Sam had never made any decisions in her life that had not been subjected to the activation of this relational constellation in her mind, not least the decision to terminate a pregnancy—a decision that she now felt she regretted.

Over the course of the sixteen sessions, Sam was able to explore this repetitive pattern through some of the current interpersonal difficulties she was facing in her relationship with her boss at work where she felt at the mercy of his bullying manner and never stood up for herself. In the therapy too, Sam's therapist was able to illustrate how Sam never allowed herself to voice her disappointment with her, as she anticipated that the therapist's agenda would always win the day and she simply had to comply with what was offered and be grateful for it. Yet behind the accommodating facade, the therapist noted Sam's anger. This dynamic, as it unfolded in the therapeutic relationship, also shed light on how Sam's 'insignificant' self-representation protected her against recognizing her own angry feelings.

By the end of the therapy, Sam had managed to give expression to her feelings of loss, guilt, and anger about the termination and took ownership of her difficulty in finding her own voice generally in her relationships with others. She had also made progress in standing up to her boss, whom she realized was not so much of a bully after all but was simply very assertive in his manner, which she invariably experienced as hostility. Once she could begin to integrate her own aggression into her representation of herself, Sam was able to divest others of her projection into them of this split-off aspect of her affective life.

Case two

Tony shared some features in common with Sam, but, as will become clear, his IPAF was nuanced slightly differently and hence provides a good example of the idiographic nature of the formulation within DIT.

Tony was an 18-year-old man who sought help after he left home for the first time to go to university. Up until then, he had enjoyed a close relationship with his mother who had been his main confidante. His father had left the family home, when he was aged eleven. He had no siblings and had a very strained relationship with his father and his new family.

When Tony started university, he became depressed. He struggled to form friendships with his peers. He was rather anxious around girls, whom he felt were either 'too superficial' or 'too intrusive'. With his male peers, he also seemed ill at ease, feeling they were 'domineering'. It seemed as though Tony could just not find the right pitch in his relationship to women in particular, and, with men, he appeared to feel he was not 'big' enough.

At first, he was very protective of the relationship with his mother—a woman who had clearly devoted herself to her son, depriving herself of a great deal to put him through a private education. However, she had also, it seemed, curtailed her own personal life, fostering what struck the therapist as a kind of Oedipal illusion (see ➲ The Oedipus complex in Chapter 2, p. 22) that had led to Tony feeling he was very special, but also feeling the burden of guilt. It did not seem insignificant that he became depressed once he left home, leaving his mother behind and feeling guilty for doing so. He was very caught up in taking care of his mother, feeling he needed to go home every weekend to be with her, as she had never remarried and hence was now living alone.

In the initial phase of the therapy, a pattern (the eventual IPAF) emerged—Tony repeatedly experienced himself as 'small', in relation to others who felt, to him, to be 'demanding' and whose needs crushed him. In these scenarios, he then started to feel a sense of rising panic. His smallness, in other words, was not related to shame, but to fear of being taken over by the needs of the other, leaving him always in a dependent, 'small' position.

His perceived 'smallness', relative to the other, contributed to him feeling a pressure to appease the other person, so as to assuage the fear that he would be abandoned if he did not satisfy their demand. Feelings of guilt featured largely in his emotional landscape. This was apparent in the way he assiduously attended sessions, in his excessive wish to please the therapist, and his tangible anxiety on the one occasion early on in the therapy when he arrived late.

In the middle phase, this pattern became the focus. As the therapist and Tony looked at what was happening at university and when he went back home, it was possible to discern how he found it very hard to assert himself and how he related to his mother in particular with a toxic mixture of dependency, guilt, and suffocated rage about her felt-to-be dependency on him which literally crushed him—an image that featured prominently in his narrative of relationships. Several sessions were devoted to helping Tony to reflect on his anxiety about what growing up and being independent meant to him emotionally and why this was so challenging. His depression appeared to serve—at least partly—the function of appeasing his mother (and hence his guilt) so that, even if he had geographically separated, he was still emotionally dependent on her, as he could not function away from her without breaking down.

It was during the middle phase that the therapist and patient also began to address Tony's relationship with his father who was conspicuous through his absence. His father emerged as a large figure in his life, whose loss had been very painful. His father had, in fact, made several attempts to engage Tony in his new family, but Tony had shunned this, retreating into an identification with his depressed abandoned mother. The pay off was that he became her special one, but this was achieved at the cost of being castrated and not able to become a man in his own right.

Tony and his therapist were able to link a different facet of his experience of himself as 'small' to the relationship with his father *in his mind* where 'small' was not linked so much there to fear, but to shame that resulted, in his mind, in him feeling castrated. This helped them to think together about how he related to his male friends at university, and one particular relationship was focused on, with the aim of helping Tony to begin to challenge his interpersonal pattern of avoidance of contact with his male peers who 'domineered' (in his mind largely), just as his father had done. This also opened up the possibility for Tony to approach his father to reignite contact, even if only tentatively at first.

In the final phase of the therapy, Tony's anxiety about losing his relationship with his therapist was intensified. He became more symptomatic again and feared that the therapy had been too brief, given how unwell he had been. His decline was marked and had a somewhat histrionic quality to it. This helpfully highlighted another dynamic hitherto inaccessible—namely, the way that he could be very 'demanding' in his own right and the pressure this put the therapist under in the transference. It was possible to raise this with him, and, although there was more productive exploration and working through of his identification with the 'demanding/dominating' other that would have been desirable, it was nevertheless helpful enough to enable Tony to recognize this tendency in himself. This, in turn, enabled him to acknowledge that he had been given something by the therapist and that, even if not perfect, it was good enough and paved the way for further exploration at a later stage. By the final session, his scores on measures of depression and anxiety were again well within the normal range.

Recommended reading

Luyten P, Van Houdenhove B, Lemma A, Target M, and Fonagy P (2013). Vulnerability for functional somatic disorders: a contemporary psychodynamic approach. *Journal of Psychotherapy Integration*, **23**, 250–62.

Dialectical behaviour therapy

(See ➔ Dialectical behaviour therapy in Chapter 2, pp. 63–6.)

Key techniques and competencies

Standard DBT involves the use of five treatment modalities, which serve different functions:

- *Individual therapy*—each patient has an individual therapist who is responsible for increasing motivation to change and helping the patient replace maladaptive responses with adaptive, more skilful responses
- *Group skills training*—the skills training is conducted in a psycho-educational format designed to enhance the individual's behavioural skills. Four modules of skills are taught: mindfulness, distress tolerance, emotion regulation, and interpersonal effectiveness
- *Telephone consultation*—many BPD patients have difficulty seeking help effectively, and the telephone consultation between an individual therapist and a patient is designed to provide practice in changing these dysfunctional patterns (in inpatient settings, nurses or other staff members can substitute for the phone consultations)
- *Consultation team*—treating clients with suicidal behaviours and/or BPD is enormously stressful, thus an integral part of DBT are the consultation team meetings designed to allow therapists to discuss their difficulties in a supportive, non-judgemental environment and also to help to improve motivation and capabilities. DBT assumes that effective treatment of BPD must pay as much attention to therapists' experience in therapy as it does the patient, as this helps to maintain effective therapeutic relationships
- *Skill generalization to the social milieu*—generalization of skills to the 'natural' environment.

DBT employs four sets of treatment strategies:

- *Dialectical strategies*:
    - Dialectic of the relationship—how the therapist structures interactions within the therapeutic relationship. A dialectical therapeutic position is one of constantly combining acceptance with change, flexibility with stability, and nurturing with challenging, and a focus on capabilities
    - Teaching dialectic behaviours—the therapist defines skilful behaviours. Behavioural extremes and rigidity (whether they are cognitive, emotional, or behavioural) are signals that synthesis has not been achieved. Instead, a middle path must be advocated by

direct teaching, offering alternative ways of thinking and behaving, and modelling dialectical behaviour
- Specific dialectical strategies—these are eight specific techniques that target the therapist/patient relationship: (1) entering the paradox, (2) using metaphor, (3) playing devil's advocate, (4) extending, (5) activating 'wise mind', (6) 'making lemonade out of lemons' (turning negatives into positives), (7) allowing natural change, and (8) dialectical assessment (asking 'what's been left out?')
- Validation strategies:
  - These form the core acceptance strategies in DBT and are fundamental to developing and maintaining an effective therapeutic relationship. Validation communicates to the patient that their responses make sense and can be understood within their current situation. There are three steps in validation:
    —Active observing—the therapist actively observes the thoughts, emotions, and behaviours of the patient
    —Reflection—the therapist, in a non-judgemental stance, reflects back to the patient their thoughts, emotions, and behaviour
    —Direct validation—the therapist identifies and reflects back to the patient the wisdom or validity of their response and communicates that this is understandable
- Problem-solving strategies:
  - These form the core change strategies in DBT. In DBT, all dysfunctional behaviours (suicide attempts, parasuicidal behaviour) can be seen as problems to be solved. DBT promotes patients having an active role in problem recognition and solving their problems effectively/appropriately, as opposed to adopting an avoidant or aggressive response. The effectiveness of problem-solving approaches is dependent upon the clear identification of what is causing the problem and maintaining this behaviour. Behaviour chain analyses are adopted throughout therapy to explore dysfunctional behaviours. Problem-solving has two stages:
    —Stage one—understanding and accepting the problem
    —Stage two—attempting to generate, evaluate, and implement alternative solutions
- Stylistic strategies:
  - This refers to the style a therapist applies during therapy, such as their tone, speed, and responsiveness. DBT balances two different styles of communication:
    —Reciprocal communication—characterized by responsiveness, self-disclosure, warmth, and genuineness, and requires taking the client's agenda and wishes seriously
    —Irreverent communication—the aim of irreverence is to tip the patient 'off balance' and to encourage them to adopt a more flexible approach, and it is often used when a patient is immovable or when the therapist and client are 'stuck'
  - The two communication styles are used in synthesis and with speed, and it is imperative that the patient and therapist have maintained a therapeutic alliance, prior to these strategies being adopted.

- *Case management strategies*:
  - When there are problems in the environment which interfere with the patient's functioning or progress, the therapist moves to the case management strategies. There are three case management strategies:
    —Consultation to the patient—this requires the therapist to be a consultant to the patient, rather than to the patient's network; the result of this is that a therapist will not intervene to adjust the patient's environment and nor will the therapist consult with other professionals about how to treat the patient, unless the patient is present
    —Environmental intervention—the approach in DBT is towards teaching a patient how to interact effectively with their environment; however, there are times when intervention is necessary (i.e. substantial harm may occur to the patient, if the therapist does not intervene), and this strategy is used over consultation to the patient
    —Consultation team meeting—this strategy balances the consultation to the patient; from this perspective, it is defined as a treatment system, in which therapists apply DBT to the patients and the consultation team applies DBT to the therapists.

What changes?

DBT provides a targeted and staged approach to treatment that enables the needs of the individual to be systematically addressed.

The four main stages, as referenced by Linehan, are:
- Pre-treatment: orienting the patient to the programme and identifying treatment targets
- Stage 1: establishing a therapeutic alliance, in order to promote safety and stabilization when addressing primary treatment targets (including parasuicidal and suicidal behaviour)
- Stage 2: emotional processing of the past to reduce post-traumatic stress
- Stage 3: setting and achieving personal goals and increasing self-respect.

Primary treatment targets
- Decreasing suicidal, parasuicidal, and violent/homicidal behaviours
- Decreasing therapy-interfering behaviours
- Decreasing quality of life-interfering behaviours
- Increasing behavioural skills (mindfulness, interpersonal effectiveness, emotion regulation, and distress tolerance).

Secondary treatment targets
- Increasing emotion modulation and decreasing emotional reactivity
- Increasing self-validation and decreasing self-invalidation
- Increasing realistic decision-making and judgement, and decreasing crisis-generating behaviour
- Increasing emotional experiencing and decreasing inhibited grieving
- Increasing active problem-solving and decreasing active passivity
- Increasing accurate communication of emotions and competencies, and decreasing mood dependency of behaviour.

Clinical populations and context

DBT was originally developed for women in the community displaying chronic suicidal and parasuicidal behaviours, and who also meet criteria for BPD. DBT has been further developed for a number of co-morbid and other clinical conditions, including alcohol and substance dependence, eating disorders, and depression. Although initially developed for the community, DBT is now widely used in a variety of settings, including inpatient and forensic services.

Case vignettes

Case one

Jane was a 25-year-old white female who had a history of self-harming behaviours and suicide attempts, and who was well known to the local CMHT. Jane had a history of planned and impulsive self-harming behaviour, suicide attempts, violence, alcohol misuse, difficulties in relationships, including the breakdown of her marriage, and having witnessed domestic abuse and experienced physical abuse and sexual assault in her childhood and early adulthood. Jane was admitted to low secure services following 33 previous psychiatric admissions.

Factors relevant to the development and maintenance of Jane's interpersonal and emotion regulation needs

Relevant childhood/early adulthood experiences:
- Invalidating environment characterized by:
  - Experiencing and witnessing abuse
  - Sexual assault
  - Bullying at school.

Additional relevant factors:
- Physical illness
- Alcohol misuse
- Breakdown in marriage
- Chaotic lifestyle.

Main presenting problems on admission
- Mood instability—difficulties controlling/modulating feelings of sadness, anger, anxiety, fear, shame, and guilt
- Negative core beliefs—including difficulties in being able to trust others, to have emotional needs met such as to experience and deserve genuine love
- Relationship instability—breakdown in relationship with husband and family
- Self-harm and suicidal behaviours—including overdoses, cutting, jumping off bridges, lying on train tracks
- History of alcohol misuse—increased risk of self-harming
- Impulsivity problems—managing anger, self-harming, alcohol use, absconding.

Treatment targets

Primary treatment targets The overall goal of the DBT programme was to assist Jane to increase her dialectical patterns of thoughts, feelings, and behaviours in response to past and current experiences, including distressing events, in order to reinforce adaptive coping to replace extreme behavioural responses, including self-harm and suicidal behaviours. The following treatment hierarchy was devised, in consultation with Jane, and identified the relevant targets for intervention, along with the proposed order in which to address these areas of need:

- *Stage one targets*:
1. *Life-threatening behaviours*:
    - Effective management of suicidal urges/behaviour
    - Effective management of self-harming thoughts/urges/behaviour
    - Effective management of violent and aggressive behaviours.
2. *Therapy-interfering behaviours*:
    - Mental state—unsettled behaviour may result in restrictions which impact on my therapy
    - Avoidance of attending therapy and not being fully engaged in the session
    - Difficulties communicating thoughts and feelings to others and limited interactions with others.
3. *Quality of life-interfering behaviours*:
    - Refusing help when required, 'fighting against support'
    - Not filling time well
    - Alcohol misuse.
4. *Skills deficits*:

Behaviours to decrease:	Behaviours to increase:
Impulsive self-harm	Mindfulness
Impulsive anger, shame, guilt	Emotional regulation
Relationship problem	Interpersonal effectiveness
Cognitive rigidity	Distress tolerance

- *Stage two targets*:
    - Addressing alcohol misuse
    - Decreasing post-traumatic stress
    - Bereavement.
- *Stage three targets*:
    - Increase self-respect
    - Achieving personal goals.

Secondary treatment targets Secondary targets refer to the hypothesized response patterns that may be functionally related to the primary target problems identified above. A number of secondary targets are proposed below. These factors are considered relevant for inclusion in the formulation and are addressed in treatment, in order to facilitate change in the primary targets:

Polarities:	Strategies:
Unrelenting crises	Problem-solving
Emotional avoidance	Exposure
Emotional vulnerability	Exposure–response prevention
Self-invalidation	Behaviour rehearsal
Active passivity	Functional analyses
Apparent competence	Feedback

Working hypothesis

Jane's experiences had led her to a point where she was unable to regulate and manage her emotions effectively, resulting in a chaotic lifestyle, characterized by self-harming behaviours, suicide attempts, difficulties within relationships, and excessive alcohol usage. She found it difficult to accept help and support, believing that her behaviour was acceptable, therefore contributing to her invalidating experiences. Jane had been making significant changes to address the above, her current controlling variable being her vulnerability, as she missed her family. This was also a motivator to her to re-establish her role within her family. Jane's preferred behaviour would be to acknowledge responsibility for her behaviour which led to self-destructive behaviours, and to be able to ask for, and accept, help.

Table 5.3 highlights how the above treatment hierarchy remains important, even after the commencement of therapy. Following the commencement of the programme, Jane was unable to identify appropriate strategies to manage her emotional responses, which resulted in her attempting to cut off her airway by ligation. The completion of a chain analysis with Jane identified her vulnerability factors, the precipitating factors, and the links that resulted in the problem behavior, along with the consequences. Doing this enabled Jane to break down the incident and closely examine each area, and she was able to identify that her current difficulties remained due to the initial identified deficits, which, in this case, acted as a reinforcer to be fully engaged in the therapy to address her difficulties.

Case two

Vera was a 40-year-old female with a long-standing history of self-harm, offending, and alcohol abuse. She had a long and extensive history of abuse between the ages of 5 and 20 at the hands of several family members. After leaving home at the age of 20, Vera lived a chaotic lifestyle and was frequently imprisoned for offences usually committed under the influence of alcohol and substances. Her offending behaviour included acquisitive offending, criminal damage, harassment, threats to kill, sexual offending, arson, and being drunk and disorderly, and she had spent the majority of her adult life in prison. Vera had one long-term relationship that resulted in her giving birth to a daughter. The child was taken into care shortly after her birth.

Prior to her admission to a medium secure psychiatric hospital, Vera was serving a prison sentence for arson. Whilst in prison, she received an Imprisonment for Public Protection (IPP) sentence for making threats to kill and harassment. An additional 8 months were also added to her sentence, due to a conviction for a sexual assault on a fellow inmate. Vera's mental health deteriorated in prison, and she engaged in life-threatening self-harm, resulting in her referral to medium secure care.

Relevant childhood experiences

Invalidating environment characterized by:

- Physical abuse within the family
- Sexual abuse within the family

Table 5.3 Chain analysis and task analysis snapshot for stage one target: life-threatening behaviours at 3 months

Vulnerability factors	Precipitating events	Links	Problem behaviour	Consequences
Could not get in touch with mum when I telephoned her Feeling lonely	Ward dynamics upsetting Not slept well Everyone appeared busy	Sadness and anger—'No one cares about me', 'I'm going to be alone' Rumination—'Things will never get any better', 'What is the point?', 'I may as well not be here', 'I always get treated this way'	Attempted to kill myself by ligating with socks	Tearful, guilty, emotions still around, restricted access to items, missed therapy session due to high risk, anger decreases—short-term immediate gain

Initial task analysis: Remove means, restrict access	Treat key links: Increase distress tolerance skills to manage immediate emotion response Increase interpersonal effectiveness skills—seeking support when required Treat rumination and judgements (cognitive restructuring to modify automatic thoughts)

Reduce vulnerability factors:
Assertiveness
Self-validation
Rehearsal—asking for support
Increasing sense of self to increase independence

- Neglect/lack of nurture
- Domestic violence
- Substance misuse (within the family and Vera)
- Lack of affection
- Running away from home.

Additional relevant factors:
- Death of Vera's mother
- Substance misuse
- Adoption of daughter
- Chaotic lifestyle and relationships
- Criminal behaviour.

Main presenting problems
- Mood instability—difficulties controlling/modulating feelings of anger, sadness, anxiety, fear, shame, and guilt
- Negative core beliefs—including a belief that she deserves to suffer and to be punished
- Relationship instability

- Grief and loss (death of mother, adoption of daughter, personal loss of appropriate relationships with family members)
- Self-harm and suicidal behaviours—including cutting, ligating, choking, burning
- Substance misuse
- Anger and impulsivity problems
- Arson
- Index offence: threats to kill.

Treatment targets

Primary treatment targets

- *Stage one targets:*
1. *Life-threatening behaviours:*
   - Effective management of suicidal urges/behaviour
   - Effective management of self-harming thoughts/urges/behaviour.
2. *Therapy-interfering behaviours:*
   - Non-completion of diary card
   - Not respecting the rules of the contract
   - Self-harm during the session.
3. *Quality of life-interfering behaviours:*
   - Inappropriate expression of anger
   - Impulsiveness
   - Judgemental responses
   - Problematic relationships (unbalanced priorities and demands—development/maintenance of unhelpful relationships, foregoing of self-respect).
4. *Skills deficits:*

Behaviours to decrease:	Behaviours to increase:
Impulsive self-harm	Distress tolerance
Impulsive anger, shame, guilt	Emotion regulation
Relationships problems	Interpersonal effectiveness
Cognitive rigidity	Mindfulness

- *Stage two targets:*
  - Decreasing post-traumatic stress.
- *Stage three targets:*
  - Increase self-respect
  - Achieving personal goals.

Secondary treatment targets

1. *Reducing emotional vulnerability*

The aim is to assist Vera to modulate her impulsive emotional reactions to events by promoting the use of mindfulness—particularly non-judgemental observation of factors that precipitate emotional responding, distress tolerance, and emotion to facilitate acceptance of distressing events and management of emotions to reduce Vera's vulnerability to experiencing intense (negative) emotions.

2. *Increasing self-validation*

Vera's self-invalidation includes a belief that she deserves to suffer and to be punished, because she feels she is a 'bad' person. These negative self-judgements are suggested to be a significant contributory factor to Vera's self-harm and suicidal behaviour. The aim is to improve Vera's distress tolerance skills and to reduce negative self-judgements, in order for Vera to validate herself and feel able to choose effective coping skills when distressed, including self-acceptance and self-soothing.

3. *Decreasing crisis-generating behaviour*

Vera's crisis-generating behaviour can be seen in the extent of the difficulties she experiences prior to distressing events such as an upcoming anniversary of the death of her mother. Vera's mood-dependent behaviour and mood-dependent decision-making result in a belief that she will not be able to cope with the distressing event. This precludes effective problem-solving and decision-making, and the aim therefore is to promote effective problem-solving, alongside the development of a non-judgemental approach to solving problems.

4. *Decreasing inhibited grieving*

The aim for this behavioural pattern is to support Vera in tolerating negative emotions, in order to learn how to reduce them. This requires exposure to negative emotions, using a carefully guided approach that allows Vera to learn that she can experience negative emotions without needing to respond to them with self-destructive patterns of behaviour.

5. *Decreasing active passivity*

Vera has shown an ability to ask for support in coping with distressing events; however, further support is required to assist her in developing a more active problem-solving style, in which she can use the resources and support available to her in a more effective manner.

6. *Increasing accurate communication of emotions and competencies*

The aim here is to assist Vera to accurately communicate (verbally and non-verbally) her feelings and her need for support. Vera has demonstrated on the ward and during her DBT sessions that her fear of not coping, or lack of belief in her ability to achieve goals, can be misleading and can prevent her from attempting new activities. Also, Vera often makes the judgement that she should be able to cope or should be feeling OK when she is not, and therefore does not ask for help when it is needed. Skills from the Interpersonal Effectiveness and Emotion Regulation modules are designed to address these particular difficulties.

Working hypothesis (synthesis statement)

Vera's childhood was characterized by an invalidating environment of abuse and neglect that significantly impaired her ability to understand and modulate her own emotional responses to internal and external experiences, to validate her own decision-making, to trust her own abilities, and to recognize helpful and hurtful behavioural patterns in her interpersonal relationships. This invalidating environment further exacerbated Vera's inherent emotion regulation problems, leading to difficulties in identifying and modulating her responses to emotional cues. Erratic, inconsistent, and harsh responding by the invalidating environment led Vera to generate extreme emotional reactions to distressing events, in order to elicit help from others and to self-validate such extreme responses as self-harm and suicide attempts. Alongside normal grief responses to the death of her mother, Vera's conflictual relationship with her mother appears to have led her to believe that she should punish herself and deserves to suffer. This is hypothesized to be due to Vera internalizing comments made by her family in relation to being inadequate, incompetent, a burden, and with the implicit or explicit suggestion that she should be a better, more acceptable person. Resulting emotional responses include guilt, shame, anger, and loneliness. Vera's experience of having her daughter adopted is likely to have strengthened her negative beliefs that she is incapable of coping effectively and managing on her own. It is suggested that these experiences led to the development of Vera's unrealistic belief that she should already be able to cope with all her problems, resulting in her reluctance to ask for help when needed, a weak or absent belief in her ability to solve her own problems, and a continuing belief that support is only deserved if she suffers significantly first. Vera also described a childhood in which she experienced frequent abuse and lived in fear of the next incident. It is hypothesized that an important function of Vera's self-harm is related to gaining control over anticipated fearful events such as attempting to cope with the anniversary date of the death of her mother. Vera reports that she does not feel pain at the time she self-harms (e.g. burning herself with a cigarette), but instead she knows that the pain will come later and be present for a couple of days afterwards.

Vera's ongoing cognitive, behavioural, emotional, and interpersonal difficulties are hypothesized to result from the above experiences and the resultant core beliefs that perpetuate her problems. Vera's participation in the DBT group skills and individual therapy sessions may enable her to further explore the development and maintenance of these problems and provide her with the necessary skills and validation needed to accept her current situation and achieve her individual goals.

Recommended reading

Dimeff L and Koerner K (2007). *Dialectical Behavior Therapy in Clinical Practice: Applications across Disorders and Settings.* Guilford Press,: New York/London.

Linehan M (1993). *Cognitive Behavioural Treatment of Borderline Personality Disorder.* Guilford Press: New York/London.

Mentalization-based treatment

(See ➜ Mentalization-based treatment in Chapter 2, pp. 66–70.)

Key techniques and competencies

Structure of therapy

MBT is structured around a trajectory which is divided into three main phases: engagement and pre-treatment, intensive treatment, leaving treatment, and follow-up:

- In the engagement phase, the patient's diagnosis, capacity for mentalizing, interpersonal functioning, risk assessment, and integration with other agencies are evaluated. Together with this, the patient is offered psycho-education and engagement in the production of a personalized formulation of their relevant personal sensitivities and mentalizing deficits, and their effects on personal functioning and in their relationships/attachment patterns. The formulation is relevant to setting goals for the treatment plan and can include a shared crisis plan.

- The work of intensive treatment requires adherence to the treatment model and periodic reviews of progress. In a population where frequent breakdowns and impulsive acts can result in dropouts from treatment, a multidisciplinary approach helps to set up and maintain adequate measures to ensure the possibility of early attention to breakdowns, and works to re-establish the treatment alliance, which may include admissions of errors on the part of the therapists.
- The end of the therapy is anticipated and worked at early on, to prepare patients who have chronic difficulties in leaving relationships and being alone. Liaising with other agencies and follow-up may be required, in order to provide adequate support outside of the psychotherapeutic programme.

Therapeutic stance

One of the most important aspects specific to the MBT therapist's approach is that it should be characterized by a '*not knowing stance*', with an authentic and genuine interest in the patient's predicament. This is possibly the most challenging aspect of the work for a clinician, as it requires an openness and personal availability that is not always a feature of other models and which needs careful monitoring, so as to maintain an optimal affective distance from the patient, without the therapist becoming too personal or, at the other extreme, pretentious.

The not knowing stance is a delicate, balanced position, in which the therapist accepts his own beliefs and values, whilst openly making room for the shared work of mentalizing aspects of the patient's experience, accepting differences, and the 'work-in-progress' nature of the task. By avoiding assumptions, mentalization is fostered through the use of the therapist's genuine inquisitiveness, acceptance of the patient's level of mentalization, and openness to learning from the encounter with the patient's experience. Leading interpretations of the clinical material, according to the therapist's preferred personal theoretical models (e.g. cognitive or psychoanalytic), are best avoided. A supportive, empathic style, focusing on the patient's mentalizing capacity and arousal, should result in an optimal regulation of the attachment system and the possibility of open, shared enquiry of the patient's experience.

Specific interventions

Spectrum of interventions

MBT comprises a spectrum of interventions of increasing complexity:
- Reassurance, support, and empathy
- Clarification, challenge, and elaboration
- Basic mentalizing—'stop, listen, look', 'stop, rewind, explore'
- Interpretive mentalizing
- Mentalizing the transference.

Principles of treatment/interventions
- Focus on the patient's mind (not behaviour)
- Simple and short interventions
- Affect-focused (love, desire, hurt, catastrophe, excitement)
- Relate to current event or activity
- De-emphasize unconscious concerns in favour of near-conscious or conscious content.

Which intervention to use when?
• Start at the surface—support and empathy
• Move to 'deeper' levels only after performing earlier steps
• If emotions become overwhelming, take a step back towards the surface
• Type of intervention inversely related to emotional intensity
• Intervention must be in keeping with the patient's mentalizing capacity.

In order to avoid the possibility of pseudomentalization in the pretend mode (see ➔ Mentalization-based treatment in Chapter 2, pp. 66–70) by getting lost in inconsequential talk and to keep a focus on the current affective state of the patient, a focus on more recent events is given priority over historical issues. For example, a patient may justify an incident on the bus that morning by reference to the impact of childhood traumatic experiences. Whilst this may be relevant, it may be more helpful to concentrate on what just occurred on the bus, enquiring about the patient's and the other's possible states of mind at the time. This could lead to a more flexible 'mentalizing' of their mental state and emotional responses, challenging prementalizing modes of explanation, and exploring together their impact on the patient's mental state and experiences.

Given the issues with interpersonal sensitivity in patients with BPD, the therapeutic work can be daunting. The therapist is invited to monitor her response and be prepared to acknowledge her failures, whilst continually redressing attention to the task of mentalizing. This can happen, for example, by stopping an increasingly heated exchange, diffusing the aroused response, taking responsibility for what may have upset the patient, and proposing to go back to examining the topic in hand from the start. This close attention to the process involving the therapist and the patient offers the possibility of recognizing and exploring together particular sensitivities which can lead to frequent breakdowns in mentalizing and leave room for prementalistic modes of relating, whilst fostering a reparative process of the collaborative efforts.

Supervision
Regular supervision is essential to set up the programme, to review clinical assessments and formulations, to support members of the team, to keep communication between different parts of the programme, to instigate review meetings on patients' progress, and to provide 'intervision' or supervision of the working of the team as a whole. A specific aspect of MBT supervision relates to joint evaluation of video and audio recordings of the clinical sessions, in order to understand the clinical progress and address any failure in the therapeutic interaction.

A comprehensive list of 17 aspects and seven competency areas of MBT can be found in the MBT-ASC. This can be used both as a form of self-directed learning or in supervision.

What changes?
The main aim of the therapy is a stabilization of affective control, maintaining and reinstating mentalizing when cooperation breaks down. This gradual increase in the capacity to mentalize, with concomitant

improvements in impulse control and emotional regulation, facilitates positive changes in the patient's behaviours, relationships, and functioning in their external life, according to the stage of treatment:

- At the beginning of treatment, the main changes relate to an increase in the patient's safety, reduction of impulsive acts, improvement in the treatment alliance, and regular attendance.
- In the middle phase, problematic behaviours and self-harm, as well as relationships, are discussed and may benefit from an increased ability to mentalize and to find alternative ways of expressing emotions and associated thoughts.
- Improvements in social inclusion, personal relationships, vocation, and planning may become more prominent towards the end of the treatment.
- The end of treatment marks the beginning of further changes in personal rehabilitative efforts and the integration in the external world.

Clinical populations and contexts

The main population studied and treated with MBT, to date, consists of patients with BPD.

More recently, MBT has been applied to the treatment of patients with other disorders, including:

- ASPD (see ➔ Antisocial personality disorder in Chapter 8, pp. 396–401; Forensic psychiatry: forensic psychotherapies, applications, and research in Chapter 12, pp. 550–6)
- Eating disorders (see ➔ Eating disorders in Chapter 7, pp. 334–8)
- Depression (see ➔ Affective disorders in Chapter 7, pp. 326–31)
- Trauma (see ➔ Trauma-related conditions in Chapter 7, pp. 355–9)
- Drug addiction (see ➔ Substance misuse in Chapter 7, pp. 338–45; Psychiatry of addictions: psychotherapies, applications, and research in Chapter 12, pp. 574–6)
- Adolescents with emerging BPD
- At-risk mothers.

Following the first long-term studies, which took place in a day hospital and later in an outpatient department, other settings and modifications of MBT, such as inpatient, family therapy, and brief therapies based on mentalization, are being increasingly described and studied.

Case vignettes

Case one

Debbie is a 34-year-old woman referred by her GP after having received counselling and CBT for depression, as she is experiencing ongoing difficulties. Clinical assessment reveals long-standing dysthymia with severe anxiety and depersonalization, problems at work, with a recent dismissal after a row with her boss, difficulties in intimate relationships, problems with impulse control and self-harm (cutting), binge eating, and excessive spending. She suffers with irritable bowel syndrome and complains of premenstrual symptoms of increased irritability. She lives on her own and is currently receiving benefits after leaving the last job. She has recently quit her smoking habit, after giving up drinking thanks to

Alcoholics Anonymous, and is feeling helpless to get on with her life on her own. She refuses antidepressants.

A psychodynamic psychotherapy assessment finds features compatible with a personality disorder. The assessor fears that the patient's tendency to be self-destructive will hinder recovery but is impressed by her ability to engage in discussion of difficult past experiences such as her disruptive family environment or her crushed dream to become a writer.

Debbie is referred for outpatient MBT and is invited for early evaluation and treatment planning. The programme is explained, and, after testing that DSM diagnostic criteria for BPD are satisfied, the diagnosis and risk assessment are discussed. A care plan is formulated which includes steps in case of increased risk to self, continued care by the GP, and the basic rules of the participation in the MBT programme.

The first phase of therapy includes an educational, 'explicit mentalization' group and individual therapy. In the explicit group, the patients are invited to discuss themes such as 'what makes me me'. Debbie voices discomfort at the irrelevance of these 'class exercises' to her problems and misses sessions. Her symptoms of depression worsen; she becomes withdrawn, and her eating deteriorates. Both Debbie's group and individual therapists discuss her case and decide to see her outside the session time to review the situation. At the joint meeting, they acknowledge her difficulties and discuss them and the importance of continuous attendance.

Debbie starts attending the programme again. The group has now progressed to 'implicit mentalization', and the topics are chosen according to the patients' own recent life events or the life of the group. An agenda of topics is set and discussed in the group where others offer support, promote questioning, and share similar doubts. In individual therapy, Debbie talks more of her partner and, at times, links this to her relationships with her family. A careful exploration of the transference and countertransference feelings in the therapist reveals similar links to the relationship with the therapist, which is used to clarify recurrent conflicts in her relationships and explore alternative solutions.

At 1 year, Debbie has stopped self-harming, and she is looking into help for her eating disorder and discussing taking antidepressants with her GP. She engages in a new relationship and discusses this in the group. Through relating episodes of their life together, she reveals her ongoing struggle to make room for her partner's strengths and limitations, instead of feeling that he is unfathomably fantastic or horrible to her, as she has previously experienced. She starts volunteering for a charity. At the end of the 18 months of therapy, she is offered follow-up meetings 6 months later, and eventually further group therapy.

Case two

Mark is a 42-year-old homosexual man who has diagnoses of ADHD and OCD, and is HIV-positive. He frequently enters intense, passionate relationships which end abruptly and lead to suicidal gestures and repeated presentations to A&E. After one of these presentations, he is referred for an MBT assessment. He undergoes a detailed assessment and psychometric testing. On discussing the results with the clinician, he talks of his relief at being diagnosed with BPD—his long-standing difficulties started to make sense to him, as he had felt that for years no one was really interested in him.

He is articulate and keen to receive treatment and engages well with the preliminary phase of treatment. He works well in individual therapy, but, whilst he enjoyed the explicit tasks set at the beginning of the introductory group, he soon finds interactions in the implicit, open group too upsetting. He becomes increasingly agitated and verbally aggressive at perceived slights, tends to dominate in the group, and threatens the therapists with complaints. The group therapists try to re-establish a climate of safety, and one of them asks Mark to leave and take time out during a particularly difficult session. After threatening to leave the programme and missing a couple of sessions, Mark talks to his individual therapist of his distress at feeling kicked out of the group and mistreated by one of the group therapists.

The therapists discuss what is going on in both the group and individual sessions during their joint supervision. The group therapists speak of their growing frustration at Mark and the relief at not seeing him in the group over the last couple of sessions, and link this to the possibility to review with him what can be planned to help diffuse unhelpful and unsafe interactions. In the next group session, the therapist facilitates a tactful discussion of the issue and acknowledges his sense of helplessness and frustration at seeing Mark getting angry again. The therapist adds that he is not sure whether he could have done something else to diffuse the anger and keep Mark in the group, and asks for help in thinking of alternative strategies. Mark readily recognizes his anger and links it with his attempts to evoke attention and a response at home and in intimate relationships. This time, he agrees to a plan where other group members can stop him with a special hand signal and help him notice his growing arousal. Review of Mark's feelings and behaviour in the group leads to expressions of satisfaction by other group members at their increased sense of establishing safety together.

Recommended reading

Allen J, Fonagy P, and Bateman A (2008). *Mentalizing in Clinical Practice*. American Psychiatric Publishing: Washington, DC.

Bateman A and Fonagy P (2006). *Mentalisation-Based Treatment for Borderline Personality Disorder. A Practical Guide*. Oxford University Press: Oxford.

Bateman A and Fonagy P (eds) (2012). *Handbook of Mentalizing in Mental Health Practice*. American Psychiatric Publishing: Washington, DC.

Fonagy P, Gergely G, Jurist EL, and Target M (2002). *Affect Regulation, Mentalization and the Development of the Self*. Other Press: New York.

Karterud S, Pedersen G, Engen M, *et al.* (2013). The MBT Adherence and Competence Scale (MBT-ACS): development, structure and reliability. *Psychotherapy Research*, **23**, 705–17.

Schema therapies

(See ➋ Schema therapy in Chapter 2, pp. 70–3.)

Key techniques and competencies

Several interventions with a focus on change of emotional memories are combined in schema therapy. The therapist identifies the unmet childhood needs and meets these unmet emotional needs in the therapy. The therapist does this through an intervention called *partial re-parenting*.

Partial re-parenting requires the therapist to be authentic in looking after the childhood modes of the patient. The therapist uses emotional atunement to attend to the mode flipping of the patient. Moment to moment, the unmet need arising from childhood neglect is traced and attended to in a compassionate fashion. Good parenting and healthy adult functioning are modelled continuously to embody an alternative healing emotional experience to the patient.

Other interventions include using cognitive therapy techniques, e.g. the cost and benefit of a schema can be discussed, toxic beliefs can be challenged.

Behavioural techniques in sessions include playing out different modes explicitly through 'putting each mode on a chair'. By using the chair techniques, previous intertwined modes can talk to each other. These chair conversations are coached and facilitated by the therapist, in order to create an emotionally safe experience.

Emotion-focused techniques are key in schema therapy; going back to toxic childhood situations in imagery, unmet childhood needs are met by giving the toxic memory an emotionally healing outcome (*re-scripting*). The therapist, through imagery techniques, provides a healing experience via emotional validation and support. The aim is to update the emotional content of the memory to correspond to the patient's adult and mature reality in the here and now. The schema can heal and ultimately drive more adult, healthy behaviours and adaptive emotional and cognitive responses to previously distressing triggers.

What changes?

The overall aims of therapy are, in sequence of therapeutic phases:
- To help the coping modes to step aside to allow the needs of the child modes to be acknowledged
- The support and meeting of the needs of the child modes through partial re-parenting and emotion-focused therapy techniques of imagery and chair work
- The fighting and elimination of dysfunctional parent modes
- To build or strengthen the *healthy adult mode*. This is conceptualized as acting as an adult individual, being able to take responsibility for self and others. The healthy adult mode is able to integrate and care for the child modes, and deal with unhelpful coping modes.

The patient's unhelpful, but understandable, attempts to respond to a sense of overwhelming emotional distress perpetuate the schemas. Schemas are less accessible to cognitive work. Schemas are held as toxic emotional memories associated with unmet childhood needs. When triggered, the emphasis is placed on devising treatment for the emotional memories through more emotionally impactful interventions.

In general, individual schema therapy extends over 2 to 3 years.

Clinical population and contexts

Because of its roots in CBT for personality disorders, the best evidence exists for the use of schema therapy in people with BPD where large

RCTs have been done to show its efficacy (see ➔ Borderline personality disorder in Chapter 8, pp. 390–6). There is now a noticeable trend to use schema-based interventions for a range of mental disorders, e.g. narcissistic personality disorder or obsessive–compulsive personality disorder (see ➔ Narcissistic personality disorder in Chapter 8, pp. 415–22; Obsessive compulsive (anankastic) personality disorder in Chapter 8, pp. 412–15). A lot of interest is emerging out of promising studies of schema therapy in forensic populations. More recently, schema-based interventions have been used for anxiety disorders and depression. These studies are still at a pilot level and will require replication in larger trials.

Schema therapy is a complex intervention with significant training requirements for the therapist. The overall availability of schema-focused techniques may be restricted by the number of available trained therapists. Nonetheless, mental vulnerabilities are often predisposed by childhood adversity and unmet childhood needs. Therefore, it is likely that schema-based interventions will be tested for a range of mental disorders in the future.

Case vignettes

Case one

Julie was a 41-year-old beautician, mother of two boys, aged 7 and 10. She came to therapy, because of recurrent breakdowns in her relationships, often triggered by intense anger outbursts, with a tendency to use physical and emotional violence towards partners. When feeling abandoned, she often superficially self-harmed, as well as engaged in casual sexual relationships in order to self-soothe. She wanted therapy, as she felt she could not cope with the 'up and down' of her emotions and wanted to stabilize her relationships, as well as become a mother who was better able to tolerate her sons' emotional expressions.

From her childhood history, it became apparent that she had a range of unmet childhood needs. Her mother was a severely emotionally and physically abusive woman, who sometimes left and abandoned the family for several days without prior warning. This led to a sense of instability, triggering schemas of emotional deprivation in Julie. Julie's mother used to manipulate emotional validation and love between Julie and her sister, and withdraw affection if one of the girls did not want to do what the mother demanded. This led to a mistrust and abuse schema, teaching Julie to 'hit people before they hit you'. The Young Schema Questionnaire (YSQ) showed that Julie suffered from a range of other schemas, including a defectiveness schema and an abandonment schema, as well as schemas around social isolation, entitlements, and grandiosity, as well as punitiveness.

The therapist established a mode model with her, highlighting her prominent modes. These included coping modes of cutting herself off emotionally from partners (*avoidant protector mode*), engaging in extreme clinginess and jealousy (*overcompensating over controller mode*), as well as attacking partners and also making false allegations against partners (*bully and attack mode*).

With regard to her child modes, she had a very underdeveloped vulnerable child mode (VCM), a very prominent *angry child mode*, and a

demanding and punitive parent mode, which constantly made her feel inferior, but also led to her being very critical of others. Overall, she tried
to look after her sons well, so there was evidence of some healthy adult
modes, but overall these were very underdeveloped.

The therapist used the first five to ten sessions to build Julie's trust, also
explaining the schema model to her. In the first of three stages, the costs
and benefits of the coping modes were analysed, and, to some degree,
the role of the coping modes were empathically challenged in chair work.
In order to provide this, the therapist supported and coached Julie to see
the somewhat unhelpful role of all the coping modes.

In the second step, Julie went back to her childhood and gave an
account of multiple episodes of very painful memories where she was
abandoned by her mother and felt unsupported by a weak and absent
father. Memories involving emotional and physical abuse were brought
up in imagery, and the therapist entered the imagery as a good parent,
in order to keep 'Little Julie' safe and to banish the abusive mother from
the image. In a homework exercise, Julie was encouraged to engage in
exercises of self-soothing, using safe place imagery, and developing compassion for the part of her that has been severely abused.

Once the vulnerable child Little Julie was strengthened and soothed,
the therapist used multiple exercises to challenge and banish the punitive parent mode. This mode was associated with toxic messages about
Julie being useless, unloved, and deserving to be punished. Partial re-
parenting involved chair work, as well as imagery work, where the therapist answered back on Julia's behalf, and banished the punitive parent in
multiple locations.

In the last stages of the therapy, the therapist encouraged Julie's
healthy adult mode to take over—to look after her own vulnerable child
and also to look after the angry part of the self in a better and soothing
way. She was encouraged to value her relationships and resolve conflict
in a more adult way. Julie and her therapist also thought about letting go
of jealous and over-angry behaviour, and to allow her partner to have
more space. Julie learned to trust that, just because her partner was not
there all the time, that did not mean that she will be abandoned.

Julie's overall functioning improved significantly—she was able to chan-
nel her anger and express her worry about being unloved or abandoned
in a healthier way. She was able to refrain from using impulsive anger
against her partner and no longer resorted to self-harming to regulate
previously overwhelming emotions. She was also able to become a more
loving mother towards her children and to tolerate their expression of
sadness or anger in a healthier adult way.

Case two

Thomas was a 40-year-old gay man from white British background.
He worked as a light engineer at a local theatre. He presented with a
long history of turbulent relationships, often intensely passionate at the
beginning of the relationship, but then resulting in increasing irritability,
arguments, and domestic violence, followed by separation and periods
of depression with heavy drug and alcohol use.

In schema therapy, schemas around mistrust and abuse were identified. These arose from being brought up by an alcoholic mother and a

range of changing paternal figures where some of his core childhood needs, including acceptance, safety, and healthy boundaries, were not met. This led to low self-esteem, fear of abandonment, emotional deprivation, unrelenting standards, and a significant degree of subjugation of his own needs in relationships.

After a period of engagement in the schema therapy model, including the therapist needing to reach out to Thomas on several occasions after he did not attend the sessions (identified as part of the avoidant protector mode), Thomas was able to come up with a schema formulation and set his own goals of therapy. Thomas identified that he used a range of coping modes, including overcompensating controlling mode by being very clingy and jealous towards partners, avoiding protector mode by staying indoors and not seeing any friends for several weeks, and compliant surrender mode by engaging and staying in abusive relationships.

After starting to manage these coping modes more assertively, Thomas was able to do meaningful work around his punitive parent mode, which was embodied in a punitiveness schema and, at times, cruel attitude towards himself and others.

In the later part of the therapy, more work was done with the VCM. The VCM arose when he often felt very lonely and abandoned, e.g. when a text message was not replied to by a friend within a short time period. Thomas was able to absorb a healthy adult mode message that he developed jointly with his therapist, and, through imagery work, he was able to feel emotionally protected when his childhood traumatic memories were triggered.

A lot of work went into behavioural experiments and behavioural interventions, with regard to changing his maladaptive patterns of forming and maintaining relationships—Thomas changed his habit of engaging in casual sexual relationships and experimented with taking a slower pace, focusing on the kindness of the other person, rather than their physical attractiveness. With time, he managed to direct more kindness towards his momentary feelings of loneliness and sadness, and to look after his own needs better, rather than cutting these feelings off through self-destructive patterns or maladaptive self-soothing with drugs and alcohol.

After 38 sessions of individual schema therapy, the regular weekly therapy was phased out, and Thomas maintained occasional email and text contact with his therapist, as well as follow-up sessions about once every 3 months over the next 2 years.

Thomas is now in a civil partnership with a man his age. Occasionally, his angry child mode arises, but he is able to express and communicate his needs more openly and in a way that does not damage or jeopardize his relationship with other people.

Recommended reading

Arntz A and van Genderen H (2009). *Schema Therapy for Borderline Personality Disorder.* Wiley-Blackwell: Chichester.

Behary WT (2008). *Disarming the Narcissist-Surviving and Thriving With the Self-Absorbed.* New Harbinger Publications: Oakland.

Van Vreeswijk M, Broersen J, and Schurink G (2014). *Mindfulness and Schema Therapy: A Practical Guide.* Wiley-Blackwell: Chichester.

Mindfulness-based interventions and therapies

(See → Mindfulness-based interventions and therapies in Chapter 2, pp. 73–5.)

Key techniques and competencies

The format of mindfulness-based interventions

MBI are generally delivered in an eight-week group programme, with 12 to 20 members in the group.

MBI serve as paradoxical interventions. Western medical and psychological approaches are targeted towards changing the way we feel. Mindfulness, on the other hand, widens our approach to suffering by opening a path towards experiencing *non-change and acceptance* as another way of dealing with both physical and mental difficulties. In this sense, MBI promote fundamentally different ways to approach discomfort, distress, and pain. Just as regular physical exercise can promote cardiovascular fitness, meditation practices may be conceptualized as exercises, in order to develop that type of *quality of mindfulness*. As an analogy, regular running or exercising would contribute to the development of the quality of cardiovascular fitness. Regular use of meditative practices promotes mindfulness.

Almost all MBI teach a variety of meditation techniques, in order for patients to learn the mental quality of mindfulness. Practising and experiencing different meditation techniques are some of the goals of the programmes. Meditation sessions, as well as daily homework meditation exercises, are considered essential for participants to engage with. Although there is no unambiguous scientific evidence that the duration of meditation practice makes a difference to the development of the quality of mindfulness, most facilitators of MBI agree that a regular and consistent practice of meditation is required. Between sessions one and four, several different meditation techniques are introduced. Meditation starts with a brief meditation exercise on an object, e.g. a raisin, which is observed in a different way.

Great emphasis is put on meditation on the body. The body is perceived to be the mirror of emotional experience and sensory physical sensations. Meditation in movement, e.g. mindful stretching, as well as mindful walking, are further opportunities to explore directing attention to the body and the moment. Sitting meditation, in a chair or on the floor, is another way of exploring the *habits of the mind* and dealing with the reactions of the body to posture, whilst embodying stillness and observation.

Brief meditation practices, e.g. the *breathing space*, offers the possibility of short focus points of attention, in addition to the longer, more formalized meditation sitting practices.

Psycho-education

Psycho-education is an important component of all MBI. Depending on what the focus of the MBI actually is, a significant amount of sessional time will be spent on psycho-education about, e.g. depression, alcohol use, eating disorder, or other elements. As an example, MBCT for relapse prevention of depression places great emphasis on recognizing triggers and symptoms of a depressive episode. It helps to become familiar with the kindling effect of ruminative processes on depressive relapse. The facilitators propose developing alternative strategies to help avert a further depressive episode. Ultimately, mindful awareness may facilitate relapse prevention through wise choices of alternative ways of dealing with early relapse signs.

Homework exercises

The use of homework meditation and other exercises are recommended by all MBI. Prior to starting in a group treatment programme, the participants are encouraged to create time for homework practice. This serves, on the one hand, to empower patients to take more care of themselves in the home environment, and, on the other hand, it gives the participants opportunities to take skills learnt in sessions into their daily lives. Developing the daily ritual of a brief meditation practice may serve as a focus point to be reminded of skills learnt in the programme.

The relapse prevention plan

The programme finishes with a written individualized development of a relapse prevention plan for the condition. The patients value the empowerment that the programme provides, as it is an intervention where patients can take control of their vulnerability. In this sense, MBI promote patient independence. Participants in MBI appreciate the responsibility that each of them can take to deal with their own health conditions in a different and self-compassionate way.

What changes?

On a general level, mindfulness can introduce a new aspect to Western clinical practice, as it is, to some degree, revolutionary—whilst Western medicine is very much focused on *changing* the condition that the patient finds herself in, mindfulness is substantially different. Mindfulness opens the option of *accepting* the condition as it is, without needing to change it at all. This may seem counterintuitive. Ultimately, mindfulness encourages the stance of observing difficulties with interest and curiosity, rather needing to alter them. This option of moving towards difficulties, without the pressure or option to change, is particularly helpful for chronic conditions, both physical and mental.

The earlier studies conducted into the effects of mindfulness promoted the ability to step back from one's own thoughts process. This can help develop a slightly more distant, less attached position towards the content of one's thoughts. This process is called meta-cognitive awareness and has been shown to be generally beneficial for a range of mental health symptoms. Empirical studies have identified a range of mediators that may facilitate an overall improvement of most measures of psychological well-being. These include higher levels of satisfaction with life, conscientiousness, self-esteem, empathy, competence, optimism, sense of autonomy, and pleasant affect.

Mindfulness induces brain changes, which can be shown through functional neuroimaging and other techniques. These biological changes include reduced bilateral amygdala activation, as well as more widespread prefrontal cortical activation. This suggests that mindfulness is associated with a better ability to regulate amygdala responses.

Clinical populations and context

MBI have been successfully used for a range of clinical and non-clinical populations across the range of physical, as well as mental, health conditions.

Many chronic physical health conditions have been investigated, with clinical trials looking into the effects of MBI, mostly mindfulness-based stress reduction. These include populations of patients with cancer, fibromyalgia, chronic pain, and multiple sclerosis. There is good evidence that MBI are helpful in patients with hypertension. MBCT has the best and most compelling evidence, with regard to preventing relapse of depression. In patients who have had three or more depressive episodes in the past, MBCT has been shown to be as good as antidepressant medication in preventing relapse. MBCT has also been used for other mental health problems, including bipolar disorder, social phobia, and GAD. Elements of mindfulness-based techniques are used in DBT for BPD, and ACT for addiction problems.

Case vignettes

Case one

John was a 38-year-old white Irish social worker who presented to his GP with a history of several depressive episodes. These went back to the age of 20 when he first became depressed, whilst being at university. In his third episode of depression, he presented with low mood, low energy levels, and having had to take time off work for 4 weeks, as he was unable to concentrate. He wanted to get better, but, as he had experienced side effects on antidepressant medication, he was reluctant to start an antidepressant.

After six sessions of guided self-help with the help of a therapist from the primary care psychological service, his depression went into remission. Nonetheless, because of past recurrent patterns, an eight-week course of MBCT was recommended.

Although John initially struggled to do the homework for the MBCT programme, he eventually managed to do a daily practice of 20 minutes of meditation. Initially, he felt slightly worse, as he became aware of the negative thoughts still going through his mind about himself, his past failures, and his worries about the future. Nonetheless, after about 3 weeks, he experienced the quality of being able to direct his attention more to his present moment experience. Through understanding the signs and the pattern of his depressive relapses, he began to develop an awareness of his mood changing, e.g. when he started to ruminate and worry. He began to experiment with using activities that he enjoyed, in order to influence how he felt emotionally. With the help of the breathing space, he found it easier to deal with situations where frustration is triggered, e.g. reading emails in his workplace. Rather than following his previous pattern of getting anxious and then ruminating about the stressful moments, he became aware of attending to his body in those situations and taking the moment to observe his emotional reaction, without needing to follow this up with rumination or expressed irritability. Towards the end of the programme, John was ready to make a plan over how to stop when he experienced certain triggers that, in the past, led to him getting depressed. He also developed his own relapse prevention plan; this involved monitoring his own mood and becoming aware of when his mood changed. He was more aware of the symptoms of depression and able to identify more subtle signs of those symptoms returning, e.g. when withdrawing from his friends.

His relapse prevention plan included making contact with people that he trusted, in order for them to be able to reach out to him when he was afraid of spiralling into depression. He listed cooking a healthy meal for himself, doing some running with his dogs three times per week, and meeting up with friends to watch football together at least once per week. He also developed his own habit of using meditation techniques on a daily basis, which included 20 minutes of sitting meditation in the morning and a breathing space after each meal, as well as having his breakfast in a mindful way, enjoying it bite by bite and without distraction.

He shared his relapse prevention plan with his partner, who agreed to do some meditation jointly with him, but also to remind him when she observed early signs of him relapsing, e.g. when he became unnecessarily irritable and withdrawn.

John has now been depression-free for 2 years and attends regular meditation sessions offered at his local GP practice with an experienced mindfulness teacher. He is very pleased that he has found a way to take control over his own emotional well-being, and he feels empowered to manage his life without needing to resort to medication.

Case two

Patma was a 57-year-old mother of two adult daughters, who was widowed 3 years ago. She had a South Asian background. Two years ago, she was involved in a serious road traffic accident which left her with chronic pain in her back and legs. She was also overweight and suffered from type 2 diabetes. She presented with a long history of recurrent depression and anxiety, preceding her bereavement and chronic illness, for which she had been treated with antidepressant medication since her twenties. She continued to be on antidepressants, as well as analgesics, antidiabetic medication, and an antihypertensive.

She had long-term psychodynamic therapy for 3 years in her twenties, as well as two subsequent courses of CBT for anxiety and depression. The most recent course of CBT finished 3 months ago, and she was recommended to engage in MBCT for relapse prevention of her depressive and anxious vulnerability.

As part of the MBCT programme, Patma developed a new relationship with her chronically aching body—through the *body scan* meditation, she became aware of how aversive her own body had become to her. Initially, she struggled to develop a kinder relationship with her body and found it almost impossible to lie still.

In order to be able to do the sitting meditation, she decided to sit upright in a chair and noticed how much her mind was distracted by body sensations. She became aware that she worried more about the future of her symptoms and their inescapability than about the pain itself, which was bearable with the help of painkillers.

Understandably, she found it difficult to deal with both physical and mental symptoms of her presentation. As the MBCT programme progressed, she understood that directing interest towards physical sensations, as well as having an open mind with regard to exploring symptoms, offered a completely new opportunity to relate to her chronic condition. She noticed that, at times, she was able to approach pain in a completely new way and realized how much her physical pain was perpetuated by the worry about the pain itself. She noticed that walking meditation, as well as mindful movement, seemed to be the most gentle and nourishing way of focusing attention on the present moment.

As part of the cognitive behavioural element of MBCT, she became more aware that she experienced moments of pleasure and satisfaction, especially when she was with her daughters. These were the moments of quality in her life that seem to have been completely missed, because of her chronic pain condition in the past.

With developing a behavioural plan of how to bring more quality of life into her daily experience, she found the courage to expand her range of activity, even though this was sometimes limited by physical pain. She is now able to register for some voluntary work and experiences increasing excitement about her daughter having her first child, and is committed to supporting her daughter with some childcare, despite being limited by her physical condition.

As part of having introduced mindfulness into her life, her use of analgesics has drastically reduced, and she has noticed a significant reduction in her depressive ruminations and levels of anxiety, which has been maintained. Mindful eating has also helped her to lose weight and improve her diet.

Recommended reading

Halliwell E (2015). *Mindfulness: How to Live Well by Paying Attention*. Hay House Basics: London.
Williams JMG and Penman D (2011). *Mindfulness: A Practical Guide to Finding Peace in a Frantic World*. Piatkus: London.
Williams JMG, Teasdale J, Segal Z, and Kabat-Zinn J (2007). *The Mindful Way Through Depression: Freeing Yourself from Chronic Unhappiness* (includes Guided Meditation Practices CD). Guilford Press: New York.

Therapeutic communities

(See ➔ Therapeutic communities in Chapter 2, pp. 75–80.)

Key techniques and competencies

The following competencies were developed by Nicholson for the Consortium of Therapeutic Communities in 2014.

Role-related competencies
- *Understanding of role*:
  - Better understand the boundaries of the therapist's role, the place this has within the wider organization, and the outcomes it is designed to achieve
- *Understanding of client group*:
  - Provide responses of understanding to the particularity of the client within the context of the community

- Show developing insight into the clinical issues extent within the client group
- Relate to others as human beings, not as diagnoses or labels
- *Clinical observation*:
  - Able to accept 'not knowing' and allow time for understanding to emerge
  - Capacity to observe behaviour/mood/interactions and notice the internal and external dynamics involved
  - Capacity to formulate a hypothesis
- *Capacity to acknowledge and use the boundaries of the TC*:
  - Developing awareness and capacity to regulate boundaries
  - Ability to share authority with all members of the community— 'dispersed authority'
  - Capacity to own and use one's own authority
  - Recognizing the significance of space and time, and how therapeutic structures are established
  - Creative/flexible use of TC structures.

Practice-related competencies
- *Understanding of TC methodologies*:
  - Show a willingness to learn and engage with 'methods'
  - Emotionally open within a 'culture of enquiry'
  - Developing knowledge and understanding of psychodynamic ideas
  - Desire to acquire both academic and experiential knowledge in a 'living–learning environment'
  - Desire to be a part of a containing matrix of relationships and use the community to address and solve problems
- *Communication skills*:
  - Openness to both conscious and unconscious communication, and recognize behaviours and affects are communications
  - Communicate in a clear, direct manner, and actively listen and engage with others to further their understanding
  - Ability to adapt the mode of communication appropriate to the audience
  - Avoid telling others what to think, but provide/create opportunities for understanding to grow/develop/emerge
- *Use of self*:
  - Sensitivity—attuned and receptive—can takes things in
  - Capacity to use one's interactions with others therapeutically
  - Ability to monitor the thoughts and feelings evoked by others and link these to underlying issues of the client
  - Genuineness—congruence—authenticity—not hiding behind professional status/role
- *Capacity to work both reflectively and reflexively*:
  - Ability to think about one's own capacities and deficits in relation to the work
  - Ability to work by continually being aware of one's responses to others and one's self
  - Self-reflection/awareness—desire to know why one is drawn to this work
  - Self-knowledge—able to self-talk and adopt a third position

- *Capacity to contain anxiety*:
  - Ability to tolerate 'not knowing'
  - Ability to tolerate stress and recognize personal limits
  - Ability to notice and sustain feeling difficult feelings long enough to understand from where they derive and to take appropriate action
  - Self-contained—ability to contain one's own anxiety
  - Owns one's mistakes
  - Capacity to retain one's identity and strength of character.

Organizational-related competencies

- *Recognize the importance of the environmental setting and external environment*:
  - Use 'daily living' as opportunities for learning—'opportunity-led work'
  - Acknowledge the symbolic nature of the environment
  - Understand 'corrective emotional experience', primary care, and therapeutic adaptation
  - Political/social awareness—ability to challenge the status quo
- *Understanding of organizational dynamics*:
  - Ability to understand and acknowledge issues of authority, power, and leadership
  - Ability to understand the varied reasons for organizational anxiety, the defences which operate to avoid this, and one's own role in managing this
  - Awareness of one's own valency—the tendency to take up a familiar defensive role in a group context
- *Participant observer*:
  - Can observe self and others, without being compelled to act before reflecting
  - Can wait, think, talk with others before acting
  - Capacity to learn from direct experience—capacity to explore and be vulnerable, not defensive/avoidant
- *Recognize the primary task*:
  - Boundaried—able to acknowledge one's own place in the organizational structure
  - Clarity about one's role—engage directly in the key tasks defined in one's job description and its relation with the primary task of the community.

There are usually four distinct, but overlapping, phases in a member's journey to, and through, a TC:
- *Engagement and stabilization phase*:
  - Referral, preparation, and selection procedures are an integral part of TC practice, involving both the prospective member and existing residents as active participants in the process, which start with referral or self-referral. Many prospective members of TCs are wary or fearful of the forthcoming therapy, and need support and encouragement to persist. This is often effectively delivered by current or ex-members, arranged in partnership with voluntary agencies or with Internet support groups. During this time, any

regular support from mental health teams or other agencies should continue.

- *Assessment and preparation phase*:
  - When a decision to proceed towards formal treatment has been made, several arrangements may need to be made. These include formal assessment processes, practical planning, and agreeing a treatment contract. This work is frequently arranged through the use of an 'assessment and preparation group', which is also designed to be a time-limited foretaste of what the treatment phase entails. The assessment process can be undertaken in this group itself, in smaller groups, or with individual appointments. The practical planning involves matters such as arranging childcare, securing stable accommodation, and agreeing plans for medication and risk management. It also includes an explicit treatment contract, which may be a verbal agreement about understanding the community rules or a formal written and signed agreement.

- *Intensive treatment phase*:
  - This usually begins with a formal 'case conference' or 'selection panel' including current community members with a decision made by voting. Subsequent therapy programmes vary considerably: from one day per week to whole-time residential; from predominantly sociotherapy to a range of psychoanalytic, cognitive behavioural, humanistic, and interpersonal and systemic groups; from a few weeks' duration to several years, either time-limited to open-ended; from group size of fewer than six to more than 50. Some communities include individual therapy, but others consider this inimical to the group dynamic process.

A typical programme would be for between 2 and 5 days per week, with all interventions delivered in groups, comprising a mixture of community meetings, small therapy groups, shared lunch, and informal time together. Such a community might have 18 members, divided into three small groups, who would stay for 12 to 18 months. Suitable arrangements would be in place for crisis meetings to be called at short notice, as well as a system for members to support each other out-of-hours.

During the first few weeks of treatment, the new member will be feeling his or her way, forming attachments to one or two others, but still wary of the groups. After the first month or two, he or she will begin participating more actively in the groups, taking part in the full life of the community with certain role responsibilities, helping and supporting other members. This will probably include experience of situations similar to those triggering referral such as having to deal with authority, fear of failure, feeling rejected or abandoned, situations evoking rivalry and competition, or many others. As before, these may trigger destructive or violent impulses towards the self or another person, or the experience of other symptoms of distress. Through the group meetings, the member is confronted with the effects of their behaviour on fellow members, and the meaning of the behaviour or symptoms is explored, making full use of the insights and understanding of fellow members. Through this repeated process, the member gradually comes to experience himself and others differently. As one member wrote: 'Bit by bit, almost grudgingly, the fact dawned on me that I wasn't surrounded by forty sticks of furniture, but by Jim, Gary, Jane . . . '.

- *Recovery and rehabilitation phase*:
  - Until recently, many TCs had a 'cliff-edge' ending where, one day, members are able to have the community's full emotional and practical support, and the next are not allowed to contact any other members. Although this has some theoretical justification, in terms of 'coming to term with endings', and has strong advocates amongst ex-members of TCs, it is now generally considered better practice to support members over the leaving process, and then into re-establishing mainstream social networks. This can be done with a specific 'leavers group' that members join, whilst in the full treatment phase, and continue afterwards, for either a fixed or indefinite period. These groups normally include a practical focus and are social and supportive, rather than exploratory and therapeutic. For those who are ready and able, they can have objectives of securing employment or education for members.

As well as planned endings, there are various other types of ending. Some members may leave prematurely, unable to cope with therapy; some may be 'voted out' by the community for a serious or repeated transgression of community rules. Such endings do not necessarily indicate a treatment failure, although the longer members remain, the more likely they are to benefit.

What changes?

TCs do not have a symptom focus, and the outcomes and changes expected are complex and operate in many different areas of a person's life over prolonged time periods.

For those who complete a treatment programme, the following improvements can be expected:

- Better general health and well-being
- More willing and able to take care of themselves
- Seeking professional help in a mature, rather than chaotic, way
- Reduced suicidality
- Reduction in other psychological symptoms
- Reduction or cessation of the need for psychotropic medication
- Improved self-esteem, confidence, and sense of purpose
- Generally improved relationships with family and friends
- Cessation of self-harm
- Reduced addictive behaviour
- Better social and community engagement
- More likelihood of long-term education and employment.

Clinical populations and context

Those likely to benefit from TC treatment usually have a number of the following characteristics:

- Marginalization from mainstream society
- Severe emotional and behavioural difficulties
- Criminal behaviour with persistent petty offending

- Dangerously reckless and impulsive behaviour
- Unstable housing
- Loneliness and isolation
- Unemployability and long-term unemployment
- Low self-esteem
- Extreme sensitivity to rejection
- Lifelong pattern of intense and unstable relationships
- Child protection issues (many people have children in care)
- Anxiety and depression
- Suicidality and self-harm
- Drug and alcohol problems.

Universal indications for TC treatment are difficult to give. Individuals of all ages, from young children to elderly members, can show benefit. Modified TCs have been developed for people with different types and levels of psychiatric disorder, and even the same TC may fluctuate in its capacity to absorb difficult members. An individual's suitability will need to be judged in relation to a particular TC at a particular time. Having made this caveat, the general indications and contraindications will usually apply.

Diagnostic indications
- Personality disorders
- Self-harm
- Adjustment disorders
- Recurrent depressive disorders
- Bipolar disorder
- Intractable anxiety disorders
- Eating disorders
- Addictions.

Indications for specialized therapeutic communities
- First-episode psychosis
- Serious and enduring mental illness
- Less than 18 years old
- Predominant addiction problems
- Learning disabilities
- Perpetrators of sexual abuse.

Contraindications
- Physically dependent addictions (generally needs acute detoxification first)
- Current manic episode
- Depression with severe retardation
- Dementia
- Dangerously low weight
- ASPD with a history of intimidation and deception
- No capacity for social involvement
- Inability to see problems in terms of relationships
- Unwillingness to engage in informal, intimate, and open style of relating with professionals
- Belief that only experts can help.

Case vignettes

Case one

Robin was the only child of 'rather distant' parents who ran a success-ful publishing firm. He was 43 when referred to a 'mini-TC' (one whole day plus one therapy group per week), soon after his mother was diag-nosed with Alzheimer's disease. Since leaving home at 25, he failed to establish a career for himself, had been twice divorced, and had spells of excessive use of alcohol and street drugs. He had lived most of his life on benefits, with considerable financial help from his parents. He had been prescribed different antidepressants by his GP over the years, with only limited success. He had numerous aches and pains, mostly related to his neck and back.

He denied any traumatic or abusive experiences in his life, but did remember being looked after by a succession of different nannies, before being sent to boarding school at about eight. He did reasonably well at school and went on to university, but dropped out of an engineering degree in his first year. He remembers feeling 'different' from the others at school and university, and spending much of his time alone. When he did socialize, he tended to drink, until he became quite drunk. Both his marriages lasted less than 5 years, and he had no children.

Within a month of joining the TC, he became enthusiastic about how 'nice it was to be able to talk to people who understood'. In the weekly analytic small group, he discussed deep feelings of abandonment he felt as a child—and how he never felt really loved or valued. He started see-ing Zoe, a female group member, outside the group—but this was picked up by another member and challenged. It was difficult for him to agree to 'stick to the boundaries', and he had an angry and difficult 3 months, with much absenteeism and occasional drunken abusive phone calls to other members. Whilst in the TC, he attended medication consultation groups and succeeded in coming off all his psychotropic and pain-killing drugs. He was supported strongly, as well as being vigorously challenged, by the group, and, as his leaving date approached, he became chair of the community and was increasingly attentive and caring to others. He was sad to leave, and the others were sad to see him go.

He re-contacted group members after the recommended 6-month break and informed them he was working for a local children's charity, and was in what he described as a 'fairly stable' relationship with Zoe. He came back for the annual Christmas party and summer outing, and made good friends with several other ex-members.

Case two

Neelema was a British-born 23-year-old with first-generation Asian parents, who was referred to a 3-day per week TC by her social worker, after having had three abortions and one child taken into local authority care. She was on a suspended sentence for repeated shoplifting and had a history of two admissions to the local mental health ward following serious overdoses. She was on a mixture of medications, including ben-zodiazepines, antidepressants, neuroleptics, and carbamazepine, which she often forgot to take, especially when she had been out drinking.

She had a personal history of persistent sexual abuse between the ages of 10 and 14, including regular rape, from a cousin 5 years older than her. It stopped when he moved away. Before that, she remembered little of family life, except being expected to look after her two younger sisters from a very early age. She was rebellious as a teenager and left school and home at 16 to live with a boyfriend of whom her parents strongly disapproved.

She was very reluctant to believe that a therapy programme would help her but was persuaded to return by an 'expert by experience' (a graduate of the programme who now worked as an assistant therapist there), who befriended her and explained how she was in a similar situation before her own therapy started. In the early phases, she often missed groups, and, at one point, her continuation was 'put to the vote'—and a decision was made to suspend her for 2 weeks, then return to decide whether she was willing to give the required commitment. She came back and made the commitment, and soon was voted into the intensive phase of the programme where she often used psychodrama sessions to understand her intense feelings about her past abuse. In the small analytic therapy groups, she eventually found what she called 'the family I never had'—although it was not without many family fallouts and squabbles. A month before her planned leaving, she came in one morning after a heavy night's drinking—still obviously intoxicated and abusive to everybody. She was sent home and returned to following groups to explain the fear and loss she was feeling about having to leave.

She did leave as planned, with the traditional ceremonial 'goodbye lunch' and exchange of gifts. She joined the 'next steps' group and had a very difficult 6 months, during which time she was very low in mood and frequently asked the others if she should go back onto her antidepressants. She managed without doing so, and her mood improved over the following months as summer came, and she re-established contact with some members of her family. She joined an access to education course and is now undertaking an undergraduate course to become a social worker. She keeps in contact with other ex-members of the TC and understands that she remains vulnerable—but she now has a very different outlook on life and, for the most part, enjoys being alive. She has a good network of friends to call on for help when things are more difficult.

Recommended reading

Haigh R (2013). The quintessence of a therapeutic environment. *Therapeutic Communities*, 34, 6–16.

Haigh R and Tucker S (2004). Democratic development of standards: a quality network of therapeutic communities. *Psychiatric Quarterly*, 75, 263–77.

Johnson R and Haigh R (2011). Social psychiatry and social policy for the 21st century—relational health. *Journal of Mental Health and Social Inclusion*, 15, 57–65.

Jones M (1968). *Beyond the Therapeutic Community; Social Learning and Social Psychiatry*. Yale University Press: New York.

Rapoport R (1960). *Community as Doctor*. Tavistock: London.

Art psychotherapy

(See ➔ Art psychotherapy in Chapter 2, pp. 81–83.)

Key techniques and competencies

The art psychotherapist will meet with the client for an initial assessment, which may take place over several sessions. They will discuss the presenting issues and the hopes for treatment. The art therapist will address key points about art therapy, e.g. that there is no right or wrong way to use the art materials and that artwork will not be 'analysed'; it is a collaborative process where both parties reflect on the work together. If art therapy seems potentially helpful, the therapist will offer a series of sessions, possibly time-limited, individually or in a group.

The art therapist will introduce the art materials, which may include paper, paint, drawing materials, inks, collage material, textiles, clay, modelling materials, and, more recently, digital media.

The components of art therapy vary according to the client and the setting. The work may focus mostly on the artwork and art making, with very little interpersonal relating, or may be quite verbal, with less focus on the art. The therapist may use transference and countertransference to inform the work. There may be a review of the work and then a planned ending, with reflection, evaluation, and the taking away or disposal of the artwork.

Art therapy may be offered in individual, open-studio, or closed group sessions. It may also be offered in theme-based groups, e.g. Art therapy and conflict.

What changes?

The provision of a safe space, art materials, and a therapeutic relationship can enable:

- The discovery of a sense of mental space
- Relaxation/tension reduction/self-soothing
- The experience of 'flow': the exhilaration of being absorbed in a creative process
- Experimentation and risk via the art making
- Problem-solving
- Emotional regulation: improved expression, containment, and processing of feelings
- Increased confidence and self-esteem
- Increased self-awareness and reflection
- Increased cognitive fluidity
- Catharsis
- The opportunity to telling one's story/'narrative competence' and to be heard.

Clinical populations and contexts

Art psychotherapists work in the NHS, in inpatient and community settings, social services, primary care, and in education, charities, drug and alcohol, and forensic settings. They also work in TCs, palliative care, and private practice. They have also sited their practice within arts settings, in art galleries, and in the workplace. They may work internationally in conflict areas and war zones.

Art therapists have developed specialisms to work with psychosis, eating disorders, depression, dementia, bipolar disorders, bereavement, dissociative identity disorder, BPD, learning disabilities, trauma, and PTSD (see ➔ Psychoses in Chapter 7, pp. 331–4; Eating disorders in Chapter 7, pp. 334–8; Affective disorders in Chapter 7, pp. 326–31; Dementia in Chapter 7, pp. 372–6; Borderline personality disorders in Chapter 8, pp. 322–3; Intellectual disability in Chapter 7, pp. 368–71; Trauma-related conditions in Chapter 7, pp. 355–9). They work with mothers and babies, children and adolescents, adults of working age and older, and carers.

Case vignettes

Case one: community-based weekly art therapy group for people with a history of psychosis

This was a new group of four members, all quite withdrawn and isolated. We used themes for initial cohesion, which the group chose by first making doodles. This week, the doodles suggested the theme of 'boats'. We then drew boats and decorated them in various ways, a process in which everyone engaged.

As we reflected on the various artwork, one person told a story about someone who had built up a business making boats. This person had been highly successful, only to later commit suicide. The emergence of this theme facilitated the sharing of group members' own occasional thoughts and feelings about suicide. Although this may seem a depressing turn for the group to have taken, members seemed relieved to be able to share feelings that can be hard to talk about and went on to share various resources that they used for support.

Case two: open-studio group in a large psychiatric hospital, shortly to close

John had been on a rehabilitation ward for a year and now awaited discharge. He attended the Art Therapy Department regularly.

On this occasion, he worked intently in pencil, with a lot of pressure and scribble. The drawing process had been intense, yet at first glance, his image seemed to show a tranquil scene: a carefully ordered park, with grass and benches, a lake, and ducks.

Then he drew the therapist's attention to the vandalized house in the corner. He talked about his anxieties about being discharged and about care in the community, which was then being introduced, and whether he would be maintained, like the park, or be neglected, like the house, or even vandalized/harmed.

The therapist thought of her first impression of a calm picture and about how we may think that everything is all right with someone when it is not. There may be real fears and anxieties underneath, and valid doubts about support and provision in the community. These had been brought to the surface in John's picture, and he could articulate them. His anxiety could be acknowledged in the therapy and also fed back to his care team, and he and his therapist could think together about what might help to 'maintain' him in the community.

Case three: individual art therapy session
Paula was having speech therapy for stammering. As she was also suffering from chronic depression, her speech therapist referred her to psychological services. At assessment, she communicated via a notepad, and art therapy was considered.

Fig. 5.3 shows someone drowning. A lifebelt is available, although to reach for it feels like giving up dignity. This reflected Paula's initial ambivalence about therapy, sense of stigma, and doubt about accessing help from mental health services.

Paula did engage in art therapy and use it to explore her difficulties in speaking. Via the artwork, she was able to express how silenced she felt in the face of workplace bullying, exploitative practices, and an environment that sounded unsupportive of mental health issues (Fig. 5.4). Successive attempts to return to work had failed.

Fig. 5.5 conveyed her depression, which she described as like wearing a diving suit. It is very heavy, so one can only move or think very slowly. The view of the outside world is restricted, and there is little contact to the person inside. There is a sense of detachment from the rest of the world. The drawing also expresses her increased engagement in art therapy. She is no longer drowning but has equipment (the diving suit), even though it is weighty. She is working on a deeper level. There is some communication between the diver and the surface, and some potential to navigate the waters. Paula has also been able to explore a highly critical/perfectionist aspect of herself, as well as a playful aspect, and to speak of the need to develop more some aspects in between. She has also found great enjoyment in making art and has started drawing in her own time.

Although Paula occasionally still stammers and becomes barely audible when stressed, she speaks fluently, at normal volume, in the sessions. The work is continuing. Meanwhile, she has been able to negotiate retirement from work and contemplate a more creative life for herself.

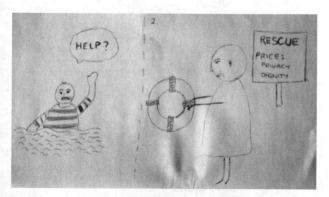

Fig. 5.3 Artwork allows the expression of ambivalent feelings at the start of therapy.

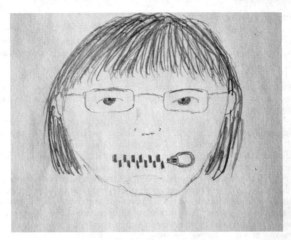

Fig. 5.4 Unable to speak.

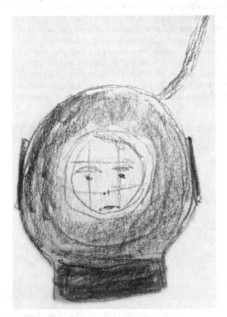

Fig. 5.5 The metaphor of a diving suit portraying the experience of depression.

Recommended reading

Case C and Dalley T (1992). *The Handbook of Art Therapy*. Routledge: London.
Gilroy A and McNeilly G (eds) (2000). *The Changing Shape of Art Therapy: New Developments in Therapy and Practice*. Jessica Kingsley: London.
Hogan S (2001) *The Healing Arts: The History of Art Therapy*. Jessica Kingsley: London.
Killick K and Schaverien J (1997). *Art Psychotherapy and Psychosis*. Routledge:London and New York.
Skaife S and Huet V (eds) (1998). *Art Psychotherapy Groups, Between Pictures and Words*. Routledge: London.

Dramatherapy

(See ⭢ Dramatherapy in Chapter 2, pp. 83–5.)

Key techniques and competencies

Dramatherapy sessions provide a real place where the imagined can be brought to life through action. Life experience is projected through fictional characters and make-believe situations, creating 'dramatic distance'. Stories essentially reflect and contain the way we, as human beings, think and experience life. With distance from the *actual*, difficult ideas or experiences can be explored with psychological safety. Patients work with resonant material of any form, e.g. literature, film, or theatre, that have meaning for them. Myth, folk, and fairy tales offer exploration of archetypes, inviting focus on aspects of self, the persona, and shadow aspects of personality. Work with small objects is a method to symbolize and characterize troublesome internalized objects by using actual objects to represent these aspects. Dramatic exploration can be formed of intrapsychic material or external situations of a patient's life. Internal conflicts or ambivalence can be dialogued between chosen objects or characters. Through role play and dramatic enactment, established societal and familial roles may be questioned. Situations that feel immovable can be rerun to consider other possible responses or outcomes. Even the telling of stories stimulates the imagination and gives us a similar sensation of that experience, as areas of the brain are stimulated by words that describe action.

Assessment techniques inform the dramatherapist of a patient's needs and capabilities, so that the therapist can adapt their approaches accordingly. Assessment presents a starting point for discussion between the patient and dramatherapist, and supports the development of aims and objectives, and duration of therapy. Aims are reviewed in collaboration with patients throughout dramatherapy treatment, as progression may require refocusing of specific aims, although overall treatment targets remain the same. Patients are assessed in the areas of embodiment, projection, and role, the ability to symbolize and mentalize, the ability to maintain boundaries, and cognitive and physical capability. Consideration will be given to themes arising throughout the therapy.

Creative expression is an intrinsic element of dramatherapy. Games in drama and play aim to improve confidence and skills in creative and dramatic expression, encouraging active and authentic involvement in personal process. Developing competencies and rehearsal in dramatherapy enable an accumulation of new skills; courses of action in sustained practice create neural pathways that continue to develop and extend.

In embodiment, the patient is adopting the felt sense of the character physically and psychologically. In enactment of story or myth, patients embody the scene, and empathy and mentalization are brought into focus, using techniques such as role reversal and 'hot seating' whereby clients hear characters express emotion and explain motivations for their actions. This illustrates a person's point of view, perspective taking, and understanding of others' behaviours and parts of themselves.

Dramatherapy is effective in both groups and with individuals, both formats applying similar principles.

Group dramatherapy

- Collaborative play and creativity increase socialization and spontaneity within the group, and help to build relationships and trust in the beginning phase of the dramatherapy.
- The use of metaphor creates a unique method by which to meet others and share experiences; in telling and sharing stories, patients find universal themes and common ground. In drama, there is playful connection with others. Working together creatively gives opportunities to improve communication, build relationships, and engage ambivalent participants. Through fictional stories, personal material is shared through the mask of metaphor, which can lessen initial fears of exposure and trust.
- There is a wide range of activities available whereby the group can craft images, verbalize stories, and explore sharing physical space and proximity to each other. In these activities, empathy, tolerance, and control can be explored, the emotions and thoughts these activities give rise to, and possible solutions to difficulties, but all within the metaphor.
- Facilitated by the dramatherapist, patients realize, direct, and role play their own drama or scenario within the containment of the group. Group members provide active support in playing parts/characters and help with setting or any aspect of a dramatic enactment. Directing one's own drama gives patients control and empowerment. Self-esteem and confidence increase, as patients share their narratives and are witnessed and accepted by others.

Individual dramatherapy

- Focuses on the building of relationships: the dramatherapist 'comes alongside' the patient in their therapeutic process, both in their imagined world and in their reality. This revisits early play and dramatic development, as the dramatherapist meets the patient through embodiment, metaphor, and symbol, mirroring the infant/caregiver dyad. Congruence in play mirrors maternal attunement, allows a shared understanding of the patient's personal material, and builds trust.
- Crafting personal drama, the dramatherapist employs creative techniques to enable the drama or narrative to be realized, whilst witnessed by the dramatherapist.

What changes?

- Ability to access and extend the range of social roles, flexibility in response to events, situations, and relationships
- Decrease in rigid thoughts and beliefs, and increased ability to provide necessary and helpful security and spontaneity for oneself in everyday life
- Patient gains understanding of mental processes and gains empathy for oneself and others
- Understanding of one's own roles and patterns of behaviour in the context of one's history and upbringing. Through drama, and narrative and creative expression, finding new roles and ways of being in the world
- Expansion of ability in the ranges of self-expression, leading to improved self-esteem and confidence. Increased expressivity reduces symptoms and anxiety and enables catharsis and letting go of emotional blocks. Creative expression introduced as a way of helping patients to manage emotion and symptoms in the long term
- Improved relationships, trusting behaviour, and acceptance of self.

Primary treatment targets
- Increased ability to be 'in relationship' with others and increased socialization
- Increased expressive flexibility within embodiment, projection, and role
- Understanding of personal history, how this may influence behaviour and emotional responses, and an ability to make alternative strategies and choices
- Assimilation of aspects of self—working towards an integrated sense of self
- Increased ability to perspective take and understand mentalization processes.

Secondary treatment targets
- Increased autonomy and responsibility
- Increased creativity
- Increase in psychological resourcing
- Overall sense of well-being and acceptance, confidence, and self-esteem
- Increased role repertoire in everyday life.

Clinical population and contexts

The versatility of the dramatic form—whether through using dramatic/theatrical metaphor to understand the process or the literal application of dramatic methods—means that dramatherapy can be applied in various settings. Dramatherapists work in adult mental health and other health contexts; educational contexts of all kinds, from mainstream schools to emotional and behavioural difficulties (EBD) and pupil referral unit (PRU) provisions; child and adolescent mental health, disability services, and forensic settings; as well as specialized services such as work in hospice care, adoption, or with refugees and asylum seekers. The nature of dramatherapy enables therapists to apply the creative methods suited to the needs of the patient. Within these contexts, dramatherapy can be applied to brief and long-term treatment, and used in assessment and evaluated, e.g. with outcome measures.

Case vignettes

Case one

Peter was in his late 30s and lived with a psychotic disorder. He started sessions playfully, thinking about favourite childhood books, scenes, and characters. At the beginning, Peter was mistrusting of the dramatherapist. The use of story metaphor created an intermediary focus between the therapist and patient, lessening the potential intensity of a one-to-one relationship. Peter used the metaphor to indirectly communicate parts of himself. He chose stories and characters that he knew from his early years and young adulthood. He portrayed children, alien creatures, wise and knowledgeable people. Themes of different worlds, being trapped, finding a way home, and judgement were reflected through the metaphoric material. The next phase moved into embodiment through music and movement. The focus now on physical presence put aside the screen of metaphor to being in the 'here and now', creating more immediacy in the relationship. Peter expressed polarities of emotion in his choice of music, movement and vocalization. Congruency and attunement developed in the non-verbal exchanges in the movement and paralleled the early non-verbal mirroring of a caregiver and child. The use of music introduced opportunities to expand the expressive range from role play to embodiment.

Later in the dramatherapy, Peter turned to words, interweaving his everyday experiences with story and metaphor, to understand themes in his life. Whereas Peter had previously used metaphor to maintain distance, the metaphor now became a bridge connecting the imagined to his real life experiences and painful childhood memories. The initial storytelling and movement phases could be seen as a way through to the pivotal material of Peter's past. Peter used the metaphor and versatile methods of dramatherapy to find his own way to access psychologically hidden material. A later part of the work was bringing the internal exploration of the dramatherapy into his external everyday life, e.g. Peter's experience of autonomy in the therapy showed him how to craft his life and make choices for himself. There was a sense of Peter growing up in the dramatherapy, working through developmental stages in play, drama, movement, and metaphor; from the child to the adult Peter.

Primary treatment targets
- Increased knowledge of past relationships, how they influence his life now, and understanding other available options
- Encourage honesty and self-expression in everyday interactions with others
- Increase confidence and self-belief
- Increased autonomy in decision-making
- Exploration of predominant and hidden social roles.

Case two

Mary had a complex mental disorder and cognitive difficulties, aged 40. At the start, Mary regularly declined sessions, making it difficult to build a therapeutic relationship. In order to build familiarity and safety in the therapeutic relationship, the therapist scheduled shortened, consistent meetings. During these early sessions, in informal conversation, Mary began storytelling, casually recounting memories from her life. With story as a mainstay of dramatherapy, the therapist then brought the focus onto the stories. This gave Mary control over the content during the sessions and through being heard, she was experiencing validation and worth. She recounted life stories in fragments, with no chronological order and the therapist, in response, brought materials and other fiction (stories, poetry, images) that linked to the themes in Mary's stories. Mary considered characters from stories and high profile people that she admired, exploring what made these people admirable. By identifying the qualities, she was, in part, identifying qualities that she wished for herself. Relationships with others were viewed through the use of spectograms (creating a visual picture of the client's relational world).

Mary was telling the therapist who she was. Words can transport us into the sensation of an experience and for Mary, there was an embodied 'aliveness' that came with the storytelling. Mary talked about her past, the therapist holding a balance by encouraging stories from the 'here and now' of her life. Fictional stories were devised using Mooli Lahad's six-piece story-making method. This technique employs a structure which breaks the story into six separate parts, based on the basic monomyth pattern. The six-piece story can be used as an intervention, for assessment, or as a core subject in the dramatherapy sessions. Stories can be realized in differing ways and scale, depending on a client's abilities or preferences, by drawing, using picture cards, with small toys or objects in a sand tray, or can be created dramatically in performance. The stories begin with creating a hero or protagonist and lead into what the hero wants, what help the hero needs, how the hero overcomes obstacles, and the conclusion to the story. Mooli Lahad has developed an assessment technique that helps the therapist to interpret, through the story, how clients perceive the world through the headings belief, affect, social, imagination, cognitive, and physiological (BASIC Ph). The structured parts of the story offer a contained way to work with imagination and the improvised nature of constructing a story. The devised story is formed directly from the client's imagination and the metaphor creates a fictional distance from the real material.

Dramatherapy can be said to treat the whole person and other areas of focus were understanding emotions, sensory experience and physical movement. It was apparent that Mary struggled to make sense of her inner world and identify emotions, words, colours, and images. This created a visual vocabulary that enabled Mary to begin developing the ability to symbolize.

Warm up theatre games such as touching corners of the room, noticing and finding different textures, colours, and temperatures helped Mary to become familiar with the work space and stimulated physical movement. Playing football with a large, soft ball simply enabled reciprocity, in kicking the ball back and forth. The ubiquitous action of football, or throwing a ball gives opportunity for clients to be in relationship to others; it can serve as a relaxant and distraction in a session and clients can experiment with rhythm and pace according to their mood. Mary also enjoyed playing percussion instruments to sound out a rhythm and she found sensory experiences by touching different natural objects and materials. Creative exercises focusing on sensory, cognitive, and imaginative play enabled Mary to begin making order of the world through symbolizing—from not knowing to acknowledgement of some understanding.

Primary treatment targets

- Enable a sense of worth and self-esteem through active listening from the therapist and encouraging storytelling
- Build a narrative that contains positive memories, as well as come to terms with difficulties, with the use of drawing, small objects, and writing
- Challenge historical negative thinking towards self and learn to overcome fear of failure and self-criticism
- Imbue positivity into the work that is completed in sessions, giving a sense of achievement and ability
- In story, metaphor, and character work, consider Mary's future and her aspirations
- Develop an ability to symbolize, to understand the bodily location of emotion as it happens, and to comprehend emotion through identity with images, colours, and textures
- Connection to whole self, body, and mind through applicable methods.

Recommended reading

Casson J (2004). *Drama, Psychotherapy and Psychosis: Dramatherapy and Psychodrama With People Who Hear Voices*. Routledge: Hove and New York.

Dokter D, Holloway P, and Seebohm H (eds) (2011). *Dramatherapy and Destructiveness: Creating the Evidence Base, Playing With Thanatos*. Routledge: Hove and New York.

Lahad M, Ayalon O, and Shacham M (eds) (2013). *The 'BASIC Ph' Model of Coping and Resiliency: Theory, Research and Cross-Cultural Application*. Jessica Kingsley Publishers: London.

Lewis L and Read Johnson D (eds) (2000). *Current Approaches in Drama Therapy*. Charles C Thomas Publishers: Springfield, IL.

Pearson J, Smail M, and Watts P (2013). *Dramatherapy With Myth and Fairytale*. Jessica Kingsley Publishers: London.

Music therapy

(See ➔ Music therapy in Chapter 2, pp. 86–91.)

Key techniques and competences

There are five main models of music therapy:

- Improvisational music therapy
- Analytical music therapy
- Creative music therapy
- Guided imagery and music (GIM)
- Behavioural music therapy.

Music therapists work across a spectrum of approaches which may incorporate elements from the five main music therapy models, according to the therapeutic needs of the client.

The music therapy spectrum of approaches;

- *Psychodynamic*:
  - Mind/body
  - Psychoanalytical
  - Transference relationship
  - Unconscious processes
  - Defence mechanisms
- *Humanistic*:
  - Self/environment
  - Holistic
  - Here and now
  - Self-growth
- *Developmental*:
  - Biological
  - Individual/separation
  - Developmental psychology
  - Cognitive
- *Physiological*:
  - Body-based
  - Biochemical
  - Medical
  - Neurological
- *Transpersonal*:
  - Integrative
  - Mind/body/spirit
  - Beyond time/space
  - Peak experiences
  - Soul.

Improvisational music therapy

Improvisational music therapy is a comprehensive approach to music therapy incorporating:

- Free musical improvisation
- Listening
- Performing
- Notating

- Composing
- Moving.

The client is given freedom for self-expression by the *absence* of rules in:
- Tonality
- Rhythm
- Beat
- Meter
- Melody
- Form and structure
- Musical technique
- Ways of playing instruments.

Free improvisation can be both:
- An active technique—the client improvises alone, with the therapist or with the group
- A receptive technique—the client listens, whilst the therapist improvises.

Musical instruments are at the centre of improvisational music therapy for:
- Free improvisation
- As objects for client projections.

There are many clinical techniques commonly used in improvisational music therapy that include:
- *Techniques of empathy*:
  - Imitating
  - Synchronizing
  - Incorporating
  - Reflecting
- *Structuring techniques*:
  - Rhythmic grounding
  - Tonal centring
  - Shaping
- *Techniques of intimacy*:
  - Sharing instruments
  - Bonding
- *Techniques of emotional exploration*:
  - Holding
  - Doubling
  - Contrasting
- *Elicitation techniques*:
  - Repeating
  - Modelling.

Analytical music therapy
Analytical music therapy is based on psychoanalytic concepts of Sigmund Freud, Carl Jung, and Melanie Klein, and focuses on the:
- *Intrapersonal*: inner parts of the self:
  - Ego 'thinking', superego 'moral', id 'instinctual'
  - Conscious, preconscious, unconscious

- *Interpersonal*: relationships with other:
  - Defence mechanisms
- *Transpersonal*: transcending the personal:
  - 'Receptive creative experience' (in the music).
- Dynamics of the therapeutic relationship
  - Transference
  - Countertransference
  - Resistance
  - Working alliance.

In analytical music therapy, the way to the unconscious is through impro-vised music. Improvised music is 'projective', in that it is a manifestation of the unconscious. The aim of music therapy is to break down defence mech-anisms, to create new emotional options and healthy responses. Different types of relationships are developed within the context of the music expe-rience shared by the client and music therapist, in which transference, pro-jective identification, and countertransference are able to develop.

Clinical objectives
- To contain the transference
- To help the client recognize the transference
- To re-experience and work through the transference.

Treatment procedures developed by Priestly incorporating psychoana-lytic concepts with musical improvisation:
- Holding
- Splitting
- Investigation of emotional investment
- Entering into somatic communication
- Guided imagery, myths, and dream work
- Reality rehearsal
- Wholeness
- Exploring relationships
- Affirmations
- Sub-verbal communication for free association
- Patterns of significance
- Programmed or spontaneous regression.

Creative music therapy—the Nordoff–Robbins model
Developed from the ideas of Paul Nordoff and Clive Robbins, creative music therapy is based on the understanding that human beings are made up of rhythm, melody, harmony, and form that are important elements in our physiological and psychological process. We can be considered as 'symphonic' beings. Nordoff–Robbins music therapy is grounded in the belief that everyone, no matter how ill, disabled, or traumatized, can respond to music.

As musical beings, our bodies have:
- Pulse
- Tone
- Tensions and resolutions
- Phrasing of actions
- Bursts of intensity

- Repetitions
- Developments.

Therefore, music accesses our whole world of experience:
- Bodily
- Emotionally
- Intellectually
- Socially.

Characteristics of Nordoff–Robbins music therapy
- Music is at the centre of the experience
- Musical responses are the primary material for analysis and interpretation
- The therapists use creative musical improvisation
- Use of a harmony instrument—piano—central to the working style
- Sophisticated use of the piano in improvised music making
- Strong encouragement for clients to use their voice.

Guided imagery and music
GIM is:

> 'A music-centered, transformational therapy which uses specifically programmed classical music to stimulate and support a dynamic unfolding of inner experiences in service of physical, psychological and spiritual wholeness.'

(AMI, 1990)

A GIM session consists of five sections that last from one and a half to two hours:
- *Prelude*: verbal start of the therapeutic encounter. Themes may arise that are drawn upon during the listening and imaging
- *Induction*: relaxation techniques used to move the client from the here and now into an altered state of consciousness (ASC). The client may be sitting down or lying on a couch
- *Listening and imaging*: the heart of the session. The client/traveller is invited to share experiences of listening to the music and to report any images to the therapist/guide. The term 'image' is used generically to refer to:
  - Visual images
  - Symbols
  - Feelings
  - Memories
  - Bodily sensations
- *Return*: the therapist assists the traveller to return to the 'here and now'
- *Postlude*: the therapist/guide helps the client/traveller process the experiences.

What changes?
Music therapy can benefit people with a wide range of difficulties or challenges, including:
- Mental health problems
- Dementia and other neurological conditions

- People experiencing serious illness such as cancer
- People who have experienced trauma
- Learning disabilities and autism.

Bruscia (1989) lists the many areas of therapeutic change commonly targeted in music therapy that can be viewed as primary goal areas for clinical practice:

- *Physiology*: heart rate, blood pressure, respiration, reduced risk of stroke, and other health issues
- *Psychophysiology*: pain, levels of arousal, levels of consciousness, state of tension/relaxation, level of energy/fatigue, feeling more relaxed, less stressed or depressed
- *Sensorimotor schemes*: reflexive responses and their coordination, fine and gross motor coordination
- *Perception*: figure ground, part-whole, and same-different perception
- *Cognition*: attention span, short- and long-term retention, level of learning capability, helping recreate memories
- *Behaviour*: patterns, activity level, morale
- *Music*: preferences, vocal range and technique, instrumental technique, ensemble skills
- *Emotions*: range, variability, appropriateness, reactivity, expressivity, defences, aggressiveness, depression, motivation, commitment, participation, raised self-esteem
- *Communication*: receptive and expressive abilities in speech, language, and other non-verbal modalities, including music, dance, drama, poetry, and art
- *Interpersonal*: awareness, sensitivity, intimacy, tolerance of others, interactional skills, relationship patterns
- *Creativity*: fluidity, divergence, originality, inventiveness.

Clinical populations and contexts

Music therapists work in a wide range of health, social care, and educational settings. Areas of work cover:

Mental health

Music therapists in the field of mental health work with patients suffering from the following conditions:

- Psychosis (see ➔ Psychoses in Chapter 7, pp. 331–4)
- Anxiety and depression (see ➔ Anxiety and anxiety disorders in Chapter 7, pp. 324–6; Affective disorders in Chapter 7, pp. 326–31)
- Alzheimer's disease and other forms of dementia (see ➔ Dementia in Chapter 7, pp. 372–6)
- Eating disorders (see ➔ Eating disorders in Chapter 7, pp. 334–8)
- BPD (see ➔ Borderline personality disorders in Chapter 8, pp. 390–6)
- Bipolar disorder (see ➔ Affective disorders in Chapter 7, pp. 326–31)
- Forensic patients (see ➔ Forensic psychiatry: forensic psycho-therapies, applications, and research in Chapter 12, pp. 550–6)
- Addictions and substance misuse (see ➔ Substance misuse in Chapter 7, pp. 338–45).

Dementia
(See ➲ Dementia in Chapter 7, pp. 372–6.)

In music therapy, people with dementia can be encouraged to participate in a shared musical experience involving:
- Listening
- Singing
- Moving
- Making music freely with percussion instruments.

This enables and supports:
- Participation
- Coordination
- Choice making
- Short-term memory skills
- Relief of anxiety and distress
- Enhancement of emotional well-being.

The use of familiar songs has also been a marked feature of music therapy sessions. Songs can often lead to reminiscences and discussions on past life events, and therefore promote the exploration of inner feelings.

The major concerns are the behavioural and psychological symptoms of dementia (BPSD):
- Apathy
- Anxiety
- Restlessness
- Depression.

Music therapy can help to minimize BPSD by encouraging basic and active involvement in musical interaction and socialization. It provides time and space to establish possible causes of BPSD which can be physical, social, or environmental:
- It promotes verbal and non-verbal expression
- It increases opportunities for meaningful social interaction
- It increases levels of cognitive stimulation
- It promotes the use of unimpaired cognitive functions
- It enables reminiscence and strengthens self-identity.

Neurodisability
Music is processed in many parts of the brain, which makes it an excellent tool for people living with an acquired brain injury or a neurodegenerative condition. Individual and group programmes can be devised for assessment and neurorehabilitation.

Three approaches are followed:
- Compensatory: using music to compensate for losses, in conjunction with tools such as memory/communication aids
- Psycho-socio-emotional: using music to enable emotional expression, engagement in social interaction, and adjustment to disability
- Restorative: using music to regain skill and function, e.g. through neurologic music therapy (NMT).

NMT is a neuroscientific model of practice, which consists of 20 standardized research-based music therapy techniques, designed to improve

the lives of people with neurological disabilities. The techniques cover three overarching rehabilitation domains, including:
- Sensorimotor training
- Speech and language training
- Cognitive training.

Music therapy can help neurodisability in maintenance and improvement of skills, including:
- Physical skills
- Cognition and thinking skills
- Emotional expression
- Communication skills
- Relating to others.

Benefits of music therapy for someone living with a neurodisability include:
- Improved engagement and motivation to participate
- Decreased anxiety
- Improved upper and lower limb function
- Improved communication and mood.

Adult learning disabilities
(See ➋ Intellectual disability in Chapter 7, pp. 368–71; Psychiatry of intellectual disability: psychotherapies, applications, and research in Chapter 12, pp. 562–4.)
 Areas of work include:
- Communication issues
- Emotional difficulties
- Relationship issues.

Music therapy for people with learning disabilities can help to:
- Increase motivation
- Empower people by offering choices
- Encourage and stimulate physical movement and coordination.

Music therapy can help with:
- Developing a clearer sense of identity and autonomy
- Increasing self-esteem and confidence
- Encouraging greater integration with other people and the community
- Increasing skills and abilities in communication and interaction with others, thereby reducing the need to use behaviour as a way to communicate distress or frustration
- Facilitating personal and emotional development by supporting the expression of difficult feelings and emotions
- Increasing the ability to reflect on, and process, feelings.

Music therapy supports the four guiding principles from the Department of Health paper *Valuing People: A New Strategy for Learning Disability for the 21st Century* (2001), giving attention to the areas of rights, independent living, control, and inclusion.

Autism

Music therapy can offer the following benefits:

- Social interaction: music therapy is based on forming a relationship between the client and therapist. This can be a way to explore the idea of relationship in a safe place.
- Communication: music provides an additional form of communication. The therapist attends closely to, and responds to, the client in a way that encourages further communication.
- Imagination: the use of music encourages the client to engage in a creative, imaginative process, with the support of the therapist. They can often move away from a ritualistic use of instruments to a more flexible, creative use. This can also lead to the development of less rigid thought and behaviour patterns.

Preschool children

(See ➜ Child and adolescent psychiatry: child and adolescent psycho-therapies, applications, and research in Chapter 12, pp. 556–61.)

Music therapy with young children promotes the development of both verbal and non-verbal communication skills. Essential aspects of non-verbal communication are encouraged such as:

- Turn taking
- Eye contact
- Anticipation
- Listening and concentration
- Awareness of self and others.

Reasons for referral for music therapy include:

- Communication difficulties
- Emotional distress
- Relationship difficulties
- Developmental delay.

Education and special education

Music therapy can help children with a variety of:

- Learning difficulties
- Behavioural problems
- Social problems
- Psychological difficulties.

Music therapy can have a positive impact on:

- Self-esteem
- Sense of identity
- Communication skills
- Social skills.

Music therapy contributes to musical development by encouraging:

- Awareness of pitch and rhythm
- Vocal confidence
- Spontaneity and creativity
- Improved listening skills
- Greater concentration.

Case vignettes

Case one: individual music psychotherapy
Patient: Harry.
Setting: residential nursing home.
Music therapy location: small lounge in the home.
Period of music therapy: 18 months.
Frequency: weekly sessions (same day and time each week).
Duration: 1 hour.

Instruments used in the sessions
- Digital piano
- Trombone
- Snare drum
- Cymbal and brushes
- Range of small percussion instruments.

Diagnosis: mixed dementia—Alzheimer's disease with vascular dementia.

Presenting problems
- Short-term memory loss and memory lapses
- Language: struggling to find the right word in a conversation, repeating himself
- Visuospatial skills: problems judging distance
- Orientation: becoming confused or losing track of the day or date
- Changes in mood: becoming anxious, irritable, and depressed, at times becoming withdrawn and losing interest in activities
- Delusions: believing things that are untrue
- Hallucinations: seeing and hearing things which are not really there.

Harry was a 76-year-old man suffering with dementia. He was a family man with two children, a son and daughter. He had one brother who he had not seen for many years. Harry had spent his life as a musician and teacher. He had been a professional jazz trumpeter, but now he had lost his ability to play the instrument. At the first meeting with the music therapists, he proudly, and sadly, showed him the trumpet that he could no longer play. This poignant moment was the beginning of the therapeutic relationship. When the therapist met Harry in the communal lounge at his home at the start of each session, he would often be sitting on his own, not talking or connecting with anyone else.

During the course of the music psychotherapy, a range of situations and scenarios arose from Harry's memories and experiences that were enacted in the music therapy sessions:
- *A music lesson*: in one session, as Harry and the therapist improvised together on the tune *Blueberry Hill*, a transformation took place, and they found themselves in a teacher–pupil relationship. The therapist was playing piano, and Harry was playing the cymbal with brushes. As they played, Harry became a caring and nurturing music teacher, sharing his knowledge of musical phrasing and swing rhythms. The therapist was the pupil, as Harry showed him how to shape the phrases of the melody using his voice to sing the lines. He played them back to Harry who was encouraging, supportive,

and complimentary. Harry was enjoying passing his knowledge and expertise on to the therapist, who, in turn, was enjoying receiving his advice. In this transference relationship, Harry was in touch with himself as an experienced and skilled musician. He had authority and wisdom. In this moment, Harry the musician and teacher materialized out of the darkening isolation and fragmentation of his dementia.

- *Rehearsal for a gig*: in another session, they were immersed in a twelve-bar blues improvisation. The therapist was playing trombone, and Harry was playing snare drum with brushes. As they improvised together, they were transported to a pub where Harry used to play with his own jazz band. They became band members, together preparing for a gig, and talked about what music would go down well. Harry drew on his memories and experience to advise on the repertoire and what songs to play or not to play. They worked on tunes, trying to 'get it right', how to begin and how to end, who would sing, and who would do a solo. They were bonding as musicians and friends, and Harry was regaining creativity, spontaneity, and self-esteem.

In one of these 'rehearsal' moments, as the therapist played a tune on the trombone, Harry made the remark 'I hope Mum doesn't catch us here!' As the therapist was thinking about what this remark could mean, it occurred to him that Harry was experiencing something special and precious that he did not want to lose, something that he feared could be stopped by his mum. He wanted to keep hold of this precious moment and not lose it, because that is what happens in dementia, in the struggle to keep hold of things that are being lost. He was also struck by Harry referring to 'Mum'. Did he mean his mum or their mum? The therapist's interpretation of this was that it reflected attachment anxieties, brought about by an underlying unconscious fear of fragmentation and falling apart. For Harry, the experience of playing music with his therapist gave rise to feelings of connection, relatedness, and bonding. It was as if he were Harry's brother. It may have been that the tune was significant, because it reached an early level of development in Harry's infancy, of attachment and bonding with his mother. The unconscious process that was at work through the transference relationship in this moment enabled Harry to feel safe and secure with his therapist in the music, counterbalancing and putting at bay fears of detachment and abandonment.

Summary

Music psychotherapy had a huge impact on Harry's quality of life. He began to relive his love of music and playing the trumpet—by listening to the therapist as he played piano and trombone to him, by playing percussion instruments as they improvised together, and through talking about the experience. During the music psychotherapy sessions, Harry was able to enjoy many things, the social and interactive experience of making music with his therapist, recalling familiar songs and melodies from his past, and experiencing a more integrated sense of himself, and his wisdom, expertise, and skills as a musician. In the moment and in the music, Harry left behind the frightening chaos and isolation he was experiencing, as his life was becoming fragmented and falling apart. He was able to have glimpses of the past, as memories emerged through the sounds and rhythms of music and songs, and he had moments of feeling whole again.

Case two: a music psychotherapy group
Setting: NHS hospital inpatient unit for patients suffering from mental illness.

Aims
- To help patients express themselves through music making
- To provide a creative space for patients to express their feelings and thoughts about their illness and their current situation in hospital
- To help patients prepare for discharge from hospital and to go back to life in the outside community.

Location: therapy room in the inpatient unit.
Period of music therapy: 12 weeks.
Frequency: weekly sessions, the same day and time each week.
Duration: 90 minutes.
Size of group: six patients.
Age range: between 45 and 60.

Patients' illnesses
- Depression
- Bipolar affective disorder
- Parkinson's disease and associated dementia
- Psychotic illness with delusional beliefs
- Huntington's disease.

The patients: Mark, Tommy, Dennis, Steve, Judy, April.

Instruments used
- Guitar, digital piano, trombone, piano accordion, melodica
- The human voice
- A range of pitched and non-pitched percussion instruments, including: xylophone, metalophone, glockenspiel, thumb piano, timpani drum, two djembe drums, buffalo drum, ocean drum, cymbal, tambourine, maracas, and shakers.

Forms of music therapy interactions with instruments and voices
- Structured musical improvising using a musical framework
- Playing and improvising on songs
- Free musical improvisation.

Examples of themes that were explored in the sessions
- Being in the group, identity, and acceptance

In the first session, the introduction session, when the group were finding out what people's names were and getting to know each other, Tommy called the therapist 'the piano man'. This name seemed to resonate with the other group members, and it stuck for the course of the therapy. Although the therapist felt some internal resistance to this label, he decided to go along with it. In the therapeutic dynamic, he interpreted this 'naming' of him as a process in which the group, represented by

Tommy, were coming to terms with being in the group, with who they were, and with how other group members saw themselves as they tried to understand their role and purpose in the group. The group started to come together musically, as they played around with the song *Piano man*, using various instruments.

'Sing us a song, you're the piano man'

(Billy Joel, 1971)

They talked about what this song meant for people, about personal identity, and about how they felt about the sessions and being in the group. The group members gave the therapist the role and identity of the piano man, in the search for their own roles and identities. One of the aims of the music psychotherapy group was to help prepare the patients for leaving hospital. In this process, the patients were struggling to find out how they fit into the world, whether it is the world on the ward or the world outside in the community.

• *Feeling lost and being trapped*
Session three started with a free improvisation, using both pitched and non-pitched percussion instruments. The music was unstructured with no set musical theme, form, or rules. The therapist waited to see who would start to play. Dennis began by beating the timpani drum, and the therapist joined in, supporting him on a djembe drum. Other members started playing—Mark on djembe, Steve and Judy on maracas; Tommy played the xylophone, whilst April played the tambourine. As they played, an uneasy feeling seemed to spread around the group, a sense of not knowing what they were playing, where they were, or where they were going. After a few minutes, the music broke down, and they all sat looking at each other. Their anxiety increased in the short silence, as they stopped playing. In an attempt to reassure the group, the therapist started playing a steady pulse on the djembe drum to act as a musical 'anchor', to hold the group music, and to provide a container for the patients' difficult feelings of anxiety. Dennis and Mark started playing again. As the three of them were beating in time together, the therapist had a feeling of relief, which appeared to be shared by the others. At this moment, an unexpected thing happened. Judy started singing:

'We're lost in music, caught in a trap, No turning back, we're lost in music'

(Sister Sledge, 1979)

In the chaos of the free improvisation, people had felt lost and stuck. There seemed to be no framework, no directions about where to go in the music. There was freedom, but what could they do with it? Tommy said he was no good at playing his instrument (xylophone). This statement resonated with some other group members who felt they were not musical and had no musical skills, which contributed to their feeling of being lost and out of their comfort zones.

Steve described feeling trapped. It felt like there was no way out of this music. During the short improvisation, the music became stuck, blocked, repetitive, and unchanging. It seemed in the improvisation like they were going round in 'musical circles'. The therapist and patients started to touch on talking about these feelings in relation to people's experiences of their illnesses where they can become 'stuck' in a pathological state, such as depression or anxiety, and caught up in unchanging patterns of behaviour. They began to play again. Judy carried on singing lines from *Lost in Music*, whilst the rest of them were the backing band, supporting on their instruments. In this improvisation, the group had the experience of being held by the music. Judy said that she felt safe as she sang. They started to make connections between the sense of safety and the previous anxiety about being trapped. Perhaps this can be thought of in terms of a patient who cannot leave hospital, someone who is trapped yet, at the same time, is held by the ward staff with thought and care. This same theme emerged in a later session in relation to thoughts of leaving hospital and going home and having a new life in the community.

- *Coming to terms with illness and disability*

The song *Anything you can do I can do better*, from the musical *Annie Get your Gun*, was introduced by April in session seven. She spontaneously sang this line, as Mark and Dennis seemed to be competing with the therapist to see who could play fastest on the drums. By this stage, the group members were fairly familiar with each other and were able to have playful moments that seemed to come out of, and transcend, the difficulties with which people were struggling. April was struggling to come to terms with Huntington's disease. She was finding it more difficult to walk, and, in the music psychotherapy sessions, she became distressed, as she started to realize that she was losing her guitar-playing skills. She could not remember some chord patterns for songs she had played for years. She told the group that she was worried about the effect her illness was having on her family and how upset they were, saying they were losing her and they 'want the old April back.' This only added to April's anger and frustration. In one remarkable improvisation, April played the tambourine. She played standing up with great energy and passion. She shook the tambourine, as she beat it with her hand, elbow, and shoulder. She became a virtuoso performer, as the rest of the group played along on percussion instruments. They sang lines from the song, as they improvised:

> 'Anything you can do, I can do better, I can do anything, better than you.'

The mood became high-spirited, as they sang *No you can't! Yes I can!* There were outbursts of laughter. In this musical improvisation, there was conscious and unconscious competing between group members, as they were getting to know each other on a deeper level. They were struggling to hold onto abilities and skills that they felt they were losing due to illness, and keeping alive a positive attitude in their struggle to come to terms with illness and loss.

- Other themes that arose in the sessions:
  - Intense feelings: loneliness, isolation, shame
  - Self-esteem and self-image
  - Family, friends, relationship issues
  - Bonding and rivalry
  - Communicating.

Summary
During the course of the music psychotherapy, group individual members who were initially feeling vulnerable, insecure, and unsafe were able to find a means of creative expression through the music, improvising and singing. They discovered ways of communicating and of being together, which hopefully gave them some inner resources to draw on in their future lives outside hospital. All of these patients have now left hospital and are living in the community.

Recommended reading

Ansdell G (1995). *Music for Life*. Jessica Kingsley Publishers: London.
Bruscia KE (ed) (1998). *The Dynamics of Music Psychotherapy*. Barcelona Publishers: Gilsum.
Bunt L and Hoskyns S (2002). *The Handbook of Music Therapy*. Brunner-Routledge: Hove and New York.
Wigram T and De Backer J (eds) (1999). *Clinical Applications of MT in Psychiatry*. Jessica Kingsley Publishers: London.
Wigram T, Pederson IN, and Ole Bonde L (2002). *A Comprehensive Guide to Music Therapy*. Jessica Kingsley Publishers: London.

Counselling

(See ➔ Counselling in Chapter 2, pp. 91–94.)

Key techniques and competencies

Key techniques
These will vary, depending on the model to which the counsellor adheres. Some of the most commonly used are:
- Allowing the client time and space for their story, and for thoughts and feelings to unfold
- Suspending judgement or comment, until the client has been able to fully tell their own story
- Listening to what is being said and also what is not being said; tuning in to all levels of communication, including unconscious, and watching out for clues
- Rephrasing, reflecting back, or clarifying what the client is trying to communicate in a way that brings insight and understanding. This needs to be done tentatively, giving the client permission to disagree, if necessary
- Offering interpretations, making links or using metaphor to help the client make sense of what is going on and why
- Asking pertinent questions at appropriate times
- Eliciting solutions or interpretations from the clients themselves and helping them to tap into their own strengths and resources
- Challenging to enable the client to recognize blocks, difficulties, unhelpful beliefs, etc.
- The counsellor tuning into their own feelings about the client, being able to identify countertransference, in order to gain further understanding of the client, which can help guide the direction of therapy

- Keeping the client (their needs, story, and solutions) at the centre of the counselling, and the counsellor keeping themselves (needs, opinions, solutions, and story) out of it. Even when CBT techniques are being suggested, these are unlikely to succeed without client buy-in
- In brief therapy, helping the client to identify a focus and to acknowledge that it is unlikely that everything can be addressed in this contract; often the counselling contract is to get the client on the right track and identify ways in which he or she can help herself, to recognize and draw on their own inner resources
- Using a range of interventions, depending on the counsellor's training and personal preference, e.g. exploring the impact of the past; incorporating CBT techniques and increasingly use of mindfulness; modelling with shells and stones, using drawing or writing; hypnotherapy; EMDR, and so on. The skill is to know when and how to use each intervention and to ensure that it is done confidently and competently. For example, if a client is highly anxious, it might be appropriate to use some anxiety-reducing techniques (mindfulness, calming breathing) to help them come to a place where they can start to engage with the counselling process effectively
- Being clear, explicit, and transparent about what the expectations and boundaries of the counselling will be, in both practical, including confidentiality, and therapeutic terms. This can help the client feel 'held' and safe, important ingredients in creating the right environment for therapeutic change to take place. Most counselling sessions last 50 minutes. It is important to start and finish on time, and to be clear about the kind of contact that might be acceptable between sessions.

Key competencies
These again will often be specific to context and counsellor orientation. Those that are general and applicable to all counsellors include:
- An ability to form a good working relationship with the client. Being able to gauge what might work best for each client—some appreciate a more directive approach, others need more space to explore for themselves
- Having a broad enough knowledge and awareness, not only of the counselling model, but also of the issues specific to the context in which the counsellor is working. For example, in the context of student counselling and counselling junior doctors, there will be additional competencies expected in terms of awareness of the client group, the pressures under which they are, and knowledge of the practicalities and procedures specific to the organization
- An ability to contain the client's distress within the contract and not to leave them in a worse place than when they started
- The counsellor being self-aware, in particular being able to recognize when their own material is getting in the way of working effectively or ethically, either in terms of past problems or memories which the client's presentation may evoke or current pressures and stresses. Being self-reflexive is essential, and being able to own up to, and

explore, one's shortcomings with peers or in supervision is a key
competency
- An ability to manage boundaries, confidentiality, and have a full
knowledge and awareness of the BACP ethical framework
- Being organized and able to keep up with paperwork, notes, and
records, etc.

What changes?

Counselling does not set out to be a treatment; it aims to help the client
to help themselves through gaining greater insight and awareness of their
feelings, thoughts, behaviour, and impact on others. Through understanding why they feel and behave as they do, counselling can empower
people to make the necessary changes to get their life back on track.

Given the wide range of issues that the counsellor is dealing with, it is
difficult to generalize on what changes. The hope is that the client will
leave feeling better than they arrived, and evidence from the use of outcome evaluation tools, such as the CORE, which is routinely used by
many counselling services, suggests this is true (see ➲ What can be the
measured outcome? in Chapter 4, pp. 143–5; Outcome research in psychotherapy in Chapter 11, pp. 518–9). The BACP research conducted
in 2012/2013 and involving over 5000 respondents from 65 institutions demonstrated 'increased confidence, increased understanding of
self and problem, increased hope for the future and improved ability to
cope'. A measure of change may be successfully supporting the client's
return to work or enabling a student who is considering leaving university to continue with their training.

Sometimes just talking things through in a safe environment with a non-
judgemental counsellor who is able to hear what is felt to be unhearable
is enough; sometimes more proactive strategies are needed. Answers
and solutions that come from the clients are usually more effective than
those suggested or imposed by the counsellor.

Clinical population and contexts

Although there is evidence to demonstrate the efficacy of counselling
for specific problems, as it is usually an intervention aimed at working
with the person as a whole, rather than just addressing symptoms or
specific behaviours, it is perhaps more helpful to think more about who
counselling can help, rather than what it can help with. It is always worth
remembering that even people with severe and enduring mental health
problems or personality disorders can benefit from counselling to deal
with managing difficult life events or feelings. It is therefore more helpful
to think about the kind of people who might benefit from counselling or
not, as shown in Fig. 5.6.

If the client comes with a specific problem, e.g. concern about drug
use, an eating disorder, a bereavement, or recent trauma such as sexual
or physical assault, a road accident, the sudden death of a close friend or
relative, or an incident at work, then counselling would be used to alleviate the symptoms or reduce the problematic behaviour. This is often
not possible in brief therapy, and the counsellor's task might then be to
assess and facilitate a referral to more specialized services. In reality,

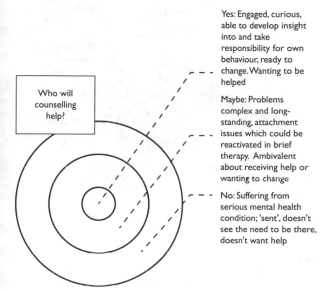

Yes: Engaged, curious, able to develop insight into and take responsibility for own behaviour, ready to change. Wanting to be helped

Maybe: Problems complex and long-standing, attachment issues which could be reactivated in brief therapy. Ambivalent about receiving help or wanting to change

No: Suffering from serious mental health condition; 'sent', doesn't see the need to be there, doesn't want help

Who will counselling help?

Fig. 5.6 Who will counselling help?

the referral options can be limited, and, on occasions, the brief therapy might be extended with successful outcomes, as it is usually the constraints of the brief contract, rather than the skill of the counsellor, which limits the intervention. Where counselling is not appropriate, this will be discussed and the client referred on.

Student counselling services are well placed to provide effective interventions for students, as they are designed to accommodate the academic cycle. This can be difficult in NHS settings, as students usually go home for the academic breaks, unless they attend a local university. Medical students also have less flexibility if they are on placement, and, although, in theory, they should be allowed time off to attend appointments, this can be difficult to arrange or the student might feel embarrassed to ask. Another important factor is that, on the whole, the student will be seen much more quickly by the student counselling service than in primary care. This is important for students where life can move very quickly. In-house counsellors will also be aware of the specific pressures under which students are and the most effective interventions, as well as the organizational systems and appropriate referral pathways to other support services within that particular university. Fig. 5.7 demonstrates the range of the kind of problems that present at the University of Leeds Student Counselling Centre and are fairly typical of what would present at any counselling service in higher education.

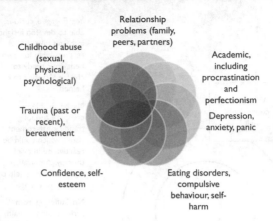

Childhood abuse
(sexual,
physical,
psychological)

Relationship
problems (family,
peers, partners)

Academic,
including
procrastination
and
perfectionism

Trauma (past or
recent),
bereavement

Depression,
anxiety, panic

Confidence, self-
esteem

Eating disorders,
compulsive
behaviour, self-
harm

Fig. 5.7 Presenting problems in the University of Leeds Student Counselling Centre.

Case vignettes

Case one: student counselling centre

Josh, a second-year medical student, was recommended counselling by his tutor after missing a deadline and concerns about attendance. In the assessment session, he spoke of being apathetic about his course, lack of motivation, and feeling that nothing mattered very much. He had been very motivated and did well in his first year. What caused things to change? Josh said he was not sure. The counsellor probed and discovered he had been violently assaulted and mugged in the first week of his second year. It was very upsetting, and things seemed to go downhill after that.

The counsellor enquired about his family background. He was an only child; his parents divorced when he was young, and he did not have much of a relationship with his father. His mother struggled to cope as a single parent, and Josh felt he had to be a good boy. He worked hard at school, which he liked. He developed a strong sense of responsibility, especially for his mother and her feelings, and found that, if he worked hard at being good, academically and behaviourally, he could feel in control of outcomes. Like many medical students, he put a lot of pressure on himself to be perfect.

It became apparent that the experience of being mugged and of being completely out of control had destabilized him, unravelling his precarious sense of safety and of self. The tasks of counselling were to enable him to understand how his early experiences could make him vulnerable to this kind of response, to help him deal with the trauma of the mugging, and to get him back on track with his studies. He was offered a counselling contract of four sessions, in which the primary focus identified by the counsellor was to get him back on track with his work.

With Josh, the counsellor wondered whether a further contract to do some EMDR (see ➲ Trauma-related conditions in Chapter 7, pp. 355–9) on the mugging might be indicated as the most efficient way of processing it but, given the time pressure, decided to see how they got on without it in the first instance. The first session was spent looking at childhood factors and helping him recognize how he had developed ways of coping and beliefs about himself. The counsellor endeavoured to help him view both himself as a child and his mother struggling in difficult circumstances with realistic compassion. She also, however, addressed the issue of his lack of motivation in the current context of the demands of the course.

They spoke about the mugging in the second session. Josh described it in some detail, saying how stupid, out of control, and humiliated he felt, blaming himself. He had become paralysed and unable to fight back. The counsellor challenged his beliefs about this but also stayed with his pain at the loss of a sense of an ideal self, one that seems particularly present in medical students and junior doctors—the figure of the heroic healer. This session was again spent allowing him to tell his story, but also to give him space to see it from a different angle (through challenging and reflecting back). Becoming too directive too early may be counterproductive in brief therapy, although the counsellor did spend some time at the end of the session on helping with motivation and getting a realistic sense of where he was with his work. She also raised the question as to whether he was depressed and would benefit from antidepressant medication. Josh was initially resistant to this, again seeing it as sign of weakness and failure, but, by the end of the session, he was able to agree that it would be worth at least visiting his GP to see what they felt.

The final two sessions were used to pull it all together. As his sleep had been affected and he was experiencing high levels of anxiety, the counsellor taught him some simple mindfulness techniques and gave him a couple of links to audio files of meditation and mindfulness practices. By this time, Josh said he was feeling much better and was pleased that he had felt more enthusiastic about his lectures, recognizing that he did want to do well on his course. They also looked at how he could put some more boundaries in place with his emotionally demanding mother.

By the end of the contract, he had developed a better understanding of himself and why the mugging had felt so particularly traumatic. He was able to be more forgiving of himself and recognize that there was nothing else he could realistically have done (which is what his friends had told him but he was not able to hear). They had also started to look at his perfectionism in the sessions (something he had not thought about) and how he set unrealistically high standards for himself, leading him to an all-or-nothing attitude to his work. He had not missed any more lectures and managed to recapture his sense of purpose. He had seen his GP, and they both felt that medication would not be indicated at this point, but to keep an eye on it. He seemed more open to this approach, especially as he had a positive experience with the GP. As the post-traumatic symptoms relating to the mugging seemed to have calmed down, the counsellor decided not to mention the possibility of EMDR at this point but reassured him that, if they continued to affect him, he could return to the service.

Case two: confidential counselling service for trainee doctors and newly qualified dentists

Emma was a young woman who had recently started her GP training and was currently working in A&E. She had been a very able student, a high achiever. She struggled during her foundation year and now had come to a point in her training where she was feeling so overwhelmed and lacking in confidence that she was seriously questioning whether medicine was for her. She had been signed off work for 2 weeks and prescribed antidepressants. Her educational supervisor suggested *Take Time*, a confidential service for trainee doctors and newly qualified dentists in the local Deanery, which offered assessment and, if appropriate, five sessions.

During the assessment, Emma was tearful and anxious. She described how hard it was for her to fit everything into her working day and frequently stayed on late, neglecting to take breaks because she had so much to do. She was terrified of making a mistake, which meant she checked and double-checked everything. Her fear of asking seniors for help, in case they thought she was stupid, led to huge anxiety. This led to her not sleeping and neglecting her own down-time. She was worried her relationship would suffer, as she thought her boyfriend was getting fed up with her crying all the time, in turn, leading to more anxiety and fears of abandonment.

A bit of exploration revealed that she had coped with a difficult upbringing by working hard and trying to maintain control. Emma, the oldest of three, took a lot of responsibility both for the care of her younger siblings and her mother's emotional well-being. Despite being bullied at school, she worked very hard, achieved excellent grades, and got into medical school, although she felt she did this more to please her teachers than herself. She had a period of depression as a student but managed to power on through, feeling that to ask for help would be seen as 'pathetic'. She had not been good at recognizing her own needs and asking for help, but had just about managed to keep a sense of control by working hard. Coming into her foundation year felt overwhelmingly stressful, as suddenly she was in an environment she could not control, and, no matter how hard she worked, there was always more and more to be done. The terror of possible consequences further drove her anxiety, and the feeling of never feeling quite good enough further eroded her precarious sense of self. This all came out in her first session. In addition, she revealed that her grandmother had died nearly a year ago.

In the second assessment, Emma and the counsellor looked further at the impact of her grandmother's death. Her grandmother had been a stable influence during her childhood and had always been there for Emma; it was her grandmother who had given Emma a lot of love, support, and validation growing up. Emma felt bewildered by the impact of her death. By the end of the assessment, she was able to get some sense of context and understanding of why she was feeling so overwhelmed. The counsellor felt that *Take Time* would be helpful and contracted for a further five sessions.

During the course of the counselling, the counsellor explored her childhood relationships, in particular being the oldest child and having to take on more responsibility than was appropriate, and how these were being played out in her current situation. Her fear of getting things wrong, as her stressed father would rage at her unreasonably and unpredictably, and being bullied at school had led to an internalized sense of shame and feeling that things were her fault. With Emma, the counsellor looked at when these feelings were being activated and helped her to recognize this and remember that she was no longer a powerless child and that the people around her were not her father or classmates. The counsellor helped her stabilize her anxiety with some gentle breathing and mindfulness exercises, and to work on giving herself permission to take appropriate breaks and hand over at the end of her shift. Emma looked at how her peers managed and conceded that some were able to do this, and no one thought any less of them. When she finally returned to work—her sick leave had been extended a further 2 weeks—the counsellor encouraged her to start taking little risks in being more assertive and not being so perfectionist. She was able to do this and see the benefit. Part of the work was also to give her permission to feel some buried feelings, grief for her grandmother, and anger with her parents and the bullies at school. Importantly, she was also able to feel sympathy and compassion for the little girl that she had been, and admiration for how well she coped.

Unfortunately, her inability to prioritize herself meant that her attendance at the counselling sessions was sporadic, but this was able to be addressed. She began to regain her perspective and see that self-care was also an important skill in being a doctor. She also changed her rotation and found that her new environment was much more supportive, which helped her regain her confidence. However, the counsellor sensed that there was still much more work to be done. She was resistant to considering longer-term psychotherapy but felt reassured that she could return to *Take Time*, if she needed to.

The work with Emma demonstrates a typical contract, using an integrative counselling model (supported by antidepressant medication) combining a psychodynamic awareness of how the past impacts on the present with a more cognitive behavioural approach—challenging her beliefs and experimenting with different behaviours. The counsellor also did some psycho-educational work and skills development. Most important of all, perhaps, was being attuned to her, being with her, and allowing her the time and space to meet herself in the presence of a non-judgemental other—a stance borrowed from the person-centred model.

Recommended reading

Claringbull N (2010). *What is Counselling and Psychotherapy?* Learning Matters Ltd: Exeter.
Dryden W (2011). *Counselling in a Nutshell*. Sage Publications Ltd: London.
Mcleod J (2009). *An Introduction to Counselling*, fourth edition. Open University Press: Maidenhead.

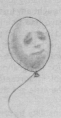
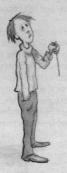

Problems through life

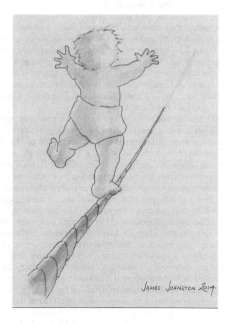

JAMES JOHNSTON 2014

Life: cradle to grave

Infants

The first months of a baby's life are full of challenges, changes, and, if negotiated well, developmental achievements. Winnicott's quote 'there is no such thing as a baby' refers to the idea of a merged experience of a baby with the mother/caregiver at the beginning of its life. The well 'held' baby will experience being thought about and understood in the mother's mind. Bion described the 'containment' of the mother who takes in her baby's feelings and anxieties, tries to understand or 'digest' them, and communicates a response that helps the baby feel understood. A baby may experience a range of unpleasant feelings: hunger, wind or dirty nappies, distress on waking, or the terror of being alone. A baby also experiences good feelings: satisfaction after being fed or changed, and positive emotional interchanges with an attuned parent. Eventually, the baby will progress from this stage of intense 'holding' to that of an increasing awareness of being a distinct individual (see ➔ Donald Winnicott and Wilfred Bion in Key contributors in Chapter 2, pp. 25–8).

Babies enter life primed to seek affective interaction with others, and these interactions impact upon the way the baby's brain connections develop and grow. The parents and the baby will gaze at, smile, and vocalize towards each other. Well-attuned parents will note when the baby wants to initiate interaction or when the baby needs a break, and will modulate their interactions accordingly.

The relationship that develops between baby and caregiver is the 'attachment relationship', and it can be defined as secure, insecure, or disorganized (see ➔ Theories of personality development: attachment theory in Chapter 8, pp. 380–1). A parent who can provide a secure relationship for the developing baby will be one who can tolerate the baby's dependency needs and respond in a timely and sensitive manner, i.e. not leaving the baby too long in a distressed state. The result is an emotionally and physiologically regulated baby.

In the interaction between baby and caregiver, the baby needs to feel that the caregiver's responses 'fit' what he is feeling. Research finds that, at best, infant–mother attunement occurs only 30% of the time. This research supports Winnicott's ideas of a 'good enough' mother. In a well-functioning infant–mother pair, mismatches are common. What is critical is that mismatches are repaired. It has been estimated that mismatches in communication are effectively repaired about a third of the time on the first attempt and that a third of the remaining mismatches were repaired by the second interaction. The purpose of 'mismatch and repairs' is believed to include: (1) promoting self–other differentiation, (2) encouraging the infant to develop interactive skills, (3) creating opportunities for the infant to feel effective by his participation in the repair, and (4) allowing the infant to learn self-regulatory skills. However, if mismatches are abnormally prolonged, the self-regulatory function can be derailed into a defence or retreat from ordinary social interactions.

A distressed baby seeks out his mother for her help in regulating his emotions and restoring him to a calm physiological state. If the baby sees fear or anger in his mother's face, he will look away. He may develop gaze avoidance, and he may stop communicating his distress to his mother. He may be mistaken as a 'good baby', when, in fact, he has developed a defensive way of dealing with distress. This is an effective short-term adaptation but risks derailing healthy emotional development in the long run. In later life, the child may struggle to understand and regulate his own distress, and not know how to let others support him.

Children

From the extreme dependency of infancy, a child moves to a more independent existence via numerous developmental stages. One of the first of these is weaning, which may happen at different ages, depending on the child, parents, or culture. The significance of weaning is the experience of separation from the mother, and this experience will be echoed through life in future separations. If a child has had enough positive experiences with the mother as a baby, then the loss experienced during weaning has a better opportunity to be mourned and successfully negotiated by the baby. Klein described this as the early Oedipal situation, when the baby begins to feel rivalry for the father—to whom the mother is also giving her time and love (see ➔ Melanie Klein in Key contributors in Chapter 2, pp. 25–8).

A child with a store of good experiences can begin to tolerate periods of absence by the caregiver and longer waits for relief of discomfort. As the baby's innate capacities for agency develop, he begins to express his wishes more clearly. The toddler stage of the 'terrible twos' refers to the ability of the child to begin to explore his world and express an intention to separate from his parent's wishes. Being able to accept or refuse food and control of the bowels and bladder are all important, as a child's development progresses. Similarly, a child with a secure attachment will begin to use his parents as a secure base from which to explore his surroundings. The 'Strange Situation' (Main) procedure shows if a child is securely or insecurely attached to parents when parents leave the room and return. Securely attached children will show distress but can be comforted by the returning parent. Insecurely attached children show avoidant or anxious behaviour on reunion with their caregiver. A further category of disorganized attachment has been associated with abuse from caregivers and can include dissociative responses, such as freezing and rocking on reunion with parents, the child simultaneously feeling the need to approach and to flee (see ➔ Theories of personality development: attachment theory in Chapter 8, pp. 380–1).

Freud's developmental stages of childhood focused on the underlying psychosexual phases and erotogenic zones (see ➔ Psychoanalytic psychotherapy in Chapter 2, pp. 22). The oral stage is a key part of infancy, and it is easily observed in that babies explore the world by putting things in their mouths. The anal stage is not only driven by the internal experience of the child's erotogenic zones, but also by the experience of taking control of defecation. The phallic stage is the psychosexual stage of genital awareness, of awareness of sexual difference, castration anxiety, and penis envy. This was interpreted by Freud as the Oedipal stage—a key developmental stage for a child; in classical Freudian terms, it is the time when the child wants to get rid of the same-sex parent who is experienced as a rival for the affections of the opposite-sex parent. This is the positive Oedipus complex; the negative Oedipus complex is rivalry for the affections of the same sex parent. Latency refers to the time when sexuality 'goes quiet', and this occurs between the Oedipal stage and adolescence, when sexuality again dominates as a focus for the individual. The latency period is generally when children begin 'proper school', and a child who has successfully negotiated the Oedipal stage will be much freer to explore the social world of peer relationships and demonstrate intellectual curiosity.

Winnicott identified the capacity to play as a key developmental achievement in childhood. Play involves creativity, and the ability to bring together separate things, to link them, and to symbolize through the use of imagination (see ➔ Donald Winnicott in Key contributors in Chapter 2, pp. 25–8).

Family

In infancy, the emphasis is on the baby's relationship with the main caregiver, due to its high level of dependency. As a child moves forward in life, other relationships in the family become increasingly significant in shaping the developing personality. A crucial role for the father is that of increasing the space between the baby and the mother when it is developmentally appropriate; when the father reasserts his crucial bond with the mother, he creates a three-person relationship (which is the basis for the Oedipal conflicts). The baby, who, if conditions were positive, was so used to being the centre of the mother's world, now has to recognize that the mother also has a relationship with the father and that he may come and 'claim' the mother for himself. In the early stages of life, the baby or toddler is not competing for the same-sex parent, but competing for the main caregiver of whichever sex. The parent who 'takes away' this main caregiver is a rival that the baby or toddler hates and wishes to get rid of. Yet, the existence of the father who takes the mother away also creates space for the baby to develop. If the mother never left the baby's side, the need to walk and be independent would be less strong. As the child with a secure base explores, going away and coming back to the parents, he begins to develop a sense of his own capacity to affect his environment.

With the arrival of a new baby, a different kind of rivalry is created, and, if the new baby comes too early in the older child's development, it can impinge on his developing independence and lead to regression to an earlier stage. This is common in many children, e.g. a child who is dry at night may begin to wet the bed; however, if a baby is very young, their own dependency needs may feel neglected too soon. Some children learn to discard these dependency needs and grow up prematurely. This can lead to a child who tries very hard to 'be good' and creates what Winnicott called a 'false self' (see ➔ Psychoanalytic psychotherapy in Chapter 2, pp. 20–30). Such children may get stuck in latency and struggle to undertake the more rebellious role of adolescence. Other children may develop severe separation anxiety or school phobia.

When faced with such difficulties, some families have resources, such as grandparents, who can provide comfort to a child feeling displaced by a new baby. Alternatively, older siblings may take on the role of carer. Whilst this can be a positive experience if taken up when a sibling is old enough, the internal resources needed to look after a younger sibling may impinge upon the older one. Other important issues in family life can include the death of a parent, migration, and cultural and identity issues specific to that family.

Parents' own attachment issues and experiences of being parented inevitably have an impact on their capacity and style of parenting their children, and this, in turn, can lead to the repetition of family dynamics (see ➲ Theories of personality development: attachment theory in Chapter 8, pp. 380–1).

Recommended reading

Freud S (1905). Three essays on the theory of sexuality. In: Strachey J, ed. *The Standard Edition of the Complete Psychological Works of Sigmund Freud*, volume 7. pp. 125–245. Hogarth Press and the Institute of Psychoanalysis: London.

Tronick E (2007). *The Neurobehavioral and Socio-Emotional Development of Infants and Children.* Norton: New York.

Waddell M (1998). *Inside Lives: Psychoanalysis and the Growth of the Personality.* Karnac Books: London.

Winnicott DW (1949). The ordinary devoted mother and her baby. In: *The Child and the Family.* 1957. Tavistock Publications: London.

Winnicott D (1958). *Collected Papers: Through Paediatrics to Psycho-Analysis.* Tavistock Publications: London.

Adolescence

Adolescence (from Latin *ad* meaning 'to' and *alescere* meaning 'grow, grow up') can be defined as a discrete transitional period of life, usually spanning from about thirteen to twenty-one, during which a number of maturational changes emerging from the so-called latency stage enable progress into young adulthood. Adolescence is an important developmental stage, enabling transition from childhood to adulthood, from childhood dependence on parents to adult autonomy, independence, and responsibility. The struggle for autonomy includes a reactivation of rebellion against caregivers and a search for new, often idealized, role models.

Freud took the view that, during puberty, there is a struggle between the urges of the early years and the inhibition of the latency period. Indeed, adolescence has later been described as a second individuation process, allowing for a reworking of earlier unresolved conflicts. These changes starting at puberty rely on a gradual reorganization of the mental structure along the various developmental lines, including physical and sexual maturation, identity formation, and the establishment of social and meaningful relationships.

Whilst adolescents have their own unique mode of developing, enabling them to negotiate physical and psychological expectations, it is during this time that adolescents become the sole guardians of their sexually mature body. For the young adolescent, their developing sexual body evokes anxiety and confusion. During the mid or later part of adolescence, the young person has to psychically integrate their new sexual identity in order to form a stable sense of self, with consequent object choice. In addition, adolescence is often a disturbing process, as it involves not only coming to terms with, and integrating, the developing sexual body, but also managing an increased aggressive potential. Consequently, conflicts around hostility, depression, and anxiety are common features amidst the oscillation between dependence and independence.

This is also a period of multiple transitions, stress, and an increasing sense of responsibility. Indeed, the adolescent has to grapple with a number of adjustments, starting from his physically maturing body to becoming independent from parental figures, whilst searching for relationships with contemporaries, as well as experimenting with sexual intimacy and social identity. However, the choice between social and intimate relationships can be a source of conflict of loyalty in those adolescents who find it hard to negotiate over whom to give priority.

For adolescents, the way they experience themselves and the world around them may take different routes according to where they are along the continuum from early, middle, to late adolescence. Adolescence can also reactivate a shame-inducing process, during which the young person has to come to terms with their origins and the renunciation of what he would have liked to be. The experience of loneliness in adolescence is an important maturational step during the process of separation from parental figures. This can be harder to bear for a young adolescent, as opposed to an older adolescent who may have begun to establish a peer group to relate to. Individual variations between adolescents, their family, social status, and culture of origin make it at times difficult to properly evaluate whether loneliness can be considered as a normal temporary process for that particular adolescent or the prodrome of a more ominous sense of isolation and vulnerability. If it is the latter, the combination of withdrawal, possible pent-up aggression, and impulsivity may give way to suicidal ideation or an actual act of self-harm as a solution to unbearable feelings of failure or an inability to negotiate frustration, distress, and disappointments. Consequently, a careful diagnostic evaluation is required, in order to distinguish the onset of serious pathology from a more transitional developmental phase.

In summary, the most important developmental task during this stage of growth consists of negotiating the separation–individuation process, at times a painful process, which allows transition into early adulthood, leading to a stable sense of identity and a realistic expectation of one's own abilities.

Recommended reading

Blos P (1962). *On Adolescence*. Free Press: New York.
Caparrotta L (2003). Oedipal shame, rejection, and adolescent development. *American Journal of Psychoanalysis*, 63, 345–56.
Erikson E (1968). *Identity: Youth and Crisis*. WW Norton: New York.
Laufer M and Laufer E (1984). *Adolescence and Developmental Breakdown. A Psychoanalytic View*. Yale University Press: New Haven.

Young adulthood

The young adulthood stage usually refers to the time between late teens and middle to late twenties. It may be regarded as another developmental phase in that the psychic structure continues to evolve 'from the cradle to the grave', as Jung pointed out, but it can also be considered as a phase of adaptation from previous established psychic changes. There is no doubt that these 'emerging adults' have to manage a number of important tasks and responsibilities, ranging from financial independence to rearing a family.

Erikson helpfully divided the art of negotiation in young adulthood (between ages 18 and 40) into opposing polarities of a psychosocial or developmental crisis, namely intimacy versus isolation. They include the capacity to form and maintain friendships, as well as to commit to intimate and meaningful sexual relationships, which may lead to pregnancy and parenthood, along with the ability of finding a satisfactory career and working life. During this time, sex and love are supposed to be mutually integrated, rather than kept separate. In addition, social and cultural elements, underpinning a clear sense of self-worth and belonging, tend to consolidate. In the pursuit of these tasks, the young adult requires the capacity to sustain their sense of identity and psychic stability in the face of successes, frustrations, failures, or adversities.

During this process, earlier life experiences and the quality of family life may foster, threaten, or disrupt self representation and integration. Hence the potential for a breakdown should not be underestimated. Indeed, it is well known that mental illness, psychological symptoms, and personality disorder diagnoses often emerge during the young adulthood phase, with ensuing negative outcomes for future life. After leaving school or university, or whilst entering a work environment, these young adults may require encouragement, validation, and possibly mentoring, in order to ease their way into the difficulties and various stresses of their working and family life. It could be argued that their future resilience in adulthood depends greatly on their successful negotiation and integration of past and new experiences during these highly important years.

In summary, the period of young adulthood represents a vital bridge to final maturity and satisfactory entrance into the adult world. If inner and external past and present tensions and conflicts have not reached an acceptable resolution, it is possible that the young adult will find it harder to withstand the pressures of the future.

Recommended reading

Arnett JJ (2004). *Adolescence and Emerging Adulthood: A Cultural Approach*. Oxford University Press.

Erikson E (1959). *Identity and the Life Cycles Completed. Psychological Issues, Monograph 1.* International University Press: New York.

Jung CG (1933). *Modern Man in Search of a Soul*. Harcourt: Brace.

Westen D and Chang C (2000). Personality pathology in adolescence: a review. In: Esmar A and Flaherty LT, eds. *Adolescence Psychiatry: Developmental and Clinical studies.* pp. 61–100. Analytic Press: Hillsdale, NJ.

Adults

After the period of adolescence, adulthood follows whereby the personality has stabilized and identity is more certain. At least, this is the hypothetical norm. In reality, human beings continue to struggle with many of the same issues that had become so important during adolescence once again, having been reawakened, perhaps for the first time, since infancy.

A number of themes emerge as being important to adults: relationships, career, the decision whether or not to have children, and a narrowing of choices, as the person makes decisions as to which path their life is going to take.

Relationships outside of the birth family become of central importance during adolescence and, during adulthood, continue to play an important role, as the person creates around them a potentially new family—both in the traditional sense, but also in terms of friends and other significant platonic relationships. Despite the way in which adulthood is portrayed and enshrined in law as being a period in which the individual makes rational choices and is responsible for these, many people can feel that their life is still not entirely their own. The unconscious mind persists in its timeless fashion, not disappearing in favour of the conscious, rational mind. What determines the level of influence the unconscious exerts is the extent to which earlier unconscious conflicts have been resolved and their interactions with stressors in the outside world (the relationship between internal and external worlds). It is the normal state of affairs that people tend to 'regress' to earlier ways of behaving and responding or reacting emotionally when under significant stress.

However, if early experiences and adolescence have been negotiated relatively well, adulthood is likely to be a relatively stable period, in which an individual can begin to realize some of their childhood wishes, but, of course, not all. The reality principle is all important, of course, and dreams and wishes may have been, and continue to be, modified as per the constraints or opportunities present in the external environment. The amount of still unresolved internal conflict carried through into adulthood depends on the individual, but everyone will have something left over, which has the potential to present a difficulty if the external circumstances are particularly challenging.

Adulthood may be the first time in their lives in which people experience significant loss in the external world, e.g. in the death of parents or other relatives, and the disillusionment of wishes which have not come to fruition. There is loss of an adolescent omnipotence which, if worked through successfully, can lead to a more realistic set of expectations of themselves and of others. Sometimes it can be difficult, for a number of reasons, for the person to give up a need for omnipotence, which can lead not to gradual disillusionment, but to accumulating dissatisfactions as disappointments which build up in number as grievances, so that mourning and loss are not experienced. The difficulty lies in not being able to face or metabolize loss; this may be one of the crucial ways in which unresolved issues from earlier in the person's life continue to exert their disturbing influence in adulthood from the unconscious mind.

Midlife

Midlife can be a particularly stable period in a person's life, perhaps because a home has been set up, a partner chosen, a career decided upon and well settled into, and children had or not. Whether or not these things have been felt to be important to the individual person, major choices will have been made, either actively or relatively passively, as to what kind of lifestyle the individual is going to be leading for the greater part of their life. Productivity, in terms of work or contribution to society, may be at its greatest during this period of life.

For those individuals who have not, for whatever reason, been able to realize their potential in life, however, this phase can be particularly challenging and painful. Some may have experienced significant illness and have gone through many bereavements by this point in life, whereas others may have experienced relatively little in this sphere. The likelihood of experiencing external losses of many kinds increases and can once again reawaken conflicts from earlier in the individual's life which have not yet been worked through satisfactorily.

In modern, westernized culture, the concept of the 'midlife crisis' may be used to refer to individuals who appear to be reworking some aspects of their youth which they had not been able to work through during their adolescence. As with all crises, there can be an opportunity for psychological growth if the crisis can be weathered. This depends on the level of resilience built up within the individual and their emotional support network. A decline in productivity may have to be faced and worked through during the later part of this period of life, and alternatives sought to previous occupations.

Regret about what has not been achieved in life, balanced with what may still be possible or what alternatives there are, is another issue to be faced, particularly in later midlife, as old age approaches. Towards the later part of midlife, illnesses may appear for the first time; a further loss of an individual's own omnipotence is inevitable, as well as the increased chance of being part of the oldest generation in one's family or network.

Some people find this to be an enriching period in life and a chance to take part in activities which a busy work or family life may have precluded them from partaking in. For others, however, the working identity, or identity as a parent, can be tricky to forgo. This links back to Freud's seminal paper on *Mourning and Melancholia* (1917) and the difficulty in moving from one phase of life to the next if early infantile losses have not been worked through successfully. Freud's thinking was that the feeling of ambivalence about who or what is lost hangs like a shadow of gloomy hatred over the self, self-recrimination being an unconscious complaint about those others by whom one feels badly let down.

As with all stages of life, the factors determining whether a new period of life can be enjoyed are the extent to which losses can be mourned, the support structures in the individual's internal and external world, and the quantity of loss to be worked through.

Recommended reading

Freud S (1917). Mourning and melancholia: In: Strachey J, ed. *The Standard Edition of the Complete Psychological Works of Sigmund Freud*, volume 14. pp. 237–60. Hogarth Press and the Institute of Psychoanalysis: London.

Later life

(See ➲ Dementia in Chapter 7, pp. 372–6; Psychiatry of old age: psychotherapies, applications, and research in Chapter 12, pp. 565–7.)

In the course of an individual's life, moving towards later life, or simply being older, brings with it the developmental task of accommodating the physical and psychic reality of the end of life through death, the readjustment of expectations, and 'constructive resignation to shortcomings' (Jacques, 1965) (taken literally, the 'shortly coming' or reduction in time available). This adjustment is often invisible, with the character of a 'smooth enough' transition and a kind of acceptance. However, an unplanned event, such as loss or illness, may precipitate a crisis, bringing about a collapse of the self and revealing the existence of a more fragile internal world, based on an emotional constellation of defensive structures and identifications, with which the individual has got by, rather than fully lived.

These responses in later life centre around an attitude to loss—loss of time, opportunity, significant persons, or work—but also convey the unique nature of the meaning of the loss for the individual. Change and loss at any stage of life demand the psychological and emotional work of mourning, and the working through again and again—or not—of the depressive feelings encountered in infancy and the associated defences against separation. Loss in later life also brings with it the complication of the personal nature and meaning of mortality.

Those who come for psychotherapy in later life often do so with difficulties or failures of mourning, and concomitant problems of stuck idealizations (e.g. work as the antidote to all ills) or identifications.

Psychotherapy with older adults both differs from, and is similar to, psychotherapeutic work undertaken elsewhere in the life course. It differs in that the therapist's associations and attitudes matter and are inexorably part of the psychological encounter. For example, a therapist starting out on a professional career, with a life to build, may not wish to encounter the finite nature of life as it has to be encountered in the older patient; equally, the older patient may find it impossible to believe a 'young' therapist can understand or help. It also differs in that the work reflects the world of, and around, the patient in ways which can intrude forcefully on the setting—bodily, environmental, and mental containment may be compromised through illness, changing living and social circumstances, and psychological coping strategies.

Davenhill, in acknowledging that the internal constellation and external life of the therapist matter and are nowhere more demanding than in the psychotherapeutic encounter with a patient in later life, advises acknowledgement of these aspects and freeing up of the treatment setting. She emphasizes the pressure to become something other than the therapist when working with so much reality, as one meets in the long life of an older patient, e.g. social worker, offspring, or physician.

These exigencies make it of real importance to hold the boundaries of the setting firmly and to maintain a focus on the patient's internal world in relation to the therapist. Time is a very important concept in therapy—because time can be experienced as more persecutory than helpful, particularly in later life, and the secure time frame of the setting provides an important aspect of physical, and thus psychic, reality, allowing the past to be distinguished from the present and the future.

Recommended reading

Davenhill R (2007). *Looking into Later Life: A Psychoanalytic Approach to Depression and Dementia in Old Age*. Karnac: London.

Evans S and Garner J (eds). *Talking over the Years: A Handbook of Dynamic Psychotherapy with Older Adults*. Brunner-Routledge: Hove.

Jacques E (1965). Death and the mid-life crisis. *International Journal of Psychoanalysis*, **46**, 502–14.

King P (1999). 'In the end is my beginning'–TS Eliot. In: Bell D (ed). *Psychoanalysis and Culture: A Kleinian Perspective.* Duckworth: London. Reprinted Karnac: London, 2004.

Martindale B (1998). On ageing, dying, death and eternal life. *Psychoanalytic Psychotherapy,* **12,** 259–70.

Lived experience

Love

Love of oneself—a primary narcissism (i.e. that existing from the beginning)—is, as Freud postulated, necessary for the subsequent development of love for others. He expounded that, even though the child appears to love others from early on, at first, this is a love in the service of the child getting their needs met. In *Instincts and Their Vicissitudes* (1915), Freud said that, in infant development, hate is older than love. This ambivalence about dependence, vulnerability, and helplessness is understandable, given that the human infant is helpless and in need of others for its own survival (both physically and psychically, for the two are intrinsically linked) for a relatively long period of time, when compared with infants of other species. In normal development, there comes a point where the child begins to love others, independent of his need for them in survival terms. Freud explained that this was indicative of a portion of the child's ego being given over to the other, rather that it being kept all to his or herself (a portion of narcissism turned outward) (see **⟶** Developmental approach in Chapter 2, p. 22).

Melanie Klein did not agree with the idea of primary narcissism and differed in her view on the developmental route by which the love of an individual for another individual can be formed. The infant struggles with intense life and death anxieties about love and hatred towards his or her mother, and later on significant others. Klein states that the love of the baby for his mother is when she is satisfying his or her bodily needs and giving sensual pleasure. However, when these needs are not being met, hateful and aggressive feelings are turned against the mother. The baby splits their love from their hatred and splits their mother (object) in two—into a good object and a bad object. The anxiety of annihilation is that hatred will overwhelm love and destroy the good object. Klein wrote that 'the feelings of love and gratitude arise directly and spontaneously in the baby in response to the love and care of his mother' (see **⟶** Melanie Klein in Key Contributors in Chapter 2, pp. 25–8).

Klein considered that the capacity for love can only emerge if 'persecutory' and 'depressive' anxieties (i.e. anxieties about one's own survival in the former, and anxieties about damage done to a significant other in the latter) have been sufficiently allayed and dealt with. In practice, this means that, if an individual is in a state of chronic anxiety, the capacity for love is impaired by unconscious hatred. The mitigation of anxieties, of hatred mitigated by love, is vital, before a child's love for themselves can be extended to those around him or her.

Freud also explored human societies and their structures. He described how love within groups bonds the group and therefore means that survival of the group is given the best possible chance. However, this necessarily means that hatred is seen as coming from outside of the group; in psychoanalytic terms, the hatred of the group is *projected*.

Winnicott described a primitive love ('id') impulse, and saw aggression as being part of an early expression of love and 'use of the object' as a separate other. His theory is that the meaningful use of the object (the first object being the mother) requires the object to survive the efforts of the infant to destroy it. He uses the idea of an excited, early love, with which the infant seeks to destroy his love object without realizing that this is the same object which satisfies him. Winnicott himself makes an assertion about his view of the development of the next stage, in which the child can feel concern (concern or *ruth*, as opposed to ruthlessness) about what he or she does to his object when excited, as being comparative to Melanie Klein's concept of the 'depressive position' (see ➔ Donald Winnicott in Key Contributors in Chapter 2, pp. 25–8).

Recommended reading

Freud S (1915). Instincts and their vicissitudes. In: Strachey J (ed). *The Standard Edition of the Complete Psychological Works of Sigmund Freud*, volume 14. pp. 117–140. Hogarth Press and the Institute of Psychoanalysis: London.

Freud S (1930). Civilization and its discontents. In: Strachey J (ed). *The Standard Edition of the Complete Psychological Works of Sigmund Freud*, volume 21. pp. 57–146. Hogarth Press and the Institute of Psychoanalysis: London.

Klein M (1997). *Envy and Gratitude and Other Works 1946–1963*. Vintage: London.

Klein M (1998). *Love, Guilt and Reparation and Other Works 1921–1945*. Vintage: London.

Winnicott D (1984). *Through Paediatrics to Psychoanalysis: Collected Papers*. Karnac: London.

Hatred

Hatred can be viewed not as the corollary of love, but as its close relation. In order to hate, one has to have already attached a great deal of significance to the object of one's hatred. So actually, the opposite of both love and hatred is indifference. Hatred of another can represent a projected part of the self which feels unacceptable, or as the feeling engendered by a profound or overwhelming disappointment by the loved 'object'.

Melanie Klein often discussed hatred in terms of it being mitigated by love, if enough love is allowed to exist in the developing individual and at times when hatred is evoked. In this way, she argued the 'good' can mitigate against the 'bad', and the individual can continue along the path of life, rather than veer towards the destruction of others and themselves. This is a dynamic process whereby the capacity of the individual to love is constantly being tested. She argued both for the presence of innate factors which affect the individual's capacity for love, and thereby the ability to mitigate against hate, but also recognized the importance of environmental factors (see ➔ Melanie Klein in Key Contributors in Chapter 2, pp. 25–8).

Winnicott argued that hate itself is sophisticated in emotional development terms, and that it therefore is not present in pure form in early infantile life. He described how, in the course of working with people in analysis, the analyst themselves has to be able to objectively hate the patient, when appropriate, in order to be able to help the patient to struggle with this feeling within themselves. In his paper *Hate in the*

Countertransference (1947), he described his work with a child who had antisocial tendencies and who would wreak havoc in the external world. Winnicott bravely relates how he had struggled with his countertransference feelings of hatred in regard to this boy, and how his recognition of these feelings, as opposed to his struggle to rid himself of them, led to him furthering his understanding of the internal world of the child. This is an example of how one of the most intense and difficult-to-accept feelings in the human emotional repertoire can be borne and understood and put to good use in the service of furthering the understanding of the human mind (see ➔ Donald Winnicott in Key Contributors in Chapter 2, pp. 25–8).

Hatred is also a group phenomenon. As alluded to in the section on love, when love is seen as coming from inside of the group, hatred can also be seen as being located outside of the group and being aimed at the group. This is the basis of the hatred and prejudice between groups which has developed between different groups of people since time immemorial, i.e. it is a projection of the hatred within the group, which feels to be more dangerous if it remains in the group than if it is felt to be coming from outside, as there is solidarity in number. This phenomenon helps to explain the solidarity described as existing amongst members of the same group during periods of unrest, particularly during major wars. When the war has passed, the group in question is forced to take back some of its projections of hatred, the recovery of which can lead to national shame and guilt, the large group equivalent of humiliation in recognition of the attack for which the self/group is responsible.

Recommended reading

Freud S (1916–1917). Introductory lectures on psychoanalysis. In: Strachey J (ed). *The Standard Edition of the Complete Psychological Works of Sigmund Freud*, volume 16. Hogarth Press and the Institute of Psychoanalysis: London.
Klein M and Riviere J (1964). *Love, Hate and Reparation*. WW Norton and Company: New York.
Winnicott D (1984). *Through Paediatrics to Psychoanalysis: Collected Papers*. Karnac: London.

Sexuality

Freud and his colleagues put forward a controversial theorem about sexuality, namely that there is an infantile sexuality which precedes full adult sexuality. Fundamentally, Freud challenged the rather fixed and narrow view of sexuality of the day and elucidated the complexity of the process of development of sexuality. He thought that sexuality developed very early on in each individual, but that this sexuality was immature by definition, i.e. the sexuality of infancy and childhood is not the same as the sexuality of adulthood. This distinction is important, because children cannot be seen to possess mature adult sexual feelings or the physical or psychological equipment to deal with them (see ➔ Developmental approach in Key Contributors in Chapter 2, p. 22).

Following on from Freud's work, Melanie Klein continued to elucidate the developmental origins of childhood sexuality and described the central importance of the infant's relation to the mother's breast and the pleasure felt by the infant in feeding which went over and above that of a pure need for food. She postulated that this initial relationship is so important that it sets up patterns, which are, mostly unconsciously, adhered to in later life in adult relationships. She also pointed to the importance of the infant's relationship with the father, but that this, in itself, was, in some way, predicated on the relationship with the mother. These early established patterns can be helpful or unhelpful, in terms of the individual's later relationships; for example, a person may be able to recognize that they repeatedly enter the same kinds of unsatisfactory adult relationship, but they may not be able to explain why and may feel confused as to why this keeps happening (see ➔ Melanie Klein in Key Contributors in Chapter 2, pp. 25–8).

Classic psychoanalytic theories have been criticized for being normative; nevertheless, it is helpful to know about these. The 'Oedipus complex', as described by Freud and named after the mythological legend of Oedipus who unknowingly killed his father and married his mother, describes a process whereby the child, between the ages of 3 to 6, forms an intense desire for the parent of the opposite gender, and a rivalry with the parent of the same gender. Gradual resolution, through reality testing, should result in the child being able to resolve this rivalry and identify more strongly with the parent of the same sex, thus giving up their desire for the parent of the opposite sex. The complex was described first in relation to male children and castration anxiety, with the corollary for female children being the 'Electra complex' and penis envy. Melanie Klein thought that the Oedipus complex began much earlier for children of both sexes than Freud had postulated. Both Freud and Klein saw the resolution of the Oedipus complex as central to the development of identity in relation to sexuality and gender (see ➔ Developmental approach in Chapter 2, p. 22; Melanie Klein in Key Contributors in Chapter 2, pp. 25–8).

In contemporary psychoanalytic theory and research, Alessandra Lemma and others have written on gender and identity issues, particularly in relation to adolescents. These include reference to the sociological literature on sexuality, gender, and identity, which has sought to explore the societal origins of these characteristics, as well as the source of prejudices and injustices towards people who do not fall into 'traditional' or expected categories in these regards, e.g. transgender individuals (see ➔ Sexual dysfunction in Chapter 7, pp. 345–9; Gender dysphoria and intersex conditions in Chapter 7, pp. 364–8).

Other contemporary psychoanalytic writers, e.g. Dinora Pines and Estela Welldon, have explored female sexuality, in terms of women's views and use of their bodies, and have sought to expand on Freud's limited understanding of the subject.

Recommended reading

Freud S (1905). Three essays on the theory of sexuality. In: Strachey J (ed). *The Standard Edition of the Complete Psychological Works of Sigmund Freud*, volume 7. pp. 123–231. Hogarth Press and the Institute of Psychoanalysis: London.

Klein M (1998). *Love, Guilt and Reparation and Other Works 1921–1945*. Vintage: London.

Lemma A and Lynch P (eds) (2015). *Sexualities: Contemporary Psychoanalytic Perspectives*. Routledge: London.

Pines D (1993). *A Woman's Unconscious Use of Her Body*. Virago: London (reprinted Routledge: London, 2010).

Welldon E (1988). *Mother, Madonna, Whore: The Idealization and Denigration of Motherhood*. Other Press: New York.

Ethnicity and culture

Culture can be defined as learnt thoughts, attitudes, and customs shared by a particular group of people, which are generally passed on from generation to generation. Culture may or may not include different ethnic groups. In order to establish a rapport with members of different ethnic groups, appropriate understanding of verbal and non-verbal communication is paramount. This is even more so within the realm of mental health issues. Certain traditional cultures with strong family and community values may have a better impact on mental health than more modern cultures defined by anomie. However, mental health stigma still remains a problem both for traditional and modern cultures.

Whilst there may be a host of overt and subtle differences amongst western and non-western cultures in the way they deal with mental health and mental distress, the relatively easy mobility of racially diverse groups migrating from their country of origin to another country means an ever increasing population of new settlers with various degrees of adaptation and integration into the accepting society. Generational differences may occur, according to the different degrees of tension between adaptation and integration of different ethnic communities who may be struggling to preserve their sense of identity. However, some ethnic communities with a strong sense of identity, such as the Chinese community, tend to deal with mental health issues within their own group and resort to their own traditional methods and helping agencies in aid of their own mentally ill members.

Sudden and traumatic displacements and immigration of various ethnic communities, along with language barriers, may cause mental health and social suffering related to the loss of community, family members, and language. During this process, cultural beliefs and values may become lost, altered, or even distorted. Hence, there is a need for understanding and being open-minded in learning about experiences of immigration.

It is clear that diverse ethnic groups are now part and parcel of any modern society, and therefore cultural factors have to be taken into account in any form of psychotherapeutic intervention. In the last decade, the introduction of IAPT in the UK has gone a long way in meeting the needs of the local population, including ethnic minority groups, in improving access to psychological therapies and psycho-education and in reducing stigma. The employment of interpreters and mental health workers with knowledge of a particular culture has facilitated this process. However, despite better language and ethnic matching, miscommunications can still be a source of misunderstanding. This is particularly so in those patients (or therapists) who have rejected or developed a highly ambivalent relationship with their culture or country of origin. Nowadays, it is vital for any therapist to be fully aware of the implication of working with ethnically diverse patients. Akhtar, for example, gives an interesting illustration of the tasks facing the immigrant analyst, whilst Bhui and Morgan address the importance of cultural and racial awareness in practising psychotherapists (see ➲ Improving Access to Psychological Therapies services in Chapter 10, pp. 463–4).

In summary, the role of culture and ethnicity needs to remain in the forefront of any psychotherapeutic relationship, and its absence will inevitably affect communication and therapeutic engagement.

Recommended reading

Akhtar S (2006). Technical challenges faced by the immigrant analyst. *Psychoanalytic Quarterly*, **75**, 21–43.

Bhui K and Morgan N (2007). Effective psychotherapy in a racially and culturally diverse society. *Advances in Psychiatric Treatment*, **13**,187–93.

Department of Health (2009). *IAPT Black and Minority Ethnic (BME) Positive Practice Guide. January 2009*. Available at: ℛ http://www.iapt.nhs.uk/silo/files/black-and-minority-ethnic-bme-positive-practice-guide.pdf.

Hayward P and Bright J (1997). Stigma and mental illness: a review and critique. *Journal of Mental Health*, **6**, 345–54.

Transitions and disruptions

Loss

Loss is encountered from the beginning of life until the end of life, i.e. from the cradle to the grave. Loss is not only a normal part of life—it is fundamental to emotional development. Losing that which holds us, the womb, the breast, the mother's arms, home, youth, health, and life itself in death are the very essence of what it is to be human.

Loss is a central theme in the psychotherapies, which can be seen as relational methods to help people to face and bear the losses in their lives, and to process them in a way which can help development in terms of personal growth and understanding.

Loss through absence

From a psychoanalytic perspective, the absence of care or the experience of failing care is a leitmotif which invokes the experience of mental pain. One aspect of the pain of being let down is to feel aggrieved, to replace grieving with grievance. This implies an inability to mourn that which was lost. Loss experienced as absence of love and care in childhood, whatever its cause, is at the heart of significant emotional distress and disorder or impoverishment later on in, or throughout, life. The absence of that love and care is experienced as a presence, as a tormenting experience, a trauma in the sense of an assault on the mind by a persecuting experience of suffering and pain. The psychoanalyst and paediatrician Donald Winnicott, in his work with delinquent youths, distinguished between experiences of 'privation' and 'deprivation'. In the former, there have never been any good objects or experience, which can only lead to hopelessness and psychic death, whereas, in the latter, there have been some early good experiences, but these have been subsequently lost to give rise to 'antisocial tendencies' of anger, resentment, and violence, which are a more hopeful attempt to regain the lost object (see ➔ Donald Winnicott in Key Contributors in Chapter 2, pp. 25–8).

Losses can therefore be thought of as traumas, but hopefully traumas that can be worked through as long as they are not overwhelming (see ➔ Adults in Chapter 6, pp. 289–90; Midlife in Chapter 6, pp. 290–1;

Later life in Chapter 6, pp. 291–3). One of the factors which contributes to an ability, or inability, to mourn a loss is the help and understanding available, both internal and external, to the person suffering from the loss, at the time of the loss and at times of previous loss.

Loss through death

The loss of a loved one through death can be complicated by feelings associated with the hidden resentments and hostility that are not acceptable, unconscious grievances which block the path to grieving.

The experience of the actual death of a person towards whom one feels both love and hatred may be an echo of the experience of losing someone through the end of a relationship or being let down in a relationship. The experience of hatred might be felt as endangering the love for the person who has disappointed us or has let us down, including by dying. The hateful feeling in this ambivalence towards the person who has gone (by disappearing from our lives, or by disappointing us in not being the person we thought they were or by dying) is then turned inwards, against the self, in the way that Freud described as 'the shadow of the object falls on the ego.' Freud used this poetic phrase in his seminal paper *Mourning and Melancholia*, describing how the two processes of grieving and depression can appear to be similar, but how, in melancholia (or what we might call clinical depression), the 'object' which is mourned is confused at an unconscious level with the drive towards life of the subject themselves, as if pulled into the deadened place with the dead object. Instead of feeling anger towards the lost 'object', as would be a normal aspect of mourning, the anger is felt to be towards the self—hence, the often referenced self-deprecation of the clinical state of depression, in which the reproach towards the self is unconsciously a reproach towards the internalized other. This is in contrast to mourning whereby the object becomes separate from the subject in the unconscious mind and is gradually separated further with the work of mourning, without depleting the subject, and, in fact, enriching the subject through the resolution of the process (see ➜ Defence mechanisms in Chapter 2, pp. 22–4; Affective disorders in Chapter 7, pp. 326–31).

Some of Melanie Klein's writings describe and discuss the repeated loss of the good object and the reinstatement of that object (the prototype being the breast in the infant's early feeding relationship) as central to the development of an ability to process losses later on in life. A concept which was developed by Klein in relation to the ability to process loss is the oscillation between the so-called 'paranoid–schizoid' and 'depressive positions.' In the first instance, the infant human being is said to be in the 'paranoid–schizoid' position whereby he or she feels persecuted by his or her emotional state, and by the external world. A huge amount of emotional support is required at this stage, but the course of development also depends on the emotional make-up of the individual tiny human being. In normal or good enough circumstances, the infant gradually develops a capacity to withstand losses such as a loss in the absence of the 'good breast' if food does not arrive quite quickly enough. Klein proposed that the frustration of the experience of absence evokes paranoid or persecutory anxieties of annihilation. The experience of being overwhelmed by feelings of persecutory anxiety is mitigated by a relationship in which such primitive fears can be received and contained. If the baby receives enough maternal containment of their anxieties, he or she will recognize that the hated absent object which deprives is the same as the loved present object which feeds, and may then integrate their loving and hating feelings and move into the 'depressive' position. This integration of loving and hating impulses in the depressive position can be described as a transient state of mind, at least at first, whereby the infant can bear to feel guilt for feeling destructive anger at the object which was not there and did not satisfy their needs straight away, and wishes to make amends and to make reparation. As experiences of deprivation and loss are intrinsic to life and facing reality, there is an oscillation between the paranoid–schizoid and depressive positions throughout life, but the prototype for this oscillation moment by moment is formed in early life (see ➔ Melanie Klein in Key Contributors in Chapter 2, p. 26; Love in Chapter 6, pp. 293–4; Hatred in Chapter 6, pp. 294–5).

The ways in which loss can be experienced in psychotherapy are in the moment-by-moment interaction of being understood or not being understood, of feeling held or of feeling dropped, of being offered help in a series of appointments, or of being hindered in being offered only a series of disappointments. The capacity to face loss includes what Winnicott described as the process of disillusionment in psychotherapy—he once said 'we have to learn to be able to fail in the patient's way.'

The very human need to take flight in manic defences from what is painful in facing a fight with damaged or lost objects and in facing the reality of our limits, of limitations, and loss becomes an experience in which both the therapist and patient turn not to finding a solution, but to seeing the problem for what it is. It is in this experience of trying to face reality that loss is given a human face, in which development involves acceptance of what is, rather than what is wished for.

Recommended reading

Brenman E (2006). *Separation: A Clinical Problem in Recovery of the Lost Good Object*. Routledge: London.

Freud S (1917). Mourning and melancholia. In: Strachey J (ed). *The Standard Edition of the Complete Psychological Works of Sigmund Freud*, volume 14 (1914–1916). pp. 237–58. Hogarth Press and the Institute of Psychoanalysis: London.

Klein M (1940). Mourning and its relation to manic-depressive states. In: *Love, Guilt and Reparation and other works 1921–1945*. pp. 344–69. Vintage: London.

Winnicott DW (1951). Transitional objects and transitional phenomena. In: *Through Paediatrics to Psychoanalysis*. pp. 229–42. Karnac Books and the Institute of Psychoanalysis: London.

Winnicott DW (1956). The antisocial tendency. In: *Through Paediatrics to Psychoanalysis*. pp. 306–15. Karnac Books and the Institute of Psychoanalysis: London.

Trauma—acute and cumulative

(See ➔ Trauma-related conditions in Chapter 7, pp. 355–9.)

Traumas can be viewed as those which are a part of normal development and lead to growth, and those for which the impact is so profound as to change the stable adult personality.

Freud described some individuals with neurotic disorders as being 'fixated' to past traumas, which reside in the unconscious, but the influence of which is so powerful as to produce physical or psychological symptoms in that person. He was referring to traumas of childhood but struggled with his own view on whether neuroses were caused, in the main, by actual trauma or imagined trauma. However, one of the ways in which this was, in part, understood was that the power of the child to imagine frightening scenarios could have a profound bearing on later psychological health or illness if the fantasized nature of the imaginings could not be separated from reality. Hence, in effect, what is real and what is imagined cannot be separated so neatly. This is one of the complex ways in which the internal and external worlds of the developing human being become entangled (see ➔ Sexual abuse in Chapter 6, pp. 303–4).

In relation to individual traumatic events in a person's life, Freud described trauma as an economic process in which a large portion of the energy of the mind is taken in by the traumatic experience; hence, the experience is repeated over and over in dreams and in what we might now call 'flashbacks'. He thought that the overwhelming stimulus of the trauma caused a disturbance in the way in which psychic energies were normally processed, and that the return to the traumatic event would suggest that working through was being curtailed. Moreover, the traumatic effects of events in early childhood may not emerge until later, in adolescence or adulthood. This is Freud's concept of 'après coup' or 'afterwardness' (from the German word 'nachtraglichkeit') in which there is a belated understanding of the meaning (retroactive attribution) giving rise to a deferred action of sexual or traumatic events that occurred earlier in the person's life.

Klein talked about what she conceptualized as necessary developmental traumas, e.g. the frustration of bodily impulses such as those which occur during weaning or toilet training (see ➔ Melanie Klein in Key Contributors in Chapter 2, pp. 25–8).

Winnicott described what he thought of as the amplifying effect of an occurrence in external reality to a circumstance which had already been imagined in the child's mind. A remark which may otherwise go unnoticed may cause the child great distress, if it is seen to act as confirmation of a dreaded occurrence the child had already thought of (see ➔ Donald Winnicott in Key Contributors in Chapter 2, pp. 25–8).

Contemporary psychoanalysts have talked about 'encapsulation' as a concept which helps to explain and think about how the mind of a traumatized individual might attempt to wall off and encapsulate the trauma, but, in doing so, it makes the processing of the traumatic event almost impossible, if not intervened upon.

A series of traumas that, on their own, may not be sufficient to cause a breakdown in the individual's psychological functioning can accumulate if, for example, they occur at the same time or act in quick succession. In effect, a series of relatively minor traumas can have a similar effect as a single, major trauma.

An individual's ego can only process so much psychological distress at once, so there is always a theoretical line which can be crossed in terms of a sheer quantity of trauma that needs to be processed at any given time. In a usually psychologically healthy individual, it is at the times when this line is crossed that more mature ego defence mechanisms, such as sublimation, give way, and more primitive defence mechanisms (such as splitting) are employed to try to mitigate against the ego being over-whelmed. Masud Khan, a controversial figure in psychoanalysis, used the term 'cumulative trauma' to describe a process whereby the maternal shield which usually protects the infant, or infantile part of the self, is broken by the sheer weight of traumatic experience. He postulated that this occurred due to multiple, perhaps imperceptible, failures on the part of the mother (or other substitute) to process traumas for the child. Subsequently, under pressure from acute trauma, the internalized shield can break down in adulthood.

Recommended reading

Earl Hopper E (1991). Encapsulation as a defence against the fear of annihilation. *The International Journal of Psychoanalysis*, **72**, 607–24.

Rayner E (1991). *The Independent Mind in Psychoanalysis*. Free Association Books: London.

Emotional abuse

Emotional abuse of a child during development can come in different forms and may be actively committed or passive, but, in either case, it implies that there is a developmentally corrosive process occurring. In order to develop into psychologically healthy adults, children require psychological understanding and support which meets them at their developmental level and encourages their innate strengths, whilst mini-mizing the negative effects of their innate weaknesses as individuals. Everybody is born with a genetic predisposition in terms of charac-ter, e.g. how aggressive or not an individual is innately, but the exter-nal environment's ability to support the development of a particular child is going to have a large bearing on their personality within certain bounds.

Passive emotional abuse can occur if a primary caregiver is not, for whatever reason, emotionally responsive to the infant or developing child. There are many reasons why this may be, e.g. parental mental ill-ness and/or lack of social support, but, for the infant, the experience of being taken in and understood psychologically is of fundamental importance.

A child may be treated as too old or too young for their actual or developmental age, and this can be a form of abuse in itself. Both extremes would have the effect of curtailing development, e.g. by encouraging unhelpful overdependence at an age when the child should be supported in having more independence in some spheres of their life, or by expecting the child to understand adult issues before they are emotionally ready.

Emotional abuse may be overtly active, in the form of deliberate and cruel neglect of the child when they are needy or in the form of bullying and undermining. The child may be confused if their primary caregiver is also their abuser, as they may have a parent to whom they cannot expect to be able to turn to in times of need, and yet they do have needs; this could have a lasting effect on the individual's ability to form trusting rela-tionships with others, as well as their ability to recognize their own needs and find appropriate ways of getting these met.

Sexual abuse

Freud, through his analysis of adult patients, as well as some children, came up with the theory that neurosis is caused by childhood sexual trauma. He later revised his theory to neurosis being caused by the repression of unacceptable sexual wishes from childhood. This remains controversial, because of the issue of what was being attributed to child-hood fantasy and what was being attributed to childhood sexual abuse. Freud's change of mind over his theories has been explored in contem-porary culture in the play *Hysteria* by Terry Johnson, for example (see ➋ Developmental approach in Chapter 2, p. 22).

Towards the end of Freud's life, his contemporary Sandor Ferenczi revised his own views on the relative importance of fantasy and real-ity when working with traumatized people. Having previously been of the opinion that fantasies were likely to be causal in a majority of cases (including those in which the person had talked about having been sex-ually abused), he decided that this view, in itself, may be contributing further to the trauma of individuals who had, in fact, experienced real sexual abuse.

One of the reasons why childhood sexual abuse has such profound consequences is because of the way it forces the developing mind to deal with adult sexuality a long time before it is ready. This is notwith-standing the fact that children do not possess the necessary psychologi-cal maturity or independence from trusted adult figures to be able to make informed judgements; this is reflected in the law in general in that children do not have 'capacity'.

The individual who has suffered sexual abuse may, for the sake of psychological survival, deny the occurrence to themselves or justify the abuse in some way, until such time as they are in an environment which is sufficiently understanding for them to be able to start to process the psy-chological consequences of the abuse. However, for some people, this environment never materializes, perhaps because they had experienced a generally negating environment, and they may continue, unconsciously, to seek this kind of negation. Unconsciously driven, the recurring seeking of this nature can be viewed as an expression of the repetition compul-sion. That is, human beings will tend to seek out similar circumstances, particularly traumatic ones, which they have not been able to process during development; perhaps with the (unconscious) aim of being able to master the situation. However, this can lead to an unhelpful repetition of traumatic relationships which the individual can feel doomed to continue (see ➋ Repetition compulsion in Chapter 2, pp. 24–5).

Another way of managing the trauma of sexual abuse may be for individuals to dissociate, i.e. to appear and to feel cut-off from external reality. In this way, overwhelming feelings associated with the abuse are anaesthetized, but, along with this, the person's connection to reality in general may be greatly impoverished in the longer term as well as in the short term. Therapy aims to gradually reconnect the person with their feelings and with their reality in a piecemeal way that gives them the best possible chance of being able to process the intense and terrifying emo-tions associated with the abuse.

Recommended reading

Ferenczi S (1994). Confusion of tongues between adults and the child (1933). In: Ferenczi S. *Final Contributions to the Problems and Methods of Psycho-Analysis*. pp. 157–67. Karnac Books: London (reprinted in *International Journal of Psychoanalysis*, 1949, **30**, 225–30).

Violence and aggression

Definitions and epidemiology

Violence has been recognized by the World Health Organization as a major public health priority, and the UK's Department of Health has endorsed a public health approach to violence prevention. Violent crime is associated with a range of negative and costly impacts on health and the wider society, including emotional and physical damage to victims, damage to property, greater police time, involvement with the criminal justice system, and increased use of health-care facilities. Physically abused children are at higher risk of developing aggressive behaviour, as well as depression, suicidal behaviour, substance misuse, and other emotional and interpersonal difficulties, in adolescence and adulthood.

Violence is usually defined as 'the deliberate infliction of physical harm with intent to cause fear, injury, and distress'. Violence needs to be distinguished from aggression, which is found in all mammals and usually linked to anger, competition, or defence against perceived threat. All humans have aggressive impulses, but very few of us will ever be criminally violent. Aggressive behaviour amongst adults is sanctioned in certain social situations such as contact sports, and personal violence is usually distinguished from state-sponsored violence in war. Even in war time, some acts of violence are recognized as falling outside what is legally sanctioned; such acts are deemed to be military atrocities or war crimes.

Mildly aggressive behaviour is not unusual in children under 5 years, but, by school age, most children have learnt to sublimate and control aggression. Persistently violent behaviour in children between the ages of 5 and 10 is unusual and associated with significant psychosocial disturbance. Young people (15–21) are most at risk of being both victims and perpetrators of violence.

Violence is an unusual form of criminal behaviour in adults, especially in women and older people, accounting for only 20% of recorded crime, and there is evidence that, in most democratic societies, levels of violence are falling. It is a behaviour most commonly perpetrated by young men who are socially isolated and antisocial, and who abuse substances. Family violence is the second commonest form of violence, including both intimate partner violence and violence to children. Sexual assaults on adults by other adults are comparatively rare (see ➔ Antisocial personality disorder in Chapter 8, pp. 396–401).

The United Nations divides homicidal violence into three groups: violence associated with crime and masculine dominance rivalries, violence associated with close relationships and attachments, and terrorist violence. In most countries, homicide remains the rarest form of violence, but the overall homicide rate varies from country to country and is influenced by political and social structures. In all societies and cultures, men account for the majority of violence perpetrators.

Psychoanalytic accounts of aggression

Human aggression and violence are vast and complex topics. Investigation of their aetiology, development, prevention, and management has gained the interest of many disciplines, including criminology, sociology, ethology, psychiatry and psychology, political science, and gender studies. Psychoanalytic and psychodynamic theories of violence and aggression aim to enhance, rather than replace, the contributions from these other fields of research.

Freud's views on aggression were complex, and his views changed over time. He initially saw aggression as being a component of the sexual instinct used in the service of mastery but later saw aggression as a response to both internal and external threats, such as loss, and used in the service of self-preservation. In 1920, he suggested that aggression was an instinct in its own right that he called 'the death instinct'— an insidious destructive force that operates in opposition to the life instinct (see ➔ Models of the mind in Chapter 2, p. 21).

Klein developed Freud's notion of the death instinct by suggesting that it was manifested by innate envy and destructiveness which she proposed predominated in early life. Klein hypothesized that unconscious infantile envy gave rise to persecutory anxieties of annihilation and primitive defences, unconscious phantasies, and an archaic harsh superego (see ➔ Melanie Klein in Key Contributors in Chapter 2, pp. 25–8).

In contrast, Winnicott saw aggression as a creative force necessary for healthy development (which included a central role for the mother) in his concepts of the 'facilitating maternal environment' and the maternal 'holding' functions. Winnicott in particular argued that hatred was a normal part of a caring relationship, and that tolerating hatred made close bonds possible, especially between the mother and child. Based on his work with children in care during the war, Winnicott believed that pathological aggression and antisocial behaviour arose as a reaction to early deprivation and trauma (see ➔ Donald Winnicott in Key Contributors in Chapter 2, pp. 25–8).

More recent psychoanalytic writers have emphasized the role of the maternal object and object relations in the genesis of aggression, but also accept that aggression may have an instinctual component. This can be seen as a move away from an unhelpful polarization towards a more coherent and flexible theoretical approach that embraces both biology and psychology. The research on attachment by Bowlby and his followers has increasingly influenced thinking on the aetiology of aggressive behaviour, leading many to conclude that the capacity for aggression is innate, but that aggressive behaviour or violence occurs in response to threats that the self perceives in relation to internal or external objects (see ➔ John Bowlby in Key Contributors in Chapter 2, pp. 25–8).

Different types of violence

(See ➔ Relationship between mental disorders and violence in Chapter 8, p. 428.)

It is also now recognized that there are different types of violence, based on different underlying types of aggression and mediated by different intrapsychic factors. Glasser proposed a useful distinction between what he called 'self-preservative violence' (sometimes called affective or reactive violence) where the person acts in self-defence in response to a perceived threat, and which is often triggered by powerful negative affects, such as anxiety, shame, and humiliation; and 'sado-masochistic violence' (sometimes called proactive, psychopathic, or instrumental violence), which is used to achieve violent purposes, including to torture and control victims, but ultimately preserve the object of the violence. Sado-masochistic violence is commoner in so-called psychopathic individuals who describe a lack of experienced anxiety, and show deficits in empathy and tend to deny the need for emotional attachments to others.

However, although most violence perpetrators are assumed to be lacking in empathy or concern for others, the evidence suggests that they are not a homogenous group in these terms. Not all violence perpetrators are psychopaths, and not all violence perpetrators are antisocial (e.g. some domestic homicide perpetrators). A group of violence perpetrators may be understood as having perverse states of mind which are encapsulated from general social functioning (see ➲ Antisocial personality disorder in Chapter 8, pp. 396–401).

Pathways from aggression to violence

The pathways that lead from aggression to violence are not linear but are dependent on several factors. Violence involves multiple dimensions and is mediated by a number of different intrapsychic risk factors which interact with specific external and situational factors to cause different types of violence. These factors include:

- The internal object world and the importance of the maternal object
- The role of the father and the development of superego
- Attachment, trauma, and loss
- Representation and mentalization of negative affects
- Primitive defence mechanisms
- The role of unconscious fantasy
- The external world and situational factors
- Gender role demands
- Sexuality.

Many psychoanalysts have located the origins of some types of violence in a pathological early relationship between the mother and infant, which prevents the child from developing a sense of separate identity. In these cases, violence can be seen as a desperate measure to create space between self and other. In some violent individuals, there may be core unconscious fantasies of the primal scene and an experience of a maternal object as overwhelming and intrusive, so that the violent act can be seen as an unconsciously motivated fantasized attack on the mother's body.

The role of the father in separating the child from the dyadic relationship with the mother is also important in the normal development of aggression and superego functioning, deficits in which can predispose to violent behaviour. Most violence perpetrators are males who have childhood experiences of absent, emotionally unavailable, or violently abusive fathers, which impedes this fundamental process of triangulation. They may also have grown up witnessing severe violence perpetrated on a helpless mother who could not protect herself or her children.

Such early exposure to violence is an example of the type of childhood abuse, trauma, and loss that can cause pathological attachment relationships in the infant, which, in turn, lead to difficulties in affect regulation and a deficient capacity for representation and mentalization. This lack of mentalization makes it difficult for the child to modulate feelings of fear and hostility, especially in response to malevolence and threat from a caregiver or attachment figure which jeopardizes the child's developing reflective process. Reactive hostility and aggression towards others help the child to defend their fragile psychological self from the assumed hostility of the other. Aggression and self-expression may become associated so regularly in the mind that there is a pathological fusion between the two, especially at a time of dependency and need.

Gilligan proposes that violence is commonly precipitated by feelings of shame and humiliation, which trigger previous childhood traumatic memories of being rejected, abused, or made to feel as if they did not exist. Fonagy and Bateman propose that the capacity to mentalize protects against violence, but that a loss of mentalization capacity increases the risk. They suggest that violence perpetrators have a fragile sense of self, which is easily destabilized by perceived 'threats'. When such individuals feel threatened, mentalization collapses, and feelings of vulnerability, weakness, humiliation, and shame must be defended against at all cost. Such unbearable feelings cannot be dealt with by representational and emotional processing in the mind but have to be projected by controlling the physical environment, including physical action to repel threat, and displacing the vulnerability and weakness into another person's body (see ➲ Mentalization-based treatment in Chapter 2, pp. 66–70).

Violence is also more likely to occur as the result of a failure in the normal defensive mechanisms against aggression. Violent individuals tend to use primitive defence mechanisms such as projection, splitting, and projective identification. These primitive defences may lead to the formation of defensive pathological organizations in the mind, which increase the internal sense of distress and threat, thus increasing the risk of violent enactment (see ➲ Defence mechanisms in Chapter 2, pp. 22–4 and Table 2.1, p. 23).

Sex differences

There are marked sex differences in violent behaviour, with the majority of violence committed by men. The ratio of male to female violent incidents is 4:1, and the ratio of male to female homicide is 10:1. However, the proportion of recorded domestic violence incidents in which the offender is female is increasing, and membership of all female gangs is on the rise. There are also differences in the targets of male and female violent behaviour. Most victims of male violent perpetrators are not known to the offender, whereas the victims of violent women are most often close family members—their partners or children. Rates of self-harm, i.e. violence directed against the self, are also much higher in females than males.

The reasons for these sex differences are not clear. Most sociologists have argued that masculine and feminine gender role expectations and stereotypes have significant influence on violence perpetration. It has been argued that women's potential for violence is the same as men's, but that women require more risk factors to be in place for violence to be enacted, because of social sanctions on female hostility. In anthropological terms, humans with a Y chromosome may be particularly vulnerable to stressors that make violence more likely such as dominance competitions and child maltreatment.

Psychoanalysts have suggested that some women tend to direct their aggression towards their own bodies, including their reproductive systems, to be used as vehicles for the expression of unconscious conflicts, often stemming from a neglectful or abusive relationship with their mothers and leading to transgenerational patterns of abuse. Some cases of infanticide and maternal child abuse may occur when the mother views their baby or child as a narcissistic extension of themselves and uses them for the expression of their own unconscious needs and unresolved conflicts. In some situations of domestic abuse where the man is the identified 'perpetrator', the woman may be unconsciously enacting underlying dynamics in the couple that contain dependent, aggressive, and sadomasochistic elements in both partners. Casting the woman solely as the 'victim', rather than acknowledging her own, albeit unconscious, aggressive participation in such relationships, denies women a sense of agency for their actions.

Aggression also plays an integral part in all sexual activity. Although one might think of sexual intimacy as being the expression of loving feelings and the wish to be truly close to the other, aggressive impulses are necessarily involved to facilitate separation and to manage anxieties about being both overwhelmed by, and losing, the other person. However, when aggressive impulses become prominent in sexual relations, with conscious or unconscious wishes to hurt, control, or dominate the other person, sexual perversions may develop. Here, activities that appear to be predominantly sexual in nature may conceal underlying hostility and fears of intimacy, and function as a defence against aggression and unbearable anxiety.

Recommended reading

Cartwright D (2002). *Psychoanalysis, Violence and Rage-Type Murder*. Brunner-Routledge: Hove and New York.

Gilligan J (1996). *Violence: Our Deadliest Epidemic and its Causes*. Grosset/Putnam: New York.

Glasser M (1998). On violence: a preliminary communication. *International Journal of Psychoanalysis*, **79**, 887–902.

Perelberg R (ed) (1999). *Psychoanalytic Understanding of Violence and Suicide*. Routledge: London.

Yakeley J (2010). *Working with Violence: A Contemporary Psychoanalytic Approach*. Palgrave Macmillan: London.

Suicide and self-harm

(See ➜ Affective disorders in Chapter 7, pp. 326–31; Borderline personality disorder in Chapter 8, pp. 390–6.)

Suicide prevention has become a national priority for all health and social services; although suicide rates have fallen since 2000, suicide remains one of the leading causes of premature death. Self-mutilation is also common, especially among younger people. For the majority of people who self-injure, their actions are an attempt to cope with the stress and difficulties they face; their purpose is not killing, but torturing the body. However, some people who self-harm may commit suicide, either deliberately or accidentally as the result of their actions.

People will self-mutilate or become suicidal for many different reasons, encompassing a range of social, psychological, and biological factors. A psychoanalytic understanding of suicide and self-mutilation aims to explore the meaning for the individual of these self-destructive acts, specifically focusing on unconscious meanings. As with any form of acting out, self-mutilation and suicide are driven by multiple unconscious purposes, some of them mutually contradictory—the wish to die or the wish to survive or be rescued, the wish to relieve others of the burden they are imposing, or the wish to inflict pain and guilt in others.

The foundations of the psychoanalytic understanding of suicidal acts was laid down in Stekel's 1910 paper:

'No one kills himself who has never wanted to kill another, or at least wished the death of another. The child now wants to rob his parents of their greatest, most precious possession: his own life. The child knows they thereby inflict the greatest pain. Thus the punishment the child imposes on himself is simultaneously the punishment he imposes on the instigators of his sufferings' (p. 87 and p. 89).

Suicide is a form of acting out. Freud originally used the term as a clinical concept related specifically to psychoanalytic treatment, to describe how patients carry out an action that, in symbolic form, represents an unconscious wish or fantasy but cannot be expressed by the patient in conscious memory or words. Since then, the concept has been widened to describe a general character trait in which a person tends to relieve intrapsychic tension by physical action.

Acting out is the substitute for remembering a traumatic childhood experience, creating an internal drama which unconsciously aims to reverse that early trauma. However, this drama passes directly from an unconscious impulse to action, bypassing conscious thought and feeling, so that the conflict is resolved, albeit temporarily, via the use of the person's body, often in a destructive or erotized way. Others in the person's current life will inevitably be involved in the person's enactment, who unconsciously represent significant figures from the person's past implicated in the original trauma. This is a manifestation of Freud's repetition compulsion which is the person's unconscious tendency to repeat past traumatic behaviour by creating the same scenario in different settings and relationships (see ➋ Repetition compulsion in Chapter 2, pp. 24–5).

As for all acting out, suicide and self-mutilation may be viewed as equivalent to symptoms in which the action is the symbol of unconscious conflict. A close examination of the external facts of a suicidal act and analysis of their symbolic meaning are the clearest pathways to the fantasies that motivate it. Five main fantasies may be identified which drive suicide and which will be largely unconscious but may become manifest in the course of treatment:

- The wish to merge with a loving object in oceanic bliss
- Revenge for the trauma of childhood, particularly rejection (so well described by Stekel)

- To kill off a thinking, feeling part of the self
- Dicing with death—leaving one's survival in the hands of fate. No means of killing one's self is infallible
- To assuage one's guilt for sins of commission or omission.

The psychological structure of those who carry out suicidal acts may fall into three groups:
- Those prone to depressive episodes, which may be psychotic
- Those with a borderline personality structure who act out excessively in response to any psychic pain
- Those with a schizoid personality structure in whom the suicidal act often 'comes out of the blue'.

The fundamental problem for the suicidal individual is their inability to trust. It is as though they are saying 'all my life I've been let down because others leave me. I thought I could trust you, but you've done it too'. The longed-for object customarily is a sexual partner, but it may be something less obvious like academic or business success which is longed for and represents being loved.

The descent into suicide when customary defences fail follows an identifiable common pathway. The starting point is that of the 'core complex', as described by Glasser. This is a constellation of interrelated feelings, ideas, and attitudes in which there is a conflict between the longing to merge with the object and a fear that the object will be overwhelming and obliterating. The person oscillates between the desire for contact and union with the object and flight from the object, with concomitant feelings of emotional isolation and abandonment, leading to desire for contact once more. The fear of being overwhelmed by the object and loss of separate existence provokes an aggressive response in the subject towards the object.

In the person who becomes suicidal, the core complex is initially in a state of equilibrium, albeit unstable, in which the individual and their partner are locked in mutual distrust. However, at some point, an event occurs, often a disengagement or a renouncement of affection by a significant other, which is perceived by a suicidal individual as an act of betrayal. The relationship now enters the pre-suicidal state, in which the suicidal person feels themselves to be in a vulnerable state—an accident about to happen. It may last hours or days, and it is in this state that the individual consciously formulates a suicide plan and prepares the means for their own execution. Eventually, they experience the final trigger—the 'coup de grace' (see Fig. 6.1). This propels them into a state of confusion, in which they breach their own 'body barrier', and the suicidal act ensues.

This can be represented diagrammatically, as shown in Fig. 6.1.

Suicide therefore exists in the context of a dyadic relationship, or rather its failure. This highlights the inherent relational component in all acts of suicide and self-harm, in which both may be seen as communications to significant others, historical and current, and in which unconscious wishes, fantasies, and feelings stemming from childhood conflicts are communicated in action, rather than being consciously thought and felt.

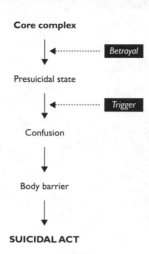

Fig. 6.1 'Coup de grace' culminating in a suicidal act.

Recommended reading

Briggs S, Lemma A, and Crouch W (eds) (2008). *Relating to Self-Harm and Suicide: Psychoanalytic Perspectives on Practice, Theory and Prevention*. Routledge: Hove.

Glasser M (1998). On violence: a preliminary communication. *International Journal of Psychoanalysis*, **79**, 887–902.

Maltsberger JT and Goldblatt MJ (eds) (1996). *Essential Papers on Suicide*. New York University Press: New York.

Stekel W (1910). On suicide. In: Friedman P, ed. *On Suicide*. pp. 33–141. International University Press: New York, 1967.

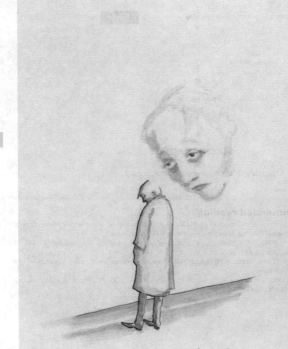

JAMES JOHNSTON 2014

Psychotherapy and psychiatric disorders

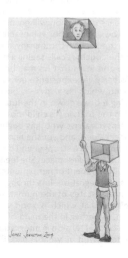

JAMES JOHNSTON 2014

Integrating psychotherapy in psychiatry

(See ➲ Chapter 1, Psychotherapeutic medicine: *thinking cradle to grave*, pp. 8–12; General adult psychiatry: medical psychotherapies, applications, and research in Chapter 12, pp. 544–50.)

Songs of innocence and of experience

Showing the two contrary states of the human soul

So wrote William Blake in the eighteenth century. An artist, poet, and visionary, he considered the contrary aspects of love, life, loss, destructiveness and sorrow to be the quintessence of being human.

What have the songs of innocence and of experience to do with integration?

Imagine a sixth-form student at their interview to get a place at medical school. He feels embarrassed, as he says he wants to be a doctor because he wants to help people. He has in mind people with physical illnesses. He is silent on the matter of his depressed mother but is desperate for her to be well, and feels helpless in the face of her mental pain and shameful about his anger towards her.

Imagine a medical student in a Balint group who, when recounting a recent contact with a patient, bursts into tears, as she realizes she was reminded of the death of her mother.

Imagine a foundation doctor who feels the consultant paediatrician is cold in relating to the death of a child. In his Balint group, he is very critical of the consultant. His own vulnerable feelings about having been admitted to hospital with illness as a boy remain distant for him, as if he cannot remember being ill or the fear he felt on the wards.

Imagine a core trainee in psychiatry, who has felt very disturbed being on call, and a relationship breaking down has led her to seek help in the sick doctor's service, as she feels she cannot cope as a psychiatrist. In facing this loss, she fears depression will envelop her and completely destroy her capacity to be useful to her vulnerable and sick patients.

Imagine an advanced medical psychotherapy dual trainee in personal therapy who, lying on the couch, recalls seeing a psychotic patient in the prison the night before and fears that he may be on the cusp of a psychotic breakdown. His early life experience involved profound deprivation and disturbance with which his analysis is beginning to allow him to be in touch, both fearing a breakdown in the future and realizing that a breakdown happened in the past, in his childhood.

Imagine a consultant psychiatrist who has begun to feel disillusioned with her work and undervalued, and yet she finds her disillusionment in the NHS goes hand in hand with a stronger and deeper relationship with why she became a doctor in the first place. She feels more in contact with the mental pain and disillusionment of her patients.

Imagining is the basis of integration. It is through the work of imagination that the 'two contrary states of the human soul' or mind, of integrating conflicting feelings, that which is good with that which is bad, may or may not happen. Whether in the mind of the individual or in the minds of a profession, a central tension in integration is that the good will be undermined, even destroyed by what is bad. Blake's *innocence* lay in celebrating being human; his disillusioned *experience* lay in an ironic pain-ful recognition of social injustice and neglect. He introduced the grave problems of poverty and maltreatment to idealized notions of the cradle of infancy and childhood (see ➲ Chapter 1, Psychotherapeutic medicine: thinking cradle to grave, pp. 8–12). Integration involves working through disillusionment in fantasy, i.e. facing psychic reality before external reality can be recognized for what it is.

Integration of psychotherapy in psychiatry

In each example of the development of a doctor from cradle to grave, they faced an emotional struggle, a process of coming to terms with some aspect of their experience they do not want to integrate because it is painful. This is the problem of integration for the individual mind; disintegration, in matters of degree from psychosis to disavowal, allows reality not to be faced. This is because reality is painful.

What is painful about reality?

Reality confronts us with limitations. When we face reality, we face our personal limits, of who we are, what we can have, where we are allowed, and when. There are boundaries and separateness and loss to be borne in reality. This is harder than imagining we can be who we want to be, believing we can have what we wish and go where we wish at any time of our choosing. Psychoanalysis calls this state of mind omnipotence. Psychiatry calls it psychosis. They have different languages for similar phenomena. The different languages that psychotherapy and psychiatry speak are important, as recognizing and tolerating difference is at the heart of facing reality and accepting not only our limits, but also tolerating others without wanting them to be more like us.

Hell is other people

Human beings cannot be conceived in isolation; the human mind devel-ops in relation to the other. The problem about the other is that they are not us. The existentialist philosopher Jean-Paul Sartre said 'Hell is other people.' Freud said, in terms of the development of love and hate, that hate is older than love. We suspect the other first and have to learn to love. So when we come across the alien, we tend to feel threatened, and this is the basis of xenophobia, the fear and hate of strangers and aliens. If you are not for me, you must be against me.

Psychiatrists used to be called *alienists*—the alienists were those who specialized in treating those deemed alien in society, those people who were alienated and excluded.

Psychotherapy and psychiatry

To learn the language and ways of a different culture, you have to visit and spend time and effort learning to listen and see how far you can assimilate this alien way of speaking and being. Unlike in the USA where psycho-analysis and psychiatry were, for many years, married and went through a divorce, in the UK, psychoanalysis and psychiatry have not been very close, barely on speaking terms for long periods. However, this more distant British relationship with emotions, the stiff upper lip of 'we don't really do all that soft squidgy feeling stuff', has allowed distinct identities for psychoanalytic psychotherapy and psychiatry to develop, without too much cross-fertilization. British psychiatry remains predominantly biological, but also distinctively social and ambivalent about medication, with a touch of the RD Laing style anti-psychiatry cropping up in some places over the years. So psychotherapy of the psychoanalytic variety has remained a somewhat alien and eccentric activity—in psychological terms, *ego dystonic* for many psychiatrists.

Other models of psychotherapy, without notions of an unconscious or a tendency to think about destructiveness and resistance and how these are manifest in the patient and professional relationship, are more palatable. Therefore, a more positivistic mental health zeitgeist has found a more accommodating *ego syntonic* relationship between psychiatrists and CBT and systemic family therapy, for example. However, where psychoanalysis runs into problems of integration because it is too different, a bit too odd, and alien, when therapies are familiar and safe and feel the same as us, they can run into a different set of problems in terms of integration.

The three 'mother models' of medical psychotherapy training in the UK are psychoanalysis, CBT, and systemic therapy. What are the different challenges of integration in psychiatry for each? Some reflections on the different challenges of integrating psychotherapy in psychiatry through the lenses of these three mother models are laid out below.

Psychoanalysis: couched in ambivalent terms

(See ➲ Psychoanalytic psychotherapy in Chapter 2, pp. 20–30, and in Chapter 5, pp. 163–72.)

Sigmund Freud said that it is not psychiatry, but psychiatrists who are opposed to psychoanalysis; William Blake saw that the human soul required two contrary states, which he described in *Songs of Innocence and of Experience*. These two views reflect a single human idea that opposition is both deeply personal and profoundly necessary for life. Hell is what other people think or believe is wrong, misguided, heresy, or simply not evidence-based, and we need it to be so. But as Blake suggests, contrariness is vital for progress in a discipline as much as in personal development, the quest for unattainable integration creating the vitality of ambiguity in which the conflict between what and who we love and hate brings to being human.

That ambiguity of humanity, that everything has two sides, loving and hating in conflict, of living with, and trying to unravel, ambivalent complexity is reflected in a history of ambivalence between psychiatry and psychoanalysis. This ambivalence dates back to the famous psychiatrist Eugene Bleuler who wrote both critically and in defence of Freudian psychoanalysis (1913) and was attacked by fellow psychiatrists for including psychoanalysis in his book *Schizophrenia* (1914), the term he invented and in which he described the importance of what he called *ambivalence* in the psychotic disturbance of the mind. Freud began to use Bleuler's term ambivalence in his writings in different ways, most often to describe the conflict between love and hate. Freud described Bleuler's ambivalent relationship with psychoanalysis as a psychiatrist in *On the History of the Psychoanalytic Movement* (Freud, 1914) and later wrote that it was not psychiatry which had a problem with psychoanalysis—it was psychiatrists. In his introductory lecture *Psycho-Analysis and Psychiatry* (1917) in which he writes this, Freud describes the relationship between psychiatry and psychoanalysis as analogous to that in medicine between anatomy and histology—the one studies the external forms of organs, the other studies their construction out of tissues and cells. Freud's metaphor of anatomy and histology nearly 100 years ago encapsulates the split between the inner world and outer world today between psychoanalytic thinking and psychiatry—a potentially complementary relationship using the body as a metaphor for the mind which remains split between what goes on invisibly inside (unconscious) and what is more evident and obvious in a concrete sense from the outside (conscious). Such splitting might be conceived as primitive ambivalence as distinct from the mature ambivalence of moving nearer to the painful challenges of integration of the opposing feelings of love and hate and of what is seen and unseen within the same subject.

For some psychiatrists, psychoanalysis has represented a bad object, one that is experienced with intense ambivalence, an alien outsider, a contrary unconscious beast which, if allowed into the tent, would leave psychiatrists feeling a sense of loneliness—an embattled uncertain science set against Freudian mumbo jumbo and witchcraft, or conversely, when the Freudian slipper is on the other foot, an embattled uncertain science set against Bleulerian brain spotters. But intense ambivalence is better than indifference.

Cognitive behavioural therapy: how's the water?

(See ➋ Cognitive behavioural therapy in Chapter 2, pp. 30–4, and in Chapter 5, pp. 172–84.)

In the story of the two young fish swimming along, they encounter an older fish swimming towards them who asks: 'Morning boys: how's the water?' When the two younger fish swim a little further along, one turns to the other and asks, 'What the hell is water?'

A senior psychiatrist said that the problem with CBT is that it is in the water. Psychiatrists, he explained, see so much of it they do not any longer see it as in any way sustaining or special, or even see it at all, as if it is see-through as water.

In terms of the therapeutic cultural zeitgeist, CBT has found ways of colouring the water to ensure it remains visible and attractive to psychiatrists. The language of second and third waves of CBT may be evocative of water, if not tsunamis of therapeutic excitement, as reinvention and recycling meet invention, rapprochement, and collaboration with other models. The use of Buddhism in DBT is an example of such creative intercourse, unions from which paradigm shifts can emerge.

Such unions have fostered ideas in CBT which have surfaced above the waves, not drowning but waving, mindfulness being one. In terms of the ontology of therapeutic modality, many psychiatrists feel comfortable offering CBT as an intervention, rather than a professional identity. In as much as it is associated with any particular professional identity, that profession is clinical psychology. In the world of defending a distinct professional identity, the lack of a clear ontological distinction may be a barrier for medical psychotherapists specializing in CBT, as it lacks a unique selling point (USP) (see ➲ Mindfulness-based interventions and therapies in Chapter 2, pp. 73–5, and in Chapter 5, pp. 239–43).

In relation to the question of defending the professional identity, medical psychotherapy has begun to see its distinct contribution in medicine as being a bridge spanning the professions of psychiatry and psychology.

The use of CBT as an application in psychiatry would therefore require it to become more than an intervention. The distinct ways it might be used in consultation between doctors would act as a Trojan Horse that carries the 'enemy' of medical perspective, experience, and credibility which is not available to clinical psychologists. This is a challenge for revitalizing CBT in psychiatry—devising a CBT application model which is able to address the professional experience in consultation and reflective practice which is not directed towards case management and formulation but engages the emotional struggle of the clinician in a manner analogous to countertransference work.

Systemic therapy: phantom limb pain

(See ➲ Systematic family and couple therapy in Chapter 2, pp. 34–42, and in Chapter 5, pp. 184–8.)

There is a common complaint in the heartland of family therapy, the country of the mind called schizophrenia, which is to ask why is systemic family therapy not given prominence in medical psychotherapy training as a major mother model, alongside psychoanalysis and CBT? It is there, but always as a minor model.

As dual training in child and adolescent psychiatry and medical psychotherapy becomes established, it is hoped that systemic therapy will secure a more prominent place as a major mother model. But father psychiatry still tends to turn a blind eye to family therapy. It is still thought to be there, and people may even cite some evidence they have heard that family therapy is effective in relapse prevention in schizophrenia, but no one ever does it, despite this evidence, they will say. It is a shame, a source of psychiatric pain that this therapy has become like a phantom limb; it is no longer there, but amputated part of us, but its memory still causes us to feel it as if it were still there.

The cutting off from sensibility, an obliviousness which leads to oblivion in organizations, requires a way of recognizing the amputation of parts of the institution to be borne from profound anxieties. The containment of anxiety in institutions is a psychoanalytic theme that systemic organizational perspectives readily integrate with and enrich. The application of a therapeutic principle in non-therapeutic settings is a strength of systemic approaches, which, along with the other models, tends to be overlooked, with an emphasis on direct therapeutic intervention. In thinking of therapy as only being for patients, not for us professionals, we cut ourselves off at the knees. The fragmentation of teams, of services becoming silos, and of managers and clinicians operating in different worlds with different systems of thought are fields ripe for the sowing of systemic seeds.

In terms of training experience, senior systemic colleagues may say that they can easily influence the CBT trainees, but psychoanalytic trainees are too wedded to a world view to be influenced by a systemic perspective. For their part, some psychoanalytic trainees may say they find systemic therapy a little too nice for their taste, and, contrary to this contempt for positivity, perhaps some systemic colleagues might suggest that this is the bad taste that comes from dwelling too long in the infantile world of Klein, suffused as it is in its paranoid–schizoid vision with grotesque phantasy in union with profound despair, reminiscent of Hieronymus Bosch meeting Charles Baudelaire on an off day.

Dual training in medical psychotherapy as a model of integration

(See ➲ General adult psychiatry: medical psychotherapies, applications, and research in Chapter 12, pp. 544–50.)

Dual training in medical psychotherapy represents an attempt at integrating psychotherapy in psychiatry by bringing together two (or three?) contrary states of the human soul, mind, and brain. Dual training offers a dialogue between the psychiatrist, who is in two minds about the inner world of feelings, and the psychotherapist for whom the material world of neuroscience is a 'no brainer'. It offers a biological and psychological interface in which to encounter difference and prejudice, and hopefully to learn another language. In dual training, the ambivalent psychiatrist and psychotherapist is the same person, and the integrative conversation occurs first of all in their own mind, before it can take place meaningfully with their colleagues. This ambivalent conversation begins not interpersonally, but intrapsychically. The engagement with ambivalence about the odd other world is essential, in order to achieve integration. Dual training in medical psychotherapy with other subspecialties of psychiatry (forensic, general adult, and child and adolescent psychiatry) is informed by the evolutionary principle of hybrid vigour; it is in the connection between contrary experiences that evolution occurs in the tension between two paradigms that the trainee, it is hoped, develops. The notion of integrating psychotherapy in psychiatry cannot be achieved by welding them together or blending them like tea or whisky, but by a recognition of their differences with sufficient clarity to draw out the contrary life in their opposition, a profound challenge of integration for the psychiatrist becoming a psychotherapist.

Freud held on to this dualistic way of thinking, manifest eventually in the controversial theory of the dual life instinct in conflict with a death instinct, if this can be concluded on a psychoanalytic note. It is, after all, a psychoanalytic note which acknowledges difference and rivalry amongst psychoanalysts, some of whom cannot accept a death instinct. See ➲ Models of the mind in Chapter 2, p. 21.

The quotidian fantasy that other people are all one, in heaven, agreeing in harmony. The derivation of the word *alone* is from old English, from putting together the two words 'all one' which is probably closer to the truth, that the perception of integration in others, in groups, or individuals is an illusion. The other people (hell) may be feeling more alone than we imagine. As EM Forster recommends, only connect.

Integration and the sense of loneliness

In her last paper, published after her death, *On the sense of loneliness* (1963), Melanie Klein describes the lifelong tension between the urge towards integration and the impossibility of sustaining a state of integration. She writes: 'Integration is difficult to accept. The coming together of destructive and loving impulses, and of the good and bad aspects of the object, arouses the anxiety that destructive feelings may overwhelm the loving feelings and endanger the good object. Thus, there is conflict between seeking integration as a safeguard against destructive impulses and fearing integration lest the destructive impulses endanger the good object and the good parts of the self.' She writes: 'I have heard patients express the painfulness of integration in terms of feeling lonely and deserted, through being completely alone with what to them was a bad part of the self.' She continues: 'And the process becomes all the more painful when a harsh superego has engendered a very strong repression of destructive impulses and tries to maintain it.' This is Klein's key contribution: *paranoid defences are raised against the painful experience of guilt* (see ➲ Melanie Klein in Key contributors in Chapter 2, pp. 25–8).

What does Klein's view of paranoid defences against experiencing guilt, meaning integration is near impossible to hold on to, even if achieved, have to offer the question of the challenge of integration of psychotherapy in psychiatry? Quite a bit, or rather bits.

First of all, integration is sometimes perceived as a *good thing*—as something we should strive to achieve to be better people, and, in this light, it can be heralded as an ideal, the goal of mental health through bringing together different conflicting states of mind—a *nirvana*. But what Klein recognized is that this integrated state of mind is painful, precisely because it entails *not* being able to split off bad parts of one's mind and *not* projecting bad parts of the self into others. Disintegration is appealing, however disturbing or disturbed the individual may be, because they are *not* functioning as an individual. Their divided self allows for a broken connectivity with the world of others, even if it is a paranoid or persecuted state of connectivity.

The problems for integration in the individual mind, of a sense of loneliness if we recover our projections of the bad parts of our minds, apply equally to groups and ideologies, in that they also require other groups or ideologies to whom they can project disowned aspects of their identity. To paraphrase Klein, the individual is not alone in the absence of a good object, as it is felt as a persecuting presence; one is never alone in the company of a bad object. Whilst hell might be other people, as Jean-Paul Sartre suggested, humans try to make a heaven by projecting their personal hell; they are not alone in the universe, as they are stalked by the ever present shadow of their projected hatred. This state of mind in its primitive developmental expression of being haunted and hunted by persecution is known as splitting and, in its extreme forms of fragmentation of self, is manifest in psychosis.

Integration is a painful challenge, as it involves mourning one's enemy in the recovery of hatred and a capacity to be alone with a mind of one's own. This state of mind is, in its mature form, experienced as ambivalence—loving *and* hating, facing separateness, accepting the responsibility for damage done, and bearing the painful limitations of who one is, what one can have, and what one can achieve.

Extinction, evolution, and hybrid vigour

(See ➲ Medical psychotherapy modalities in Chapter 2, pp. 14–20.)

In terms of the three major mother models used by medical psychotherapy in psychiatry, there has been a tradition in which eclecticism rules for some, and clear blue water between islands of therapy for others. Observing psychotherapists arguing over what, to them, are fundamental differences will seem like bickering over how many angels dance on the head of their particular therapeutic pin and might be interpreted as enacting what Freud called 'the narcissism of minor differences'. When neighbouring countries go to war, their projected bad objects are going to seem much bigger to them than to those from another country.

Ideological differences are vital to life, and contrariness is not to be calmed or relinquished with sophistry. The underpinning passions are to do with survival and, at the root, the love of one's good object, a way of thinking about being human which is deeply sustaining and profound.

Extinction anxiety, the loss of a loved object, the castration of an existential pillar of belief, can therefore lead to hatefully embattled positions and silos. These polarized and potentially murderous positions run counter to an integrating principle in evolution which requires intercourse and difference for strength and development. Xenophobia breeds only a kind of Armageddon of the creative life. Engagement in life and living involves meeting with what is contrary and novel, with the inherent risk of facing the unknown and feeling potentially out of control, enraged in the face of impotence—if not out of control, certainly painfully uncertain, the vital basis of achievement.

The relationship between psychiatry and psychotherapy is a competition; two very different ideologies are at variance in various degrees, one more closely aligned with the paternal function and structure of science in medicine, the other more closely aligned with a maternal function of the feminine in creative work.

A psychoanalytic view would consider a triangulation, in which a third position between the science of psychiatry and the art of psychotherapy might be found. This third perspective might be an unknown patient with an unfamiliar problem who confronts each paradigm with a problem of uncertainty.

The rivalry between psychiatry and psychotherapy cannot be helped by pretending it does not exist, to fuse one with the other as if they are the same or to turn a blind eye to the existence of the other paradigms and carry on head down regardless. Obliviousness fuels oblivion.

The only certainty we can have is that, in developing, we will have to compete, and, though integration may not mean psychotherapy and psychiatry becoming all one, it may mean having a capacity to be alone in the presence of other people whose different ways of thinking may sometimes feel like hell, but with whom there might be some dialogue and learning from experience. This connection of the contrary has a well-established evolutionary history, known as hybrid vigour.

Recommended reading

Blake W (1967; 1789–1794). *Songs of Innocence and of Experience: Shewing the Two Contrary States of the Human Soul.* Oxford University Press: Oxford.

Freud S (1914). On the history of the psychoanalytic movement. In: *The Standard Edition of the Complete Psychological Works*, volume 14. pp. 6–66. Hogarth Press: London.

Freud S (1917). Psycho-analysis and psychiatry. In: *The Standard Edition of the Complete Psychological Works of Sigmund Freud. Introductory lectures on psycho-analysis (Part III)*, volume 16. pp. 254. Hogarth Press: London.

Klein M (1963). On the sense of loneliness. In: *Envy and Gratitude and Other Works 1946–1963*. pp. 300–13. Vintage: London, 1997.

Sartre, J-P (1984; 1943). *Being and Nothingness: An Essay on Phenomenological Ontology.* Philosophical Library: New York.

Psychotherapy and medication

The relationship between psychotherapy and medication

The interface between psychotherapy and medication has been a point of contention for a long time. In the past, many psychotherapists and psychoanalysts were resistant to the use of pharmacological agents. Some would feel humiliated at the idea of having to resort to medication, as such action might indicate that the therapeutic process was failing. In addition, it was felt that psychotropic medication would interfere with motivation and transference or block the emergence of meaningful affect in the psychotherapeutic process, and therefore should be avoided. Nowadays, however, the combination of psychotherapy and medication has not only become a common practice, but there is evidence that it may improve the therapeutic alliance and reduce dropout. A number of studies have reported an increase in positive effects in mental disorders, such as anxiety, depression, and BPD, when medication and psychotherapy work synergistically.

Principles of prescribing

However, this combination still presents a number of challenges, particularly if the place and role of medication and prescriber have not been made explicit in the first place. Prescribing, like any other form of treatment, is highly specific and individualized. As in any psychotherapeutic contract, when the use of medication is clearly required, it is essential to clarify it from the outset and be specific about its duration, i.e. whether or not it is on a short- or long-term basis. It is equally important for the prescriber to give reassurance and a full explanation of the advantages and disadvantages of medication, including its short- and long-term side effects. This information should also be communicated to the psychotherapist, particularly if he/she is not familiar with the relevant medication.

Prescribing during psychiatric crises

When the need for prescribing arises in the midst of a psychotherapeutic process, including during a crisis, the pros and cons of the use of medication have to be properly considered. In conditions such as BPD, crises are a common occurrence, and any pharmacological intervention has to be introduced with caution and be embedded into the treatment plan, whilst the patient and therapist will continue to explore other ways of dealing with the crisis. This means a well set-out level of coordination between the prescribing clinician, the psychotherapist, and, when appropriate, the multidisciplinary team.

In BPD patients, NICE guidelines recommend that the need for medication should be only confined to co-morbid conditions. Other clinicians, however, advocate the use of antidepressive, antipsychotic medication or mood stabilizers, particularly in order to regulate hostility, impulsivity, hypervigilance, and interpersonal hypersensitivity in BPD patients (see ➜ Borderline personality disorder in Chapter 8, pp. 390–6).

Split treatment model

Although some medical psychotherapists may consider being the prescribers of medication in their own clinical practice, it has become increasingly commoner to allocate a different prescribing doctor, be it a GP or a psychiatrist, who is not the psychotherapy clinician at the same time. This widely accepted 'split treatment' enables the treating clinician to continue the therapeutic process, so long as the function of medication is suitably explored during therapy, whilst the prescribing—and preferably psychotherapeutically minded—psychiatrist applies his mind to medication. This is a sensible practice, because the latter is also usually better informed and more up-to-date with regard to advances in psychopharmacology. It is worth remembering, however, that transference and countertransference issues are phenomena which should not be underestimated by the prescriber. For example, when the patient shows a poor response, the prescriber's frustration, anxiety, and despair may account for irresponsible dose escalation, as well as polypharmacy. Consequently, effective and regular communication between the prescriber and the psychotherapist is essential. In order to avoid unnecessary splitting, the patient should be informed that such communication is regularly taking place.

Patients' use and experience of medication

There are many reasons why a patient may accept or take against medication, which are important to identify and explore with the patient, if possible. For some patients, symptom relief is essential, before commencing a course of psychotherapy. Others may prefer to secretly use illicit substances, in order to 'medicate' their unsettled mind. There is also a subgroup of patients who are particularly suspicious of all medication, its side effects, and its long-term effects on their overall health. Their suspiciousness can, at times, be justified, if they suffer from long-term medical conditions, which often require a variety of medications with very limited results. Some other patients may (unconsciously) prefer to hang on to their psychotic beliefs or overvalued ideas, or continue to deny the severity of their illness. Hence, they resist the use of medication, since it may signify they are more ill. Other patients, particularly those suffering from chronic conditions, may resent the withholding of medication on the part of the therapist who may advise against its use in the name of maintaining a 'pure' psychotherapeutic relationship. Conversely, other patients view medication as an intrusion in their psychotherapeutic work. Finally, those who do take medication may secretly develop problems with compliance, whilst patients with a tendency to splitting may use medication defensively by attributing all the improvement to medication, whilst denigrating the therapist and the ensuing psychotherapeutic work.

Summary

In summary, good psychotherapy and good prescribing are not nowadays mutually exclusive. Indeed, the integration of psychopharmacology and psychotherapy can prove to be useful and effective in clinical management, particularly in highly disturbed patients, so long as this integration is set out for the right reasons, and it is well coordinated and includes the patients' collaboration.

Recommended reading

Bateman A and Kravitz R (2013). *Borderline Personality Disorder. An Evidence-Based Guide for Generalist Mental Health Professionals*. Oxford University Press: Oxford.
Cuijpers P, Sijbrandij M, Koole S, Andersson G, Beekman A, and Reynolds C (2014). Adding psychotherapy to antidepressant medication in depression and anxiety disorders: a meta-analysis. *World Psychiatry*, **13**, 56–67.
Gabbard G and Kay J (2001). The fate of integrated treatment: whatever happened to the bio-psychosocial psychiatrist? *American Journal of Psychiatry*, 158, 1956–63.
Kandel E (1998). A new intellectual framework for psychiatry. *American Journal of Psychiatry*, 155, 457–69.

Anxiety and anxiety disorders

Anxiety

Anxiety (from latin *angere*: to cause pain) is an unpleasant emotional state or affect, characterized by tension, guardedness, and apprehension, in the face of imagined impending danger and doom. It typically involves a sense of helplessness in its most acute form, i.e. panic, which is usually accompanied by a number of physical concomitants such as tachycardia, sweating, dryness of the mouth, and tremor.

Psychoanalytic perspectives

(See ➲ Psychoanalytic psychotherapy in Chapter 2, pp. 20–30.)

Within the psychoanalytic perspective, the term anxiety is viewed as central to mental distress. The onset of neurotic symptoms is understood as a way of avoiding the distressing experience of anxiety. Hence, one of the aims of any psychoanalytic endeavour is that of trying to uncover the unconscious motivation lying behind anxiety symptoms.

In trying to explain the origin of anxiety, Freud moved from his first theory of anxiety (1895), in which the anxiety, which he called *aktual neurosis* ('aktual' meaning current) was the result of transformation of undischarged libido, to his second theory of anxiety (1926) whereby the anxiety was conceptualized as a response to a threat to the individual. Freud distinguished different types of anxiety:

- *Realistic anxiety* (akin to fear)—a response to real external danger
- *Neurotic anxiety*—a response to internally perceived danger

- *Signal anxiety*—a less intense form of anxiety that is developmentally normal and which tends to arise in anticipation of danger, as opposed to being its result. Signal anxiety may be adaptive by mobilizing ego defences to ward off danger and may lead to fight-or-flight responses.

Developmental classification of anxiety

One of the main psychotherapeutic tasks in dealing with anxiety is to increase its *tolerance*, in order to explore the underlying conflicts. From the developmental point of view, there are a number of levels of experience of anxiety—a developmental hierarchy of anxiety, which can create a variety of conflicts for the patient. These include:

- *Separation anxiety.* This is evoked by situations of actual, anticipated, or imagined loss of a significant relationship. The consequent helplessness may pave the way to an ensuing depressive reaction. Separation anxiety can manifest itself at any stage of life.
- *Fragmentation or disintegration anxiety.* This involves a more profound disturbance of self-cohesion than separation anxiety, and originates from the fear of the sense of self merging with the other or when others do not respond with the necessary form of positive support.
- *Paranoid or persecutory anxiety.* This occurs when the patient feels persecuted by external forces invading the inner self.
- *Superego anxiety.* This generally refers to not being able to live up to the internalized standards set up by parental figures.

DSM-5 anxiety disorders

Anxiety disorders, as defined in DSM-5, include GAD, agoraphobia, specific phobia, panic disorder, separation anxiety disorder, and selective mutism in children. The global prevalence of anxiety disorders is about 7%, and they are commoner in women and in developed countries. These disorders can be debilitating and enduring, and can be co-morbid with other mental disorders, in particular substance misuse and depressive conditions. Predisposition to anxiety is overdetermined and includes biological and environmental factors, whilst life events and adverse circumstances can often act as precipitants.

Psychological treatments for anxiety disorders

A wide range of therapeutic interventions can be effective at various levels. In deciding the most appropriate therapeutic intervention in the treatment of anxiety disorders, it is important first to evaluate the degree of severity, as well as the duration of the condition. A stepped-care approach will be applied, according to patients' preference and whether the severity and duration are considered mild, moderate, or severe.

Following the initial screening, the NICE guidelines (2014) suggest therapeutic interventions varying from simple self-help aids and psychoeducation, facilitated relaxation and mindfulness groups, and short-term CBT to more sophisticated types of psychotherapy such as psychodynamic psychotherapy delivered on a more long-term basis either individually or in groups. Medication, such as selective serotonin reuptake inhibitors (SSRIs), may need to be considered as an adjunct, particularly in poor responders, to the above described interventions.

Advantages of structured and stepwise therapeutic progression are:
• It may help some patients to normalize their symptoms within the context of their life
• It provides patients with some simple and understandable tools which they can use in case of relapses
• It reduces the number of inappropriate referrals to tertiary services, thus enabling more sophisticated psychotherapies to deal with increasingly more appropriate clinical conditions
• It reduces the burden of patients' presentation in general practice.

Disadvantages of structured and stepwise therapeutic progression are:
• The relative inexperience of the young mental health practitioner who may underestimate or overestimate the level of severity
• The lack of time, minimal training, and/or insufficient supervision can limit the professional's capacity to elicit the correct history and precipitating and perpetuating causes
• It may involve multiple assessments, which can be detrimental for the patient and may led to poor engagement and dropout
• It may neglect the detection of morbid and pre-morbid personality traits or disorders underpinning the original presentation
• It may be of limited value in preventing relapses and a chronic trajectory.

Therefore, in order to consider the most suitable way forward, it is always advisable to elicit a careful history, which includes predisposing, perpetuating, and precipitating factors. Given the vast number of anxiety disorder presentations, the usefulness of NICE recommendations should not be underestimated. Therapists should be aware of how debilitating and interfering an acute anxiety state can be in establishing and maintaining the therapeutic relationship. Hence, when considering psychodynamic or psychoanalytic therapy, a previously well-conducted more basic psychological intervention or a sensible use of medication aimed at reducing the level of anxiety can be of clear value, both to the patient and psychotherapist. A more manageable level of anxiety can not only foster a better therapeutic alliance, but it may also allow for a better unravelling of the underlying unconscious factors.

Recommended reading

DSM-5 (2013). *Diagnostic and Statistical Manual of Mental Disorders, fifth edition.* American Psychiatric Association: Washington DC.

Freud S (1926). Inhibitions, symptoms, and anxiety. In: Strachey J (ed). *The Standard Edition of the Complete Psychological Works of Sigmund Freud,* volume 20. pp. 75–175. Hogarth Press: London, 1959.

Gabbard G (2005). *Psychodynamic Psychiatry in Clinical Practice.* American Psychiatric Publishing: Washington DC.

National Institute for Health and Care Excellence (2014). *Anxiety Disorders. NICE Quality Standard [QS53].* Available at: ℜ https://www.nice.org.uk/guidance/qs53.

Affective disorders

The idea behind the concept of a group of affective disorders rests upon the observation that some mental disorders are primarily disorders of mood, whilst others mainly affect thinking. This distinction holds only up to a point. Depression and mania are, in fact, combinations of thought *and* feeling *and* behaviour.

Diagnosis and classification

DSM-5 describes three main types of depressive *disorders*—major depressive, persistent depressive (formerly dysthymia), and bipolar disorder; criteria are given in terms of clinical features, severity, duration, and effects on functioning. Genetics suggest that bipolar disorders may be biologically distinct from the others. Depression, however, overlaps with other common neurotic conditions. For example, half of individuals diagnosed with depression will also fulfil diagnostic criteria for GAD. Clinical presentations change over time, with the features of depression, anxiety, phobic disorder, or OCD alternating. Depression and anxiety share the same environmental risk factors and respond to the same classes of medication. These findings cast doubt upon the existence of these as distinct conditions and have led to the proposal that they should be replaced simply by the descriptive generic term 'common mental disorder'. Depressive mood occurs frequently as part of many mental disorders and commonly accompany physical disorders as well (see ➔ Anxiety and anxiety disorders in Chapter 7, pp. 326–31).

Prevalence

The literature is replete with references to the prevalence, the burden of disability, and the economic costs associated with depression. Depending upon the sample studied and definitions used, different surveys estimate the prevalence of mixed depression and anxiety to be anywhere between 9% and 18%, with something like 0.7% to 1.0% of the general population suffering from more severe chronic or relapsing forms. In UK depression samples, the lifetime risk of death by suicide is 4%—12 times greater than that of the general population. Depressive disorders will soon be the largest contributor to the burden of human disease in developed countries, whilst, in developing countries, only HIV/AIDS will have a larger effect (see ➔ Suicide and self-harm in Chapter 6, pp. 308–11).

Wider significance

The above facts only convey part of the significance possessed by affective disorders. A capacity for degrees of both depression and mania are elements in the normal human repertoire of mental states. They arise in connection with the central events and life experiences with which we all must struggle to come to terms. They are important parts of our adaptive responses.

According to a psychoanalytic point of view, their meaning is only partly conscious. It deals nevertheless in disappointments and triumphs, arrivals and departures, endings, absence, separations, and loss, all arising in relation to large matters of birth and death, sex, and relationships, as well as occupation or work. Freud observed how these intrinsically meaningful issues were also operating in mania, as well as melancholia too. He hypothesized that, like mourning, they both occur in response to loss, even though the individual subject might not be aware of what precisely has been lost. The model Freud proposed was that the lost object relation cannot be relinquished. Instead it is ambivalently kept alive within the person (introjected). The subject identifies with it but cannot cease the internal complaints and protests in part arising from

its absence. As a consequence, the subject's internal world deteriorates, so that, in the extreme case of melancholia, the sufferer experiences himself and the world outside as dead. This model remains at
the heart of the psychoanalytic account of depression, although it has
been much further developed. Psychoanalytic approaches to the treatment of affective disorders depend upon developing a specific kind of
therapeutic relationship, in which the individual can gain some familiarity with his or her personally central issues and with how, as well as in
childhood, they continue to operate in daily adult life and relationships
(see ➲ Psychoanalytic psychotherapy in Chapter 2, pp. 20–30; Loss in
Chapter 6, pp. 298–300).

The social scientist George Brown devised methods to empirically test
out these observations about depression's meaningfully causal connectedness with personal loss events. As a result, we now know that excesses
of adverse or stressful life events do, in fact, precede depression, melancholia, and mania. Other researchers have investigated psychoanalytic
hypotheses about how adverse features in the baby's early relationships,
particularly with his or her mother (e.g. maternal post-natal depression),
as well as neglect and maltreatment in childhood, may give rise to a vulnerability to depression not only concurrently, but persisting later in life.

Cognitive approaches to depression, originally based upon Beck's
thinking, focus, in contrast, upon teaching sufferers strategies for exercising control over thought patterns deemed negative or maladaptive,
typically regarding thoughts as either functional or dysfunctional, rather
than upon any meaningful content they may be considered to possess
(see ➲ Cognitive behavioural therapy in Chapter 2, pp. 30–4, and in
Chapter 5, pp. 172–84).

Principles of treatment services for depression and allied disorders

(See ➲ Planning psychotherapy services within psychiatric care in
Chapter 10, pp. 462–6; Psychotherapeutic understanding of organizational processes in Chapter 10, pp. 471–5.)

The general principles of organizing psychological treatment services,
as well as the role of the medical psychotherapist in delivering them, apply
to two somewhat different kinds of task. The first is organizational—
namely, how to provide a good service overall which can form part of
a larger system, hopefully leading to an increase in mental health in our
collective community. This requires finding how to have something that
is valuable, timely, and fair to offer for usually larger numbers of patients
than the resources available can easily supply. The second principle is
that what is provided for each patient should be as good as is possible.
This depends upon provisions for the training, supervision, and ongoing
support of staff, so that their work may be sustainable and enriching for
them personally.

In relation to the wider responsibilities for the service in which he or
she works, the medical psychotherapist needs to develop a thorough
grasp of the following:
• The extent to which states of mind reflecting those of the patient
  group will unconsciously be brought to bear upon the culture and

morale of the staff of the service concerned. Depressed patients may unconsciously act upon the service to bring about feelings of failure, masochistic guilt, and sometimes destructive despair over the impossibility of the internal repair of damaged objects, as well as potentially feeling a very deep appreciation of the service for its containment of these states, particularly if sustained over the longer term. Whatever their particular approach or orientation, all services unconsciously construct defences against these states of mind. In the optimal case, the defences adopted permit sufficient openness to these states of mind and do not excessively rely upon omnipotent or bureaucratic denial, whilst still protecting staff from levels of affect or emotion which might overwhelm them.

- Depression is often regarded as a self-limiting condition when, in fact, most patients suffer from a lifelong vulnerability. Currently, 25% to 40% of patients presenting with depression in primary care will have at least one further episode within the following 2 years; 60% at least one further episode within the following 5; three-quarters of those who have had a depressive illness will suffer on average four subsequent episodes; although episodes of depression last about 3 months, in about 12%, they continue for ≥2 years, and up to 55% do not respond to antidepressants. The short-term nature of most of the treatments offered therefore is based upon a denial of these realities. However, it does not follow that short-term interventions cannot play a valuable part, e.g. within a service with an understanding of the long-term nature of the vulnerability. Nonetheless, augmented, combined, or longer psychological term treatments are still too few.
- The consequences of the fact that depression is a psychosomatic condition which has important physical, as well as psychological, expressions.
- The risks associated with affective disorders, in particular of suicide or, more rarely, of homicide or infanticide, and how a therapeutic relationship can be a valuable tool in managing these risks (see → Suicide and self-harm in Chapter 6, pp. 308–11).

Treatment provisions for depression in psychological therapy services

Necessarily, the treatments offered by any given service will depend upon local, as well as more general, factors. These will have to take into account the high- and low-intensity treatments approved by the revised NICE depression guideline, as well as the potential value of coordination with IAPT services, which, in turn, depends upon their state, level of functioning, and the attitude of the personnel involved.

Many of the treatment modalities described in detail in previous chapters can offer value for patients with depression. The following kind of provisions should form part of any service aiming to offer a good provision for depressed patients. However, as well as precisely what is on offer, how well it is done matters as much.

- An invaluable first step remains getting a sense of a person and his or her life and illness, current and past, plus the very considerable therapeutic benefits for the individual patient associated with doing so. Although belonging to a bygone era, Karl Menninger's brief paper *The Psychiatric Diagnosis* continues to give an exemplary account of how to go about this.

- Psychodynamic and psychoanalytic approaches are distinguished by the emphasis they give to the role of subjectivity, interiority, intentionality, and personal meaning in affective states. There is an increasingly strong evidence base for the efficacy of such treatments in depressive disorder for both short-term therapies, such as DIT, and longer-term therapies. For example, the Tavistock Adult Depression Study is producing evidence about the effectiveness of 60 sessions of psychoanalytic psychotherapy with chronically depressed patients. A German trial used the same manual to compare the effects of longer psychoanalytic treatments with those of an augmented form of CBT, also with chronically depressed patients. The Tavistock treatment approach authorizes psychoanalytically trained clinicians to use their skills to 'follow the patient', rather than to apply a simplifying structure or predetermined focus, as is the case in most manualized approaches to psychodynamic or psychoanalytic forms of therapy (see ➲ Psychoanalytic psychotherapy in Chapter 2, pp. 20–30, and in Chapter 5, pp. 163–72; Dynamic interpersonal therapy in Chapter 2, pp. 61–63, and in Chapter 5, pp. 215–20).
- Whilst psychoanalytic or psychodynamic approaches match the preferences of many patients, they are by no means wanted or liked by all. Many patients prefer and value a cognitive behavioural approach, and may gain more benefit from it (see ➲ Cognitive behavioural therapy in Chapter 2, pp. 30–4, and in Chapter 5, pp. 172–84).
- Group therapy: in NHS settings, individual treatments currently are time-limited. In this context, psychodynamic group therapy following on individual treatments offers the advantage of therapy continuing for longer than otherwise could be the case. It also provides a chance for the patient to work with the anxieties involved in moving from the shelter of illusory, exclusive one-to-one relationships (such as may be sought through individual treatments) to a social world involving the benefits, as well as the difficulties, of identification with peers. The ability to feel personal in the company of others has often presented difficulties for many depressed people. Groups offer an opportunity to transfer into the social sphere what was initiated in a one-to-one setting (see ➲ Group therapy and group analysis in Chapter 2, pp. 42–7, and in Chapter 5, pp. 188–94).
- Family and/or couple therapies: the designated patient's depression is sometimes sustained by an interpersonal systemic situation operating either in a family or a couple setting. Moreover, one individual's depression often has—or, in the case of suicide, will have—long-term effects on spouses, parents, children, and others. In these situations, family or couple therapy may be indicated (see ➲ Systemic family and couple therapy in Chapter 2, pp. 34–42, and in Chapter 5, pp. 184–8).
- Medication: results from studies of combined drug and psychological therapy are mixed, but there is evidence of 'extra value' from adding

psychodynamic or cognitive treatments to medication. Also, adding medication to psychotherapy, especially where vegetative symptoms are pronounced, should not be forgotten (see ➔ Psychotherapy and medication in Chapter 7, pp. 322–4).

Conclusion

Depression and its meaning are intimately concerned with central features of the human life cycle. It is principally for this reason, not cost-economic ones or for the production of a vacuous form of happiness, that the quality of what mental health services offer to those who are depressed is so important. As a result of it, those involved in trying to help understand and alleviate depression and its extremely painful suffering often feel privileged to have had the opportunity to do so.

Recommended reading

Harris T (ed) (2000) *Where Inner and Outer Worlds Meet: Psychosocial Research in the Tradition of George Brown.* Routledge: London.
Hill J (2009). Developmental perspectives on adult depression. *Psychoanalytic Psychotherapy*, **23**, 200–12.
McQueen D (2009). Depression in adults: some basic facts. *Psychoanalytic Psychotherapy*, **23**, 225–35.
Menninger K (1959). The psychiatric diagnosis. *Bulletin of the Menninger Clinic*, **23**, 226–40.
Rosenfeld H (1959). An investigation into the psycho-analytic theory of depression. *International Journal of Psychoanalysis*, **40**, 105–29.

Psychoses

In recent years, there has been increasing interest in the psychological therapies of people who have experienced psychoses. This stems from the increasing realization that: (a) there will be no single biological or genetic explanation for the aetiology of psychoses, (b) adverse nurture and trauma considerably increase vulnerability to the psychoses, (c) adverse nurture and trauma alter the developing brain structure and functioning, and (d) medications and their side effects are unacceptable to a considerable percentage of patients. The voice of experts by experience and families has grown louder, requesting listening/talking therapies. Most importantly, there is increasing evidence of the effectiveness of several modalities of psychotherapy for psychoses.

Psychotic illnesses are classified in DSM-5 under the category of 'Schizophrenia spectrum and other psychotic disorders', which includes schizophrenia, schizotypal personality disorder, delusional disorder, brief psychotic disorder, schizophreniform disorder, schizoaffective disorder, and other specified and 'unspecified schizophrenia and other psychotic disorder'. They are defined by abnormalities in one or more of five domains: delusions, hallucinations, disorganized thinking or speech, grossly disorganized or abnormal motor behaviour, and negative symptoms. Although DSM-5 has dropped the narrower subtypes (e.g. paranoid, disorganized, catatonic), due to their clinical unreliability, DSM-5 introduces only modest changes to the conceptualization of psychotic illness, and the current categorical diagnoses remain limited in that they are based on phenomenology, rather than aetiological factors or underlying dynamic processes, and do not accurately capture the variability of symptomatology, response to treatment, and social functioning. For example, it seems that, if services are organized to treat psychosis soon after onset, patients are more likely to receive a diagnosis of brief psychotic episode, rather than schizophrenia which requires the presence of symptoms for 6 months.

Family interventions

(See ➲ Systemic family and couple therapy in Chapter 2, pp. 34–42, and in Chapter 5, pp. 184–8.)

Family interventions have the best evidence base of all the psychological therapies for psychosis and have long been firmly advocated by NICE guidelines which recommended, in 2014, that a family intervention be offered to all patients and families for at least ten sessions or for up to a year. The evidence is best for family interventions in reducing the relapse of psychoses, though there are many ways in which families can be helped and no evidence that a particular orientation is superior. Multifamily groups have also been shown to be effective, though the uptake is lower.

Cognitive behavioural therapy for psychosis

(See ➲ Cognitive behavioural therapy in Chapter 2, pp. 30–4, and in Chapter 5, pp. 172–84.)

CBT for psychosis (CBTp) has been well researched, especially for its effectiveness in reducing distressing psychotic symptoms in spite of adherence to medication. The more recent application of CBTp to a wide range of problems suggests that CBTp should no longer be regarded as an equivalent to medication and that it should be considered clinically and in further research more, according to the specific cognitions and emotions being targeted. CBTp therapists have increasingly recognized the link between disturbing emotions and psychosis, as well as the secondary affective consequences of psychosis. CBT has led the way in shifting professional 'beliefs' that delusions were not amenable to reason. Current research has indicated that CBT may well benefit a useful number of patients who, for whatever reason, do not take neuroleptic medication.

Psychodynamic therapy

(See ➲ Psychoanalytic psychotherapy in Chapter 2, pp. 20–30, and in Chapter 5, pp. 163–72.)

There was a period of time after the introduction of neuroleptics when some suggested that psychoanalytic or psychodynamic therapies were no longer indicated. Much of the research from those times was of poor quality, e.g. in using unskilled therapists or only evaluating shorter-term outcomes. In other studies, the techniques used may well have been those suited for people with non-psychotic conditions. Modern psychodynamic techniques for people with psychosis are very different, incorporating more supportive elements and greater therapist flexibility, and less exclusive emphasis on interpretation.

There are a few contemporary RCTs in psychodynamic therapies for psychoses. A recent trial of weekly therapy indicated considerable superiority over standard care. Many psychodynamic practitioners, however, question the ethical status and validity of RCTs for psychosis on the grounds that individual people with psychosis have such different individual needs from one to another that it is inappropriate to treat them with the same single intervention and that a needs-adapted approach offers better outcomes. Successive cohort outcome studies of the needs-adapted approach give these views support.

The Open Dialogue approach

This approach emerged from the needs-adapted one and is based on fundamental changes in the way general psychiatric care is organized and provided. In its original location, nearly all the mental health providers of care are trained to a national standard in family therapy, and all psychiatric referrals are met, usually in their own homes, within a working day or two of referral, together with key persons in the patient's lives, with a focus more on understanding the problems, rather than the symptoms; these meetings take place as frequently as needed and for as long as needed. The long-term outcomes for psychotic conditions are outstanding, with particularly notable features being the high rate of return to work and study, the low rate of need for long-term neuroleptics, and the reducing rate of schizophrenia in the community, but a corresponding increase in transient psychosis. In the UK, there are now training programmes in Open Dialogue, as well as research initiatives.

Other psychological approaches

(See ➔ Art psychotherapy in Chapter 2, pp. 81–83, and in Chapter 5, pp. 251–5; Music therapy in Chapter 2, pp. 86–91, and in Chapter 5, pp. 261–74; Group therapy and group analysis in Chapter 2, pp. 42–7, and in Chapter 5, pp. 188–94.)

Though not yet subject to satisfactory research, art therapies (art, music, dance, and related therapies) and other group therapies are widely valued by many patients. An increasing number of people with psychosis are turning to peer groups for effective support, especially in finding alternative or additional ways to medication, in understanding and managing voices. The use of a computer avatar to modify unpleasant voices shows great promise in early trials.

Common features

(See ➔ Medical psychotherapy modalities in Chapter 2, pp. 14–20; Research in psychotherapy in Chapter 10, pp. 154–63.)

It is likely that successful psychological therapies have a number of important features in common (erroneously called non-specific factors). Most important of all will be the capacity of the professional to gradually form a solid relationship with the patient and his family. Research has shown that patients repeatedly attempt to talk about the content of their psychotic symptoms, but this is a source of noticeable interactional tension and difficulty for experienced psychiatrists. Other research has long shown how few teams in the UK have organized themselves to provide psychosocial therapies, especially family therapy, in spite of the evidence of effectiveness being available for three decades. Since psychosis, by definition, implies an altered relationship to reality (and the creation of a new reality), it may require particular skills to understand the contextual issues that provoked the psychosis and the reality that the psychosis is disguising.

Recommended reading

Alanen Y (1997). *Schizophrenia: Its Origins and Need-Adapted Treatment*. Karnac Books: London.
Birchwood M and Trower P (2006). The future of cognitive -behavioural therapy for psychosis: not a quasi-neuroleptic. *British Journal of Psychiatry*, **188**, 107–8.
Hagen R, Turkington D, Berge T, Grawe RW (eds) (2010). *CBT for Psychosis*. Routledge; London.
National Institute for Health and Care Excellence (2014). *Psychosis and Schizophrenia in Adults: Prevention and Management*. NICE guidelines CG178. Available at: ℜ https://www. nice.org.uk/guidance/cg178.
Rosenbaum B, Harder S, Knudsen P, et al. (2012). Supportive psychodynamic psychotherapy versus treatment as usual for first episode psychosis: two-year outcome. *Psychiatry: Interpersonal and Biological Processes*, **75**, 331–41.
Seikkulaa J, Alakareb B, and Aaltonena J (2011). The Comprehensive open dialogue approach in Western Lapland. *Psychosis*, **3**, 179–204.

Eating disorders

Introduction

Eating disorders—anorexia nervosa (AN), bulimia nervosa (BN), binge eating disorder (BED), and 'other specified feeding or eating disorder' (OSFED)—comprise a group of multi-determined syndromes encompassing physical, psychological, and social features. Eating disorders have the highest mortality rates of any psychiatric disorder, with a reported six-fold increase in mortality, compared with the general population.

Epidemiology

About one in 250 females and one in 2000 males will experience AN at some point in their lives, whilst five times that number will suffer from BN. BED and OSFED are commoner still, making up to 50% of cases seen in clinical settings. Onset is usually between 12 and 25 years. Whilst previously thought to be a group of conditions limited to young, western, Caucasian women from higher socio-economic backgrounds, recent findings suggest that eating disorders are increasing in men and older people, and have become a global phenomenon affecting people from all socio-economic backgrounds.

Diagnosis

DSM-5 criteria

Anorexia nervosa

- Body mass index (BMI) <18.5 kg/m^2
- Intense fear of gaining weight or becoming fat, even though underweight
- Disturbance in the way in which one's body weight or shape is experienced, undue influence of body weight or shape on self-evaluation, or denial of the seriousness of the current low BMI
- **Subtypes**: restricting type, binge eating/purging type.

Bulimia nervosa
- Recurrent episodes of binge eating characterized by both:
  - Eating a large amount of food within a 2-hour period
  - Recurrent inappropriate compensatory behaviour to prevent weight gain (e.g. self-induced vomiting)
- Binge eating and compensatory behaviour both occur, on average, ≥1×/week for 3 months
- Self-evaluation unduly influenced by body shape and weight.

Binge eating disorder
- Recurrent episodes of binge eating ≥1×/week for 3 months
- Binge eating not associated with the recurrent use of inappropriate compensatory behaviours as in BN.

Other specified feeding or eating disorder
A group of disorders where eating behaviours cause clinically significant distress and impairment, but full criteria for AN, BN, and BED are not met. Examples include:
- Atypical AN: all criteria for AN are met, but BMI >18.5 kg/m²
- Atypical BN: all criteria for BN are met, but binge eating and compensatory behaviours occur at a lower frequency
- Atypical BED: all criteria for BED are met, but binge eating occurs at a lower frequency
- Purging disorder: recurrent purging behaviour to influence weight and shape, without binge eating.

Differential diagnosis

Organic disorders
- Hyperthyroidism
- Diabetes mellitus
- Chronic infection (tuberculosis, AIDS, fungal infection)
- Inflammatory bowel disease (Crohn's disease, ulcerative colitis)
- Malignancy (lymphoma, stomach cancer)
- Hypothalamic lesion or tumour
- Chronic respiratory disease (cystic fibrosis, bronchiectasis)
- Chronic pancreatitis.

Psychiatric disorders
- Depression
- Somatoform disorders
- OCD
- Schizophrenia.

Aetiology
The following factors have been implicated in the aetiology of eating disorders.

Biological
- Concordance rates MZ:DZ = 65%:32%
- Obstetric complications
- Recent studies suggest a close association between psychological experiences and specific alterations in brain function and

neuropsychological deficits. Such findings have questioned the validity of the old dichotomy of physiological and psychological events, and include:
- Insular dysfunction and hypoperfusion of the anterior cingulate
- Serotonin and noradrenaline dysregulation
- Reduced attention and visuospatial abilities
- Poor executive functioning and set-shifting.

Personality and environment
- Personality traits (anankastic, anxious/avoidant, perfectionism)
- Adverse life events (e.g. physical/emotional trauma, neglect, bereavement, bullying)
- Culture of thinness promoted by the media and peer influences
- Adolescent obesity
- Occupation (e.g. dancing, athletics).

Psychodynamic
- Family pathology and early attachment difficulties—overinvolvement/ enmeshment, overprotectiveness, lack of conflict resolution, perfectionistic, focus on success
- Psychoanalytic theories—regression to childhood, fixation at oral stage
- Lack of personal identity or autonomy.

Clinical features
Core psychopathology
- Fear of normal body weight
- Pursuit of thinness
- Body dissatisfaction
- Self-evaluation solely in terms of weight and shape
- Body image distortion.

General psychopathology
- Depression
- Anxiety
- OCD symptoms
- Paranoid ideation
- Suicidal ideation
- Social isolation
- Cognitive impairment.

Behavioural features
- Calorific restriction (daily intake <1000 kcal/day)
- Avoidance of 'fattening' foods
- Prolonged fasting
- Excessive exercise
- Binge eating
- Purging (e.g. self-induced vomiting, laxative misuse)
- Excessive fluid intake
- Food rituals (e.g. cutting food into small pieces, hiding food)
- Substance misuse
- Deliberate self-harm
- Avoidance of treatment
- Body-checking.

Physical complications

The range of physical complications seen in eating disorders is extensive, and knowledge of these is essential when assessing physical risk.

A screening assessment of physical risk should include a minimum of:
- BMI = weight (kg)/height (m)^2
- Blood pressure, pulse, temperature
- Tests of proximal myopathy (the stand-up/squat test)
- Full blood count, urea and electrolytes, bicarbonate, phosphate, magnesium, calcium, glucose, thyroid function, and liver function
- Electrocardiogram
- Dual-energy X-ray absorptiometry (DEXA) scan.

Evaluation of physical risk should be seen as a longitudinal process, with medical monitoring being a cornerstone in longer-term care, alongside standard psychological and social interventions.

Co-morbidity

Co-morbidity is seen in 50% of cases, with co-morbid depressive disorders, anxiety disorders, substance misuse, PTSD, and personality disorder being common.

Management

General principles

There will often be a number of people involved in the care of patients with eating disorders, including the patient, family and carers, primary and secondary care services, hospital physicians, and specialist eating disorder services. Therefore, care coordination and communication are essential in achieving successful outcomes, and there should be clarification of roles and responsibilities amongst all health professionals involved in the patient's care. Most patients will be treated as an outpatient; however, in severe cases, some patients may require inpatient treatment on a medical unit for nasogastric feeding and/or stabilization of physical risk. Effective treatment requires a combination of both nutritional rehabilitation and psychological intervention, and the best services are those which provide an eclectic mix of treatments which encompass these areas.

Treatment of anorexia nervosa

(See ➔ Cognitive analytic therapy in Chapter 2, pp. 47–52, and in Chapter 5, pp. 194–202; Cognitive behavioural therapy in Chapter 2, pp. 30–4, and in Chapter 5, pp. 172–84; Interpersonal psychotherapy in Chapter 2, pp. 52–5, and in Chapter 5, pp. 203–7; Psychoanalytic psychotherapy in Chapter 2, pp. 20–30, and in Chapter 5, pp. 163–72; Systemic family and couple therapy in Chapter 2, pp. 34–42, and in Chapter 5, pp. 184–8.)

NICE guidelines in the UK recommend the use of CAT, CBT, IPT, focal psychodynamic therapy, and family interventions for the treatment of AN. Moreover, the aims of psychological treatment in AN should be to reduce physical and psychological risk, to encourage weight gain and healthy eating, and to facilitate psychological and physical recovery. Such change will require a core therapeutic understanding of the meaning of food and body image for the patient and support from the therapist to help the patient explore more functional ways of self-expression and self-soothing. The therapist should be aware of the characteristic ego-syntonic self-starvation, denial, and minimization often seen in AN, and they may need to consider the need for consolidation of object constancy to resolve splitting which is commonplace. Treatment of AN is often long-term, and the therapist will benefit from an understanding of psychodynamic processes, such as transference and countertransference, that are often experienced during intensive therapy.

Treatment of bulimia nervosa and binge eating disorder

(See ➲ Cognitive behavioural therapy in Chapter 2, pp. 30–4, and in Chapter 5, pp. 172–84; Interpersonal psychotherapy Chapter 2, pp. 52–5, and in Chapter 5, pp. 203–7.)

Treatment approaches for BN and BED are very similar, and NICE guidelines in the UK recommend the use of an evidence-based self-help programme as a possible first-line intervention for both conditions. Furthermore, CBT for BN (CBT-BN) and CBT for BED (CBT-BED), specifically adapted forms of CBT, should be offered to adults with BN and BED, respectively. The course of treatment should be for 16 to 20 sessions over 4 to 5 months. CBT models for BN and BED are based on the principle that disordered eating and weight and shape concern originate from a cycle of binge eating (in BN and BED), followed by extreme compensatory behaviours (in BN) which exacerbate the core psychopathological features and, in turn, reinforce disordered eating behaviours. Hence, the rationale for CBT is first to address the starve/binge/purge cycle by the use of behavioural and dietary interventions, followed by the use of cognitive techniques to address the core psychopathological features, thus promoting the 'normalization' of eating patterns and achieving a more balanced relationship with food and body image. When patients with BN or BED have not responded to, or do not want, CBT, then IPT should be considered as the alternative.

Medication

Research does not support the use of psychotropic medication in AN; however, antidepressant medication may be justified in cases where there is co-morbid depression or anxiety. Fluoxetine 60 mg is recommended for BN and BED as an adjunct to psychological intervention.

Recommended reading

Hay PJ and Claudino AM (2010). Evidence-based treatments for the eating disorders. In: Agras WS (ed). *The Oxford Handbook of Eating Disorders.* pp. 452–79. Oxford University Press: New York.

Jones WR, Schelhase M, and Morgan JF (2012). Eating disorders: clinical features and the role of the generalist. *Advances in Psychiatric Treatment*, **18**, 34–43.

Royal College of Psychiatrists (2010). *MARSIPAN: Management of Really Sick Patients with Anorexia Nervosa, Council Report CR162.* Royal College of Psychiatrists: London.

Substance misuse

(See ➲ Psychiatry of addictions: psychotherapies, applications, and research in Chapter 12, pp. 574–6.)

Substance misuse has been around for centuries, and, although significant progress has been made in understanding its aetiology, it still presents with many therapeutic challenges. Recreational use of psychoactive substances is fairly common. Surveys show that, in 2012, more than one in four schoolchildren were offered drugs; around 17 in 100 secondary school pupils had tried drugs at some point. The total number of deaths related to drug misuse in England and Wales was 1496 in 2012. According to the latest British Crime Survey, around 36% of the population has used an illegal drug at some point in their lives; cannabis use accounts for 77% of all drug use.

Clinical definitions

The main classification systems ICD-10 (Disorders due to psychoactive substance use) and DSM-5 (Substance use disorders) describe the core features of addiction to a particular substance as a cluster of cognitive, behavioural, and physiological symptoms, in which the individual continues using the substance despite experiencing significant substance-related problems. There may be evidence of return to substance use after a period of abstinence, leading to rapid reappearance of the other features of the syndrome that occurs with non-dependent individuals.

Diagnosis is made on the basis of an assessment, comprising a combination of self-reported data, evidence of clinical signs and symptoms, collaborative information, and objective analysis of biological specimens—urine, blood, saliva, and hair analysis.

Theories of addiction development

Addiction may be viewed as a chronic neurobiological disease state, produced by repeated exposure to a drug that activates the brain reward systems and produces loss of control over the drug of use. Addictive drugs act through the reward circuits located in the mesocorticolimbic dopamine systems that include projections into the nucleus accumbens, amygdala, and prefrontal cortex. The underlying change in brain circuitry may persist beyond detoxification or abstinence from the drug, particularly in individuals with severe disorders. The behavioural effects of these brain changes may be exhibited in the repeated relapses and intense cravings when the individuals are exposed to drug-related stimuli and repeated relapses or continued use despite physical and mental health problems produced by the drug. These persistent drug effects may benefit from long-term approaches to treatment.

The risk of addiction is associated with a number of factors:

• *Individual factors*—genetic predisposition, co-morbid psychiatric conditions, liking the substance
• *Environmental factors*—occupation, peer group, culture, and social stability
• *Substance of abuse*—availability, cost, speed of entering the brain and causing euphoria, efficacy as a tranquillizer.

The following table shows other theories about the aetiology of addiction—each model/theory lays the basis for corresponding types of therapies (see Table 7.1).

Table 7.1 Aetiological models of addiction

Theory	Rationale	Treatment approach
Biological/ genetic	Genetic susceptibility, combined with chemical changes, following exposure which lead to withdrawal symptoms	Pharmacological
Learning	Classical conditioning, e.g. pairing drug use with certain cues; operant learning, e.g. learned behaviour contingent on positive effects of drugs; social learning, e.g. peer pressure, parental drug use	Psychosocial interventions, including CBT, behaviour modification using contingency management, network therapy
Psychodynamic	Regression, emotional arrest, impulsivity, need for immediate gratification. Addiction involves impairment of the mechanisms needed to control impulses	Psychoanalytic psychotherapy, therapist-directed reflection, motivational approaches
Educational model	Lack of awareness, poor knowledge of extent of potential harm	Psycho-education, preventative approach through schools, workplaces, etc.

Treatment approaches

(See ⭍ Cognitive behavioural therapy in Chapter 5, pp. 172–84.)

Addiction disorders are chronic recurring disorders, often associated with enduring maladaptive behaviour patterns that have been developed over time; treatment involves identifying and addressing these behaviours, including factors that predispose the individual to substance use, that act to maintain substance use and are triggers for relapse. A major aspect of addiction treatment involves behaviour change.

Treatment for addiction utilizes a number of evidence-based pharmacological and non-pharmacological interventions, adhering to core basic principles: harm reduction, specific treatments, relapse prevention, and rehabilitation with individual recovery. Pharmacological interventions, where clinically applicable, are most effective when administered in conjunction with psychological interventions.

Psychosocial interventions

The main UK guidelines for management of addiction recommend formal psychosocial interventions (PSI) in the treatment of drug misuse-related problems, including co-occurring mental disorders, e.g. CBT for depression, formal PSI or discrete packages of PSI which may be delivered alongside basic key working and pharmacological interventions, if appropriate. In the field of addiction practice, PSI are used to indicate psychological therapy, with some of the psychological therapies focusing on the social network. With a majority of the drugs liable to be misused, e.g. cannabis, novel psychoactive substances, or gambling, PSI are the only treatments available. This is because there are no evidence-based pharmacological treatments or substitute prescribing available for these substances.

As per guidance from Public Health England, the interventions are categorized as either low- or high-intensity, that allow ease of application of the 'stepped approach' to care (see Table 7.2).

PSI interventions can be delivered in an individual or group setting. They can be delivered in different formats, including therapist-facilitated, using maps or computerized manuals, and self-directed homework. Factors, such as clinical competence, empathy, warmth, congruence, and the therapeutic alliance, can influence outcomes.

In a typical service model employing the stepped-care approach to treatment, clients would first be offered a low-intensity intervention. If there are no successful outcomes, in terms of addiction or co-morbid mental health, then care is 'stepped up' to high-intensity interventions.

Table 7.2 Psychosocial interventions

	Low-intensity PSI	High-intensity PSI
Delivered by	Keyworkers/clinical nurse specialists	Qualified psychologists
Training	DANOS competencies, usually level 5 counselling skills	Specific training in psychological therapies, with a focus on addiction
To address drug use	Motivational interventions Contingency management	Behavioural couples therapy
To address mental health problems	CBT by guided self-help Behavioural activation Treatment engagement	CBT for depression and anxiety Formal psychological therapies
Goals	To reduce substance use To minimize harm To address relapse prevention	To address co-morbid mental health problems To work towards recovery and abstinence To bring about motivation to change in resistant patients
Suitable for/ideal client population	Suitable to engage service users in treatment, and supporting early changes in drug using behaviour, as well as achieving harm reduction goals	Suited to service users with a sufficient degree of stability and in those who may be working towards being drug-free OR Suited for dual-diagnosis clients struggling to move towards recovery

Psychological therapies specific to addiction treatment
Motivational-based approaches

A major shift in the treatment of addiction over the last two decades has been the role that motivation plays in the individual's ability to engage and benefit from treatment, as well as the role of therapy in building up motivation to change. Prochaska and DiClemente's cycle of change (see Fig. 7.1) outlines a series of stages of change and identifies reaction tasks that an individual needs to undertake, in order for them to take action and maintain change.

This forms the basis of motivational-type psychological interventions. One way of matching the psychological therapies is based on what stage of change the individual is in the cycle of change. Someone in a pre-contemplation stage would benefit from motivational interviewing to enable them to make changes. Patients in the contemplation stage would benefit from motivational enhancement to harness that motivation further. Whilst in the action determination stage, they may benefit from CBT-type approaches and relapse prevention work.

Motivational-based approaches tend to utilize a number of interventions and strategies which focus on enabling the individual's engagement and movement through the process of recovery. The most well-known intervention is that of *motivational interviewing* which focuses primarily on preparing people for change and tackling ambivalence to change. It encompasses a model of patient–therapist interaction characterized by collaboration, evocation of ambivalence, and the promotion of autonomy to enhance decision-making and the resolution of ambivalence. *Motivational enhancement therapy* is a more formal four-session stage-based manualized treatment which utilizes adaptations of motivational interviewing.

Relapse prevention—cognitive behavioural treatments
(See Cognitive behavioural therapy in Chapter 5, pp. 172–84.)

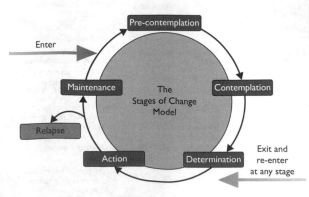

Fig. 7.1 The stages of change model.

CBT has been shown to be effective across a wide range of addictive disorders. CBT is utilized in the treatment of specific substances and the management of co-morbid psychiatric conditions, such as depression and anxiety, which occur frequently in the treatment-seeking population. The CBT approach for addiction disorders has an emphasis on understanding drug use with respect to its antecedents and consequences (functional analysis) and on skills training aimed at developing problem-solving and practising the practical application of these skills as part of relapse prevention. A key limitation in the utilization of CBT in the treatment of addiction in the UK is the limited availability of trained clinicians for substance misuse services. However, this may now be changing, as commissioners are specifically commissioning services with psychological interventions.

Contingency management
There is extensive empirical evidence showing that operant conditioning plays an important role in the development and maintenance of ongoing drug use. In contingency management, the patient receives incentives (e.g. vouchers, privileges) contingent on demonstrating or achieving predefined treatment goals (e.g. submitting drug-free urine specimens, attendance at appointments, and other favourable changes).

In order for contingency management (CM) to be most effective, it is necessary to:
• Use a written contract
• Define the therapeutic target
• Stipulate the schedule on which progress will be measured
• Schedule frequent opportunities for patients to experience the programmed consequences
• Objectively verify that the target response has occurred
• Tackle single, rather than multiple, responses
• Specify what happens when the target response occurs and when it does not occur
• Specify the duration of the contract
• Specify the consequences to follow the verification of the target response, without delay.

CM has been used extensively in the USA, especially for cocaine addiction, and shows great effectiveness in the short term. A limitation of CM is that the gains do not last very long after CM ceases.

Network therapy
Network therapy engages members of the patient's social support network (i.e. friends, family) to help them in moving towards recovery. Efforts are also made to build up 'social capital'—this could be mentors, peer support, and other sources of support from voluntary organizations or social clubs, and activities which promote a drug-free lifestyle. Patients, as well as their significant support members, are required to attend regular sessions, usually using CBT approaches. UK's NICE strongly recommends the use of behavioural couples therapy, along with CBT and mindfulness interventions. The network therapy links to further peer-supported self-help interventions, i.e. 12-step approaches,

Alcoholic Anonymous (AA), Narcotics Anonymous (NA), and Smart Recovery groups. Again there is a significant evidence base to support the efficacy of attending mutual aid groups in promoting and maintaining abstinence.

Psychodynamic psychotherapy

(See ➔ Psychoanalytic psychotherapy in Chapter 2, pp. 20–30, and in Chapter 5, pp. 163–72.)

Psychodynamic psychotherapy (insight-orientated psychotherapy) for addiction is a modified form of therapy that utilizes psychodynamic techniques aimed at increasing self-awareness, growth, and the working through of conflicts, and can be combined with other cognitive approaches such as relapse prevention. It focuses on current conflicts and the therapeutic relationship, as they relate to the past. Abstinence from the substance of addiction is essential for successful treatment.

Dialectical behaviour therapy

(See ➔ Dialectical behaviour therapy in Chapter 2, pp. 63–6, and in Chapter 5, pp. 220–9.)

Originally developed for personality disorder with chronic self-harm, DBT has also been used for substance misuse treatment. It incorporates two seemingly opposite concepts—acceptance and change. DBT sets targets that incorporate all principles of treating substance abuse. It insists on total abstinence, with a non-judgemental problem-solving approach to managing relapses. DBT is especially useful in managing substance use disorders in patients with BPD but is yet to be widely available in substance misuse services in the UK.

Acceptance and commitment therapy

(See ➔ Mindfulness-based interventions and therapies in Chapter 2, pp. 73–5, and in Chapter 5, pp. 239–43.)

ACT includes principles of acceptance and mindfulness. ACT and mindfulness have been researched in gambling, smoking cessation, and also general relapse prevention. Mindfulness incorporates Tibetan meditation principles and exercises. An example of using cognitive de-fusion is when there is craving to use. Rather than saying 'I am craving for . . . this substance', the client is taught to defuse himself from the thought by saying 'I have a thought that I am craving . . .' And then 'I noticed that I have a thought that . . .' This creates a distance between oneself and the thought, and thereby reduces the effect of that thought.

Mindfulness-based relapse prevention

(See ➔ Mindfulness-based interventions and therapies in Chapter 2, pp. 73–5, and in Chapter 5, pp. 239–43.)

Mindfulness-based relapse prevention (MBRP) helps to identify triggers for relapse and then combine those with meditative practice to deal with them better. Examples of mindfulness, which have been tried in addiction treatment, are urge surfing, SOBER space, mindful movement, and kindness or 'metta mantra'. To elaborate on one, urge surfing teaches patients to merely accept and notice the fact that they have an urge to use, rather than fighting it. This acceptance, combined with meditation, is to be continued until the urge has peaked and waned. MBRP has been trialled in RCTs and shown to have promising results in addiction treatment.

Some of the therapies mentioned above are not widely available in clinical settings in the UK, but some of the principles are used in clinical sessions. However, the paradigm shift is in focusing on psychological interventions, in addition to medications, to enable recovery from addiction. Due to this, psychological interventions increasingly form an integral part of an effective and recovery-focused treatment delivery in substance misuse.

Recommended reading

Department of Health (England) and the devolved administrations (2007). *Drug Misuse and Dependence: UK Guidelines on Clinical Management.* London: Department of Health (England), the Scottish Government, Welsh Assembly Government, and Northern Ireland Executive.

Dimeff LA and Linehan M (2008). Dialectical behaviour therapy for substance abusers. *Addiction Science and Clinical Practice,* 4, 39–47.

Miller WR and Rollnick S (2012). *Motivational Interviewing Helping People Change,* third edition. Guildford Press: New York.

National Institute for Health and Care Excellence (2007). *Drug Misuse in Over 16s: Psychosocial Interventions.* NICE guidelines CG51. Available at: ℜ http://www.nice.org.uk/guidance/cg51.

West R (2013). *Models of Addiction.* European Monitoring Centre for Drugs and Drug Addiction: Lisbon.

Sexual dysfunction

Sexual functioning is at the heart of an individual's being and their relationships with others, whether these are same sex or opposite sex. Sexual functioning can help us connect with partners in different ways. In both physical illness and psychiatric disorders, the prevalence of sexual dysfunction can be quite high as part of the symptom profile, but also as a common, but poorly recognized, side effect of medication, whether this is used for physical conditions or psychiatric conditions.

Prevalence rates of sexual dysfunction are high, though data vary, depending upon from where the sample is collected. Often clinicians do not ask the right questions, and the problems remain unexplored and undiagnosed. However, it is important to identify, as the outcomes of the therapeutic treatment of sexual dysfunction are generally positive, partly due to treatability factors, but also as individuals are likely to be highly motivated.

Sexual cycle

The sexual cycle is generally seen as having four key components, and these include desire, followed by sexual excitement and arousal, the act itself and orgasm, followed by a refractory period. For both men and women, the general components remain the same, though the difficulties may arise in one or more stages. The contexts within which dysfunction may appear vary dramatically, and clinicians need to be aware of such a variation.

Classification of psychosexual disorders

Psychosexual disorders can be primary or secondary. In both ICD-10 and DSM-5, the classification is based roughly on the sexual cycle. Libido and sexual desire can be increased or decreased, sometimes leading to a disparity in desire between the two partners. One individual may have high libido, whereas the other may have poor libido, and this can lead to demands by one partner which the other may resent, creating further tensions in the relationship. There are major issues related to challenges in classification, including definitions of what is 'normal' and how abnormality is defined.

Assessment of sexual dysfunction

The assessment of sexual dysfunction should include the following stages:
- Defining the dysfunction
- Assessing whether it is organic or non-organic, primary or secondary
- Assessing immediate or precipitating causes
- Assessing resources for dealing with the dysfunction and its impact on the relationship
- Ascertaining motivation
- Deciding on correct management and prognosis.

The aim of assessment is to ascertain whether the dysfunction is primary or secondary, to assess the relationship with the partner to determine whether strains in relationships are affecting sexual functioning or whether dysfunction is producing relationship problems. In addition, physical, psychological, and social factors must be assessed. Physical disorders, such as diabetes, hypertension, and cardiovascular, gynaecological, and urological disorders, and the iatrogenic effects of medication must be explored. Psychological factors include stress, a poor intimate relationship, clinical depression, anxiety, psychosis, past history of sexual abuse, low self-esteem, as well as other co-morbid psychiatric disorders. Social factors include interpersonal problems, poverty, overcrowding, religious and cultural differences or conflict, differences in values, and childbearing.

The quality of the couple relationship may also be assessed and information gathered regarding previous relationships, engagements, associated circumstances, courtship, if married—age at marriage(s), marriage forced by pregnancy, arranged marriage, age, occupation, health of partner, quality of relationship, fidelity, changed circumstances, dates of divorce or separation, whether the partner is a threat to the relationship, why they have come now, and who initiated the referral.

Management of sexual dysfunction

General principles

There are specific treatment strategies for specific conditions, which are illustrated in Table 7.3. However, as anxiety often causes dysfunction, it is important to use relaxation techniques, along with educational materials, to get the patients to start thinking of an anxiety cycle and how to manage and reduce anxiety. As part of the education process, it is essential to identify and address myths and stereotypes, e.g. that female sexuality does not exist and women should not make the first move or seek sex; that men do not show feelings and that they are more sexual, rather than sensual; that men automatically know what women want; that sex should not be talked about in the process; that the man always

Table 7.3 Specific interventions

Sexual dysfunction	Technique
Low desire/drive/ interest	Sensate focus
Excessive desire/drive/interest	Overstimulation
Erectile dysfunction/impaired arousal	Sensate focus
Premature ejaculation	Squeeze
Anorgasmia	Sensate focus
Retarded ejaculation	Sensate focus and overstimulation
Sexual pain/dyspareunia	Relaxation and exposure
Vaginismus	Relaxation and exposure
Sexual phobias	Relaxation and exposure

takes on the active role, etc. Often, in long-term relationships, one partner may think about the other, 'If you really loved me, you'd know how I feel without me telling you'. Often partners may not tell each other what they like or dislike, and may not communicate their feelings about the sexual act itself to each other.

As part of the first step in educating the individual or the couple, they need to learn how to communicate, recognizing and articulating actual emotional feelings which should be expressed using the first person singular. Often ignorance about the sexual act itself provides the trigger for the problems, so education is a key essential step.

Specific treatments
Behavioural therapy
Based on Masters and Johnson's approaches, these methods are today called modified Masters and Johnson where couples are given graded sexual exercises. During the first stage, all genital sexual contact is banned, but the couple is encouraged to explore each other's bodies using tactile touching and massage, taking turns to please each other. This stage is known as non-genital sensate focus, and, after two to three sessions per week for a few weeks, the couple can move to the next stage of genital sensate focus, especially if they are making good progress. In this stage, actual intercourse still remains banned, but the couple can touch each other's external genitalia. The purpose is to improve both verbal and non-verbal communication. Once the couple have learnt these strategies, they can add specific interventions, according to the underlying condition. For example, they may use the 'squeeze technique' in cases of premature ejaculation, or they could use 'overstimulation' in cases of retarded ejaculation. Throughout, cognitive elements are included to reduce anxiety, challenge stereotypes, and reduce generalizations and catastrophizing. For women with anorgasmia or vaginismus, exposure and behavioural therapies have been shown to be effective and successful. For vaginismus, using vaginal dilators, whilst managing anxiety, and then gradually increasing their size will help.

Couple therapy
Couples go through various stages through their time together, especially in long-term relationships. These stages typically are: marriage or establishment of stable sexual relationship, early parenthood (prenatal, having young children), late parenthood (adolescent children), midlife, older age, and then death. At each stage, relationship expectations may vary, and clinicians, when offering couple therapy, must take these stages into account.

Systemic therapy
(See ➔ Systematic family and couple therapy in Chapter 2, pp. 34–42, and in Chapter 5, pp. 184–8.)
Such an approach looks at the whole system. If one partner develops symptoms, the other may adjust his/her life accordingly, so that, when the symptoms are treated, this may lead to resentment on the part of the partner who has already adjusted to the symptoms. Thus unwanted gains will need to be explored and dealt with in the course of the therapy.

Cognitive behavioural therapy
(See ➔ Cognitive behavioural therapy in Chapter 2, pp. 30–4, and in Chapter 5, pp. 172–84.)
CBT is beginning to show some success rates. The focus in therapy is on challenging underlying assumptions which may be contributing to the sexual dysfunction. Patients may be asked to keep diaries and include accompanying thoughts.

Psychoanalytic psychotherapies
(See ➔ Psychoanalytic psychotherapy in Chapter 2, pp. 30–4, and in Chapter 5, pp. 172–84.)
These have been used in some cases, but there are limited long-term data indicating improvement.

Physical treatments
(See ➔ Psychotherapy and medication in Chapter 7, pp. 322–4.)
Many conditions can be treated using physical treatments such as hormones. For erectile dysfunction, medications, such as sildenafil and tadalafil, or intra-cavernosal injections, such as papaverine, can be used. For other conditions, such as premature ejaculation, antidepressants have been shown to be effective, but these should be accompanied by supportive or exploratory psychotherapy to improve therapeutic adherence.

Conclusion

Sexual dysfunction is a very common psychiatric disorder and often gets ignored, either due to lack of expertise or lack of knowledge. Co-morbidity with physical conditions and psychiatric conditions and iatrogenic onset must be remembered. Basic principles can be used to identify the degree of problems and potential solutions.

Recommended reading

Balon R and Segraves RT (eds) (2009). *Clinical Manual of Sexual Disorders*. American Psychiatric Publishing: Washington DC.

Bancroft J (2009). *Human Sexuality and its Problems*. Churchill Livingstone Elsevier: London and New York.
Bhugra D and Colombini G (2013). Sexual dysfunction: classification and assessment. *Advances in Psychiatric Treatment*, **19**, 48–55.
Crowe M and Ridley J (2009). *Couple Therapy*. Blackwell: Oxford.
Leiblum S (ed) (2007). *Principles and Practice of Sex Therapy*. Guildford Press: New York.

Paraphilias

(See ➜ Sexual dysfunction in Chapter 7, pp. 345–9.)

Diagnosis

DSM-5 defines paraphilias as conditions in which there is intense and persistent sexual interest, other than sexual interest in genital stimulation or preparatory fondling with phenotypically normal, physically mature, consenting human partners. The abnormality of the sexual interest lies in: (a) its object, (b) its intensity and fixity, (c) the process of engagement with the object, and (d) the absence of consent in practices that involve humans. The *object* of a paraphilia may be human or non-human; the *process* of a paraphilia may also involve the treatment of human persons as objects or things, rather than erotic partners.

Although most paraphilias are not synonymous with statutory crimes, and generally the overt intention of the paraphilic behaviour is to achieve sexual arousal, much paraphilic activity is also associated with an intention to cause hurt, distress, fear, or shame in others. When the paraphilic activity is associated with hostility and threat behaviours, this will bring the perpetrators to the attention of the criminal law, even if the paraphilia itself is not a crime.

DSM-5 specifies eight specific paraphilias and paraphilic disorders (see below), although many more have been described in the literature.

DSM-5 paraphilic disorders
- Voyeuristic disorder (covert observation of others in private activities)
- Exhibitionistic disorder (exposing the genitals)
- Frotteuristic disorder (touching or rubbing against a non-consenting individual)
- Sexual masochism disorder (undergoing humiliation, control, or suffering)
- Sexual sadism disorder (inflicting humiliation, control, or suffering)
- Paedophilic disorder (sexual arousal to images or contact with vulnerable or dependent children which may include involvement in child pornography)
- Fetishistic disorder (using non-living objects or having a highly specific focus on non-genital body parts)
- Transvestic disorder (engaging in sexually arousing cross-dressing)
- Other specified paraphilic disorder (includes *zoophilia* (animals), *scatalogia* (obscene phone calls), *necrophilia* (corpses), *coprophilia* (faeces), *klismaphilia* (enemas), *urophilia* (urine)).

The definition of paraphilias is essentially normative, i.e. with reference to a so-called 'normal' sexuality. For this reason, defining paraphilias has historically been fraught with ethical confusion, cultural controversy, and legal debate. There is a general lack of knowledge, as well as disagreement, about what constitutes the full range of 'normal' human sexual behaviour; it is likely that many adults participate consensually in practices that might be considered harmful or aberrant by others but never seek any psychiatric or psychological help, until/unless they become identified as deviant by others. Significant difficulties remain with the classification of paraphilias, especially the the relationship between paraphilias, criminality, and sexual offending, and the lack of good-quality empirical research to inform the validity and reliability of diagnostic systems such as the DSM.

DSM-5 differentiates between atypical human behavior, that is not associated with a mental disorder or harm to others, and atypical behaviour that is or may be associated with a range of psychopathologies and causes harm. A distinction is made between *a paraphilia* (atypical sexual interest or behaviour, which may be associated with a variety of mental disorders, or none) and *a paraphilic disorder* (which gives rise to a mental disorder).

Thus, to be diagnosed with a paraphilic disorder, the person must:
• Feel personal distress about their interest, not merely distress resulting from society's disapproval, and/or
• Have a sexual desire or behaviour that involves another person's psychological distress, injury, or death, or a desire for sexual behaviors involving unwilling persons or persons unable to give legal consent.

Prevalence and co-morbidity

Reliable prevalence studies of paraphilias are hard to establish. Studies are biased towards those individuals who are detected in behaviours that are also criminal (such as sexual sadism or paedophilia) and do not include those people who are undetected in their behaviours but who are naturally reluctant to admit to activities that are deemed criminal or shameful. For example, evidence from the so-called Dunkelfeld or 'dark-field' studies of paedophilia in the community suggest that there may be a significant subgroup of men who have persistent sexual interest in children who are undetected and untreated. These studies are consistent with studies of reported experience of child abuse, which suggest that 8–10% of boys and 12–20% of girls have been victimized by paraphilic adults, generally males.

In relation to other paraphilias, a Swedish study found that 3.1% of a large sample of adults aged 18–65 years reported at least one incident of exhibitionism; 7.7% reported voyeuristic behaviour, and 2.8% reported transvestic fetishism. These paraphilic behaviours were two to three times commoner in men and were associated with greater drug and alcohol use. Those who reported such behaviours also reported more psychological problems, same-sex sexual experiences, and childhood histories of parental separation and sexual abuse.

Paraphilias in females are rare but not unknown; perhaps the most commonly reported form is severe masochistic disorders that occur in the context of a relationship with a sexually sadistic partner. Paraphilic women who abuse children sexually usually do so in the context of a relationship with a paraphilic male partner; in these cases, sexual abuse of children is usually accompanied by severe physical abuse and neglect.

Paraphilias are associated with high rates of co-morbid mental illness, particularly mood and anxiety disorders, personality disorders, and alcohol and substance misuse. A recent study in the USA of paraphilias within psychiatric populations reported rates of 13.4% of psychiatric inpatients having a diagnosis of DSM-IV paraphilia.

Paraphilias are more likely to be associated with crime and violence, if the individuals concerned also have other risk factors for violence such as ASPD, a history of crime and violence perpetration, and a history of substance misuse. Although serious sexual violence in people with paraphilias is rare, up to 80% of sexual murderers have a history of paraphilic behaviours. Rates of paraphilias in sex offenders are reported to be much higher than for general populations, varying between 25% and 75%, depending on the study.

Aetiology

The origins of most paraphilias are thought to lie in the aberrant development of: (a) sexual and gender identity, (b) erotic object choice, (c) interpersonal closeness, and (d) negative affect management. Most paraphilic perpetrators lack the capacity to make effective and intimate adult relationships, and experience fear and hostility in the context of sexual arousal. Contempt and derogation for vulnerability, both their own distress and that of their victims, is common. Different aetiological models have different emphases, including psychoanalytic, social learning, cognitive behavioural, cultural, feminist, attachment, evolutionary, and biological theories, emphasizing genetic and neurodevelopmental factors.

Most of the research into the aetiology of paraphilias has been in relation to paedophilia and associated abuse of children. Empirical studies of men (and women) who abuse children have found that they have greater attachment difficulties, social incompetence, emotional dysregulation, and disinhibition caused by empathy deficits, compared to non-abusive populations. Sexual abusers of children frequently report histories of abuse themselves as children at higher levels than are reported in the general population (40–50%, as compared to 10–20%). They also report higher levels of substance misuse, and neurodevelopmental abnormalities appear to be commoner, although these studies are affected by detection sampling bias and the tendency of detected offenders to report potentially mitigating problems and vulnerabilities. Studies of sexual abusers of children are also complicated by evidence that not all such abusers meet the criteria for paedophilia, in terms of their sexual interest in children. There is also evidence that incestuous abusers of children may differ from abusers of children who are not related to them.

More recent multifactorial theories propose multiple pathways to paraphilic offending, based on different clusters of clinical problems which are also associated with particular risk factors for offending. These clusters include intimacy and social skills deficits, cognitive distortions, emotional dysregulation, distorted sexual scripts manifesting in atypical and deviant sexual fantasies and arousal, and sex offences associated with more general criminality.

The psychodynamic model of paraphilias complements and adds meaning to a neurodevelopmental model of paraphilias by considering notions of defence and conflict. In the psychoanalytic tradition, paraphilias are subsumed under the concept of 'perversions'. The term 'perversion' refers to both aberrant sexual behaviours, but also perverse character traits and modes of relating to others. Freud's early theories described perversion as infantile sexual instincts that had escaped repression and developed as a defence against castration anxiety. On this account, perverse states of mind and behaviours may be seen as a sexualized defence against unresolved hostility and psychotic anxieties, particularly those concerning emotional intimacy. All perverse activities contain aspects of hostility, secrecy, collusion, and self-deception that may not be conscious. In many cases of perversion, the unresolved hostility relates to childhood sexual trauma, usually at the hands of a caregiver or trusted attachment figure (see ➔ Psychoanalytic psychotherapy in Chapter 2, pp. 20–30).

Treatment
(See ➔ Forensic psychiatry: forensic psychotherapies, applications, and research in Chapter 12, pp. 550–6.)

General treatment principles
Individuals with paraphilias may initially present to mental health services with other mental disorders, such as anxiety, depression, or substance misuse, and may be reluctant to report paraphilic behaviours, due to their illegality or associated feelings of shame and low self-worth. Co-morbid disorders should be appropriately treated; however, clinicians should be aware that apparent treatment resistance may be due to undisclosed paraphilias. Issues of risk, confidentiality, and disclosure should be carefully considered, and an opinion from a forensic psychiatrist may be sought, if there is any indication of criminal rule breaking or a likely identifiable victim. Current GMC guidance should be consulted, if it appears that a child is presently at risk.

Paraphilias may occasionally be a feature of psychotic illness or organic mental disorders, resulting in disinhibition and lack of impulse control. This may occur after brain injury or in the context of dementia, or learning difficulties and developmental conditions such as an autistic spectrum disorder. In these contexts, the paraphilia needs to be managed in the context of these primary conditions, and again with reference to identified victims and risk management. In such cases, there may be a role for neuropharmacological treatments that reduce sexual arousal and libido, such as cyproterone acetate, or luteinizing hormone-releasing hormone (LHRH) agonists such as tryptorelin and goserelin. Some antidepressants, such as the SSRIs, have been shown to reduce recidivism and may be indicated for individuals who experience a strong compulsive element to their paraphilic sexual urges.

Psychological therapies are the main form of treatment for paraphilias. These offer individuals an enhanced sense of agency and well-being, as opposed to simple repression of behaviours. They also offer individuals an opportunity to be involved in their own risk management and take responsibility for their risk. Psychological therapies typically explore the thoughts, feelings, and values associated with the paraphilia for the perpetrator.

Cognitive behavioural therapies
(See → Cognitive behavioural therapy in Chapter 2, pp. 30–4, and in Chapter 5, pp. 172–84.)

Most research on the treatment of paraphilias has focused on group cognitive behavioural interventions for identified sex offenders, typically as part of a Sex Offender Treatment Programme (SOTP) for child sex offenders and rapists. Other interventions include social skills training, cognitive restructuring, development of victim empathy, imaginal desensitization, and behavioural modification techniques such as covert desensitization and minimal arousal conditioning to reduce deviant sexual arousal. Relapse prevention therapy programmes specifically for sex offenders have also been developed from CBT principles. Programmes that adhere to the 'risk–need–responsivity' (RNR) principles show the largest reductions in sexual and general recidivism.

More recent therapeutic programmes for sex offenders focus less on victim empathy and more on evidence-based dynamic factors such as intimacy, attachment, emotional regulation, and impulsivity, as well as promoting the therapeutic relationship. The Good Lives Model (GLM) has gained increasing prominence in sexual offender rehabilitation programmes and is a strengths-based approach which aims to equip offenders with the skills necessary to satisfy basic human values in personally meaningful and socially acceptable ways.

Overall, CBT programmes appear to offer a modest reduction in recidivism in men who sexually offend against children who are strangers to them. There is less convincing evidence that such programmes are effective for sexual sadists (usually convicted of rape offences) or other types of paraphilia.

Psychodynamic therapy
(See → Psychoanalytic psychotherapy in Chapter 2, pp. 20–30, and in Chapter 5, pp. 163–72.)

Very few empirical studies have examined the efficacy of psychodynamic psychotherapy for paraphilias. However, psychoanalysts and psychodynamic psychotherapists have long been interested in understanding and treating abnormal sexual fantasies and behaviours. Many patients with paraphilias describe premature sexualization via experiences of overt childhood sexual abuse or exposure to disturbing pornography in early adolescence. Such premature sexualization interferes with the normal sexual developmental trajectory, and sexual impulses may become confused with aggressive impulses arising from prior experiences of maltreatment or neglect. Paraphilic fantasies often emerge in adolescence as an escape from painful feelings and traumatic experiences, and may progress to being enacted in paraphilic behaviours, which may eventually become habitual and dominate the person's social and interpersonal relationships. Many patients with paraphilias describe a very disturbed sense of self, in which feelings of self-disgust, shame, and humiliation predominate. The paraphilic act bestows a powerful sense of excitement, control, and triumph, which may act as an antidote to feelings of helplessness, powerlessness, or inadequacy.

Psychodynamic treatment aims to explore the meaning of the patient's paraphilic behaviours and fantasies in relation to his history and current interpersonal relationships. The focus is on understanding the paraphilia(s) as defending against underlying, often unconscious, anxieties and aggressive impulses, especially around intimacy, paying particular attention to how the patient's perverse modes of relating may become manifest in the dynamics of the therapeutic relationship or transference/countertransference arena. For example, an exhibitionist's narcissistic wish to be the centre of attention may become manifest by the patient trying to impress or excite the therapist, whereas patients presenting with voyeuristic activities may be experienced by the therapist, or other patients in a group, as reluctant to reveal much about themselves but obtaining perverse gratification from hearing about others' intimate difficulties.

Psychodynamic treatment may be delivered in the form of individual, group, or couple therapy. Group psychotherapy may be considered the treatment of choice for patients whose paraphilic activities involve secretiveness and deception such as perpetrators of paedophilic sexual abuse. Here, a group can more effectively challenge and penetrate the pervasive patterns of deception, often not entirely conscious, that characterize the person's way of relating to himself and others (see → Group therapy and group analysis in Chapter 2, pp. 42–7, and in Chapter 5, pp. 188–94.)

Service provision

There are few specialized services for the treatment of paraphilias, and many individuals with paraphilias are only referred for treatment after they have offended. The majority of treatment services available for people convicted of offences related to paraphilias are located within the criminal justice system as SOTPs. These programmes are usually based on cognitive behavioural and RNR principles and delivered via group therapy, and focus primarily on the reduction of risk or rates of recidivism, rather than improvements in mental health. Some forensic mental health services offer specialized sex offender treatment services, but provision across the country is patchy.

Specific treatment services within the NHS for patients with paraphilias that do not result in offending are even more limited. Some may be treated in psychosexual clinics, others within general psychology and psychotherapy departments. A few may be referred to specialized forensic psychotherapy services such as the Portman Clinic in London, an NHS specialist psychoanalytically oriented forensic psychotherapy outpatient clinic.

Recommended reading

Glasser M (1996). Aggression and sadism in the perversions. In: Rosen I (ed). *Sexual Deviation*, third edition. Oxford University Press: Oxford.

Laws R and O'Donohue WT (eds) (2008). *Sexual Deviance: Theory, Assessment and Treatment*. Guilford Press: New York.

Yakeley J and Wood H (2014). Paraphilias and paraphilic disorders: guidance on diagnosis, assessment and management. *Advances in Psychiatric Treatment*, **20**, 202–13.

Trauma-related conditions

Diagnosis

Many psychiatric and psychotherapy patients will have a significant history of trauma in their development. There is considerable evidence that developmental trauma increases the risk of a wide variety of psychiatric conditions in adult life, including depression, anxiety, PTSD, BPD, and ASPD.

This chapter focuses on those conditions in which the experience of trauma is required to make the diagnosis and a particular symptom profile linked to the trauma is present. These conditions are:

- Acute stress disorder (ASD)
- PTSD
- Persistent complex grief disorder
- Complex trauma.

DSM-5 describes the first three disorders. It also includes adjustment disorders where a stressor causes marked distress and/or significant impairment within 3 months which generally resolves within 6 months of the stressor resolving. Current plans for ICD-11 will include all of these diagnoses. There are differences in the criteria required for PTSD between the two classificatory systems, with DSM-5 including, as a core element, disturbances in cognitions and affect. What impact this will have on the research in this area is still unclear, although one preliminary study in Australia looking at ICD-10 versus DSM-5 suggests that the narrower criteria in ICD-11 will reduce the prevalence rates. The phenotype for research in the future may be markedly different, according to the diagnostic system used.

Prevalence

ASD prevalence varies with the nature of the event and the context in which it is assessed. The rate is higher (20–50%), following interpersonal traumatic events such as an assault or rape, compared with events that do not involve interpersonal assault such as motor vehicle accidents (13–21%). Recovery for the majority appears rapid when prospective studies are reviewed. A study describing ASD symptoms in New Yorkers after the September 11 attack found that they reduced from 7.5% at 1 month to 1.6% at 4 months and 0.6% at 6 months. This has important treatment implications in these early stages.

Approximately 50% of individuals will be exposed to at least one traumatic event in their lifetime. Approximately 8% of survivors will develop PTSD. In the USA, the lifetime prevalence rates are found to be 8.7%. The 12-month prevalence rates in the USA are around 3.5%. Lower estimates are seen in Europe and most Asian, African, and Latin American countries, clustering around 0.5–1%. Rates of PTSD are higher in veterans and those vocations where traumatic exposure is increased, e.g. firefighters, police, etc. Highest rates (up to 50% of those exposed) are amongst survivors of rape, genocide, military combat, and captivity. Estimates of PTSD prevalence amongst refugee groups vary widely, with studies reporting rates ranging from 4% (Vietnamese refugees) to

79–86% (Cambodian refugees). The lifetime prevalence for PTSD for a woman (10.4%) is more than twice that for men, despite the fact that men are more likely to experience trauma than women.

The prevalence for persistent complex grief disorder is approximately 2.4% to 4.8%. The disorder is more prevalent in women than men. Complex trauma prevalence rates remain elusive, partly because it is a diagnosis yet to be given formal status within a psychiatric classification.

Treatment of acute stress reactions/debriefing

NICE guidelines in the UK suggest that, in the initial phases after a trauma, one should adopt a stance of 'watchful waiting'. This is in essence a programme of psycho-education with the recommendation to make use of current support networks. Formal psychological interventions targeted at everyone involved in traumatic events have been shown to be ineffective. Some studies have reported negative outcomes in people who receive single-episode, individual critical incident debriefing. This has led NICE to recommend that this kind of intervention should not be used.

Complex early interventions have been studied and are generally variations on the CBT models used in PTSD treatment. These are usually initiated 1 to 3 months after the event and are often shorter in duration.

Treatment for post-traumatic stress disorder

ICD-11 proposes a definition of:

> 'A disorder that develops following exposure to an extremely threatening or horrific event or series of events characterized by: (1) re-experiencing the traumatic event(s) in the present in the form of vivid intrusive memories accompanied by fear or horror, flashbacks, or nightmares; (2) avoidance of thoughts and memories of the event(s) or avoidance of activities or situations reminiscent of the event(s); and (3) a state of perceived current threat in the form of excessive hyper-vigilance or enhanced startle reactions. The symptoms must last for at least several weeks and cause significant impairment in functioning.'

DSM-5 has re-experiencing, avoidance, and hyperarousal categories that are similar, but it also includes negative alterations in cognitions and mood associated with the traumatic event as a separate category.

Psychological interventions having the best evidence for the treatment of PTSD are the trauma-focused therapies of trauma-focused CBT (tf-CBT) and EMDR. Both are individual treatments usually provided over a course of up to 12 to 16 sessions.

The cognitive behavioural approach to treatment has a number of intervention models that focus, to a greater or lesser degree, on the behavioural and cognitive components. More behavioural emphasis suggests that the original traumatic event results in a learned association of the emotional trauma that has occurred with the stimuli of the event. Future encounters with these triggers activate the traumatic experience, resulting in increased anxiety. Thus, exposure with response prevention is necessary where exposure involves re-experiencing the images for long enough that the patient habituates to the fear response and avoidance is prevented. Cognitive techniques address the dysfunctional beliefs that have arisen through the episode and work on cognitive restructuring. Ehlers and Clark (2000) describe a tf-CBT model that incorporates a number of specific interventions reflecting three targets of treatment: elaborating and integrating the trauma memory, modifying problematic appraisals, and dropping dysfunctional behavioural and cognitive strategies (see ➜ Cognitive behavioural therapy in Chapter 2, pp. 30–4, and in Chapter 5, pp. 172–84).

EMDR was developed by Shapiro (1989) and requires the patient to evoke an image of events causing them anxiety, whilst tracking the therapist's finger as it is moved rapidly and rhythmically from side to side (or other forms of bilateral stimulation such as sound or tapping). At the same time, they generate cognitive coping statements. EMDR is said to facilitate rapid, adaptive, associative information processing by integrating sensations, affects, and self-attributes. Although there is good evidence for the efficacy of EMDR, when contrasted to wait-list or non-specific treatments, within-trial contrast against exposure does not suggest any gains in relation to efficacy. Whilst dismantling studies that examine the mutative value of the eye movements do not support this theory, they all include a distraction technique and do not disprove the notion that there is a benefit to combining exposure with redirection of attention.

There is limited evidence for the efficacy of psychodynamic techniques in the treatment of PTSD. Most studies are case reports or open trials, and most of the trials have methodological problems and thus contribute to an equivocal picture. However, in an early RCT in 1989, the effects of psychodynamic therapy, behavioural therapy, and hypnotherapy were studied. All of the treatments proved to be equally effective. These results are consistent with a more recent meta-analysis that found no significant differences between bona fide treatments of PTSD.

Psychodynamic treatment models for PTSD focus on the meaning of the event for that individual, recognizing the links that may occur at an unconscious level with earlier traumatic experiences. This may then be re-enacted in the transference with the therapist through the repetition compulsion. Thus, working in the transference enables an elaboration of the meaning at an unconscious level. Recognizing that all trauma involves loss, and thus requires mourning, allows for an understanding of how mourning may be defended against and the impact of this on the mind (see ➜ Psychoanalytic psychotherapy in Chapter 2, pp. 20–30, and in Chapter 5, pp. 163–72; Loss in Chapter 6, pp. 298–300).

A number of other therapies may be used for particular symptom management in PTSD, often to allow stabilization before trauma focused-work can be used. These include using mindfulness, yoga, neuro-feedback, or relaxation therapies for hyperarousal. Various body-focused therapies have also been used, as well as energy psychology.

Treatment for persistent complex grief disorder

ICD-11 proposes a definition of:

'A disturbance in which, following the death of a person close to the bereaved, there is a persistent and pervasive yearning or longing for the deceased, or a persistent preoccupation with the deceased that extends for an abnormally prolonged period beyond expected or cultural norms and this is sufficiently severe to cause significant impairment in functioning. The response can also be characterised by difficulties accepting the death, feeling one has lost a part of oneself, anger about the loss, guilt or difficulty engaging with social or other activities.'

Although there has been some controversy over this new category in DSM-5, and the proposed one for ICD-11 linked to a concern of pathologizing grief, there is evidence of reliability and validity of the diagnosis, distinct from depression or PTSD.

An RCT conducted in 1990 showed that short-term psychodynamic group therapy was significantly superior to a waiting list. In a second RCT study in 2001, the same researchers looked at psychodynamic group therapy and found a significant interaction. For grief symptoms, patients with a high quality of object relations improved more with interpretive therapy, whilst patients with a low quality of object relations improved more with supportive therapy (see ➔ Psychoanalytic psychotherapy in Chapter 2, pp. 20–30, and in Chapter 5, pp. 163–72; Group therapy and group analysis in Chapter 2, pp. 42–7, and in Chapter 5, pp. 188–94).

Treatment for complex trauma

ICD-11 defines complex trauma as:

'A disorder which arises after exposure to a stressor typically of an extreme or prolonged nature and from which escape is difficult or impossible. The disorder is characterized by the core symptoms of PTSD as well as the development of persistent and pervasive impairments in affective, self and relational functioning, including difficulties in emotion regulation, beliefs about oneself as diminished, defeated or worthless, and difficulties in sustaining relationships.'

The clinical picture thus entails PTSD core features alongside affect dysregulation, somatization, dissociation, revictimization, and identity disturbance. This diagnosis would include many traumatized refugees and asylum seekers, as well as victims of domestic violence or other situations of repeated or prolonged trauma or captivity. It may also include victims of childhood physical and sexual abuse.

The absence of complex trauma as a diagnosis until ICD-11 has meant that research into treatment is limited. Many different treatment modalities have been described with this group, including CBT, EMDR, psychodynamic and psychoanalytic adaptations, narrative exposure therapy, and body-focused therapies. However, the different treatment modalities tend to have a number of common themes. CBT therapists describe three stages in treatment: stabilization, trauma-focused treatment, and reintegration. A psychodynamic approach emphasizes safety, remembrance and mourning, and reconnection. Thus, the therapeutic alliance is emphasized in the first stage, trauma work in its different forms, and then reconnection with the external world.

Treatment of complex trauma in asylum seekers and refugees, in particular, also requires close attention to the psychosocial factors that may limit engagement. Thus, the early phase of safety and stabilization may require considerable psychosocial intervention, attending to status, housing, finances, and occupational and educational needs.

Psychoanalytic and psychodynamic therapies stress the need to attend to the often difficult transference and countertransference experiences in working with complex trauma patients, linked to unconscious repetition of previous traumatic experiences enacted in the therapeutic space. Coupled with this is the frequency of dissociation as a part of the presentation, which may require adaptations such as CBT grounding techniques.

Many therapeutic approaches emphasize the importance of the narrative and link this to the need to change traumatic memories from the procedural to the declarative memory system. This enables emotional processing of the fear/trauma structure or, put in a psychoanalytic frame, it enables symbolic functioning, to bring words to what has been nameless terror.

Clearly, more research is essential in this area to elucidate evidence-based treatments that address the complexity of this presentation. With the advent of inclusion in ICD-11 imminent, this will pave the way for a better recognition of the diagnosis and appropriate research.

Recommended reading

Benish S, Imel Z, and Wampold B (2008). The relative efficacy of bona fide psychotherapies for treating post traumatic stress disorder: a meta analysis of direct comparisons. *Clinical Psychology Review*, **28**, 746–58.

Ehlers A and Clark DM (2000). A cognitive model of post-traumatic stress disorder. *Behavioural Research and Therapy*, **38**, 319–45.

Garland C (ed) (1998). *Understanding Trauma: A Psychoanalytic Approach*. Tavistock Book Series: London.

Herman J (1992). *Trauma and Recovery*. Basic Books: New York.

Shapiro F (1989). Efficacy of the eye movement desensitisation procedure in the treatment of traumatic memories. *Journal of Traumatic Stress Studies*, **2**, 199–223.

Medically unexplained symptoms

Introduction

'Medically unexplained symptoms' (MUS) is not a diagnosis, but a convenient way of bringing together patients with medically unexplained symptoms. Such patients are difficult to manage and costly, and often have other psychiatric co-morbidities. They often attract negative responses from doctors and others in the caring professions. However, a growing body of empirical evidence supporting the efficacy for various different types of psychological therapy for patients with MUS has encouraged the development of specific services in both primary and secondary care, offering treatment for this 'hard-to-treat' population.

What is/are medically unexplained symptom(s)?

Freud and Breuer, in their *Studies on Hysteria* (1895), described case studies of patients, their physicians, and their families struggling with sometimes seemingly un-understandable phenomena that did not conform to any identifiable anatomy or pathology and appeared or disappeared seemingly at random. Some of such phenomena we may now call MUS. In this work, Freud developed his thoughts on a number of important psychoanalytic concepts, including catharsis, repression, and free association, as well as sexuality, symbolism, and transference, and remained interested in the importance of the body and bodily symptoms throughout his working life. This tradition—of working to understand the problematic relationship between body and mind—has continued in multiple traditions, including the psychoanalytic (e.g. in the work of Winnicott in the UK, and Aisenstein in France), the applied psychoanalytic (e.g. Brook, Guthrie), cognitive behavioural (e.g. Wessely, White, Chalder), and systemic (e.g. Launer) models (see ➲ Psychoanalytic psychotherapy in Chapter 2, pp. 20–30; Cognitive behavioural therapy in Chapter 2, pp. 30–4; Systematic family and couple therapy in Chapter 2, pp. 34–42).

MUS is not a typical psychiatric diagnosis, in that it describes medical phenomena, with no reference to the mind. In DSM-IV (APA, 1994), which is explicitly 'atheoretical', the criteria for the diagnosis of somatization disorder (SD) were entirely behavioural, with no concept of psychiatric phenomenology, of states of mind, let alone emotions. DSM-5 continues with this atheoretical stance, whilst widening the scope and introducing two new diagnoses (see later text).

Indeed, John Launer, a GP and systemic psychotherapist, has persuasively described a different decoding of MUS, closer conceptually to that of psychotherapists, describing MUS as 'medically unexplained stories', personal narratives requiring exploration.

In recent years, the term 'MUS' has taken over in popularity from other terms, such as 'hysteria', 'somatization', and 'somatoform disorders', and remains rooted in a mode of thinking derived from Cartesian dualism, i.e. a schism between mind and body. The other term, often posited as the 'opposite' is 'long-term conditions' (LTCs)—here, there is 'organic damage' to tissues and organs such as in diabetes mellitus or chronic obstructive pulmonary disease. Politicians, health economists, and researchers endeavour to differentiate between those with MUS and those with LTCs, yet, for many patients, the distinction is not tidy or clear-cut; patients often straddle both terms or oscillate between them over the years.

This Cartesian dualism was reflected in the DSM-IV classification. If no disease was found in the body, it was assumed that it was all in the mind and that symptoms that are medically unexplained were considered, by default, to be 'psychiatrically explained'. The DSM-IV classification reflected this view, with 'somatoform disorders' having, as their central concept, 'medically unexplained symptoms', and the key somatoform diagnosis 'somatization disorder' (SD) based on counting a number of MUS. MUS and SD may describe phenomena, but they explain nothing. DSM-5 contains many revisions, but few are as sweeping as those involving somatoform disorders. In the updated edition, hypochondriasis and several related conditions have been replaced by two new, empirically derived concepts: somatic symptom disorder and illness anxiety disorder.

Prevalence of medically unexplained symptoms

The prevalence of MUS is variable, depending on definition, social class, gender, age, ethnicity, and location, including primary care or secondary/tertiary care.

In a study of UK general hospital patients published in 2001, MUS were found to be common across general/internal medicine and represented the commonest diagnosis in some specialties, with the highest prevalence in gynaecology clinics (66%). MUS were associated with being female, younger, and currently employed. Those with MUS were less disabled, but more likely to use alternative treatments, in comparison with those whose symptoms were medically explained.

An American study from primary care found that 14 common physical symptoms were responsible for almost half of all primary care visits and that only about 10% to 15% of these symptoms were caused by an organic illness over a 1-year period. The study concluded that patients with MUS were frequently frustrating to primary care physicians and utilized medical visits and costs disproportionately.

Co-morbidity

Patients fulfilling criteria for SD, often overlapping with those with MUS, frequently suffer from co-morbid psychiatric conditions. A recent study from South Africa showed that a co-morbid depressive disorder was present in 29.4% of patients, and a current co-morbid anxiety disorder in 52.9%. Patients with a co-morbid depressive disorder (current or lifetime) had significantly higher physical symptom counts, greater functional impairment, higher unemployment rates, more clinician-reported difficulties, and more dissatisfaction with health-care services than those without the disorder. A larger number of co-morbid disorders was associated with greater overall disability. Co-morbidity is frequent and shown repeatedly across countries and cultures (see ➔ Anxiety and anxiety disorders in Chapter 7, pp. 324–6; Affective disorders in Chapter 7, pp. 326–31).

Personality pathology has been shown to be highly prevalent in SD, with one study showing a prevalence of 72% patients with SD having a co-morbid personality disorder, compared with 36% of controls. Certain personality disorders, including passive–aggressive, histrionic, and dependent, occurred significantly more often in the SD patients than controls (see ➔ Chapter 8).

Criticisms of the concept

The changes in DSM-5 have been described as a paradigm shift, and criticized as being overly broad and likely to lead to increased mental health diagnoses in the medically ill. In particular, the new diagnosis of 'somatic symptom disorder' is included, based not on MUS, but on the reporting of bothersome and persistent somatic symptoms, accompanied by an excessive psychological response. Thus, this new diagnosis could be given to both MUS and somatic symptoms 'explained' by a diagnosis such as cancer. The implications are that psychiatrists may well have a wider role for the management of these patients, to include those with severely troublesome symptoms from any cause. Some argue that this will lead to better detection and management of previously underdiagnosed psychological co-morbidity, whilst others argue that patients will be stigmatized by the presence of a psychiatric diagnosis unnecessarily.

Psychological therapies for medically unexplained symptoms

Many different modalities of psychological therapy are on offer, and there is growing research evidence supporting some such therapies.

Psychodynamic models

(See ➔ Psychoanalytic psychotherapy in Chapter 2, pp. 20–30, and in Chapter 5, pp. 163–72.)

A recent review of RCTs for somatoform disorders showed evidence for the effectiveness of psychodynamic psychotherapy in the treatment of irritable bowel syndrome, chronic functional dyspepsia, gastrointestinal symptoms, chronic pain, and multisomatoform disorders. A recent meta-analysis on the effectiveness of psychotherapy for severe somatoform disorder showed that psychotherapy was more effective than treatment as usual in severe somatoform disorder, particularly in terms of reduction of physical symptoms and functional impairment. Psychodynamic interventions were more effective in improving functioning than cognitive interventions, although not in improving symptoms, suggesting that other forms of psychotherapy, besides CBT, are potentially effective for severe SD. Overall, older patients benefit less than younger ones, and women improve more than men with regard to physical symptoms.

A service which uses predominantly brief dynamic models of therapy in the treatment of MUS patients in primary care is a service operating in Hackney, East London (UK): the Primary Care Psychotherapy and Consultation Service (PCPCS), as part of the Tavistock and Portman NHS Trust. A recent health economics research evaluation of the PCPCS showed that, for the 141 MUS patients studied, an average of £425/patient was saved by the PCPCS intervention, representing 32% of the treatment cost. The intervention, using the concept of 'quality-adjusted life-year' (QALY), was adjudged to be one which would be considered cost-effective by NICE.

Cognitive behavioural models

(See ➔ Cognitive behavioural therapy in Chapter 2, pp. 30–4, and in Chapter 5, pp. 172–84.)

The cognitive behavioural (CBT) model has been studied in many conditions, with chronic fatigue syndrome (CFS) being an example. An important research paper comparing CBT, adaptive pacing therapy (APT), graded exercise therapy (GET), and specialist medical care (SMC) for CFS is a good example of the work (White *et al.* 2013), indicating that CBT and GET can safely be added to SMC to 'moderately improve outcomes' for CFS, but that APT was not an effective addition.

Mentalization models

(See ➔ Mentalization-based treatment in Chapter 2, pp. 66–70, and in Chapter 5, pp. 229–34; Dynamic interpersonal therapy in Chapter 2, pp. 61–63, and in Chapter 5, pp. 215–20.)

Luyten, Lemma, Target, and colleagues have written convincingly about attachment, personality, and (embodied) mentalization in functional somatic syndromes (FSS), and are gathering data regarding the efficacy of DIT in patients with MUS.

Reattribution model

This model involves four stages. The first stage requires the GP to take a full history of the patient's symptoms, to listen to their story of how they developed, and to carry out a focused physical examination. In stage two, information is fed back to the patient, including the results of any physical examination, and acknowledging the worry and concern caused by symptoms. In the third stage, the doctor links the patient's symptoms to appropriate psychosocial issues, using a normalization approach, and provides a credible aetiological mechanism. Finally, the doctor discusses and negotiates with the patient possible treatment or management options.

Reattribution techniques have been evaluated in a small number of RCTs in primary care involving patients with MUS. One recent study reported on a definitive cluster RCT of reattribution training for GPs involving 16 practices and 70 GPs. All GPs recruited to the reattribution limb completed training and found it helpful. This suggests that reattribution is acceptable to GPs, and training can be delivered to whole practices.

Responses from health-care practitioners

MUS patients are often resistant to receiving psychological therapy, irrespective of modality, especially if they perceive the offer as an indication that the reality of their physical symptoms is not believed by their doctors. They often attract negative responses from health-care professionals, which can take the form of pejorative comments, over- or under-investigation, inappropriate discharge from services, and the like, often very similar to the responses evoked by patients with personality disorder diagnoses. In many cases, consultative work with GPs and other health care professionals, which may help their negative countertransference and propensity for ordering excessive investigations and tests, may be of as much, if not more, help as the offer of therapy to a patient who is determined to see his/her symptoms are purely 'physical'. Many modern services designed to work with MUS patients (e.g. the PCPCS service mentioned earlier) will have, as part of the service specification, work to help empower, educate, and support GPs.

Recommended reading

Carrington A, Rock B, and Stern J (2012). Psychoanalytic thinking in primary care: the Tavistock Psychotherapy Consultation model. *Psychoanalytic Psychotherapy*, **26**, 102–20.

Freud S and Breuer E (1895). *Studies in Hysteria*. Basic Books Classics.

Koelen J, Houtveen J, Abass A, et al. (2014). Effectiveness of psychotherapy for severe somatoform disorder: a meta-analysis. *British Journal of Psychiatry*, **204**, 12–19.

Parsonage M, Rock B, and Hard E (2014). *Managing Patients with Complex Needs*. Centre for Mental Health: London.

White PD, Goldsmith K, Johnson AL, Chalder T, and Sharpe M (2013). Recovery from chronic fatigue syndrome after treatments given in the PACE trial. *Psychological Medicine*, **43**, 2227–35.

Gender dysphoria and intersex conditions

(See ➜ Sexual dysfunction in Chapter 7, pp. 345–9, and Paraphilias in Chapter 7, pp. 349–54.)

The term gender dysphoria is used in DSM-5 to refer to persons whose gender identity does not correspond to that of their sex at birth. The term replaces gender identity disorder which was used in DSM-IV. Whilst gender identity disorder appeared alongside sexual disorders and paraphilias in DSM-IV, gender dysphoria appears in DSM-5 as a section on its own. The dysphoria refers to a deep sense of unhappiness experienced by the person in relation to their gender. Gender dysphoria is a condition which may affect children, adolescents, and adults, and must be present for at least 6 months for a diagnosis to be made. Prevalence rates vary according to differing studies, but it is estimated at around 20 per 100000 in the UK, with the ratio of biological males to biological females as 5:1. The aetiology of gender dysphoria is unknown at present. No biological factors have consistently been identified, and, despite numerous psychological and social theories being described over time, it is most probably that a combination of biological, psychological, and social factors all play contributory roles.

Not all people with gender dysphoria are transsexual. Whilst physical treatments (hormones and sex reassignment surgery) may be useful for transsexual patients with a fixed and binary gender identity, they are less helpful for those with more atypical gender identity conditions. Patients with gender identities, which are less fixed and have a tendency to change, are unsuitable for long-term or permanent physical interventions such as hormones or surgery. Those with more fluid gender identity conditions, which do not conform to a binary male/female gender framework, may not be appropriate for binary sex reassignment procedures. For such atypical gender identity patients, a specialist application of psychotherapy may be clinically more useful.

Such psychotherapy may be useful for a number of allied conditions, including those in whom the initial presentation is uncertain, such as patients who are unsure as to whether they are transsexual or transvestites.

Conditions treated

- Gender dysphoria (dissatisfaction/confusion in relation to gender)
- Atypical gender identity disorders
- 'Post-op regretters': transsexuals who have had surgery but no longer identify with 'trans' identity
- Dual-role transvestism (cross-dressing without wish to change sex)
- Fetishistic transvestism (cross-dressing associated with sexual excitement)
- Autogynaephilia (biological males with the sexual fantasy of having female sex organs)
- Autoandrophilia (biological females with the sexual fantasy of having male sex organs).

Specialist psychotherapy services for gender identity and intersex conditions

At present, psychotherapy services dedicated to patients with gender dysphoria are limited. Gender dysphoria remains outside of the clinical experience of many psychotherapists who often find themselves under-/over-attending to the condition where it presents. Counselling exists in many gender identity clinics, but often this is limited only to helping those patients undergoing gender reassignment to acclimatize to their chosen (usually binary) gender role, rather than an exploratory type of psychotherapy aimed at those with differing forms of gender dysphoria, for whom gender reassignment may not be an option or goal.

The outpatient specialist psychotherapy service for patients with gender identity conditions and also the specialist psychotherapy service for people with intersex conditions described here are currently unique services and are provided by the Priory Hospital Roehampton as an independent provider to the NHS. The services are open to referrals from patients across the entire UK and further if the patient is able to attend for therapy.

Aims of a specialist gender identity psychotherapy service are
- To facilitate understanding of gender and how it relates to themselves and others (e.g. what do they mean by 'always felt female'? Male/female are not feelings)
- To reduce the degree of preoccupation and accompanying distress and unhappiness associated with their gender conflict or confusion
- To enable the person to come to a specifically tailored gender identity, which they feel to be relevant to them, and help them to achieve a degree of stability in that gender identity.

Aims of gender identity psychotherapy ARE NOT
- To persuade/encourage persons to undergo gender reassignment
- To dissuade/discourage persons from undergoing physical interventions for gender reassignment (hormones/surgery)
- To help people to appear or behave or 'pass' as a certain gender.

Delivery of therapy
- *Assessment*: ascertain the type of gender identity condition, associated conditions relating to sex, gender, and sexuality, patient personal history and context of gender presentation, and any additional mental health problems.
- *1:1 sessions*: the patient is seen on an individual basis by the therapist who is later to be their group therapist in order to build a rapport before eventually joining the weekly group.
- *Group*: weekly slow-open group dedicated to patients with some form of gender identity condition.

Specially adapted therapeutic model
(See ➲ Group therapy and group analysis in Chapter 2, pp. 42–7, and in Chapter 5, pp. 188–94; Mentalization-based treatment in Chapter 2, pp. 66–70, and in Chapter 5, pp. 229–34.)
This comprises elements of group analytic psychotherapy and MBT in a slow-open small group (approximately eight patients) with one therapist.

Patients in the group may have any condition relating to their sense of gender identity and would have undergone an assessment and a period of individual sessions with the group conductor prior to their joining the group. Therapeutic interventions are directed to individuals within the group, in addition to the group as a whole. Any member of the group, including the conductor, and not merely the conductor alone, may offer therapeutic interventions to any member of the group or to the group itself. It is up to the conductor to maintain the therapeutic setting and boundaries and to ensure that the subject of gender is mentalized with the group. Patients would typically remain in the group for 2 years.

MBT-Gender: mentalizing gender

Preconceived ideas or notions of gender offered by any of the patients in therapy are open to be considered, questioned, and examined by the therapist or the group. Examples include what it means to be a male or female and what a person means by 'masculine' or 'feminine': 'I was very 'girly' as a boy . . .', 'I like wearing very feminine clothes . . .', 'I used to like boys sports . . .'

The group are discouraged from making assumptions in relation to gender, in terms of emotions, behaviour, or appearances, and are encouraged to consider a more diverse heterogeneous spectrum within gender and discouraged from restricting themselves to caricatured gender stereotypes.

Qualities of the therapist

The therapist must have the following qualities:
- Comfortable working with persons with an array of sex/gender presentations, including those who have undergone physical sex reassignment interventions
- Open-minded and accepting of persons with differing and diverse identities relating to their sex, gender, and/or sexuality
- Their understanding of gender should not be limited to binary identities or caricatured stereotypes, but be familiar with more atypical/fluid/non-binary gender identities
- Familiar with running therapy groups
- Familiar with the principles of MBT.

Common themes: 'parallel processes'

The following themes have been observed, when running a specialist gender identity psychotherapy service. The themes were observed in:
- The patients having therapy
- The therapeutic process itself/in the therapist
- As a dynamic within the organization delivering the therapy
- As an organizational dynamic between organizations involved with the gender patient.

The observed themes were as follows.

Binary rigidity (examples)
- Patients' rigid understanding of gender roles
- Patients switching between binary gender identities during the therapy

- Professionals being drawn into adversarial stances of 'for' or 'against' gender reassignment or mistakenly being perceived as occupying such positions.

Genital centrality (examples)
- 'Everything would be fine if only I had a vagina'
- Clinicians mistakenly believing 'nothing can be done' therapeutically for those who have undergone genital sex reassignment surgery
- Setting up groups for 'pre-op' or 'post-op' patients, rather than mixed groups.

Confusion (examples)
- In the patient: in relation to their identity
- In the therapist whose patient's appearance dramatically changes during the course of therapy
- Which gender pronouns to use
- In the organization: allied professionals not readily able to think about gender identity disorder/complexity.

Questioning of authenticity (examples)
- Concern whether others will perceive them authentically in their chosen gender role
- Patient feeling 'inauthentic' in original gender role, but later feeling similarly inauthentic in the post-operative transgender role
- Professionals questioning the validity of psychotherapy for gender identity patients.

Psychotherapy for intersex conditions

Approximately one in 200 live births can be classified as 'intersex', due to a disorder of sex development, resulting in a variation of physical sex characteristics, including chromosomes, reproductive organs, or body phenotype.

Intersex conditions
- Androgen Insensitivity syndrome (AIS)
- Congenital adrenal hyperplasia (CAH)
- 5-alpha reductase deficiency
- Aphalia
- Cliteromegaly
- Gonadal dysgenesis
- Klinefelter's syndrome
- Turner's syndrome.

It is common for babies known to have an intersex condition to be assigned to a male/female gender at the time of birth, and they may or may not later come to understand their intersex status. Some individuals do not find out about their intersex condition until later on or in adulthood, e.g. when unable to reproduce. Gender dysphoria is an understandable occurrence in people living with an intersex condition.

Psychotherapy in the form of a specialist gender group, similar to that outlined earlier for gender identity disorder, may be offered for persons with intersex conditions. The aim of the group is to enable the intersex person to examine what it means to be any gender at all and to come to a meaningful understanding of their sense of identity. The group may also be the only regular contact the intersex patient has with others who live with an intersex condition and where a sense of isolation may be replaced by peer support, identification, resonance, and mirroring.

Gender identity psychotherapy outcome measure

It is unusual that, in the current climate of evidence-based medicine, outcome studies in relation to gender dysphoria remain very limited, as do suitable outcome measures which may be used to measure success of interventions offered to this patient population. The Gender Preoccupation and Stability Questionnaire (GPSQ) is an outcome measure used to evaluate the effectiveness of any intervention (medical, surgical, therapeutic) offered to patients with gender identity conditions. The GPSQ is currently undergoing reliability and validity studies by Hakeem *et al.* at the University of New South Wales (UNSW).

Recommended reading

Hakeem A (2010). Parallel processes: observed in the patient, therapy and organization. *Group Analysis*, **43**, 141–54.

Hakeem A (2012). Psychotherapy for gender identity disorders. *Advances in Psychiatric Treatment*, **18**, 17–24.

Intellectual disability

Definition of intellectual disability

(See ➔ Psychiatry of intellectual disability: psychotherapies, applications, and research in Chapter 12, pp. 562–4.)

Intellectual disability (ID) is now the adopted term in DSM-5, altered from the term mental retardation used in previous editions of the DSM. The new term aims to improve patient assessment and management, encompassing three domains that mostly describe the condition such as intellectual impairment, difficulties in social functioning, and difficulties in adaptive functioning.

The revised diagnosis maintains that the impairments should be present during the person's early development shown in the addition of intellectual developmental disorder (IDD), appended to intellectual disability. It recognizes that IDD is a chronic disorder with physical and mental health consequences and significant comorbidities.

IQ tests should never be the sole source of the diagnosis of ID, which must always be supplemented by clinical assessments of social and adaptive functioning. Generally, IDD is synonymous with an IQ score below 70, which is approximately two standard deviations below the population mean.

In the UK, the term learning disability is often used interchangeably with intellectual disability.

Prevalence

The prevalence of ID is thought to be approximately 1% based on a recent review of international studies. In the UK, estimates of prevalence are suggested to be at around 2.5% including both mild and severe ID, which probably overestimates prevalence. However, only a minority are known to services at any time. Identification is usually higher during late childhood but decreases sharply following the end of statutory education and is also dependent to an extent upon the socioeconomic status of the family, that is, families of higher means may not use state resources and therefore individuals may not appear in service registers of ID. Gender differences appear more prominent in younger persons with a male to female of 1.5:1. However, this difference appears to dissipate with age.

Mental ill health and IDD

IDD is associated with the presence of a variety of mental and developmental disorders despite the difficulty in diagnosing most of these conditions in people with more severe intellectual impairments. Overall rates of mental disorders range from 40% to 80% depending on study design and population studies. Though there is a dearth of comparative studies of the prevalence of mental disorders in people with IDD and their peers of average intelligence, it is accepted that schizophrenia and psychotic disorders are up to five times more frequent in people with IDD. Other diagnoses include mood disorders, anxiety disorders, OCD, substance related disorders, delirium, dementia and other cognitive disorders, motor disorders, autism spectrum disorder, and attention deficit and disruptive behaviour disorders. It has been shown that in people with mild IDD suicidal ideation and suicidal acts are quite common.

Another important category of disorders often seen in people with IDD are challenging behaviours, which are usually defined as behaviours that may place the individual and others at risk, lead to social exclusion, and may be the result of failure of environments to respond appropriately to a person with IDD. They are found in approximately 20% of people with IDD living in the community, and are of variable severity and frequency. Episodic aggression is the commonest problem which, however, may dissipate with age.

Several chromosomal abnormalities have been associated with the presence of mental disorders, e.g. Prader–Willi syndrome, which is due to deletion of chromosome 15 and is linked to depressive disorder with psychotic symptoms, and deletion of chromosome 22 which is linked to schizophrenia.

Identification of mental disorders in IDD

Diagnosis of any mental disorder in people with IDD can be hampered by communication problems, cultural norms and actual symptom presentation. For example, psychotic symptoms can be identified in cases where developmental milestones have not yet been achieved, as in the case of young adults talking about imaginary friends, or hallucinations may be poorly formed and fleeting. A variety of other conditions may also interfere with ascertaining mental disorders in a person with IDD, such as delirium, epilepsy, sensory impairments, pain, aggression, or other behaviours. Often symptoms may be due to abuse and trauma but can be misidentified as evidence of severe mental illness.

Another issue that may lead to misdiagnosis is that of *diagnostic overshadowing*, a term that denotes the primacy placed on IDD to the detriment of identifying a mental disorder.

Psychological treatments for adults with IDD and mental ill health

The contribution of psychosocial approaches to the management of mental ill health in people with IDD has been controversial and of long standing. The overriding view for many years, leading to therapeutic nihilism, was that people with IDD were unable to participate in and benefit from psychotherapeutic approaches to mental disorders. Behavioural approaches attempting to foster pro-social behaviours became the norm across a variety of developmental disorders, mainly for challenging behaviour, including aggression.

In the present day, both in and outside the UK, several different psychosocial approaches are being considered and delivered to people with at least mild IDD, although for those with more significant impairments, behavioural approaches are mainly considered, as are staff-targeted interventions.

Considered here are current treatments that have been reported in the literature as applied to adults with IDD, including paid and family carer interventions. Such interventions are usually suggested following an assessment of the individual's presenting problems and circumstances and may be delivered in individual or group formats. Interventions can be provided by professionals working in community intellectual disability services or in generic mental health services, e.g. Improving Access to Psychological Therapies (IAPT) services or general practices (see ➲ Improving Access to Psychological Therapies services in Chapter 10, pp. 463–4).

The emphasis is on person-centred care, which promotes resilience and recovery. This is very important as people with IDD may have problems with attachments, learned helplessness, have experienced prolonged adversity and stress, and have deficits in problem solving and social skills. Despite the progress in societal attitudes to disability, people with IDD are still subject to stigma, lack opportunities, remain in social housing, have small social networks, and are more likely to be neglected or abused as recent scandals still attest to.

CBT

(See ➲ Cognitive-behavioural therapy in Chapter 2, pp. 30–4, and in Chapter 5, pp. 172–84.)

CBT is the treatment of choice for uncomplicated mild mood disorders as well as many other disorders. There is considerable literature on its application to people with IDD and a variety of mental disorders and symptoms such as anger, and it can be delivered to individuals and also to groups. The basic skills required are verbal ability at the level of a 10–11 year old, the capacity to recognize and name feelings, and to link feelings with actions and thoughts or beliefs about various situations. There has been significant discussion about the ability of people with IDD to learn appropriate cognitive skills and to respond to more cognitive aspects of the treatment. Such debate has given rise to adaptations of the treatment and increased the focus on its more behavioural aspects. Adapted manuals include pictorial materials, simplified language, support with homework tasks, and increasing awareness of paid/family carers to support the therapy.

There is emerging interest in behavioural activation as another option of short term therapy for people with IDD and mood disorders.

Psychodynamic psychotherapy and counselling
(See ➲ Psychoanalytic psychotherapy in Chapter 2, pp. 20–30, and in Chapter 5, pp. 163–72; Counselling in Chapter 2, pp. 91–94, and in Chapter 5, pp. 274–81.)

Psychodynamic psychotherapy is a recent addition to the treatments available to people with IDD, and counselling is now offered widely to people with IDD, challenging previous assumptions that psychodynamic approaches were not suitable for this population. The aims of such treatments are to promote well-being, improve functioning, and develop the potential to form loving and enduring relationships. Many patients with IDD bring stories of emotional difficulties and require support and active listening in order to learn to cope with the pain of the realization of having an IDD. Others may have experienced several losses or significant interference with childhood attachments and ongoing problems in expressing their sexuality and having their own families. Psychological support may also be required by the parents who discover that their child has IDD; feelings of grief at the loss of the "perfect child" and worry about the impact of the disability need to be discussed and understood so that parents can gain an understanding of the condition and work together in helping their child to fulfil his/her potential.

Other psychological treatments
Behavioural therapy is based on operant conditioning and is mainly used for the amelioration of challenging behaviour. It includes functional analysis of the behaviour and a treatment programme that addresses the identified area of interest. Best known versions of behavioural treatments include positive behaviour support and applied behavioural analysis.

Emerging promising interventions for challenging behaviour relate to the application of mindfulness, trauma-based frameworks, and attachment-based frameworks in the management of challenging behaviour. (See ➲ Mindfulness-based interventions and therapies in Chapter 2, pp. 73–5, and in Chapter 5, pp. 239–43.)

Finally, systemic therapy is used in complex cases in order to apply psychological thinking to the care and support network of the person with IDD with the purpose of enhancing and promoting wellbeing and inclusion. (See ➲ Systemic family and couple therapy in Chapter 2, pp. 34–42, and in Chapter 5, pp. 184–8.)

Recommended reading
Ali A, Blickwedel J, and Hassiotis A (2014). Interventions for challenging behaviour in intellectual disability. *Advances in Psychiatric Treatment*, 20, 184–92.

Maulik PK and Harbour CK (2010). Epidemiology of Intellectual Disability. In: JH Stone, M Blouin (eds). *International Encyclopedia of Rehabilitation*. Available online: http://cirrie.buffalo.edu/encyclopedia/en/article/144/ (accessed May 2014).

Morgan VA, Leonard H, Bourke J, and Jablensky A (2008). Intellectual disability co-occurring with schizophrenia and other psychiatric illness: population-based study. *The British Journal of Psychiatry*, 193, 364–72.

Taylor JL, Lindsay WR, Hastings RP, and Hatton C (eds) (2013). *Psychological Therapies for Adults with Intellectual Disabilities*. Wiley Blackwell: UK.

Dementia

(See ➔ Psychiatry of old age: psychotherapies, applications, and research in Chapter 12, pp. 565–7.)

Dementia is a term describing a range of symptoms caused by physical changes in brain cells. It is not a natural part of ageing, as it can also occur in early-onset forms, and is not a disease in its own right. There are many different forms of dementia, as well as many known causes; individuality of symptomatology is consequent upon the specific cause, location, and nature of changes in the brain. If progression is a feature of the symptom grouping for an individual, there may be changes in the structure and chemistry of the brain, which lead to damage and gradual death of brain cells.

Resulting problems associated with concentration, thinking, memory, cognition, and language may lead to difficulties in how an individual perceives what is happening around him or her. This may sometimes result in confused states and emotional instability, combinations of which may bring about changes in behaviour. Symptoms vary with individuals, as do stages of progression, and diagnosis requires detailed attention to physical, psychological, neurological, and psychic domains of functioning.

Types of dementia

In the UK, four of the commonest types of dementia, which, together with two or more of these in combination (known as mixed dementia), account for about 95% of diagnosed dementias:

- *Alzheimer's disease* is characterized by short-term memory loss and difficulties with language in the early stages, along with confusion and difficulty following what is going on, sometimes making everyday activities challenging, and gradually becoming more severe over time.
- *Vascular dementia* is the consequence of problems with blood supply to the brain, presenting with a varied clinical picture, depending on the part of the brain affected, and the cause, nature, and location of the blood supply problem, e.g. stroke-related dementia or subcortical vascular dementia.
- *Dementia with Lewy bodies (DLB)*, also known as Pick's disease or Lewy body disease, has certain mental symptoms in common with Alzheimer's disease, such as confusion and loss of memory, and physical symptoms associated with Parkinson's disease such as gait and slow movement. It is now recognized as a distinct medical condition, and not a variant of either of these two diseases with which it appears to share symptoms.
- *Frontotemporal dementia*, a less common form (also known as Pick's disease or frontal lobe dementia), has a variety of symptoms caused by damage to different areas of the frontal and temporal lobes, and covers a range of specific conditions, including behavioural variant frontotemporal dementia, progressive non-fluent aphasia, and semantic dementia.
- *Mixed dementia*, as the term suggests, refers to the existence of forms of dementia together in one individual. Alzheimer's disease with vascular dementia is a common combination; Alzheimer's disease can also exist in combination with DLB.

Under the age of 65, an individual can develop any form of dementia, (known as early-onset or young-onset dementia), though it is more likely to be a less common form than is the case with older people, e.g. frontotemporal dementia or a type of dementia with a genetic cause. Only a third of younger people with dementia have Alzheimer's disease.

Mild cognitive impairment (MCI) is diagnosed for some individuals who experience problems which are not severe enough to be dementia such as with memory, thinking, language, or visuospatial skills. Whilst a diagnosis of MCI represents an increased risk for the development of dementia, some people with MCI will not go on to develop dementia and may even get better.

These diagnostic variations are but part of the picture in a field of study under constant and increasing review.

Prevalence

Currently, around 800000 people in the UK have dementia. The chance of developing dementia increases significantly with age. One in 14 people over 65 years of age, and one in six people over 80, has dementia. Over 17000 younger people (under the age of 65) in the UK have early-onset dementia. Dementia is believed to be commoner amongst women than men—current estimates indicate that two-thirds of people with dementia are women. However, differentials between incidence (dementia has, by definition, one onset) and prevalence need to be taken into account—prevalence is affected by the length of illness and by women (at present) surviving longer than men.

DSM-5

Changes in diagnostics, as described by DSM-5, may develop the arenas of both research and care. In DSM-IV, what used to be called 'Delirium, Dementia, Amnestic, and other Cognitive Disorders' is now named 'Neurocognitive Disorders' in DSM-5 and includes three main diagnoses: mild neurocognitive disorder (NCD), major NCD, and delirium. The diagnosis of mild NCD is new and specifies the existence of changes which impact cognitive functioning, requiring an individual to adopt compensatory strategies to remain independent and manage daily living activities. 'Dementia' was a formal diagnosis in DSM-IV; this has been replaced with the term 'major NCD', although dementia is accepted as an alternative.

Care principles, diagnosis, and assessment

In the UK, NICE (2012) guidance on dementia, published in association with the Social Care Institute for Excellence (SCIE), proposes a 'person-centred' approach underpinned by five specific principles which acknowledge:

- the human value
- the individuality of the person with dementia
- the perspective of the person with dementia
- the importance of their relationships and interactions in supporting well-being
- support for the person's carers, whether familial or institutional (described as 'relationship-centred' care).

Further key principles in the field are the opportunity for the person with dementia to have a say in care and treatment decisions and, where capacity affects this, to have regard for the guidance offered by the Department of Health and the Mental Capacity Act; and to involve family and carers, in line with the wishes of the individual, in the processes of information gathering, diagnosing, and care decisions. Memory services are suggested as the primary point of referral for all individuals with dementia—where dementia is suspected, structural imaging is recommended, both to help determine the aetiological subtype and to exclude other cerebral pathology. Other kinds of assessment can be considered where the behaviour of the person with a diagnosis of, or suspected, dementia causes concern; a detailed and sensitive assessment of the individual and his/her environment may reveal causes as varied as anxiety, depression, psychosocial or physical factors, undetected pain, or medication side effects. A range of pharmacological interventions and non-pharmacological interventions exist to address both cognitive and non-cognitive symptoms, co-morbid psychological or emotional conditions, and behaviour which is of concern or is challenging.

Treatment interventions: pharmacological

The main drugs developed for Alzheimer's disease are acetylcholinesterase inhibitors (donepezil, rivastigmine, and galantamine) for use in early and middle stages, or memantine for later stages. These may also be offered to someone with DLB, to improve cognition and decrease hallucinations, but could contribute to Parkinsonian-type symptoms. In contrast, no benefits of use of these drugs have been shown for people with frontotemporal dementia. The drugs developed for Alzheimer's disease are not recommended for vascular dementia, unless as part of mixed dementia, and instead the conditions which increase the risk of stroke are treated.

Treatment interventions: non-pharmacological

New ways of thinking about dementia, arising from areas of research and experience beyond medicine, encompass psychosocial, neuropsychological, and psychotherapeutic approaches.

One of the central tensions in health care over time, locating ill health or well-being in either the body or the mind, poses particular difficulties in understanding and treating the dementias, which require, of both families and health and social care staff, a willingness to understand the psychological and social dimensions of physical and neurological events. It is as important to think about the internal world of the person with dementia, as it is to consider the social impact and the physical changes. It is all too easy to focus only on one area, to the exclusion of a perspective which might provide relief and understanding for the person at the centre of the diagnostic and care process or for the carers tasked with being that person's 'auxillary mind'. Ignoring the meaning of actions and experiences of individuals in the social and care contexts can, in a very real way, compound the disabling effects of dementia. These realities of the challenges of engaging with dementia have led to what is termed 'person-centred' care, based on psychotherapeutic principles.

Accounts of psychotherapeutic approaches to people with dementia are increasing, reflecting the diversity one encounters in individuals, their diagnosis and their response, their stage of the experience, and their psychosocial and familial circumstances. The psychotherapies range from counselling, reminiscence, or life story work, 'validation therapy', and cognitive stimulation therapy to psychodynamic approaches. CBT, as used to treat depression and anxiety, is regarded as being also helpful for people with dementia and depression. Family therapy may be indicated where problems are developing because of changes in relationships and accepted family roles and structures. Couple therapy, or therapeutic couple work in dementia care, e.g. therapy with the 'carer' where one of the couple has dementia, has been shown to mitigate some of the profound and inevitable frustrations in a relationship, moderating the change from partnership to full dependency, extending the period of time spent at home, and sometimes delaying the removal to residential care, as shown by Balfour (2014) (see ➜ Psychoanalytic psychotherapy in Chapter 2, pp. 20–30, and in Chapter 5, pp. 163–72; Cognitive behavioural therapy in Chapter 2, pp. 30–4, and in Chapter 5, pp. 172–84; Systematic family and couple therapy in Chapter 2, pp. 34–42, and in Chapter 5, pp. 184–8).

Amongst the shared features of accounts of psychotherapeutic work, one finds a focus on the emotional content and personal meaning of the communications of the person with dementia, and an acknowledgement of the need for modification of technique as a person progresses through the stages of dementia, including changing frequency of sessions and recognition of time to end.

The very real difficulty of knowing what is happening in the internal world of the person with dementia will only be mitigated by the sensitive observation of the effect of the person on the people around them, whether by therapist or care worker, partner, or family member.

This kind of 'taking in', of communication without words to develop meaning, is an ordinary, but important, part of the beginning of life where a level of detailed reciprocal attention, watchful interest, and reliability afforded to infants as they develop in the good enough care of another, the primary carer, offers a template for care of people with dementia. As the physical, social, and psychic areas of functioning change in reverse, in dementia, the development of meaning from communication which seems to be incomprehensible is as important. This suggests the therapeutic focus, beyond the limits of meaningful individual or group therapy for the person with dementia, will be on the care 'environment', which may be the couple or the family, or the group of care workers around the individual. As Balfour (2014) suggests, 'the important thing is containing the container' (see ➜ Later life in Chapter 6, pp. 291–3).

Recommended reading

Balfour A (2007). Facts, phenomenology, and psychoanalytic contributions to dementia care. In: Davenhill R (ed). *Looking into Later Life: A Psychoanalytic Approach to Depression and Dementia in Old Age*. pp. 222–47. Karnac: London.

Balfour A (2014). Developing therapeutic couple work in dementia care: the living together with dementia project. *Psychoanalytic Psychotherapy*, **28**, 304–20.

Evans S (2014). What the National Dementia Strategy forgot: providing dementia care from a psychodynamic perspective. *Psychoanalytic Psychotherapy*, **28**, 321–9.

Sinason V (1992). The man who was losing his brain. In: Sinason V. *Mental handicap and the human condition: new approaches from the Tavistock*. Free Association Books: London.

Wood H (2007). Caring for a relative with dementia—who is the sufferer? In: Davenhill R (ed). *Looking into Later Life: A Psychoanalytic Approach to Depression and Dementia in Old Age*. pp. 269–82. Karnac: London.

Personality disorder

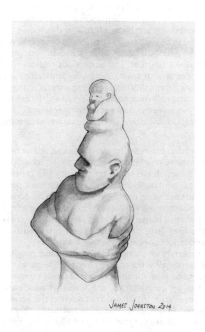

JAMES JOHNSTON 2014

Theories of personality development

Personality and personality development

'Persona' comes from the Greek word for 'mask'. The word 'personality' derives from this word, and its Greek root reminds us that our personalities are not just personal to us; they are an important part of how we relate to others. This is important when thinking about what goes wrong with personalities and how they become dysfunctional (see ➔ Personality disorders in Chapter 8, pp. 384–422).

What are you like?

Human beings have been attempting to classify each other's characters since antiquity. Early theories include the effect of the positions of the stars (astrology), the effect of different kinds of bodily fluids, and the notion of 'humours', and the effects of bodily shape. Of the many problems with these early classifications, the most important is that categorical approaches just do not reflect the realities of how people function or the sophistication of the human personality. None of the classical personality theories deal with the question of how personalities both remain stable and change over time, nor do they give any account of how 'personality' relates to concepts like 'personal identity' and the 'self'.

Questions about personality

Your personality helps you 'do' things, not just 'be'; it has a function and is therefore dynamic. However, your personality also describes the way you generally go about things and is therefore also stable over time. Your personality helps you to be recognizable to others over time, which facilitates group membership and is vital to human survival. Your personality helps you deal with novel, unusual, and ambiguous situations which require flexibility and openness to taking in new information and perspectives. A well-functioning personality includes a capacity to engage with time and the capacity to imagine how one might feel in a different time and situation. Personality includes the concept of 'temperament', i.e. the degree to which people regulate their degree of arousal and excitability.

Trait theory

Extensive theoretical and research work has been done on the 'trait theory' of personality. A 'trait' is a set of individual dispositions that people habitually use. Research based on trait theory has generated standard personality assessment tools and the theory that most people's personalities can be classified using the 'Big Five' dimensions: conscientiousness, openness, neuroticism, agreeableness, and extraversion. More recent research suggests that human personality constellations may also include traits from the 'Bad Five' of impulsiveness, suspiciousness, irritability, grandiosity, and lack of concern for others distress.

Extensive research involving twin studies and longitudinal studies suggests that personality traits are inherited via genetic transmission. However, the mechanism for this process is highly complex. Some traits are mediated by neurochemicals, the levels of which are affected by genetic subtypes. Parental behaviour can affect the genetic expression of these subtypes in offspring, who may therefore react differently to stress and display different types of trait behaviours. Personality traits are likely to reflect a complex interaction of genetic profile with psycho-social environment.

Theories of personality development

Most work on personality has focused on trait theory and the extent to which people can be classified according to traits. There is an extensive literature on the stability of personality traits across time; for example, children who are classified as extraverts tend to be classified the same way in adolescence and adulthood.

However, it is also clear that people's personalities can and do change, sometimes for the better, sometimes not. ICD-10 and DSM-5 list post-traumatic personality change as a recognized condition, and different situations can sometimes elicit different types of personality function. Gordon Allport, one of the earliest researchers into personality, described how personality traits become organized into a reasonably stable system, but how they can change when environments change. This makes sense in evolutionary terms; individuals who can change personal responses in different situations are more likely to survive that those who are rigid.

Theories of personality development include a biopsychosocial model that incorporates neurobiology and genetics, psychology (both individual and interpersonal), and sociology.

An example of the biopsychosocial: an ecological model
(See Fig. 8.1.)

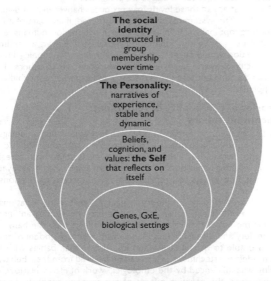

Fig. 8.1 Ecological model of the person. (Data from McAdams and Pals, 2006.)

In this model, the genetic core of the personality affects the development of neural networks and regulation of activity at neural synapses in networks that underpin affect and arousal regulation. They are the most stable and least open to change. People are not conscious of this level of personality activity.

The cognitive level is the domain of beliefs, information processing, and thinking skills, which is relatively dynamic and subject to change. Some of the activity of this level is conscious; there is evidence that many rapid-acting cognitions are not conscious, but more slow-acting ones are. Many forms of education and therapeutic techniques operate at this level (see ➔ Neuroscience and psychotherapy in Chapter 11, pp. 526–42).

The narrative level of the personality includes an interpersonal aspect, and includes what the individual calls the 'story' of his/her own life and the sense of personal identity. This level is heavily influenced by relationships with others and reflections on experience. This level of the personality can change, in response to major environmental challenges such as loss events, traumata, and sudden changes in social position. The 'dynamic' forms of therapy (both group and individual) operate at this level (see ➔ Psychoanalytic psychotherapy in Chapter 2, pp. 20–30, and in Chapter 5, pp. 163–72; Group therapy and group analysis in Chapter 2, pp. 42–7, and in Chapter 5, pp. 188–94).

The outermost level of the personality is the social where group membership is crucial. Social constructs generate 'culture', which, like the individual personality, has both stable and dynamic elements. Social constructs about gender or status are influential.

Changes at any of these levels may produce changes in an individual's personality. The system may become disordered, if any part of it is not functioning optimally. Defining 'optimal function' for humans entails considerations of values, ethics, and morality; however, a parsimonious definition would suggest that optimal human functioning involves the capacity to work, to love, and to be connected to others. Those who can do none of these things die early and experience morbidity and unhappiness.

Theories of personality development: attachment theory

Attachment theory is a neurobiological theory of how human beings use their relationships with others to manage stress, fear, and threats of loss across the lifespan. It is a theory of how humans utilize both caregiving and care-eliciting behaviours when they are stressed, and how they make and maintain psychological representations of care-giving relationships across time.

John Bowlby's original theory suggested that early relationships between mothers and babies lead to the baby developing an 'internal working model' of that relationship, which affects how the baby deals with anxiety and threats of loss. Babies with a 'secure' model of attachment are able to handle stress and loss better than babies with insecure models of attachment, which can be inferred from their behaviour. Bowlby was influenced by the ethological work of Harry Harlow, who had observed the negative effects of raising infant monkeys in social isolation (see → John Bowlby in Psychoanalytic psychotherapy in Chapter 2, pp. 20–30).

Mary Ainsworth carried out research with human infants and observed distinct patterns of behaviour in children in response to the 'strange situation' (where the mother leaves the infant for a short period with a stranger and then returns) that could be reliably identified and linked with a distinct attachment pattern. Secure and insecure patterns of behaviour could be reliably distinguished, and there were three further identifiable patterns of insecure attachment: avoidant, ambivalent, and disorganized. Mary Main and others extended Ainsworth's findings to measuring adult mental representations of attachment with the AAI. Main showed that the representations of an adult parent's own attachment experiences may have significant influence on their children's development and attachment patterns.

Longitudinal follow-up studies have found that childhood attachment patterns tend to be stable across time, especially insecure attachment patterns. Insecure children tend to become insecure adolescents and insecure adults. Insecurity of attachment in adults is manifest in social behaviours and can be reliably assessed using both self-report and interview (see Table 8.1).

Insecurity of attachment is not a psychopathology in itself, but a risk factor for other pathologies. The insecure adult struggles to manage their arousal and affective response to loss and threat of loss, or any situation where there may be uncertainty or ambiguity. However, the risk may be buffered by protective factors, such as intelligence and positive attachments in adulthood, and there may be degrees of insecurity, so that only severe insecurity is associated with psychopathology.

About 40% of the general population has an insecure attachment system. However, this figure rises steeply for clinical populations, including personality disorder. Most studies have found very high level of insecurity (60–70%) in people with BPD, and even higher in populations where personality disorder is prevalent such as offender populations (see → Borderline personality disorder in Chapter 8, pp. 390–6; Antisocial personality disorder in Chapter 8, pp. 396–401).

The links between attachment security and personality are clear. The attachment system regulates arousal and affect at times of fear and vulnerability, and an insecure system is a dysregulated system. People with personality disorders struggle to regulate affects of fear and anger, especially in interpersonal systems. Insecurity of attachment is associated with instability of personal relationships and sense of self, just as people with personality disorders describe. Personality disorder is associated with childhood abuse and trauma, which are also known to make insecurity of attachment more likely, especially disorganized attachment. Insecurity of attachment is also commonly found in people with psychosomatic disorders, who also frequently meet criteria for personality disorder (see → Medically unexplained symptoms in Chapter 7, pp. 359–60).

Personality and the self

There is remarkably little discussion about the relationship between the personality and the self. When asked to describe themselves, people

Table 8.1 Characteristics of attachment patterns

Attachment pattern	Response to separation	In adulthood	Offspring security	Relationships with caregivers	Comment
Insecure Ambivalent Category C in strange situation	Distressed on being left. Clings to stranger. A mixture of responses to mother	Oscillating emotions between positive and negative. Seeks help but then avoids. Category E on AAI	Tends to have babies rated as C on strange situation	May be compulsive care giver in adulthood but anxious about care giving role. May seek help but not be able to use it	Between 15–18% of general population. Over-represented in BPD and psychotherapy seeking populations
Insecure avoidant Category A in strange situation	Makes little protest on being left. Does not go to mother on reunion	Avoids expression of negative emotion; values independence Category D on AAI	Tends to have babies rated as A on strange situation	Avoids seeking help and may be belittling of those that do. Avoids both caregiving and care-eliciting. Denies neediness	Between 15% and 20% in normal populations. Much higher (60+ %) in offender populations. Present in some caregivers
Insecure, disorganized Category D in strange situation	Odd behaviours on being left. May 'freeze' or be aggressive on reunion	Mixture of avoidant and ambivalence as adult. Dissociative symptoms seen in adolescents. Highly incoherent attachment narratives	Some evidence that mothers with highly disorganized attachment systems and unresolved trauma have D-rated babies on strange situation	Often a mixed picture of relationships with caregivers. May present as hostile, scared, or helpless with caregivers	Rare (2%) in general populations, but commoner in clinical populations (10%). May be associated with unresolved trauma and fear experiences
Secure Category B in strange situation	Makes active protest. Clings to mother on reunion and seeks comfort	Appropriately distressed. Seeks helps and values it. Comfortable with dependency Category F on AAI	Secure	Seeks helps and utilizes it. Neither avoids nor seeks caregiving role	60% of most populations. Found in some people with poor mental health

tend to use language from the social world of how others might see them and how they interact with people. If the personality is that part of the self that interacts with others and responds to stressors in the social world, the self seems to be that private, individual experience of an observer looking at the world from their utterly particular vantage point. Many people identify their sense of self as being behind the eyes, yet separate from their bodies, and they may talk of an awareness of either 'being' themselves or 'not being' themselves at any given time.

In contrast, there is a vast literature from philosophy and psychology about the nature of the self: its actions, its choices, and its moral relevance. Many philosophers have commented that there is a relationship between the sense of self and the stream of thought and inner speech that most people experience. Indeed, disorders of the sense of self are often described in terms of disorders of action, choice, thought, and inner speech.

People with personality disorders often describe a fragmented or disorganized sense of self, although this may be most true for people with BPD, and less true for people with avoidant, narcissistic, or paranoid personality disorder. There are some forms of personality dysfunction that present with a highly organized sense of self, often either with a grievance and sense of being hard done by and/or a highly suspicious sense of self that views others as a source of threat. Such people may have sufficient sense of self to interact superficially with others and may only present in need after a major life change such as bereavement or loss of occupation.

Disorders of the self

Different clinical disorders are associated with different types of self experience. Disorders of the bodily sense of self may be seen in MUS of various sorts, body dysmorphic syndrome, and the eating disorders. Gender identity disorder appears to have benign and malignant forms; the benign forms respond to changes in the somatic self, but the more malignant ones do not.

Most people with psychotic disorders report disorders of the sense of self, especially those who experience intrusions into personal identity and agency. Some authors have suggested that the sense of being personally invaded and threatened is a psychotic experience that is highly likely to lead to violent action. Those who hear voices describe intrusions into their personal space, but not everyone feels that their sense of self is disturbed. There is some interesting research into people with paranoid experiences, some of whom feel that their delusions and hallucinations are making some comment about a 'bad me'.

Disorders of volition and the addictions impact on the sense of self; many addicts describe not being 'themselves', unless they have used their substance of choice. Some people with chronic depression have described feeling that they are now their 'real' selves when prescribed antidepressants.

Finally, the ability to engage in a process of reflection about oneself and one's thinking processes is associated with good mental health and optimal functioning. In contrast, many mental disorders are associated with a lack of reflective function and mentalizing skills (see ➔ Mentalization-based treatment in Chapter 2, pp. 66–70).

Recommended reading

Adshead G and Jacob C (2008). *Personality Disorder: The Definitive Collection.* Jessica Kingsley: London.

Livesley J (2001). *Handbook of Personality Disorders: Theory, Research and Treatment.* Guilford Press: New York.

McAdams D and Pals JP (2006). A new Big Five: Fundamental Principles for a new integrative science of personality. *American Psychologist,* **61**(3), 204–17.

Oldham JM and Skodol AE (eds) (2014). *American Psychiatric Publishing Textbook of Personality Disorders,* second edition. American Psychiatric Press: Washington DC.

Sarkar J and Adshead G (2012). *Clinical Topics in Personality Disorder.* Royal College of Psychiatrists: London.

Personality disorders

Assessment of personality disorder

Classification of personality disorder: dimensions or categories?

Classification of personality disorder is the subject of debate. There is a move away from the categorical approach of DSM-IV-TR and DSM-5 towards an integration of theory-driven and empirically derived models of personality development and psychopathology, taking into account the interactions between psychosocial and neurobiological processes. It is anticipated this will provide a more comprehensive and clinically relevant, dimensional approach to classification.

To diagnose a personality disorder according to DSM-5, the following criteria must be met:

A. Significant impairment in self and interpersonal functioning
B. One or more personality trait domains or facets
C. These impairments are stable across time and situations
D. Are not better understood as normative for the individual's developmental stage or sociocultural environment
E. Are not solely due to the direct physiological effects of a substance (e.g. a drug of abuse, medication) or a general medical condition (e.g. severe head trauma).

Clinical assessment: psychiatric

Personality disorders are common, associated with high levels of morbidity and mortality. The presence of personality disorder significantly affects the outcome of associated mental illnesses. Assessment of personality should form part of routine psychiatric assessment. Most commonly, assessment is made on the basis of clinical judgement. The use of screening tools augments the reliability of clinical judgement (see Box 8.1).

In both psychiatric and psychotherapeutic assessment, formulation can overcome some shortcomings of categorical classification, informing risk assessment, and clinical and therapeutic management (see Fig. 8.2).

Psychiatric assessment depends upon history taking. Attend to:

• *Presentation*: self-harm, suicide attempts, impulsiveness, relational context, fluctuations in mood, transient psychotic symptoms

Box 8.1 Screening tools

Self-report questionnaires
- International Personality Disorder Examination Screen (IPDE-S; Lenzenweger *et al.*, 1997)
- Personality Diagnostic Questionnaire-Revised (PDQ-R; Hyler, 1992)
- SCID-II Screen (Exselius *et al.*, 1994)

Interviewer-administered screens
- Standardised Assessment of Personality-Abbreviated Scale (SAPAS; Moran, 2003)
- Iowa Personality Disorder Screen (IPDS; Langbehn *et al.*, 1999)
- Rapid Personality Assessment Schedule (PAS-R; Van Horn *et al.*, 2000)

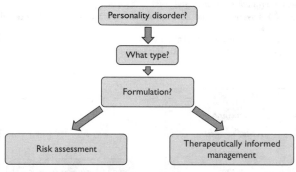

Fig. 8.2 Questions to be addressed at assessment.

- *Direct questioning*: symptoms of complex trauma, including dissociation, OCD, disordered eating, somatization, substance and alcohol misuse
- *Psychiatric history*: multiple previous diagnoses, past risk history, evidence of overprescribing, ongoing and pervasive problems rather than episodic
- *Developmental history*: childhood illness/injury, separations before the age of 5, history of childhood abuse (physical, sexual, and emotional) and neglect, relationships with both parents and between parents, sibling relationships and order, significant others, significant events, educational history
- *Current relational functioning*: important relationships, including family, impact upon day-to-day functioning, achievements, work history
- *Psychosexual history*: stability of relationships, capacity for rupture and repair, controlling abusive relationships, promiscuity

- *Forensic history*: convictions, cautions, aggression, deceit
- *Mental state*: unstable mood, impaired reality testing, self-referential, persecutory ideation, magical thinking, delusional ideas (seldom systematized), auditory, and sometimes visual, hallucinations experienced in external space (related to significant others in personal history).

Types of personality disorder

Ten types of personality disorder are identified in DSM-5. They are classified in clusters (see Fig. 8.3) and differentiated from each other, in terms of their specific pattern of clinical features (see Table 8.2).

Assessment tools

Semi-structured interviews are the preferred method, ensuring reliable, replicable comprehensive and systematic assessment. These include open-ended questions, indirect enquiries, and observations of the respondent's manner, as well as direct questions (see Box 8.2).

Psychotherapeutic assessment

(See ➔ Psychodynamic assessment and formulation in Chapter 4, pp. 122–4.)

Arriving at a formulation, rather than a diagnosis, is the central purpose of psychotherapy assessment. This requires therapeutic engagement

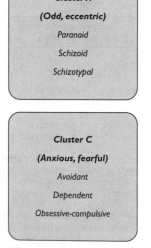

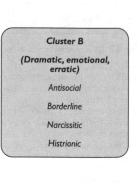

Fig. 8.3 DSM-5 personality disorders.

Table 8.2 Differential diagnosis between personality disorders

Cluster		Social withdrawal	Odd beliefs	Ego-syntonic	Anxious	Persecutory ideation	Impaired reality testing	Somatization	Perfectionism	Emotional constriction	Emotional dysregulation
A	Paranoid PD	×			×	×	×				
	Schizoid PD	×		×						×	
	Schizotypal PD	×	×	×		×	×			×	
B	Antisocial PD			× o ×	×	×					×
	Borderline PD		×		×	×	×	×			×
	Histrionic PD										
	Narcissistic PD										
C	Avoidant PD	×			×	×				×	
	Dependent PD				×					×	
	Obsessive–compulsive PD	×		×				×	×	×	

PD, personality disorder.

Box 8.2 **Assessment tools**

Interviews explicitly coordinated with DSM-IV-TR
- Diagnostic Interview for Personality Disorder (DIPD; Zannarini, Frankenburg, Chuancy, and Gunderson, 1987)
- International Personality Disorder Examination (IPDE; Loranger, 1999)
- Personality Disorder Interview IV (PDI-IV; Widiger et al., 1995)
- Structured Clinical Interview for DSM-IV Axis II Personality Disorders (SCID II; First et al., 1997)
- Structured Interview for DSM-IV Personality Disorders (SIDP-IV; Pfohl, Blum. and Zimmerman, 1997)

Diagnostic instruments, filled in by clinicians already very familiar with the patient
- Personality Assessment Form (PAF; Pilkonis, Heape, Ruddy, and Serrao, 1991)
- Shedlar Westen Assessment Procedure (SWAP-200; Shedler, 2002)

Self-report inventories
- The personality disorder scales of the Minnesota Multiphasic Personality Inventory-2 (MMPI-2; Butcher, 1997)
- Millon Clinical Multiaxial Inventory-III (MCMI-III; Millon and Davis, 1997)
- Personality Diagnostic Questionnaire-4 (PDQ-4; Hyler, 1994)
- Personality Assessment Inventory (PAI; Morey, 1991)
- Wisconson Personality Disorders Inventory (WISPI; Klein et al., 1993)

Assessments for individual personality disorders
- Revised Diagnostic Interview for Borderlines (DIB-R; Zannarini, Gunderson, Frankenburg, and Chauncey, 1989)
- Diagnostic Interview for Narcissism (DIN; Gunderson, Ronningstam, and Bodkin, 1990)
- Hare Psychopathy Checklist-Revised (PCL-R; Hare, 2003)
- Structured Interview for the Five Factor Model (SIFFM; Trull and Widiger, 1997)

with the patient in understanding their difficulties, as they arise in the transference at the assessment interview. The formulation emerges through this process and may be the basis for a trial interpretation. This brings clarity about the person's ability to use therapeutic work and the risks associated with it. To arrive at this, the structure of psychiatric assessment is complemented by a therapeutic approach adopted from the outset. When assessing people with personality disorder, splitting and projective defences dominate, so attending to countertransference is essential, as is attending to the events that follow a point of emotional contact at assessment. This can provide an indication of the risks likely to arise in therapy.

Formulation
(See ➜ Formulation in Chapter 4, pp. 122–4.)

A formulation provides a model-specific conceptual structure within which to understand the patient's narrative, facilitating the assessment of risk and therapeutic planning.

Psychodynamic formulation
(See ➜ Psychoanalytic psychotherapy in Chapter 2, pp. 20–30, and in Chapter 5, pp. 163–72; Psychodynamic assessment and formulation in Chapter 4, pp. 127–30.)

A psychodynamic formulation derives pictures of relationships with objects from a detailed relational developmental history. It finds the pattern of relating which provides a common theme and the most comprehensive explanation of these three areas (see Fig. 8.4) pointing to the point of maximum core pain against which the patient seeks to defend themselves.

Cognitive behavioural therapy formulation
(See ➜ Cognitive behavioural therapy in Chapter 2, pp. 30–4, and in Chapter 5, pp. 172–84; Cognitive behavioural assessment and formulation in Chapter 4, pp. 135–40.)

CBT formulations of personality disorder are grounded in the following concepts:

• Schemas: unconscious stable cognitive structures which organize experience and behaviour. They are triggered by events similar to those in which they originated. In personality disorder, evaluations of self and others are the dominant cognitive schemas.
• Personality disorder is characterized by reciprocal, underdevelopment, and overdevelopment of behavioural strategies.
• Cognitive distortions may be present, e.g.:
  • Schizotypal: source monitoring problems (confusions about the origin of thoughts)
  • Antisocial: attributional bias (perception and interpretation of information).

DBT of BPD proposes an invalidating environment with biologic dysfunction leading to dysfunctional coping behaviour (see ➜ Dialectical behavioural therapy in Chapter 2, pp. 63–6, and in Chapter 5, pp. 220–9).

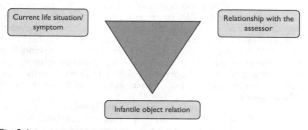

Fig. 8.4 Psychodynamic formulation.

Cognitive analytic therapy 'reformulation'

(See **➲** Cognitive analytic therapy in Chapter 2, pp. 47–52, and in Chapter 5, pp. 194–202.)

Ryle incorporated object relations theory and Vygotsky's activity theory, making CAT applicable to BPD. He proposed that faulty procedural sequences are deployed by people with BPD without revision.

Three main kinds of faulty procedure are:

- Traps—the consequences of behaviour promote its perpetuation
- Dilemmas—false choices or unduly narrowed options
- Snags—future consequences are anticipated to be so negative they halt procedures before they run.

Internalized templates and reciprocal roles are subject to deformities allocated to three levels:

- First level: small number of highly maladaptive reciprocal roles
- Second level: small stimuli evoke state changes without smooth transitions
- Third level: impaired self-reflective capacity.

These concepts can be drawn upon to arrive at a CAT formulation, following assessment.

Recommended reading

Hinshelwood RD (1991). Psychodynamic formulation in assessment for psychotherapy. *British Journal of Psychotherapy*, **8**, 166–74.

Linehan M (1993). *Cognitive-Behavioural Treatment of Borderline Personality Disorder.* Guilford Press: New York.

Ryle A, Leighton T, and Pollock P (1997). *Cognitive Analytic Therapy of Borderline Personality Disorder: The Model and the Method.* John Wiley & Sons: Chichester.

Borderline personality disorder

BPD is a common mental disorder, with prevalence rates between 1.1% and 4.6% in the adult population. Being amongst the 'dramatic, emotional, erratic' Cluster B personality disorders, presentations are common in both emergency and routine psychiatric practice.

Diagnosis

BPD is a diagnosis commonly misconceived as being associated with 'attention-seeking behaviour' and poor response to treatment. In fact, it is a serious mental disorder, with a high mortality rate (suicide rates <10%). There is a continuum of severity. A significant proportion of those diagnosed with BPD recover spontaneously with time. At 10-year follow-up in one study showed that 86% no longer meet the criteria for 'caseness'. Some use non-intensive outpatient treatment and are never hospitalized; others become severely ill and are heavy users of inpatient services.

The DSM-5 diagnostic criteria for BPD stipulate that the person must show a pervasive pattern of instability of interpersonal relationships, self-image, and affects, and marked impulsivity, beginning in early adulthood and present in a variety of contexts, as indicated by five (or more) of the following:

1. Frantic efforts to avoid real or imagined abandonment
2. Pattern of unstable and intense interpersonal relationships, characterized by alternating between extremes of idealization and devaluation

3. Identity disturbance: markedly and persistently unstable self image or sense of self
4. Impulsivity in at least two areas that are potentially self-damaging (e.g. spending, sex, substance abuse, reckless driving, binge eating)
5. Recurrent suicidal behaviour, gestures, or threats, or self-mutilating behaviour
6. Affective instability due to a marked reactivity of mood
7. Chronic feelings of emptiness
8. Inappropriate intense anger, or difficulty controlling anger
9. Transient, stress-related paranoid ideation or severe dissociative symptoms.

The ICD-10 classification uses the term emotionally unstable personality disorder, of which there are two subtypes: impulsive type and borderline type.

Why has this disorder acquired its undeserved reputation? Perhaps the answer lies in the relational nature of the disorder itself. This is perhaps best summarized through understanding BPD as an attachment disorder activated by close dependent relationships in adult life, including relations with caring professionals. Professionals may perceive that their interventions worsen the difficulties of BPD and so conclude they should withdraw. At extremes, the behaviour of people with BPD can be bewildering and demanding, and can evoke in professionals a sense of violation or exploitation which can be difficult to tolerate when it is not understood. A cycle of rejection from services can ensue. The relational nature of personality disorder requires a formulation-based approach to mental health management and effective team-based therapeutic interventions, alongside evidence-based formal psychotherapy, where indicated (see ➲ Theories of personality development: attachment theory in Chapter 8, pp. 380–1).

Co-morbidity
• Other personality disorders, especially schizotypal and antisocial (see ➲ Schizotypal personality disorder in Chapter 8, pp. 401–6; Antisocial personality disorder in Chapter 8, pp. 396–401)
• Anxiety disorders (see ➲ Anxiety and anxiety disorders in Chapter 7, pp. 324–6)
• Major depression (see ➲ Affective disorders in Chapter 7, pp. 326–31)
• Eating disorders (see ➲ Eating disorders in Chapter 7, pp. 334–8)
• Substance misuse or addiction (see ➲ Substance misuse in Chapter 7, pp. 338–45)
• Somatization disorder (see ➲ Medically unexplained symptoms in Chapter 7, pp. 359–63)
• Some reports of overlap with autistic spectrum disorder.

Aetiology
The aetiology of BPD is multifactorial, based on empirical evidence that genetic, biological, and psychosocial factors are influential in the development of the disorder.

Genetics
Twin studies demonstrate 35% concordance in monozygotic (MZ) twins and 7% in dizygotic (DZ) twins. Heritability is 0.69.

Neurotransmitter abnormalities
- Impulsiveness, self-directed aggression, and aggression to others are associated with serotonergic dysfunction.
- There is some evidence of increased dopaminergic activity associated with psychotic symptomatology in BPD.
- Noradrenergic abnormalities are thought to be associated with risk taking and sensation seeking.

Neuroscience findings
- Evidence of increased attention to emotionally salient stimuli in BPD subjects—intense, slowly subsiding amygdala activation, compared with normal subjects.
- Studies also demonstrate decreased orbitofrontal metabolism, thought to be associated with decreased frontal regulatory function.

Psychosocial influences
There is good evidence that the capacity for self-control and attention are linked and that the quality of the mother–child relationship is a further important predictor of the growth of self-control skills.
Psychosocial factors contributing to the development of BPD are:
- Prolonged early separations from parents/carers (of 1 to 3 months) or losses
- Disturbed, highly conflictual relationships with parents
- High prevalence of affective disorder and substance misuse in first-degree relatives
- Childhood histories of physical or sexual abuse, including parent–child incest.

It has been proposed that BPD is, in fact, a form of complex post-traumatic stress resulting from childhood sexual abuse. The evidence in support of the causal role of sexual abuse in BPD remains inconclusive. It is thought the biparental failure as the context within which sexual abuse can occur may be the more important factor in the development of the disorder.

Attachment theory
(See Theories of personality development: attachment theory in Chapter 8, pp. 380–1.)
Attachment theory provides a convincing aetiological framework, incorporating the role of both biological and environmental factors, particularly early childhood trauma, in the development of BPD. Bowlby's attachment theory did not, in the first instance, describe the disorganized attachment pattern commonly seen in BPD but was later described by Mary Ainsworth in some infants, who had experienced early environmental adversity. In adult BPD, it is manifest in deep ambivalence and fear of close relationships and simultaneous anxiety about abandonment. Studies using the Adult Attachment Instrument to identify styles of attachment in people with BPD demonstrate a tendency towards classification as 'preoccupied' along with indications of unresolved trauma.

Therapeutic approaches
There are a number of effective models of psychotherapy of BPD. NICE guidelines make the following recommendations for treatment of the disorder.

General principles
- People with BPD should not be excluded from services, because they have self-harmed.
- They should be actively involved in finding solutions to their problems.
- Developing a trusting relationship is important.
- The strong emotions which are likely to follow endings and transitions should be anticipated.
- Mental health professionals need training, supervision, and support to working effectively with people with BPD.

Psychological treatment
- Do not use brief psychological interventions of less than 3 months.
- Where reducing self-harm is a priority, consider DBT or MBT.
- Transference-focused therapy, CAT, and schema-focused therapy may be effective for those with less severe difficulties.
- Psychological therapies should be delivered in well-structured community-based services.
- Further trials are needed.

The role of drug treatment
(See ➲ Psychotherapy and medication in Chapter 7, pp. 322–4.)
- Medication does not treat the disorder itself but can provide useful short-term symptomatic relief.
- Antipsychotics should not be used in the medium/long term.
- The use of sedative medication should not exceed 1 week.
- Treat co-morbid depression.

Specific therapeutic models for borderline personality disorder
Dialectical behaviour therapy
(See ➲ Dialectical behavioural therapy in Chapter 2, pp. 63–6, and in Chapter 5, pp. 220–9.)

DBT was originally adapted from a cognitive behavioural model by Marsha Linehan for BPD to include:
- Dialectics (polarities without synthesis): 'getting what is desired is as problematic as being denied'
- Emotional dysregulation (biology/invalidating environment)
- Mindfulness: balancing the reasonable mind, emotional mind, and wise mind.

It is based on a biosocial theory (see Fig. 8.5).

DBT comprises both group and individual therapy. Individual therapy addresses dialectics and motivational issues; group sessions address skills training. Stage 1 of the treatment lasts 1 year and addresses treatment avoidance and self-harm. It is often used as a first-stage treatment,

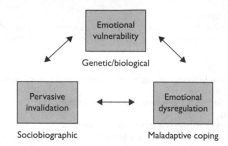

Fig. 8.5 Biosocial theory of borderline personality disorder.

before exploration of the underlying defences, and relational and attachment difficulties.

RCT evidence points to the effectiveness of DBT in BPD in reducing:
• Suicide attempts and self-injury
• Medical risk
• Premature dropout
• Inpatient/emergency admissions and days
• Drug abuse.

Mentalization-based therapy
(See ➔ Mentalization-based treatment in Chapter 2, pp. 66–70, and in Chapter 5, pp. 229–34.)

MBT was originally developed by Anthony Bateman and Peter Fonagy for BPD and is based on attachment theory. Mentalization refers to the process by which the capacity to think of mental states as separate from, and yet potentially causing, actions develops. The capacity for mentalization is conferred by a parent who allows representations of aroused self states to develop through playful interaction. The ventromedial prefrontal cortex is essential for mentalization but is switched off by high levels of arousal in an attachment context.

Important concepts in MBT are:
• *Self-agency*: a developmentally constructed capacity
• *Teleological agency*: a stage in development at which the infant can choose the most efficient way to bring about a goal from a range of alternatives. Agency is teleological in adults with BPD and restricted to surface reading of behaviour, rather than reading mental states.
• *Contingent marked mirroring*: parental mirroring enables the infant to develop a secondary representation of his own emotional state
• *Psychic equivalence*: in which the external world is felt to be isomorphic with the internal world
• *Pretend mode*: in which the child's mental state is decoupled from reality
• *The context within which mentalization fails*: preoccupied, fearful, confused, or overwhelmed attachment style—unresolved with regard to trauma and abuse.

Treatment goals in mentalization-based treatment

MBT aims to enhance the capacity for mentalization in a relational context, thereby enhancing affect regulation by:

- Appropriate expression of affect
- Establishing stable representational systems
- Formation of a coherent sense of self
- Development of a capacity to form secure relationships, via maintenance of mental closeness and attention to relationships.

MBT is a group and individual model which can be offered in day (partial hospitalization) or outpatient settings. A full programme is offered over 18 months.

RCT evidence points to the effectiveness of MBT in BPD in reducing:

- Frequency of suicide attempts and self-harm
- Hospital admissions
- Medication
- Psychiatric symptoms, interpersonal functioning, and social adjustment.

Transference-focused psychotherapy

(See ➲ Melanie Klein in Key contributors in Chapter 2, pp. 25–8.)

Transference-focused psychotherapy (TFP) is a psychoanalytic psychotherapy model based on Kleinan and object relations theory and developed by Otto Kernberg for the treatment of BPD. In this model, the internal world is made up of object relations dyads. It is proposed that excessive aggression leads to splitting and difficulty integrating positive and negative aspects of self and other in patients with BPD. This, and a lack of affect regulation termed 'effortful control', are the focus of therapeutic work.

There is a strong emphasis on maintaining boundaries in therapeutic work which proceeds in stages:

- Strategy 1: define dominant object relations, name the protagonists, attend to the patient's reaction
- Strategy 2: observe and interpret role reversal in dyads
- Strategy 3: identify defensive linkages between dyads
- Strategy 4: identify and work through the difference in the real relationship.

TFP is offered individually in an outpatient context once or twice weekly for 2 years.

RCTs demonstrate improvement in multiple domains, including suicidal behaviour, aggression, impulsivity, anxiety, depression, and social adjustment. TFP outperforms DBT in improvement in anger and impulsivity. In one study, schema-focused CBT showed greater improvements than TFP.

Therapeutic communities

(See ➲ Therapeutic communities in Chapter 2, pp. 75–80, and in Chapter 5, pp. 243–50.)

These are therapeutic programmes which offer an intensive form of treatment through provision of an environment and social milieu in

which staff work alongside patients to promote change. This is achieved through:
• Promotion of attachment and a culture of belonging
• Containment and a culture of safety
• Communication and a culture of openness
• Involvement and participation: a culture of participation and citizenship
• Agency: a culture of empowerment.

TCs can be provided in inpatient and day settings. Their principles can be applied in outpatient settings. Some offer a purely group analytic approach, whilst others also offer individual therapy. A large number of outcome studies of the effectiveness of TC treatments have been undertaken which point to improvement across a range of indicators.

Other treatments for borderline personality disorder with an established evidence base
• CBT
• Schema-focused therapy
• CAT for BPD
• Psychodynamic psychotherapy.

Recommended reading

Bateman A and Fonagy P (2004). *Psychotherapy for Borderline Personality Disorder*. Oxford University Press: Oxford.
Clarkin J, Yeomans F, and Kernberg FO (2006). *Psychotherapy for Borderline Personality Focusing on Object Relations*. American Psychiatric Publishing: Washington DC.
Linehan MM (1993). *Cognitive-Behavioral Treatment of Borderline Personality Disorder*. Guilford Press: New York.
National Institute for Health and Care Excellence (2009). *Borderline Personality Disorder: Recognition and Management*. NICE Guidelines CG78. Available at: ℘ https://www.nice.org.uk/guidance/cg78.
Zanarini MC, Frankernburg FR, Reich DB, and Fitzmaurice G (2010). Time to attainment of recovery from borderline personality disorder and stability of recovery: a 10-year prospective follow-up study. *American Journal of Psychiatry*, **167**, 663–7.

Antisocial personality disorder

(See ➜ Psychological therapy in secure settings in Chapter 8, pp. 438–9; Forensic psychiatry: forensic psychotherapies, applications, and research in Chapter 12, pp. 565–7.)

Prevalence
Antisocial personality disorder (ASPD) is common. Estimates of prevalence vary between 1% and 6%. It is commoner in men and is found in up to 70% of the prison population. The personal and financial costs of this disorder are high, in terms of harm to others, disruption of social and family function, damage to property, involvement of police and criminal justice systems, and childcare proceedings. Despite this, there is a lack of service provision and research, partly because people with ASPD do not tend to seek treatment, and professionals are unwilling to treat when a history of aggression and antisocial behaviour comes to light.

Diagnosis
The DSM-5 diagnostic criteria for ASPD are as follows:

A. Pervasive pattern of disregard for, and violation of, the rights of others since age 15, as indicated by three (or more) of the following:
  • Failure to conform to social norms
  • Deceitfulness
  • Impulsivity or failure to plan ahead
  • Irritability and aggressiveness
  • Reckless disregard for safety of self and others
  • Consistent irresponsibility
  • Lack of remorse
B. At least 18 years
C. Evidence of conduct disorder, with onset before age 15 years
D. Antisocial behaviour not due to schizophrenia or bipolar disorder.

The ICD-10 classification uses the term dissocial personality disorder.

Psychopathy and antisocial personality disorder
Cleckley was the first to describe psychopathy in 1941. Psychopathic disorder was a term used in the MHA until 2007. Now psychopathy usually refers to antisocial and behavioural personality traits, as measured by the Hare Psychopathy Checklist-Revised (PCL-R) (Hare, 2003). It is a concept used in the assessment of violent patients in forensic services; high scores are empirically associated with an increased risk of violence. Hare psychopathy is not synonymous with a behavioural history of criminality, and only one-third of individuals who fulfil diagnostic criteria for ASPD have severe psychopathy; this latter group has a significantly poorer treatment prognosis than do patients with mild to moderately psychopathic ASPD.

Co-morbidity
• Substance misuse (see ➔ Substance misuse in Chapter 7, pp. 338–45)
• >50% have anxiety disorder (see ➔ Anxiety and anxiety disorders in Chapter 7, pp. 324–6)
• 25% have depressive disorder (see ➔ Affective disorders in Chapter 7, pp. 326–31).

Aetiology
It is thought ASPD falls into at least two groups with different development pathways: those with higher levels of callousness and psychopathy, and low levels of demonstrable anxiety; and those with moderate to low levels of psychopathy, and higher levels of anxiety. The former, more psychopathic, group are thought to have more of a genetic predisposition to violent behaviour; the latter, more anxious, group are more likely to have experienced early environmental trauma, particularly physical abuse, resorting to violence to compensate for conflict or distress.

Biological and genetic factors
Twin studies show:
• Aggressive antisocial behaviour is more heritable than non-aggressive behaviour
• Aggressive antisocial behaviour in children shows strong heritability in those with callous, unemotional traits, indicating biological predisposition

- Impulsive aggression is heritable and linked with biological indices, particularly serotonergic activity
- There is significant gene–environment interaction. Children who are genetically susceptible to antisocial behaviour tend to receive harsh, inconsistent parenting.

Neuroscience findings
- Executive dysfunction: prefrontal metabolic activity is reduced with impulsive aggression in patients with BPD and ASPD
- PET studies show murderers have reduced prefrontal glucose metabolism
- Processing of input from the limbic system is dysfunctional, particularly in psychopathic ASPD individuals
- ASPD individuals display deficits of executive functions which cannot be accounted for by confounding variables such as head injury or substance misuse.

Environmental factors
These factors are implicated in the aetiology of ASPD. These are also risk factors for early attachment difficulties:
- Malnutrition
- Smoking in pregnancy
- Harsh parenting practices, including parental abuse.

Attachment and mentalization
(See ➔ Theories of personality development: attachment theory in Chapter 8, pp. 380–1; Mentalization-based treatment in Chapter 2, pp. 66–70.)

Forensic patients and prisoners have higher levels of insecure attachment than the normal population. They are more likely to report separation, abuse, and neglect from early caregivers. In psychopathy, callous and unemotional traits in children are associated with disorganized attachment, maladaptive interactive patterns in families, and severe institutional deprivation. Mentalization deficits resulting from these attachment disorders may lower the threshold for emotional reactivity. Bateman and Fonagy suggest threats to the self result in high levels of arousal and overwhelming negative affect and failure of mentalization. For those with ASPD, threats take the form of threatened loss of self-worth or respect, shame, and humiliation. These unrepresented feelings have to be expelled through violence. An increased capacity for mentalization may therefore protect against violence. See summary in Table 8.3.

Assessment
Assessment of ASPD follows these stages:
- Identify co-morbid treatable conditions such as depression or substance misuse
- Identify personality traits which might be positive indicators for the effectiveness of therapy:
  - Capacity to form an attachment and relationships
  - Anxiety
  - Willingness to seek help

Table 8.3 Characteristics of anxious and psychopathic subgroups in antisocial personality disorder

	Anxious	Psychopathic
Proportion of ASPD	2/3	1/3
Childhood antecedents	More likely to report childhood physical abuse	Maladaptive family interactions and severe institutional deprivation
Associate attachment disorder	Insecure attachment	Dismissive attachment
Precipitants of violence	Become violent in response to perceived threats to their sense of self	Planned, predatory violence
Violence	High affect, impulsive, hyperaroused	Low affect, callous, unemotional

See **➔** Violence and aggression in Chapter 6, p. 304–8.

- Risk assessment, preferably with a well-validated risk assessment tool:
  - HCR-20
  - Violence and Risk Appraisal Guide (VRAG)
- Assess severity of psychopathy using PCL-R.

Contraindications for therapy
- Sadistic, aggressive behaviour resulting in serious injury
- Complete absence of remorse or justification for aggressive behaviour
- Very superior intellect or mild intellectual disability
- Absence of capacity to form attachments
- Unexpected fear experienced by the clinician in the patient's presence
- More predatory violence is less amenable to treatment.

Treatment
(See **➔** Psychological therapy in secure settings in Chapter 8, pp. 438–9.)
  There have only been a few quality trials of the effectiveness of psychological therapies in people with ASPD. Programmes with the largest effect size adhere to the RNR model which targets those at greatest risk of reoffending, focusing attention on empirically established dynamic criminogenic risk factors. Dropout rates are high, so offender engagement is a priority.

Medication
- Evidence of the effectiveness of pharmacological treatment is limited.
- Medication should not be used routinely for the primary traits of ASPD.
- Be alert to problems of adherence and misuse.

Creating a safe setting
The safety of patients and staff must be secured, before treatment can begin. This includes not only the physical setting, but also the emotional setting in which therapy takes place. People with ASPD are less likely

than people with other mental health difficulties to engage in treatment and, when offered it, are more likely to reject it. This can provoke powerful rejecting responses in clinicians, which can lead to staff enactments, if not attended to. Risks can only be managed if the anxieties of staff and patients are managed. Supervision and reflective practice are therefore essential.

Main treatment approaches
• CBT
• DBT
• Schema-focused therapy
• MBT.

Each of these different modalities may be delivered in group, individual, TC, or family formats. Group therapies are less arousing for those with poor impulse control and offer more opportunities for mentalizing. Modelling appropriate behaviour is also important.

Engagement
Factors contributing to poor engagement are:
• Most of those with ASPD do not accept they have a problem and need help.
• Referral for therapy can be made for the wrong reasons, e.g. to reduce risk. Therapy should be aimed at addressing mental health and psychological factors, not only risk.
• Therapeutic motivation is often overestimated.
• 75% who start drop out. Treatment dropouts show poorer outcomes.

Improving engagement
• Psycho-education about personality disorder
• Goal-based motivational interviewing
• Introduce strategies to reduce factors known to reduce adherence
• Rapport and relationship are essential
• Being authoritative, not authoritarian.

Establishing a group process
Suspicion and lack of trust are likely to get in the way of forming relationships in therapeutic groups. This may be overcome by:
• The therapist actively fostering links, as those with ASPD may have little interest in each other
• Avoiding the development of a paranoid 'basic assumption' group
• Linking actions to affects and internal mental states
• Focusing on improving self-regard and social and interpersonal success
• Interventions aimed at victim empathy not likely to be successful in the early stages.

Boundaries
When establishing boundaries regarding behaviour in sessions, the following features of ASPD need to be taken into account:
• Experience of relationships in terms of power and control
• Dominance and hierarchy are likely to pervade
• Distrust of parental figures and authority

- The group may have their own strict code of conduct
- Boundary violations are likely.

Establishing boundaries
- Explore their own code of conduct first
- Recognize, at breaks in therapy and endings, there will be increased risk of acting out
- Gender: treat male and female people with ASPD separately.

Women present different diagnostic needs and profile and have a higher incidence of co-morbid BPD.

Recommended reading
Bateman A and Fonagy P (2008). Co-morbid antisocial and borderline personality disorders: mentalisation-based treatment. *Journal of Clinical Psychology: In Session*, **64**, 181–94.
Cleckley H (1941). *The Mask of Sanity*. Mosby: St Louis, MO.
Meloy JR (1988). *The Psychopathic Mind: Origins, Dynamics and Treatment*. Rowman and Littlefield Publishers, Inc.: Lanham, MD.
Meloy R and Yakeley J (2014). Antisocial personality disorder. In: Gabbard GO and Gunderson J, eds. *Gabbard's Treatments of Psychiatric Disorders*. American Psychiatric Publishing: Washington DC.
Yakeley J and Williams A (2014). Antisocial personality disorder: new directions. *Advances in Psychiatric Treatment*, **20**, 132–43.

Cluster A personality disorders
Paranoid, schizoid, and schizotypal personality disorders fall within Cluster A (DSM-5). Cluster A personality disorders are a relatively neglected subject, and there are few studies to draw on regarding the effectiveness of therapy. This is, in part, because those people who suffer from these disorders are generally disinclined to seek treatment. Tyrer (2003) described a broad classification of personality disorders into treatment seeking (Type S) and treatment rejecting (Type R) subgroups. The wish to seek help is not confined to one diagnostic category but does approximate to PD clusters:
- Cluster A likely to be Type R
- Cluster B may be either Type R or S
- Cluster C likely to be Type S.

People with Cluster A PD are less likely to come to the attention of mental health services than either the dramatic or anxious fearful clusters. If they do, they are less likely to engage in and complete therapy. The prevalence rates of Cluster A PDs are between 1% and 4% in community samples. They are commoner in men than women.

Paranoid personality disorder
Diagnosis
People with a paranoid personality disorder (PPD) demonstrate global mistrust and suspicion of the motives of others. DSM-5 diagnostic criteria describe the following features in PPD:
- Beliefs that others are using, lying to, or harming them, without apparent evidence
- Doubting the loyalty or trustworthiness of others
- Reluctance to confide in others, for fear confidence will be betrayed

- Interpreting ambiguous or benign remarks as threatening
- Holding grudges
- Believing their reputation or character is being assailed and retaliating
- Jealousy and suspicion that intimate partners are being unfaithful.

These difficulties have been present since adolescence or early adulthood, and are not part of a psychotic episode or the result of substance misuse. People with this disorder tend to be antagonistic in their behaviour, introverted, hypersensitive, and hypervigilant. They demonstrate rigidity in their thinking and patterns of relating, and a tendency to excessive autonomy. Where paranoid beliefs are based on the belief that persecution is deserved, depression may be present. A degree of suspiciousness falls within the normal spectrum of personality functioning and may confer an evolutionary advantage in detecting threat.

Differentiating PPD from other types of personality disorder characterized by social withdrawal can be difficult:
- Schizoid personality disorder (SPD)—social withdrawal is due to indifference
- Schizotypal personality disorder (StPD)—odd beliefs
- Avoidant personality disorder (AvPD)—social withdrawal is not on the basis of others' malevolence.

Co-morbidity with other personality disorder is present in over half of cases of PPD, and over 50% suffer from panic disorder.

It can be difficult to distinguish PPD from delusional disorder. Generally, people with PPD do not display persistent delusional symptoms, the degree of impairment of reality testing being the distinguishing feature. Delusional disorder may emerge in the face of a stressful event in someone who has a PPD. This is important from a legal point of view. People with PPD should not be detained under the Mental Health Act, unless there is intercurrent mental illness, and they should be held responsible for their actions. PPD appears genetically distinct from schizophrenia.

Conceptualizations of paranoid personality disorder
(See ➜ Psychoanalytic psychotherapy in Chapter 2, pp. 20–30; Cognitive behavioural therapy in Chapter 2, pp. 30–4.)

Table 8.4 outlines psychoanalytic and cognitive conceptualizations of PPD.

The risk of violence in PPD is a consequence of:
- Others' actions perceived as threatening—the risk of retaliation
- Violence generally follows provocation
- Co-morbid disorders which increase disinhibition and escalate risk
- PPD is associated with stalking behaviour, making threats, and complaining behaviour (see ➜ Violence and aggression in Chapter 6, pp. 304–8).

Therapeutic approaches in paranoid personality disorder
There have been no RCTs of therapy in PPD. If therapy is offered, a pragmatic approach is advocated, directed towards:
- Recognizing and accepting vulnerability
- Increasing feelings of self-worth
- Developing a more trusting view of others

Table 8.4 Conceptualizations of paranoid personality disorder

Psychoanalytic model	Cognitive model
Paranoid schizoid position (Klein): <ul><li>Primary part object split into good and bad</li><li>The ego rids itself of the bad object using projective mechanisms</li><li>The dominance of projective mechanisms</li></ul>	*Externalizing attributional bias:* <ul><li>Normal self-serving bias exaggerated and distorted</li><li>A default position of paranoid attribution is resorted to as cognitive load increases</li><li>Explain negative events by blaming others</li><li>Hypervigilance associated with attentional bias towards noticing threat-related information</li></ul>
Problems with introjection: <ul><li>Introjection of bad part object threatens the infant with destruction</li><li>Omnipotent attempts to ward off the bad object through splitting, idealization, and disavowal</li><li>Object constancy is not established</li></ul>	*Information processing:* <ul><li>This may include deficits in emotional and social perception</li><li>Underuse of contextual information</li><li>Perceptual deficits result in a return to the default paranoid position</li></ul>
The link with depression: <ul><li>Beneath this defensive structure lie infantile feelings of helplessness, worthlessness, inadequacy, and depression</li><li>Paranoid and melancholic defences may be resorted to as a defence against loss</li></ul>	*Interpersonal processes:* <ul><li>Normal subjects become paranoid in certain social situations:<ul><li>Feeling different from the social group, under evaluative scrutiny, uncertainty about social status</li><li>Paranoid thinking emerges in the face of sudden social loss or isolation</li><li>Acute disruption of social networks</li><li>Sensory deficits</li><li>Actual powerlessness and victimization</li></ul></li><li>Depression and low self-esteem considered secondary or co-morbid</li></ul>
Environmental failure to contain infantile feelings and aggression play a fundamental pathogenic role in paranoia. This may also reflect a developmental failure of mentalization in infancy	Deficits in theory of mind— understanding the intentions and mental states of others

- Verbalizing distress
- Avoiding counterproductive strategies
- Duration of at least 12 months.

Countertransference considerations are important and may include:
- The patient being referred for treatment by others
- Expect countertransference defensiveness, avoid reactive counterattacks
- Avoid excessive warmth or physical contact
- Do not minimize or oversimplify the risks of violence
- Avoid arousing suspicion
- An open, firm attitude may be required.

Patients struggle with any therapy, because of distrust. The following specific therapeutic approaches are thought to be effective:
- Residential therapeutic treatment
- Supportive dynamic therapy
- Schema therapy
- CBT.

If delusional symptoms develop, antipsychotics might be considered.

Schizoid personality disorder
Diagnosis
People with SPD are emotionally detached from social and personal relationships. Whilst they feel isolated, if alone for too long, close contact with others feels overwhelming, with fear of loss of identity.
   DSM-5 criteria for SPD include:
- Neither wants nor likes close relationships, counting being part of a family
- Almost constantly picks introverted activities
- Has little, if any, thought in engaging in any sexual experiences
- Seldom derives pleasure from any activities
- Has no close friends other than immediate relatives
- Appears apathetic, to the admiration or disapproval of others
- Shows emotional coldness, detachment, or flattened affectivity.

Their presentation is characterized by:
- Poor social skills
- Limited emotional range
- Limited expressions of feelings towards others
- Contact with others is painful and lacks meaning
- Internal fantasy life can be intense, but difficult to access
- Hostility is rare, but passive resistance common.

It can be difficult to distinguish SPD from autistic spectrum disorder. As a result of the difficulties with engagement, they may resort to substance misuse.

Conceptualizations of schizoid personality disorder
(See ➔ Psychoanalytic psychotherapy in Chapter 2, pp. 20–30; Cognitive behavioural therapy in Chapter 2, pp. 30–4.)
   Table 8.5 outlines psychoanalytic and cognitive conceptualizations of SPD.

Table 8.5 Conceptualizations of schizoid personality disorder

Psychoanalytic model	Cognitive model
The withdrawal characteristic of SPD is a defence against a tendency to: • Rapidly identify with others becoming transiently dependent, demanding, controlling, and devaluing • The 'claustro-agoraphobic dilemma' (Rey, 1986) • Oscillation between extremes of identification and withdrawal • The good parts of the self are projected, leading to ego depletion • Introjected bad part objects lead to persecution of the ego	SPD may exist on a continuum between: • Normality and negative symptoms of schizophrenia and • Extreme introversion, possibly linked with autistic spectrum disorder *Interpersonal processes:* • Problems understanding and experiencing emotions, social rules, and interpersonal behaviour like autistic spectrum disorder • Deficits in processing theory of mind may be crucial • Disturbed maternal relationship compounded by social learning

Therapeutic approaches

Whilst there is no strong evidence regarding effective therapeutic practice, the principles of therapeutic work are:

• Careful attention to the therapeutic alliance
• The therapist's responsiveness to psychotic anxieties
• Attention to countertransference phenomena, especially negative countertransference
• Attention to the communicative aspects of countertransference as a means of understanding and articulating the patient's unbearable states of mind.

Group therapy can help with socialization. Medication has little impact.

Schizotypal personality disorder
Diagnosis

The term 'schizotype' was first used by Rado in 1953. It indicates a pervasive pattern of social and interpersonal deficits, characterized by reduced capacity for relationships and odd beliefs. StPD has features in common with schizophrenia and schizoaffective disorder. Although its onset is in early adulthood, features may be evident in childhood. The presentation is subject to periodic exacerbations with the development of delusional beliefs. Family, twin, and adoption studies indicate it is best classified in the schizophrenia spectrum. A small minority go on to develop schizophrenia.

DSM-5 criteria for StPD include:
• Ideas of reference
• Odd beliefs and magical thinking
• Unusual perceptual experiences, including bodily illusions
• Odd thinking and speech
• Suspiciousness or paranoid ideation

Table 8.6 Conceptualizations of schizotypal personality disorder

Psychoanalytic model	Cognitive model
From an internal world perspective:	
• Strong feelings evoke intense anxiety and can threaten their hold on reality	• StPD is on a continuum between the normal range and positive symptoms of schizophrenia
• People with StPD have fragmented ego function and a precarious sense of identity	• Related experience within the normal range would include phenomena such as déjà vu
• Early fragmentation of the ego and damage to the sense of self similar to that in schizophrenia	• Odd superstitious beliefs are attributed to internal emotional and reasoning biases
• Fixation at paranoid schizoid level	
• Primitive part object relationships	
• Impoverished mental representations	

- Inappropriate or constricted affect
- Odd, eccentric, or peculiar behaviour or appearance
- Lack of close friends
- Excessive social anxiety.

Conceptualizations
(See ➲ Psychoanalytic psychotherapy in Chapter 2, pp. 20–30; Cognitive behavioural therapy in Chapter 2, pp. 30–4.)

Table 8.6 outlines psychoanalytic and cognitive conceptualizations of StPD.

Therapeutic approaches
(See ➲ Psychoanalytic psychotherapy in Chapter 2, pp. 20–30; Cognitive behavioural therapy in Chapter 2, pp. 30–4.)

- Psychodynamic: fragmentation of objects and mental functioning are a defence against making links between cause and effect which might bring painful feeling (Bion, 1967). An additional complication of therapeutic work with people with StPD is the tendency towards psychotic decompensation in the face of progress towards integration in therapy.
- CBT: particular attention to cognitive distortions and reality testing is required in StPD.

Recommended reading

Beck AT, Freeman A, and Davis DD (2004). Paranoid personality disorder. In: Beck AT, Freeman A, and Davis DD, eds. *Cognitive Therapy of Personality Disorders*, second edition. Guilford Press: New York.

Bion WR (1967). The differentiation of the psychotic from the non-psychotic parts of the personality. In: *Second Thoughts*. pp. 43–64. Heinemann: London (reprinted Karnac: London, 1984).

Rey H (1986). The schizoid mode of being and the space-time continuum (beyond metaphor). *Journal of the Melanie Klein Society*, **4**, 53.

Tyrer P, Michard S, Methuen C, and Ranger M (2003). Treatment rejecting and treatment seeking personality disorders: Type R and Type S. *Journal of Personality Disorders*, **17**, 263–8.

Cluster C personality disorders

Avoidant, dependent, and obsessive–compulsive personality disorders fall within Cluster C (DSM-5). Cluster C personality disorders generally show less impairment than personality disorders in Clusters A and B. Most treatment studies have examined the three Cluster C personality disorders together and have generally focused on individual psychotherapy and day treatment programmes. Although there are few clinical trials of Cluster C personality disorders, compared to BPD, there is evidence that both psychodynamic and cognitive behavioural approaches produce positive effect sizes. Moreover, attrition rates by the end of treatment for patients with Cluster C disorders are lower than those with Cluster A and B disorders.

Avoidant personality disorder

Diagnosis

AvPD is characterized by a pervasive pattern of social inhibition, feelings of inadequacy, and hypersensitivity to negative evaluation, beginning in early adulthood and present in a variety of contexts. People with this disorder want interpersonal relationships but, because of their extreme sensitivity to criticism, actively avoid social situations, unless total acceptance is guaranteed.

DSM-5 specifies that they present with four or more of the following:
- Avoidance of occupational activities that involve interpersonal contact, because of fears of criticism, disapproval, or rejection
- Are unwilling to get involved with people, unless certain of being liked
- Show restraint within intimate relationships, because they fear being shamed or ridiculed
- Are preoccupied with criticism or rejection in social situations
- Are inhibited in new interpersonal situations, because of feelings of inadequacy
- View themselves as socially inept, personally unappealing, or inferior to others
- Are unusually reluctant to take personal risks or engage in any new activities, because they may prove embarrassing.

Prevalence is less than 1% of the general population and around 10% of clinical populations.

Co-morbidity

People with AvPD have a high incidence of:
- Depressive episodes (see ⊃ Affective disorders in Chapter 7, pp. 326–31)
- Drugs and alcohol use to self-medicate anxiety (see ⊃ Anxiety and anxiety disorders in Chapter 7, pp. 324–6; Substance misuse in Chapter 7, pp. 338–45)
- 45% overlap with dependent personality disorder (DPD) (see ⊃ Dependent personality disorder in Chapter 8, pp. 410–12).

Aetiology
- Biological mechanisms:
  - There is evidence that a shy, reserved temperament and over-reactivity to novelty are genetically transmitted
  - Hypersensitivity of brain areas involved in the separation anxiety response and overactive limbic serotonergic circuits may be implicated
  - AvPD may have biological mechanisms in common with anxiety disorder and social phobia
- Developmental contributions:
  - Significantly greater childhood rejection and isolation in AvPD than controls
  - Children belittled, criticized, or rejected by parents, reinforced and perpetuated at school
  - Most childhood shyness dissipates in adolescence but may worsen in those who go on to develop AvPD
  - Anxious attachment: people with AvPD want attachment but are simultaneously anxious about punishment and neglect:
    —Anxious avoidant attachment corresponds to AvPD
    —Anxious ambivalent attachment corresponds to those with AvPD and DPD.

Conceptualizations
(See ➲ Psychoanalytic psychotherapy in Chapter 2, pp. 20–30; Cognitive behavioural therapy in Chapter 2, pp. 30–4.)
  Table 8.7 outlines psychodynamic and cognitive conceptualizations of AvPD.

Therapeutic approaches
Evidence suggests that:
- Those who are simply avoidant may respond better to cognitive models of therapy, whereas those with an obsessive component to their avoidance are more likely to respond to psychodynamic or interpersonal models.
- Short-term social skills training, along with CBT, increases the frequency of social encounters.
- Adding behavioural interventions has some success. Symptomatic improvement does not often lead to remission of AvPD.
- The struggle between the therapist and patient may be the common effective factor in interpersonal models.
- After 1 year of supportive expressive psychodynamic therapy, 40% still had AvPD, but depression, anxiety, and interpersonal problems improved.

Anxiolytic medication may relieve anxiety but should be combined with psychological treatment.
  The following treatments have been used:
- CBT (see ➲ Cognitive behavioural therapy in Chapter 2, pp. 30–4, and in Chapter 5, pp. 172–84)
  - Cognitive and behavioural strategies are based on:
    —Reinforcing assertiveness and self-esteem
    —Restructuring cognitive distortions between self and others
    —Addressing conscious and unconscious dependency needs

Table 8.7 Conceptualizations of avoidant personality disorder

Psychodynamic models	Cognitive behavioural models
Psychoanalytic: A defence against embarrassment, humiliation, and rejection incurred during developmental interactions (Gabbard)	*The risk resources model (Beck):* • AvPD magnifies the risks of the task and minimizes their own resources
Core conflict relationship theme (Luborski): Harsh superego projected and experienced as harsh expectations from others	*Early maladaptive rigid, chronic schemas (Young):* • Incompetent • Unlovable • Vulnerable to harm
Structural analysis of social behaviour model (Benjamin): • Relentless control in childhood to create a favourable social image • Mistakes responded to through humiliation and exclusion	*Dysfunctional cognitive processing (Newman):* • Magnifying errors of commission • Minimizing errors of omission
Defences: Paranoid schizoid position: • Projection of the bad object into an external world, then experienced as persecuting • Splitting: ideal self, loved by ideal object; bad self, rejected by bad object Harsh critical superego, experienced as the judgement of others. Ego diminished and in the thrall of superego *Object:* experienced as intolerant of difference *Self:* intolerant of loss and disappointment	*Typical beliefs:* • I can't tolerate negative feelings • If others getting close and discover the 'real me', I will be rejected • If I don't expect much, I won't be disappointed • Better not to act than act and fail • I am not good socially

- Attending to:
  - Excessive focus on risks, insufficient on rewards
  - Limited trial and error: lack of habituation
  - Limited opportunities for surprising success and peak experiences from striving to overcome
  - Regretful embitteredness about the limitations imposed by self-protective strategies
  - The reinforcing effects of disappointment and disapproval of others through avoidance
- Supportive expressive therapy (Luborski):
  - Identification of core conflictual relationship theme, describing relational style during development as manifest in the transference
  - Empathy for humiliation and embarrassment, using examples in the transference

- Attention to unconscious impulses and fears which lead to avoidance, e.g. fear of exposure of sexual interest or unconscious aggressive feelings
- Anxieties about retaliation or harm
- Exposure in psychodynamic work involves exposure to the anxiety-provoking social scenario in the transference
- Structural analysis of social behaviour (Benjamin):
  - Social relationships are complementary and polarizing
  - Avoidance elicits excessive demands and leads to conflict.

Dependent personality disorder
Diagnosis
The behaviour of people with DPD is directed towards avoiding the loss of intimate others and the need to be taken care of. To this end, they relinquish their own needs, opinions, expression of feelings, and self-identity, getting others to take over responsibility. Their self-concept is characterized by weakness and helplessness.

DSM-5 criteria for individuals with DPD include:
- Difficulty making routine decisions without reassurance and advice from others
- Requiring others to assume their responsibilities
- Fear of disagreeing with others and incurring disapproval
- Difficulty initiating projects without support
- Excessive need for nurturance and support from others, allowing others to impose themselves, rather than risk rejection
- Feeling vulnerable and helpless when alone
- Desperately seeking another relationship when one ends
- Unrealistic preoccupation with being left alone and helpless
- Passive expression of sexual or aggressive needs.

Prevalence: around 0.7% in general population.

Co-morbidity
- At higher risk of anxiety, depression and adjustment disorders following loss (see ● Anxiety and anxiety disorders in Chapter 7, pp. 324–6; Affective disorders in Chapter 7, pp. 326–31; Loss in Chapter 6, pp. 298–300)
- A significant proportion also have AvPD (see ● Avoidant personality disorder in Chapter 8, pp. 407–10)
- Dependence is a feature of other psychiatric disorders, including schizophrenia and depression.

Aetiology
Research indicates that:
- A proportion of those who go on to develop DPD show separation anxiety in childhood
- It is more likely that DPD arises from deprivation than overgratification
- Oversolicitous, controlling parents discourage getting needs met outside the family
- Families of those with DPD tend to be low in expressiveness, strong on control.

Conceptualizations
(See ➲ Psychoanalytic psychotherapy in Chapter 2, pp. 20–30; Cognitive behavioural therapy in Chapter 2, pp. 30–4.)

Table 8.8 outlines psychoanalytic and cognitive conceptualizations of DPD.

Therapeutic approaches
Whilst there have been few RCTs of therapy for DPD, those studies undertaken demonstrate that the treatment of DPD is often successful. This is the case for both CBT and psychodynamic treatments. Longer treatments may be needed for patients with DPD, compared to patients with non-dependent personality traits.

Therapy with people with DPD presents particular challenges:
• Repeated requests of the therapist for advice and help
• Succumbing to pressure to assume a directive dominant role
• Compliance to preserve the therapeutic attachment at the cost of real engagement
• The development of a punitive relationship
• Failure to mourn losses prior to termination
• Underestimating the importance of cultural context.

The following therapeutic approaches have been used in DPD:
• CBT (see ➲ Cognitive behavioural therapy in Chapter 2, pp. 30–4, and in Chapter 5, pp. 172–84):
  • Foster therapeutic alliance
  • Accept the relationship is a microcosm of the dependence problem
  • Encourage openness

Table 8.8 Conceptualizations of dependent personality disorder

Psychodynamic model	Cognitive model
Early psychoanalytic theories:	*Typical beliefs:*
• Fixation at oral stage of development (Freud)	• I am inadequate and helpless, and the world is cold, lonely, and dangerous
• Excess oral gratification (Abraham)	• If I rely on myself ,I will fail
Psychoanalytic theories of loss and separation (Freud, 1917):	• If I depend upon others, I will survive
Freud identified two defences against loss of an object from which a mature separation has yet to occur:	• The best strategy is to find someone who can deal with the world and protect me
• Melancholic—the lost object is internalized and aggression directed towards the self	
• Paranoid—blame for the loss is projected and experienced as an attack.	
Those deploying melancholic defences may treat others as part of themselves from whom they are inseparable to avoid the pain of separation.	

- Foster accurate self-appraisal, independent decision-making, and behaviour through:
  —Setting goals
  —Socratic questioning
  —Avoiding taking the lead
- Formulation of cognitive profile
- Relaxation training to reduce anxiety
- Graded exposure
- Group therapy may reduce dependence
- Taper frequency of sessions

- Individual psychodynamic therapy (see ➲ Psychoanalytic psychotherapy in Chapter 2, pp. 20–30, and in Chapter 5, pp. 163–72):
  - Address dependence directly in the transference
  - Expect high levels of dependency in the transference
  - Take up dependence to promote emotional growth
  - Promote self-expression and assertiveness
  - Promote decision-making and independence
  - Avoid taking a directive role
  - Interpret defences against loss and difficulty coming to terms with the separateness of the therapist
  - Increase moves to autonomy, in anticipation of ending
- Group psychotherapy (see ➲ Group therapy and group analysis in Chapter 2, pp. 42–7, and in Chapter 5, pp. 188–94):
  - A number of studies have demonstrated the effectiveness of group psychotherapy in DPD
- Day and residential therapies:
  - Uncontrolled studies demonstrate large effect sizes in DPD. These approaches are usually offered to treatment-refractory groups
- Family therapy (see ➲ Systemic family and couple therapy in Chapter 2, pp. 34–42, and in Chapter 5, pp. 184–8):
  - Family therapy may be effective for those with DPD who live with their families of origin and who may be participants in complex family dynamics
  - Change in the individual may require change in the family system
- Medication (see ➲ Psychotherapy and medication in Chapter 7, pp. 322–4):
  - Antidepressants, either alone or with psychodynamic supportive therapy, have been found to be effective in the treatment of depression and underlying personality traits.

Obsessive–compulsive (anankastic) personality disorder
Diagnosis

Those with obsessive–compulsive personality disorder (OCPD) present as fearful, insecure, compulsive individuals who demonstrate an exaggerated and pervasive attempt to control those who are close to them. They assert control of their thoughts and emotions and every uncertainty. They are thought to lack an internal sense of security and so attempt to make the world predictable. They are characterized by their inflexibility and stubbornness, and perfectionism and orderliness, at the cost of efficiency.

They should present with at least four of the following, according to DSM-5:

- Preoccupation with details, rules, lists, order, organization, or schedules, to the extent that the point of the activity is lost
- Perfectionism that interferes with task completion
- Excessive devotion to work, to the exclusion of leisure and friendships, without economic necessity
- Overconscientiousness, scrupulousness, and inflexibility about morality, ethics, or values outside cultural and religious identifications
- Unable to discard worn-out or worthless objects when they have no sentimental value
- Reluctant to delegate tasks or to work with others, unless they submit to exactly his or her way of doing things
- A miserly spending style towards self and others; money is hoarded against future catastrophes
- Rigidity and stubbornness.

They may be indecisive, out of fear of making a mistake, conscientious and scrupulous, and pedantic, respecting rules and authority as absolute. They tend to be humourless, lacking spontaneity, and their affect controlled and stilted.

Prevalence: 1% of the general population; 10% of depressed and anxious psychiatric patients. Males > females.

Co-morbidity
- OCD: there is overlap, but most of those with OCD do not have OCPD
- Depressive and anxiety disorders are common, as well as phobic and somatoform disorders (see ➜ Anxiety and anxiety disorders in Chapter 7, pp. 324–6; Affective disorders in Chapter 7, pp. 326–31).

Conceptualizations
(See ➜ Psychoanalytic psychotherapy in Chapter 2, pp. 20–30; Cognitive behavioural therapy in Chapter 2, pp. 163–72.)
Table 8.9 outlines psychoanalytic and cognitive conceptualizations of OCPD.

Therapeutic approaches
Studies suggests that:
- There is relatively little evidence for the effectiveness of therapy in OCPD
- Comparative studies demonstrate both short-term dynamic psychotherapy and CBT are effective, bringing symptomatic improvement in around 50% of patients, which is sustained at 2-year follow-up
- Depressed patients with OCPD respond slightly better to interpersonal than cognitive behavioural approaches
- Relatively longer periods of therapy are required than in OCD.

Table 8.9 Conceptualizations of obsessive–compulsive personality disorder

Psychodynamic model	Cognitive model
Early analytic theories: • Linked with the anal stage of development • Orderliness—a reaction formation against anal messiness • Libidinal drives in conflict with parental attempts at socialization • Self-critical internalization of maternal power struggle as a punitive superego • Catastrophic anxiety at the Oedipal stage; leads to a retreat to the anal stage *Later analytic theory:* • Autonomy versus parental wishes • Shame and criticism for expressions of anger • Praise for what the child does, rather than what he is • Feelings seen as weak and shameful • Individual emotions subordinated to the needs of the group *Object relations theory:* • Strong, unfulfilled, dependent longings; rage at unavailable parents • High expectations of parental demonstrativeness • Both dependence and anger are unacceptable, hence reaction formation and isolation • Anxious that anger will drive others away • Harsh superego expects more and more	Strong hereditary component to anankastic personality traits Compulsive behaviour learned during upbringing through: • Competitive spirit, separating winners from losers • 'Work hard, avoid mistakes' • Develops into needless self-restrictions Out of touch with their own desires or wishes, and so doubt their decisions Stimulus-bound thought processes: preoccupied with detail, rather than the bigger picture CBT approaches attend to perfectionism, scrupulousness, and intolerance of failure

The challenges of therapeutic work with people with OCPD are:
• Perfectionism in the patient
• Competitiveness with the therapist
• Enervating countertransference.

The following therapeutic approaches have been used:
• CBT (see ➲ Cognitive behavioural therapy in Chapter 2, pp. 30–4, and in Chapter 5, pp. 172–84): therapy starts with a descriptive evaluation of faulty behaviour and evaluation of maintaining factors.

- List maladaptive beliefs such as:
  —It is important to do a perfect job in everything
  —Any flaw or defect in performance will lead to disaster
  —People should do things my way
  —Details are extremely important
- Open-ended Socratic questioning
- Increase tolerance of mistakes will reduce the degree of punishment
- Interventions may be made emotionally evocative by the introduction of imagery
- Indecisiveness: counter the belief that there is an absolutely right decision to make
- Identify schemas such as incompetence, unrelenting standards, lack of individuation
- Maintaining factors: innate conservatism mitigates against change
- Psychodynamic therapy (see ➔ Psychoanalytic psychotherapy in Chapter 2, pp. 20–30, and in Chapter 5, pp. 163–72):
  - Identifying feelings underlying intellectual defences
  - Interpret defences against unacceptable feelings
  - Focus on that which interferes with enjoyment
  - Therapy aims for modification of harsh superego
- Medication (see ➔ Psychotherapy and medication in Chapter 7, pp. 322–4):
  - Benzodiazepines can reduce tension
  - Antidepressants can improve mood and global functioning.

Recommended reading

Freud S (1917). Mourning and melancholia. In: Strachey J, ed. *The Standard Edition of the Complete Psychological Works of Sigmund Freud, 1914–1916*, volume 14. pp. 243–58. Hogarth Press: London.

Leichsenring F and Leibling E (2003). The effectiveness of psychodynamic therapy and cognitive behaviour therapy in the treatment of personality disorders: a meta-analysis. *American Journal of Psychiatry*, **160**, 1223–32.

Luborsky L (1984). *Principles of Psychoanalytic Psychotherapy: A Manual for Supportive Expressive Treatment*. Basic Books: New York.

Narcissistic and histrionic personality disorders

Narcissistic personality disorder (NPD) and histrionic personality disorder (HPD) fall under the 'dramatic, emotional, erratic' Cluster B of DSM-5, along with BPD and ASPD. Both NPD and HPD have conceptual antecedents in a rich psychoanalytic literature. However, due to their poor construct validity and the lack of rigorously designed treatment trials for these disorders, particularly for HPD, the DSM-5 Personality Disorders Work Group originally recommended the deletion of these two diagnoses from the diagnostic manual. Nevertheless, the identification of narcissistic and histrionic personality traits in patients presenting for treatment may be clinically useful in tailoring therapeutic approaches, particularly where such traits influence the manifestations of co-morbid mental disorders.

Narcissistic personality disorder
Diagnosis
Narcissism ranges from healthy to pathological, with malignant narcissism and psychopathy representing its most severe forms. The boundary between normal and pathological narcissism will vary, according to the person's experiences of life circumstances and interpersonal relationships. Moreover, it is not always clear where temporary protective narcissistic strategies, which may be necessary to enhance self-esteem and self-regulation, are replaced by more stable and enduring pathological narcissistic traits that may constitute a diagnosis of narcissistic personality disorder (NPD).

DSM-5 diagnostic criteria for NPD require five or more of the following features:
• Has a grandiose sense of self-importance (e.g. exaggerates achievements and talents, expects to be recognized as superior without commensurate achievements)
• Is preoccupied with fantasies of unlimited success, power, brilliance, beauty, or ideal love
• Believes that he or she is 'special' and can only be understood by, or should associate with, other special or high-status people (or institutions)
• Requires excessive admiration
• Has a sense of entitlement (i.e. unreasonable expectations of especially favourable treatment or automatic compliance with his or her expectations)
• Is interpersonally exploitative (i.e. takes advantage of others to achieve his or her own ends)
• Lacks empathy, is unwilling to recognize or identify with the feelings and needs of others
• Is often envious of others or believes that others are envious of him or her
• Shows arrogant, haughty behaviour or attitudes.

Prevalence
The lifetime prevalence of NPD has been estimated at 1% to 6% in the general population, and 2% to 16% in clinical populations. 50% to 75% of those diagnosed with NPD are male. Narcissistic traits are particularly common in adolescents, but most will not go on to develop the full disorder; however, older adults with NPD may have special difficulties in adjusting to the ageing process. There is also some evidence that narcissistic traits in the general population are increasing over time, possibly due to sociocultural influences on parenting practices and the promotion of self-esteem independent of achievement.

Co-morbidity
NPD is associated with a number of mental disorders, including:
• Depression and anxiety (see ➋ Anxiety and anxiety disorders in Chapter 7, pp. 324–6; Affective disorders in Chapter 7, pp. 326–31)
• Eating disorders (see ➋ Eating disorders in Chapter 7, pp. 334–8)

- PTSD (see → Trauma-related conditions in Chapter 7, pp. 355–9)
- Substance misuse (see → Substance misuse in Chapter 7, pp. 338–45)
- Suicidality (see → Suicide and self-harm in Chapter 6, pp. 308–11)
- Borderline, histrionic, paranoid, and antisocial personality disorders (see → Borderline personality disorder in Chapter 8, pp. 390–6; Histrionic personality disorder in Chapter 8, pp. 420–2; Paranoid personality disorder in Chapter 8, pp. 396–401; Antisocial personality disorder in Chapter 8, pp. 396–401)

Aetiology

Like other mental disorders, NPD is best understood in a biopsychosocial model. Empirical research shows that:

- Behavioural genetic studies indicate NPD has a heritable component, accounting for about 40% of the total variance
- Narcissistic traits in children precede the development of NPD in adults
- Overpermissive parenting is associated with grandiose narcissism
- Cold, overcontrolled parenting is associated with vulnerable narcissism
- Insecure attachment styles as measured on the AAI are associated with NPD (see → Theories of personality development: attachment theory in Chapter 8, pp. 380–1)
- Rates of narcissistic traits in students are higher today, compared to 30 years ago.

Conceptualizations

(See → Psychoanalytic psychotherapy in Chapter 2, pp. 20–30; Cognitive behavioural therapy in Chapter 2, pp. 30–4.)

The origins of narcissism as a psychological construct may be traced to psychoanalytic formulations, based in Freud's concepts of narcissism and libido theory. The two main psychoanalytic theorists who have furthered the conceptualizations and treatment of pathological narcissism are Otto Kernberg and Heinz Kohut in their respective, albeit conflicting, theories—the former emphasizing conflict and aggression in the aetiology of NPD, and the latter more focused on deficit and narcissistic injury leading to poor self-esteem and depression. More recent psychodynamic conceptualizations emphasize problems in the regulation of self-esteem, with co-occurring grandiosity and vulnerability, and associated difficulties in identity, self-direction, empathy, and intimacy; and linking the development of these deficits to early disruptions in attachment and the impairment of mentalization/reflective function. Meanwhile, cognitive theorists, such as Jeffrey Young, have expanded Beck's original theories of core distorted beliefs and dysfunctional schemas in NPD via integration with interpersonal and gestalt perspectives and a particular focus on the role of early experiences and affect in the aetiology and treatment of the disorder.

Table 8.10 outlines psychodynamic and cognitive conceptualizations of NPD (see → Psychoanalytic psychotherapy in Chapter 2, pp. 20–30; Cognitive behavioural therapy in Chapter 2, pp. 30–4).

Table 8.10 Conceptualizations of narcissistic personality disorder

Psychodynamic models	Cognitive behavioural model

Kernberg (conflict model):
• Early childhood experience of cold, indifferent, or aggressive parental figures; child finds area of talent or specialness as retreat
• Grandiose self is a highly pathological structure composed of ideal self, ideal object, and real self
• Primitive defence mechanisms of idealization, denigration, and splitting predominate
• Grandiosity is defence against projection of oral rage stemming from inability to internalize good objects
• Superego pathology—deficits in capacity for sadness and mourning, experience shame, but not guilt or remorse
• Main affects are envy and aggression
 Kohut (deficit model):
• Pathological narcissism arises from failure to integrate 'grandiose self' and 'idealized parental imago' in childhood development, due to early unempathic care
• Grandiose omnipotence defence against fragmentation of self
• Main affects are emptiness and depression in response to narcissistic injury
	NPD stems from combination of dysfunctional schema and core beliefs, developed via direct and indirect messages from parents, siblings, and others that mould beliefs about personal uniqueness and self-importance.
	• Core dysfunctional beliefs:
	  • Since I am special, I deserve special dispensations, privileges, and prerogatives
	  • I'm superior to others, and they should acknowledge this
	  • I'm above the rules
	• Behaviour reinforces their superior status
	• Main affect is anger when they do not get admiration or respect they believe they are entitled to; they may also become depressed
	• Deficits in cooperation and reciprocal social interaction

Therapeutic approaches

Individuals with NPD may present for treatment for a variety of reasons related to the specific stage or circumstances of their lives; however, a common factor is that their experience of life does not live up to their internal expectations and aspirations. They may present in crisis, describing difficulties and complaints from family, friends, or employers, or legal sanctions that they do not accept; or they may be referred to mental health services due to co-morbid mental conditions or suicidality. People with NPD may be difficult to engage in treatment, which underscores the importance of gradually building a therapeutic alliance with mutually agreed goals within a clearly outlined treatment frame in the initial stages of any treatment offered.

Challenges of treatment include:
- Premature dropout
- Sensitivity to developmental life changes (e.g. marriage, childbirth) and unexpected external life events that can disrupt the treatment alliance
- Patient not accepting the diagnosis of NPD, especially features of grandiosity, entitlement, and lack of empathy
- Sensitivity to feeling blamed, criticized, and unfairly treated, including by the therapist
- Poor affect tolerance, especially experiencing underlying negative affects, e.g. anxiety, shame, insecurity, and vulnerability
- Wish to please/impress the therapist or imitation of their perspective without any real change
- Suicidal ideation and behaviour
- Secondary gain from symptoms
- Aggressive, antisocial, or psychopathic features associated with poorer prognosis (see ➔ Antisocial personality disorder in Chapter 8, pp. 396–401).

A number of different treatment approaches have been developed and advocated for patients with NPD, although none have been empirically tested for evidence of efficacy. The main approaches include:
- Psychoanalysis and intensive psychoanalytic psychotherapy (see ➔ Psychoanalytic psychotherapy in Chapter 2, pp. 20–30, and in Chapter 5, pp. 163–72): advocated for highly motivated patients with good insight and affect tolerance. More severe character pathology requires a more active inter-relational approach:
  - Kernberg's ego-psychological object relations: emphasizes role of aggression and envy in the development of pathological narcissism; focus on interpretation of grandiose self, grandiose defences, and negative transference, and use of countertransference to understand patient's split-off internal representations
  - Kohut's self psychology: emphasizes roles of self-esteem and self-cohesion in the development of narcissism; focus on mirroring, idealization, and twinship, and understanding of empathic failures in the therapeutic alliance and transference
- Psychodynamic approaches (see ➔ Psychoanalytic psychotherapy in Chapter 2, pp. 20–30, and in Chapter 5, pp. 163–72):
  - TFP (Kernberg): focus on narcissistic defences, aggression, envy, sensitivity to humiliation and shame to increase tolerance of negative affect. Technique adaptable to range and level of narcissistic pathology—less interpretive for more severe
- Cognitive behavioural approaches (see ➔ Interpersonal psychotherapy in Chapter 2, pp. 52–5, and in Chapter 5, pp. 203–7; Schema therapy in Chapter 2, pp. 70–3, and in Chapter 5, pp. 234–8):
  - Schema-focused therapy (Young): focus on early maladaptive schemas of self and others, repair and regulate narcissistic modes, and promote healthier adult mode via re-parenting in therapeutic relationship

- Metacognitive interpersonal therapy (Dimaggio and Attina): manualized step-by-step treatment, starting with shared understanding of the patient's problems, progressing to recognition of maladaptive schemas and interpersonal functioning, to promoting change through identification of normal grandiosity, distancing from old behaviour, reality and perspective taking, and building healthier schemas.

Other treatment modalities that have been used for patients with NPD include CBT, DBT, MBT, and psycho-education. Group therapy can be effective in exposing and challenging difficulties around shame, dependency, self-sufficiency, narcissistic fantasies, and contempt and envy of others, although highly narcissistic individuals may dominate or disrupt groups and compete with the therapist to be the group leader (see ➔ Cognitive behavioural therapy in Chapter 2, pp. 30–4, and in Chapter 5, pp. 172–84; Dialectical behavioural therapy in Chapter 2, pp. 63–6, and in Chapter 5, pp. 220–9; Mentalization-based treatment in Chapter 2, pp. 66–70, and in Chapter 5, pp. 229–34; Group therapy and group analysis in Chapter 2, pp. 42–7, and in Chapter 5, pp. 188–94).

Pharmacological treatment has not been shown to be effective for the specific features of NPD and should be reserved for the treatment of co-morbid mental disorders such as bipolar disorder, depression, or anxiety (see ➔ Psychotherapy and medication in Chapter 7, pp. 322–4).

Histrionic personality disorder
Diagnosis
DSM-5 specifies that people with HPD present with a pervasive pattern of excessive emotionality and attention-seeking, as indicated by five or more of the following:

- Is uncomfortable in situations in which he or she is not the focus of attention
- Interaction with others is often characterized by inappropriate sexually seductive or provocative behaviour
- Displays rapidly shifting and shallow expression of emotions
- Constantly uses physical appearance to draw attention to self
- Has a style of speech that is excessively impressionistic and lacking in detail
- Shows self-dramatization, theatricality, and exaggerated expression of emotion
- Is suggestible (i.e. easily influenced by others or circumstances)
- Considers relationships to be more intimate than they actually are.

Prevalence
Although studies have indicated that HPD has a prevalence of around 2% to 3% in the general population, and 10% to 15% in inpatient and outpatient mental health institutions, other studies in specific personality disorder populations have identified very low prevalence rates of HPD (0.4%). The diagnosis has been traditionally associated with women, due to the classical notion of hysteria as 'wandering womb'. Although it is diagnosed four times more frequently in women, rather than men, this may be partly due to cultural stereotypes, and HPD may be commoner in men than previously thought.

Co-morbidity
(See ➲ Borderline personality disorder in Chapter 8, pp. 390–6; Narcissistic personality disorder in Chapter 8, pp. 407–15; Dependent personality disorder in Chapter 8, pp. 410–12; Substance misuse in Chapter 7, pp. 338–45.)

HPD has a high co-morbidity with other personality disorders, particularly BPD, NPD, and DPD, raising doubts about its validity as a diagnostic construct. However, those who receive the diagnosis may present with problematic and distressing character traits, which are more fixed and less amenable to treatment than traits associated with other personality disorders. Moreover, co-morbid substance misuse and dependence may be particularly problematic in patients with HPD.

Conceptualizations
(See ➲ Psychoanalytic psychotherapy in Chapter 2, pp. 20–30; Cognitive behavioural therapy in Chapter 2, pp. 30–4.)

The diagnosis of HPD arises from a long psychoanalytic tradition of hysterical neurosis or hysterical personality, and most of the literature on HPD has been written from a psychoanalytic or psychodynamic standpoint. More recently, HPD has received interest from cognitive therapists, although there is considerable overlap between psychodynamic and cognitive therapeutic techniques advocated for the disorder.

Table 8.11 outlines psychodynamic and cognitive conceptualizations of HPD.

Table 8.11 Conceptualizations of histrionic personality disorder

Psychodynamic model	Cognitive behavioural model
Developmental conflicts and defences:	Core negative beliefs leading to dysfunctional behaviours:
• Poor early relationship leads child to turn to parent for nurturance, gaining their attention via flirtatiousness and dramatic displays of emotion	• If I don't engage others, they won't like me
	• Unless I entertain or impress people, I am nothing
• Adult sexual relations characterized by primitive neediness	• The way to get what I want is to dazzle and amuse people
• Sexual promiscuity substitute for longed-for maternal love—'penis–breast equation'	• In order to be happy, I need other people to pay attention to me
• Goal is to be object of desire to others	• If I entertain people, they will not notice my weaknesses
• Exaggerated theatrical behaviour defence against core childhood experience of not being recognized	• It is awful if people ignore me
• Use of repression, denial, dissociation, and suppression as defence mechanisms to reduce emotional arousal	

Therapeutic approaches
There have been no empirical psychotherapy or pharmacotherapy treatment trials specifically focused on HPD. Medication is not normally considered with this group of patients who have been traditionally treated with psychoanalytic or psychodynamic psychotherapy, and, more recently, cognitive behavioural approaches. Building a therapeutic alliance, empathic listening, and agreeing goals are important in all therapeutic approaches for HPD.

Gabbard emphasizes the importance of understanding the psychodynamic organization underlying the more overt behavioural and interpersonal characteristics of HPD. He differentiates between more neurotic or hysterical patients with HPD who may be suitable for psychoanalytic or exploratory psychotherapy and those who have a more primitive underlying personality structure who present with more florid symptomatology and interpersonal difficulties and need a more supportive, rather than insight-oriented, therapeutic approach. Individuals with the neurotic variant of HPD are able to experience more mature triangular interpersonal relationships and work within the transference, whereas those with the more primitive variant experience relationships as dyadic, suffer from overwhelming separation anxiety, and may develop primitive erotized transferences to the therapist.

Because of the entrenched nature of many of the personality traits that characterize this disorder, therapy is more likely to be effective if it is long-term. Group therapy may be particularly useful in making patients with HPD more aware of the impact of their seductive, dramatic, and attention-seeking behaviour on others.

Recommended reading

Campbell WK and Miller JD (eds) (2011). *Handbook of Narcissism and Narcissistic Personality Disorder*. Wiley: Hoboken, NJ.

Gabbard GO (2014). Histrionic personality disorder. In: Gabbard GO and Gunderson J, eds. *Gabbard's Treatments of Psychiatric Disorders*. pp. 1059–72. American Psychiatric Publishing: Washington DC.

Ronningstam EF (2014). Narcissistic personality disorder. In: Gabbard GO and Gunderson J, eds. *Gabbard's Treatments of Psychiatric Disorders*. pp. 1073–86. American Psychiatric Publishing: Washington DC.

Personality disorder services

(See ➲ Therapy in clinical practice in Chapter 5, pp. 154–63; Psychological therapy in secure settings in Chapter 8, pp. 428–39; Planning psychotherapy services within psychiatric care in Chapter 10, pp. 462–6; Forensic psychiatry: forensic psychotherapies, applications, and research in Chapter 12, pp. 550–6.)

In one form or another, patients with personality disorder have been treated by mental health services for perhaps as long as services have been in existence. Whether under the guise of the treatment of 'moral insanity' in a Victorian asylum or of severe and entrenched relational difficulties in an NHS psychotherapy unit, the treatment of what we would now term personality disorder has long been the remit of mental health services in the UK. As such, services have essentially been treating patients with personality disorder for a lot longer than there have been formal personality disorder services, and it is only relatively recently that PD-specific services have been developed. Agreement over their structure, function, and specification is continuing to develop. An understanding of the development of PD services, as well as a working knowledge of what services are—and should be—available locally, can be very helpful clinically, particularly in those (not uncommon) cases where patients can become 'stuck' within the system.

Context

Given that the key features of a personality disorder often include problems in engaging consistently with treatment and a fragmented sense of self, it is perhaps not a coincidence that services for patients with personality disorder have struggled to develop in a consistent, integrated, and coherent manner. There has been a long history of ambivalence around the development and maintenance of personality disorder services, which is perhaps not entirely unrelated to the complex way that patients with personality disorder can interact with the system. Until relatively recently, it was often a widely held view that personality disorder was not the remit of secondary mental health services and that personality-disordered patients were essentially 'untreatable'. Many therapy services would view personality disorder as grounds for exclusion. Treatment in those cases, such as it was, would often be limited to crisis interventions. The personality disorder services that did exist tended to develop in an ad hoc manner as independent 'silos'. They were often excessively dependent upon the energy and expertise of local specialists or practitioners with an interest in the area. Pathways within and between different parts of services were often rudimentary or not present at all.

The case of Michael Stone is often cited as the main reason for high-profile government intervention in the development of personality disorders services. In 1996, Michael Stone had been deemed untreatable, because of his diagnosis of personality disorder, and therefore could not be detained under the MHA at that time and was thus at liberty to kill his victim Lynn Russell. Although the high-profile and shocking nature of this case was one of the main drivers for a change in government policy, which included removing the 'treatability clause' of the MHA, there were already growing levels of awareness of (and frustration about) barriers to treatment and gaps in service provision, as well as the lack of widespread knowledge and expertise in the treatment of patients with personality disorder. Whatever the ultimate cause, it was subsequent to this highly publicized case that the government made a considerable amount of money available for the development of the 'Dangerous and Severe Personality Disorder' (DSPD) programme and launched the National Personality Disorder Development Programme.

The National Personality Disorder Development Programme was designed with the aim of shifting attitudes towards the treatment of patients with personality disorder; increasing awareness and skill levels; improving the evidence base and theoretical developmental of personality disorder treatment; and the development of more integrated treatment pathways at national and local levels for patients in the community, hospital, secure care, and the prison estate. Central to this was the release, in 2003, of the key policy documents 'No Longer a Diagnosis of Exclusion' and 'Breaking the Cycle of Rejection'. These were launched to support service development and to help set a framework for training and workforce development.

In 2004, 11 innovation projects were set up nationally in the community, with the main aim of treating patients with personality disorder, as well as providing information and outcomes to aid for future planning of services. In 2007, the Department of Health and the Ministry of Justice commissioned the development of a national framework to support people to work more effectively with personality disorder—the Knowledge and Understanding Framework (KUF). The framework comprises educational programmes that are delivered by experienced and highly trained personality disorder practitioners and service user consultants. One of the central aims of the framework was (and is) to improve service user experience through developing the skills and expertise of the multi-agency workforce (health, social care, and criminal justice) who deal with the challenges of personality disorder (see ➜ Service user involvement in Chapter 10, pp. 466–71).

The DSPD programme, which was run in medium and high secure hospitals and the prison estate, provided an essential stimulus in setting up and developing areas of expertise in the treatment and management of highly disturbed, high-risk individuals who would have previously been deemed untreatable. Following a major review, the DSPD programme is undergoing decommissioning, but there continues to be a number of patients treated within it at a reduced number of sites for the time being. More recently, the emphasis in the forensic programme has shifted from focusing on intensive treatment for the 'critical few' to attempting to make fundamental changes to the system that manages offenders/high-risk patients to ensure that all offenders within the criminal justice system who have a personality disorder are identified at the earliest opportunity and screened into the personality disorder programme, and that those working with them are offered case formulation and an appropriate pathway for treatment. In essence, this represents a switch from a low-volume/high-intensity model to a higher-volume/lower-intensity approach, with the aim of having a greater overall impact on those who suffer from the effects of personality disorder (including the victims of violent offences committed by offenders with personality disorder). Part of the rationale for this appears to have been the limited evidence for the efficacy/cost-effectiveness of the original DSPD programmes, despite the good work that was undertaken (see ➜ Psychological therapy in secure settings in Chapter 8, pp. 438–9).

Another aspect of the personality development programme which has seen important changes brought in has been the close partnership with service users. Service user involvement is now an integral part of development within the field and is now nationally coordinated by the user-led organization 'Emergence', as well as through local organizations (see ➜ Service user involvement in Chapter 10, pp. 466–71).

Organization

As part of the developments, services were organized and clustered to fit in with a national personality disorder pathway model, based on six 'tiers' (see Fig. 8.6). Tier One, with the highest volume of patients who

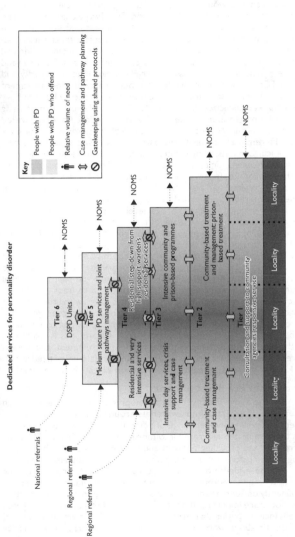

Fig. 8.6 Tiered model of personality disorder services.

have unmet needs, would be delivered through primary care, social care, specialist outreach, and the third sector. Tier Two would be delivered by mainstream mental health and specialist outreach, whilst Tier Three would see increasingly complex or high-risk patients within local specialist services. Tier Four is the level at which services become residential and involve regional and super-regional specialist services. Tiers Five and Six are essentially forensic levels, Tier Five being medium security and prison TCs, whilst Tier Six involves the personality disorder treatment units in Ashworth, Rampton, and Broadmoor High Secure Hospitals.

Recent well-publicized changes to NHS structure and commissioning processes brought about by the Health and Social Care Act 2012 have led to some uncertainty over the continued use of this tiered model, primarily as different parts of this tiered pathway are now overseen by different Clinical Commissioning Groups and bodies, leaving certain services liable to decommissioning at a local level. Tier Three services (in particular, the 11 pilot sites for specialist community-based personality disorder treatment services) had been centrally funded through the Department of Health but recently have had to apply to local Clinical Commissioning Groups for ongoing funding at a local level. This has led to some radical cuts and indeed closures of many of these units. Linked to this, Secure Commissioning Groups appear to have tightened the remit of low and medium secure provision, so that only those who present a serious risk of harm to others are admitted. In practice, this appears to mean that patients who had been referred into secure services for their capacity to provide specialist personality disorder treatment and robust relational security and understanding are being transferred to (mostly independent sector) locked rehabilitation placements, often with little specialist capacity to treat complex patients with personality disorder. Presently, there are only 60 beds in Tier Four placements, provided by four units in the London region and two in Yorkshire. Clearly, this is insufficient for the numbers of patients requiring residential treatment, and work is currently being undertaken to determine the actual level of need and to think about how this can best be provided on a local or regional level.

Further service development

Through the above initiatives and developments, there is now a much wider base of expertise and awareness around personality disorder in general, as well as a wider range of personality disorder-specific therapies that are better integrated into more coherent pathways. The issue of creating and providing national and local models and pathways that bridge commissioning interfaces (and gaps) requires ongoing work, however. As the evidence base and expertise increase, there is a growing view that no one theoretical model or mode of treatment is shown to be significantly better than another and that several factors are as important as, if not more important than, the modality of treatment itself. These factors include: having clear treatment aims; staff who are suited to, and enthusiastic about, working with personality disorder; good adherence to whatever treatment model is used; an emphasis upon the *therapeutic relationship* as the main determinant of treatment success; a good structure for supervision; and good links between management and clinicians regarding service design, treatment aims, and outcomes.

Although it appears that there is little demonstrable difference in the efficacy of the main therapeutic modalities, it may be that it is important that services are configured to allow patients to receive the most appropriate treatment at the right time, in terms of the *sequencing* of their care, e.g. offering engagement or pre-engagement work for those patients who cannot yet tolerate regular therapy, before then progressing to a therapy aimed at distress tolerance or symptom reduction (e.g. DBT). Patients could then, if required, progress to a therapy that requires more reflective capacity and is perhaps more focused on inner experience such as MBT, CAT, or psychodynamic therapy. Obviously, if patients are able to make use of such a therapy straight away, then that is what should be available for them. Ensuring that there are good links between the different treatment phases in the pathway and that endings, beginnings, and transitions can be processed appropriately should be a part of good service design.

At the time of writing, the service structure for personality disorder pathways and treatment is perhaps now less clear than it was just a few years ago. Although it could be seen that services are currently facing a period of radical change and cuts, a longer-term view is one that personality disorder and therapy services in general have a long history of struggling to define themselves and to be securely attached and well integrated—much like the patients that they try to help. Whether or not there is a link between the characteristics of patients and how the services have developed is open to opinion. What is clear is that very often the more complex and severe patients with a personality disorder often get stuck at different stages in the system, with much conflict and frustration about what the next most appropriate steps should be and where these may be available. As much as having a framework to develop a good understanding of a patient's internal world is important to assisting the patient, so too therefore is an understanding of what treatments and services are provided. This allows the practitioner to be better able to help patients and teams negotiate the inevitably difficult relationships that can develop through their treatment pathway.

Recommended reading

Department of Health (2003). *Personality Disorder: No Longer a Diagnosis of Exclusion*. Department of Health: London.

Department of Health and Home Office (1999). *Managing Dangerous People with Severe Personality Disorder: Proposals for Policy Development*. Home Office and Department of Health: London.

National Institute for Mental Health in England (2003). *Breaking the Cycle of Rejection: The Personality Disorder Capabilities Framework*. National Institute for Mental Health in England: London.

National Institute for Health and Care Excellence (2009). *Borderline Personality Disorder: Recognition and Management*. NICE Guidelines 78. Available at: ✍ https://www.nice.org.uk/guidance/cg78.

Social Exclusion Task Force (2006). *Reaching Out: An Action Plan on Social Exclusion, 2007*. Cabinet Office: London.

The Personality Disorder Knowledge and Understanding Framework. Available at: ✍ http://www.personalitydisorderkuf.org.uk.

Psychological therapy in secure settings

Forensic patients

(See ➲ Forensic psychiatry: forensic psychotherapies, applications, and research in Chapter 12, pp. 550–6.)

Patients detained in secure hospitals and prisoners with psychiatric disorders often have complex mental health needs. They typically present with a complex constellation of issues that together increase their risk of behaving violently towards others. These may include a combination of an underlying mental illness, dysfunctional personality traits, and substance misuse problems. The overwhelming majority of forensic patients have experienced some form of early life trauma or disadvantage. A proportion will have a learning disability.

The role of forensic mental health services is to provide treatment interventions which address offending behaviour and reduce the level of risk associated with antisocial behaviour. A crucial component of forensic services is to develop a working partnership with criminal justice agencies, including multi-agency public protection panels[1] (MAPPPs). The prison service also offers a programme of psychological interventions designed to reduce offending and promote risk reduction.

Relationship between mental disorders and violence

(See ➲ Violence and aggression in Chapter 6, pp. 304–8.)

This is a complex area of debate. Both violence and mental disorder are caused by multiple risk factors operating simultaneously. Mental disorders are common, but most mentally ill people are not violent, and repeated studies have shown that there is only a small, albeit significant, association with mental illness, particularly schizophrenia. The principle risk factors for violence are male gender, substance misuse, and a diagnosis of ASPD. However, if these risk factors are combined with paranoid states of mind, then the risk of violence is increased, although, every year in the UK, there are a small number of homicides where none of these risk factors were identified beforehand.

Psychopathy

(See ➲ Antisocial personality disorder in Chapter 8, pp. 390–6.)

The DSM-5 criteria describe ASPD as 'a pervasive pattern of disregard for, and violation of, the rights of others that begins in childhood or early adolescence and continues into adulthood'. Of those individuals with ASPD, a smaller group has been identified as demonstrating psychopathy. The key feature of psychopathy is a diminished capacity for empathy or remorse.

Psychopathy is commonly measured against a validated risk assessment tool called the Psychopathy Checklist-Revised (PCL-R), which was developed in the 1980s by Robert Hare, a Canadian researcher. This is based on four facets, including interpersonal, lifestyle, affective, and

---

[1] Multi-agency public protection arrangements (MAPPAs) were established in 2001 in England and Wales to oversee statutory arrangements for public protection by the identification, assessment, and management of high-risk offenders.

antisocial features, to create a score out of 40, which is used to predict future risk. It is, however, largely based on historical data, carrying an implication that previous offending behaviour is associated with high risk despite treatment intervention.

The treatment of psychopathy is an issue of continuing debate, which is a politicized and highly emotive issue in the public eye. In the past, psychological interventions for psychopathy have been criticized, due to a lack of evidence for their effectiveness. However, a number of treatment programmes have been established for which there is a growing evidence base.

Types of security

Forensic patients and prisoners are detained in buildings that are categorized as providing low, medium, or high security measures. These measures are designed to ensure the safety of patients and the public, to prevent escape and absconding and to reduce the likelihood of patients failing to return from agreed periods of leave. The Department of Health (DoH) and Ministry of Justice (MoJ) provide guidance and policies that govern provision at each level. Depending on individual needs, patients may go through an integrated care and treatment pathway that spans one or more levels of care.

'Security' includes a range of physical, procedural, and relational measures put in place to ensure the provision of a safe and secure environment in which treatment is delivered:

- *Physical security* refers to the environmental measures in place to keep people safe and prevent escape. It includes perimeter walls, locked doors, and personal alarms.
- *Procedural security* consists of the policies and procedures in place to maintain safety and security. This includes, for example, operational procedures for screening staff, searching patients, and having safe staffing levels.
- *Relational security* consists of the detailed knowledge and understanding staff have of their patients, including their backgrounds and their reasons for admission, and the translation of this information into appropriate responses and care. Relational security is derived from the therapeutic relationships established, as well as their wider treatment programmes.

Low secure services

Definition of low security

Low secure services are for people aged 18 years and over detained under the MHA who cannot be treated in other mental health settings because of the level of risk or challenge they present. Patients are admitted or transferred from general mental health services (including psychiatric intensive care units, PICUs), the community, courts, prison, and medium or high secure services. They usually have an offending history and may be subject to additional restrictions under the MHA, but will not require the level of physical security provided by medium secure services.

As a significant proportion of low secure patients step down from higher levels of security, often following treatment for a number of years, there tends to be a greater emphasis on rehabilitation. Patients may step down to a low secure rehabilitation ward from either mental illness or personality disorder wards in medium security.

Low secure treatment objectives

Using the Care Programme Approach (CPA), the emphasis of treating patients in a low secure setting will be on rehabilitation, with the multi-disciplinary team taking a recovery-focused approach, aimed at building the patient's resilience and preventing relapse. Broadly speaking, this will encompass the following:

• Addressing accommodation, employment, and educational needs
• Combating stigma
• Improving social support
• Encouraging effective links with community support and recreational activities to support discharge and sustainable rehabilitation
• Following the 'step-care' approach where, depending on the patient's risk and level of progress, they are either 'stepped down' to the community, with assisted support through accommodation needs, for example, or 'stepped up' to the medium secure unit if the patient displays ongoing elevated risk.

One of the stated objectives of low secure services is to provide recovery-focused care and treatment for detained patients, including transferred prisoners. Department of Health commissioning guidance states that, using the CPA, the multidisciplinary team will take a comprehensive, recovery-focused approach, aimed at building resilience and preventing relapse. This should include addressing accommodation, employment and learning needs, meaningful social contact, and combating stigma.

Psychiatric intensive care

PICUs exist in both acute and forensic services. Those in acute services provide a similar level of security to low secure units but provide care to acutely disturbed patients who present a risk of violence to others typically in the acute phase of a psychotic or manic illness. Occasionally, patients with a primary diagnosis of personality disorder will receive treatment in a PICU during crises. Patients in PICUs cannot be managed in an open (unlocked) psychiatric ward, due to the level of risk they present to themselves or others. Staffing levels are higher than on general psychiatric wards, and the patient's stay is usually short to manage the acute agitated phase of their mental illness before returning to an open ward.

Medium secure services

Medium secure hospitals

Medium secure services are for people who present a significant risk of causing harm to others. As with low secure services, they are provided by a range of NHS and independent sector organizations. Most patients will have a history of offending, and some will have been transferred from prison to receive inpatient treatment. Typically, patients will remain in treatment between 2 and 5 years. Some medium secure hospitals provide separate services for patients with a primary diagnosis of personality disorder. Where specific treatments are required for individual patients (e.g. arson or sexual offending programmes) and the Regional Secure Unit (the NHS medium secure hospital for the local area) does not provide these, out-of-area placements may need to be purchased. Some units also provide specialist services for particular groups of patients, including those with pervasive developmental disorders, acquired brain injury units, and adolescent services.

Women's enhanced medium security
In 2007, following a review of the three high secure hospitals in England and Wales by the Department of Health, three new units were set up to cater for the small number of women who had committed severe offences or who could not be managed in existing medium secure units but did not require high secure care. These units are known as Women's Enhanced Medium Secure Services (WEMSS), which, in total, provide 46 beds in the UK. The level of physical security provided at WEMSS is equivalent to that within standard medium secure services, whilst there is an enhanced level of relational and procedural security.

Adolescent medium secure units
Young people with mental disorders who have committed serious offences may be treated in medium secure adolescent units, of which there are several in the UK. These provide a range of psychological therapies, including family therapy, and other interventions similar to both CAMHS and forensic services. In recent years, provision of services in this sector has not kept pace with the growing demand.

Medium secure personality disorder services
Entry into specialist medium secure forensic services for personality disorders may follow a structured clinical assessment and careful consideration of the best treatment option for the patient. In general, the essential admission criteria to a medium secure personality disorder service encompasses the following:
• Patients aged 18 years or over as the age threshold for admission
• A diagnosis of a personality disorder that merits detention under mental health legislation (where there is a dual diagnosis of mental illness, the mental illness should be stable and unlikely to interfere with treatment focusing on personality disorder)
• The patient presents a serious physical or psychological risk to others or potential risk of a degree that requires admission to a medium secure service, and there is a link between the personality disorder and high risk that can be clinically justified
• The treatment needs of the patient are best met in a secure NHS setting.

There are a variety of psychological interventions available that are specifically tailored in a care plan approach to the individual needs of the patient. A variety of therapies are available, including DBT, CBT, MBT, and schema-focused therapy. Further evidence-based research is required into these psychological modalities in this setting, as these services are relatively new and continually being shaped under the Offender Personality Disorder Strategy (see ➲ The National Personality Disorder Offender Pathways Strategy in Chapter 8, pp. 423–4; Cognitive behavioural therapy in Chapter 2, pp. 30–4, and in Chapter 5, pp. 172–84; Dialectical behavioural therapy in Chapter 2, pp. 63–6, and in Chapter 5, pp. 220–9; Mentalization-based treatment in Chapter 2, pp. 66–70, and in Chapter 5, pp. 229–34; Schema therapy in Chapter 2, pp. 70–3, and in Chapter 5, pp. 234–8).

Private sector care

Low and medium secure hospital beds are provided by both the public and private sectors. The number of beds for people with mental illness in the NHS dropped from a peak of 148 000 in 1954 to 35 740 in 2000. As this decline accelerated, a private market has emerged for the provision of beds for long-stay patients across the UK. It is estimated that over a third of beds in England for patients in need of secure care are within privately owned institutions.

High secure services

High secure hospitals

High secure services for England and Wales are provided at Ashworth[2], Broadmoor[3], and Rampton[4] hospitals. Whilst all of these hospitals are part of NHS Trusts, their relationship to the Department of Health is unique, as the NHS Act 2006 places a specific duty on the Secretary of State to provide high secure services. The State Hospital (Carstairs) provides a high secure service for offenders requiring high secure hospital care in Scotland and Northern Ireland. High secure hospitals provide a treatment environment for patients who are assessed as presenting a serious and immediate danger to others.

High secure hospital services are divided into directorates, based on the range of services provided at each of the sites. Ashworth and Broadmoor Hospitals have mental illness and personality disorder directorates, whilst Rampton provides both of these services, in addition to a number of specialist services which include those for patients with intellectual disabilities, women, and the hearing impaired. The directorates within high secure services typically have both admission and high dependency wards, as well as wards where the primary function is rehabilitation.

Evidenced-based therapy in high security

Psychologists and psychotherapists with special experience in working with high-risk forensic patients are primarily responsible for providing the therapies in high secure hospitals. The particular modality of therapy used will depend on the primary nature of the patient's psychopathology.

---

[2] Mersey Care NHS Trust, Maghull, Liverpool.

[3] West London Mental Health NHS Trust, Crowthorne, Berkshire.

[4] Nottinghamshire Healthcare NHS Trust, Retford, Nottinghamshire.

In the mental illness directorate where the diagnoses almost always involve a psychotic component, a cognitive behavioural approach, in conjunction with antipsychotic medication, is typically used to develop coping strategies for psychotic symptoms and to improve the patient's capacity to function with them. Patients with a primary diagnosis of psychosis will also be considered for additional psychological therapies to address other aspects that might contribute to their offending behaviour such as dysfunctional personality traits and substance misuse problems. Often these treatments will take place once the patient has moved from a high dependency unit to a rehabilitation ward (see ➲ Cognitive behavioural therapy in Chapter 2, pp. 30–4, and in Chapter 5, pp. 172–84; Psychoses in Chapter 7, pp. 349–54).

In the High Secure Personality Disorder Directorates, patients will almost always fulfil criteria for ASPD, although paranoid and emotionally unstable personality disorders are also common and frequently coexist. Occasionally, patients are treated within personality disorder services where the primary diagnosis is Asperger's syndrome. At present, specific services for autistic spectrum disorders are not provided in high security, so this generally only occurs where the patient's history and index offence indicate a need for high security on the basis of risk (see ➲ Antisocial personality disorder in Chapter 8, pp. 396–401; Paranoid personality disorder in Chapter 8, pp. 401–4; Borderline personality disorder in Chapter 8, pp. 390–6).

The treatment focus is on both reducing the patient's subjective distress and improving their capacity to maintain healthy relationships, whilst reducing the risk to the public that arises directly from their personality disorder and associated behaviours. Both psychodynamic psychotherapy and CBT are currently available in the special hospitals. DBT is used in the management of self-harming behaviours and to target anger and violence in both female and male patients. Schema-focused therapy and MBT are also increasingly being used in high secure hospital settings for the treatment of BPD and ASPD (see ➲ Psychoanalytic psychotherapy in Chapter 2, pp. 20–30, and in Chapter 5, pp. 163–72; Cognitive behavioural therapy in Chapter 2, pp. 30–4, and in Chapter 5, pp. 172–84; Dialectical behavioural therapy in Chapter 2, pp. 63–6, and in Chapter 5, pp. 220–9; Mentalization-based treatment in Chapter 2, pp. 66–70, and in Chapter 5, pp. 229–34; Schema therapy in Chapter 2, pp. 70–3, and in Chapter 5, pp. 234–8.).

Dangerous and severe personality disorder units

The national DSPD programme was established in 2001 and set up two units in the prison estate, one in medium security and one in each of the three high secure hospitals in England. They were intended to provide treatment for offenders who were diagnosed with a severe personality disorder who presented a grave and immediate risk of harm to the public.

The original criteria for admission to a DSPD high secure unit included the following:

- The potential patient is more likely than not to commit an offence that might be expected to lead to serious physical or psychological harm, from which the victim would find it difficult or impossible to recover; and
- Has a severe disorder of personality; and
- There is a link between the disorder and the risk of offending.

There was considerable variation in the treatment packages delivered across the various sites. This was, in part, due to differences in the offender populations held at the different sites—those in the hospitals held proportionately more sex offenders and those in the prisons more violent offenders. Another factor was the lack of an evidence base to define a singular treatment package. Eleven main categories of similar treatments were established: psycho-education, motivation, psychological skills, sexual offending programmes, violent offending programmes, general offending programmes, psychopathy programmes, cognitive therapies, psychodynamic therapies, vulnerability to relapse, and trauma. Different sites prioritized specific types of programme. All of the sites used a mixture of individual and group sessions.

The DSPD programmes ran an SOTP for those patients whose offences involved a sexual element. These provided treatments largely on a one-to-one basis, using a cognitive behavioural approach, which combined the methods of violence reduction programmes and aimed to provide coping strategies to avoid reoffending (see ➔ Paraphilias in Chapter 7, pp. 349–54).

In 2010, a review article found that, although there had been some gains from the DSPD project during the 10 years that it was fully functioning, little benefit had been demonstrated, in terms of managing those individuals it was primarily targeting, and it may not have been cost-effective. The main advantage identified was its contribution to developing personality disorder services in general.

The National Personality Disorder Offender Pathways Strategy
The DSPD programme has recently been disbanded, in favour of the National Personality Disorder Offender Pathways Strategy, introduced in 2012. This is a reconfigured national strategy for managing high-risk personality-disordered offenders, based on a 'whole systems pathway' across the Criminal Justice System and NHS. Under this strategy, offenders with personality disorders are the joint responsibility of the National Offender Management Service and the NHS. Those who present a high risk of serious harm to others are primarily managed through the criminal justice system, with the lead role held by offender managers receiving support from mental health professionals.

This strategy is informed by a developmental model of personality disorder and recognition of the centrality of attachment experiences in the lives of offenders. It promotes education of the workforce about personality disorder through initiatives, such as the KUF, towards the goal of creating more therapeutic environments in prisons and forensic institutions, as well as prioritizing the development of specialized services for the management and treatment of neglected groups of personality-disordered offenders, including women, adolescents, and young adults, and those with learning difficulties. The importance of meaningful service user involvement in the development and delivery of services is also emphasized.

Psychological therapies in prison
Prison statistics
The number of offenders in the prison estate in England and Wales has been rising steadily over the last century. As of 16 May 2014, the prison

and young offender population stood at 84 918, including 81 052 males and 3866 females. In March 2014, the child custody population was 1177. In December 2013, there were 11 800 remand prisoners.

Categorization of prisons and prisoners

There are broadly five categories of prisons:

- Local prisons for unconvicted and short-term prisoners
- Dispersal prisons for high security prisoners
- Training prisons for long-term prisoners who do not need the highest security
- Category C prisons, which are closed but have less internal security
- Open prisons for prisoners not believed to be a risk to the public or in danger of escaping.

Prisoners are classified as either remand (pre-trial and pre-sentencing) or sentenced. Sentences can be either determinate (fixed-term) or indeterminate (IPP and imprisonment for life). Whilst women prisoners and young offenders are generally not categorized[5], following sentencing, adult male prisoners are categorized (A–D) at reception according to the likelihood that they will seek to escape and the risk that they would pose, should they do so.

Psychiatric morbidity in prisons

The Office of National Statistics study, in 1997, found that nine out of ten prisoners met their criteria for at least one mental disorder, with no more than two out of ten having only one disorder. Around 70% of prisoners suffer from two or more mental disorders. In the general population, the figures are 5% for men and 2% for women. Prisoners are more likely to be abusers of illegal drugs and alcohol than other sectors of the community. Psychosis, personality disorder, anxiety and depressive disorders, learning disabilities, and drug and alcohol dependency are grossly over-represented in the prison population. Certain prison minority groups have particular vulnerabilities, including women, black and ethnic minorities, older and younger people, and foreign nationals.

Organization of services

(See ➔ Planning psychotherapy services within psychiatric care in Chapter 10, pp. 462–6; Personality disorder services in Chapter 8, pp. 422–7.)

   Services providing mental health care in prisons are organized along similar lines to those in the community with certain exceptions. Primary care teams comprising GPs and nursing staff normally provide the responsibility for screening and the provision of treatment for conditions such as uncomplicated depression and anxiety. In some cases, there will be a dedicated mental health nurse who will provide psychological support and CBT for patients who do not require oversight by an In Reach CMHT. The In Reach team typically consists of psychiatrists and community psychiatric nurses. Some teams will also have provision

[5] Women and young offenders are only categorized if they are considered to be category A prisoners.

for a psychologist or psychotherapist who will provide assessments and therapy for a select group of prisoners.

Most prisons will have a health-care wing where prisoners suffering from either physical or mental illnesses can be transferred for assessment and, where consent is provided, treatment with neuroleptic medication[6]. Where a prisoner is identified as suffering from an enduring mental illness of sufficient severity that they are unable to manage in the prison environment or where they are non-compliant with medication, they may be transferred to an external secure psychiatric hospital for treatment under the MHA. The same is also true of a select group of prisoners suffering from personality disorders, often with mixed dissocial and emotionally unstable traits, where they present a high risk to themselves.

Prison-based treatment programmes
There are a variety of programmes designed to reduce risk that are run by the prison and probation service, and delivered by prison-based psychologists and trained counsellors. These are mostly based on a cognitive behavioural model and include enhanced thinking skills, anger management, substance misuse, and sex offender treatment programmes. Most of these programs are not accessible to those with severe mental health problems, as they are unable to cope with the group format and intensity of sessions. The SOTP run in prisons has been adapted for use in prisoners with borderline learning disabilities and for those who are considered to be at very high risk of further offending.

Psychotherapy in prisons
The underlying principle of mental health care to prisoners is that they should receive the same access to, and quality of, psychological therapy services as the non-prison population. Prison In Reach Teams should therefore be providing the same standard of care, including access to psychological treatments, as their non-prison counterparts the CMHTs. This should include at least one full-time psychotherapist providing psychotherapeutic assessments and treatment. Given the high rate of personality disorder within prison settings, the therapist should be skilled in providing treatment to this patient group and be able to offer both short- and longer-term interventions for this. It has been recommended that the provision of activity-based therapies (e.g. art therapy and dramatherapy) should also be considered as an integral part of psychological provision in prisons. Certain prisons offer psychodynamic therapy, which is often provided on a pro bono basis by honorary therapists. However, despite these recommendations, in many prisons, such psychotherapy provision is lacking (see ➲ Art psychotherapy in Chapter 2, pp. 81–83, and in Chapter 5, pp. 251–5; Dramatherapy in Chapter 2, pp. 83–5, and in Chapter 5, pp. 255–60; Psychoanalytic psychotherapy in Chapter 2, pp. 20–30, and in Chapter 5, pp. 163–72).

---

[6] Prisons are not covered by the Mental Health Act 1983 (as amended in 2007). Therefore, where a prisoner does not willingly accept medication and is deemed to require treatment, they must be transferred to hospital where this can take place under the Mental Health Act.

Addictions
(See ➔ Substance misuse in Chapter 7, pp. 338–45.)

The Drug Intervention Programme (DIP), launched in 2003, was part of the government strategy to reduce the effect of drug-related crime on the community. It aims to get offenders who misuse drugs out of crime and into treatment and other support. This scheme encourages seamless treatment by attracting drug misusing offenders into treatment, and then tracking them throughout their stay in prison and ensuring they are picked up by community services on their release.

The Integrated Drug Treatment System (IDTS) was introduced to ensure evidence-based, individual-focused, consistent care across prisons in the UK. On reception, prisoners who are dependent on substances undergo detoxification by a clinical service in a specialist facility. Substitute prescribing is then provided, alongside a range of intensive and short-term treatment psychological interventions. These include both abstinence programmes (such as TCs and twelve-step programmes) and various cognitive behavioural interventions.

Following detoxification, prisoners with addiction issues are then referred to substance misuse services that are now generally provided by contracted third sector organizations such as Rapt. The services will provide care coordination to help ensure that timely continuity of care can be provided for offenders returning to the community. They provide specialist advice and counselling and liaise with external drug rehabilitation services to secure their access to treatment on release.

The National Personality Disorder Offender Strategy and prisons
It was envisaged that the National Personality Disorder Offender Strategy would lead to a greater role for penal institutions in the treatment of offenders with personality disorders, whilst ensuring access to treatment in hospital for those who need it

Under the resulting programme, the two prison-based dangerous and severe personality disorder units at HMP Whitemoor and HMP Frankland lost their DSPD designation and became generic personality disorder units for sentenced prisoners.

A London Pathways Progression Unit (LPPU) at HMP Belmarsh opened in April 2013. This was a 41-bedded unit for men who have significant personality difficulties to prepare them for potential release into the community within 2 years. It also provided support for patients to progress through their sentence, whether downgrading from category A or by progressing into open conditions. In 2016 the Unit was moved to HMP Brixton.

Psychologically Informed Planned Environments (PIPEs) are currently being developed to reshape existing Dangerous and Severe Personality Disorder (DSPD) services in the NHS and in prisons. The aim of PIPEs is not to provide therapy as such, but to set a new, more collaborative and community-orientated direction for working with this complex group of offenders. They are designed to support and maintain existing developments, to maximize ordinary situations in the prison, and to provide education to staff to approach these in a psychologically informed way.

Prison-based democratic therapeutic communities
A number of prisons, such as HMP Grendon, in the UK provide treatment in TCs. Prison TCs are not truly democratic, because primary responsibility for certain decisions remains with staff. However, staff decisions are open to scrutiny, and the idea that certain decisions are made collectively is central. See ➔ Therapeutic communities in Chapter 2, pp. 75–80, and in Chapter 5, pp. 243–50.

Evidenced-based therapy in secure settings

Therapies for personality disorder
There is broad agreement about the basic parameters for providing services to people with personality disorder. These include:
- A service delivered over a relatively long period
- Staff who are able to work flexibly with service users, whilst ensuring the service they provide is consistent and reliable
- Therapists who have the capacity to deliver more than one intervention of varying intensity and deliver social, as well as psychological, treatment
- Therapies need to engage service users with different levels of motivation
- In addition, in forensic services, therapy for personality disorder needs to focus on improved mentalization and risk reduction.

One of the key issues in the treatment of personality disorder is addressing different levels of motivation and willingness to change. Service users with emotionally unstable traits are often more willing and able to engage in therapy (although they may be ambivalent, once engaged). Service users with antisocial traits are often difficult to engage and may withdraw from therapy prematurely.

Psychological treatments available for specific offending patterns
The Ministry of Justice has accredited certain treatment programmes on the basis of their emerging evidence base, to support their use in reducing reoffending. The programmes vary in length and complexity, as well as mode of delivery, and are targeted according to risk and need.
- *SOTPs*: these are based on a cognitive behavioural model and aim to help offenders develop an understanding of how and why they have committed sexual offences, whilst increasing awareness of victim harm. A central focus is to help the offender develop meaningful life goals and practise new thinking and behavioural skills that will lead him or her away from offending (see ➔ Cognitive behavioural therapy in Chapter 2, pp. 30–4, and in Chapter 5, pp. 172–84).
- *Democratic TCs*: these provide residential treatment programmes which operate on a participative, group-based approach to long-term mental illness, personality disorders, and drug addiction. Although a number of principles have been identified, the key concept is that as much responsibility as possible is delegated to the community as a whole. The TC with its structures of group decision-making and pro-social cooperation is intended to model a pro-social society outside

prison (see ➜ Therapeutic communities in Chapter 2, pp. 75–80, and in Chapter 5, pp. 243–50).

• *Offender Substance Abuse Programmes (OSAPs)*: these programmes use cognitive methods to address alcohol and drug misuse by targeting attitudes and behaviour to prevent relapse and reduce offending (see ➜ Substance misuse in Chapter 7, pp. 338–45).

Recommended reading

National Institute for Health and Care Excellence (2009). *Antisocial Personality Disorder: Prevention and Management*. NICE guidelines CG77. Available at: ℘ https://www.nice.org.uk/guidance/cg77.

National Institute for Health and Care Excellence (2009). *Borderline Personality Disorder: Recognition and Management*. NICE guidelines CG78. Available at: ℘ https://www.nice.org.uk/guidance/cg78.

Poole R, Ryan T, Pearsall A (2002). The NHS, the private sector, and the virtual asylum. *BMJ*, **325**, 349–50.

Royal College of Psychiatrists Centre for Quality Improvement (2012). *Standards for Low Secure Services*. Available at: ℘ http://www.rcpsych.ac.uk/pdf/Standards%20for%20 Low%20Secure%20 Services.pdf.

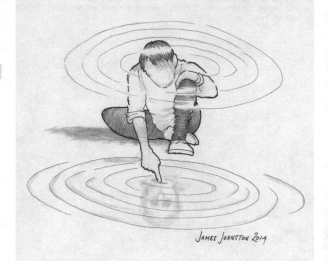

JAMES JOHNSTON 2014

Ethics and boundaries

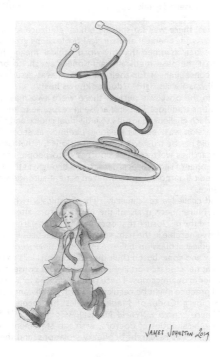

JAMES JOHNSTON 2014

Approaches to medical ethics

Ethics is the discourse of 'ought' and 'should'. It is the study of how to take right action where there are a number of possible 'good' options or where at least one of the 'good' options may also bring about some harm or wrong.

Medical ethics is the study of how to make good-quality ethical decisions in everyday clinical work. It is as much about acquiring reasoning skills and a type of intelligence as it is about determining right and wrong. Moral philosophy is the study of how we decide what is 'good' and 'bad', and medical ethical decision-making is about how that actually works in practice.

It has always been recognized that healers have increased power and authority in social groups—first, because of their specialist knowledge; second, because of their value to the group in terms of health and welfare preservation; and third, because they have to relate to others who are vulnerable. With increased power comes increased responsibilities, and healers in Antiquity devised a code of ethics to regulate the behaviour of doctors and give the profession an 'ethical identity'. This has been called the Hippocratic oath, and it has persisted as a marker of professional identity to the present day (although it is only taken by a handful of medical graduates).

For centuries, there was no specific ethical guidance for health-care professionals. As the medical and surgical professions grew and developed, it was widely assumed that the word 'ethical' meant the same as 'good' and that, because medical practitioners sought to bring about good health consequences for their patients, it was assumed that the doctor's view was always right—'doctor knows best'.

However, in the post-war period, there were two massive cultural challenges to this tradition. The first arose in response to the civil rights movement, which challenged insults to individual choice and dignity. The medical profession was seen as treating 'patients' as second-class citizens, who could not be trusted to make decisions for themselves, much as white patriarchies were seen as oppressive to people of colour and women. A number of seminal legal cases were brought at this time which challenged medical authority and privileged patient autonomy over medical beneficence.

The second challenge to 'clinically right is ethically right' arose as a result of the Nuremberg trials of the Nazi doctors after the Second World War and the disclosure that doctors had taken part in murder and cruelty to the vulnerable in the name of 'medical practice'. Forty-five per cent of the medical profession in Germany at that time were members of the Nazi party and contributed their medical clinical skills to the 'euthanasia' programme, research on live humans without consent and selection for murder in death camps. These revelations led to a sea change in how medical practice might be regulated, which is still continuing.

The Nuremberg Code of Medical Ethics has been revised and expanded. There is now a World Medical Association (WMA) declaration of the ethical duties of doctors, with sub-statements addressing various issues such as research, boundary violations, and the influence of drug companies in medicine. For psychiatrists, there are a number of particular statements that apply—mainly in relation to state-imposed detention and treatment, conflicts of interest with drug companies and families, and boundary violations.

Internationally, doctors are bound by a variety of professional ethical codes, which are enforced by their licensing authorities. In the UK, doctors are registered with the GMC, which gives ethical guidance to doctors in the form of guidelines called *Good Medical Practice* (*GMP*). This is continually being revised and reconsidered.

Psychiatrists are bound by the principles of GMP and also by the guidance given by the Royal College of Psychiatrists (*Good Psychiatric Practice*). UK psychiatrists are advised to follow the *Royal College of Psychiatrists Code of Ethics*. Other therapists are also bound by codes of ethics of their particular professional group.

Key ethical precepts are:
- Do not exploit the patient's vulnerability.
- Do no harm, and make sure you are skilled enough to provide the right help.
- Treat vulnerable people justly and holistically.

Justice and psychotherapy

Justice is a concept that can be understood in three ways. First, justice can be understood as 'fairness'—the moral obligation to treat everyone as having equal value, and avoiding bias and prejudice in social relationships. Second, justice can be understood as promoting welfare and righting wrongs—decisions about rationing and allocation of resources in health care involve thinking about justice as welfare, and justice is also the process by which wrongs are explored and retribution or reparation is mandated. Finally, justice can include those social processes that encourage citizens to behave well and develop a pro-social identity. In this sense, justice actively supports virtues of compassion and courage, rather than leaving people free to do as they please. A famous distinction is made between negative liberty (i.e. freedom from interference by the state) and positive liberty (i.e. the freedom to pursue one's own choices and vocations).

Psychotherapy and psychotherapists are not exempt from thinking about justice and considering how it applies in practice. In the first sense of justice, some schools of psychotherapy have taken up discriminatory positions with regard to sexism and homophobia. It is not so long since some psychotherapists cited conversion to heterosexuality as evidence of successful therapy or described successful women as competing with men where 'competition' seems to be a bad thing.

Justice as welfare raises issues of resources and the fact that psychotherapy may not be made available to all who need it, although all may be offered medication. However, the costs of medication, compared to therapy, have not been assessed, especially for antipsychotic drugs. When working with victims or perpetrators of violence, it is tempting to take up positions that reflect justice as retribution—being critical of perpetrators or taking up victim's experiences as a cause. Therapists have encouraged patients to bring criminal or civil cases as part of their victim identity and have given testimony against patients who have confessed to offences in therapy. These practices may not be 'wrong' in a simplistic sense, but they raise questions about the role of therapists as agents of justice.

Justice as virtue is manifested as boundary setting and maintenance; it is unjust to treat patients badly in therapy, as well as be harmful to them, because such bad treatment treats patients merely as a means to an end.

Most psychotherapy trainings encourage trainee therapists to undergo personal therapy to look at their own biases and prejudices, so they can avoid them. But there remain questions about the values of therapy offered to most patients and the ideals that underpin therapy.

Values-based practice in psychotherapy

Values-based practice (VBP) is the 'twin sister' to evidence-based practice in medicine. In particular, it is an approach to ethical decision-making in health care which acknowledges the significance of personal values for ethical reasoning. The key authors of this approach Woodbridge and Fulford argue that medical decision-making is often said to be based on facts, when actually the values of the decision-maker are also operative. Both facts and values are important for medical practice, but often the different value perspectives of the different parties involved are not explicit. Similarly, it is argued that many ethical dilemmas come down to a clash of values, which themselves arise from judgements which are ignorant of other perspectives.

VBP aims to provide a framework and skills to enable people to work in a respectful and sensitive way with those whose values and perspectives are different to their own. This framework of skills includes:

- Raising *awareness* of values and how they influence situations
- *Exploring* values using an explicit reasoning process
- Having *knowledge* of both values and facts that are relevant to the situation
- Being able to *communicate* about conflicts in values, with a view to resolution
- Being *user-centred* and seeking the user's perspective
- Working in a *multidisciplinary* way that admits multiple perspectives
- Being able to work in *partnership* with others
- Recognition of the importance of both *facts and values, and the distinction* between them.

VBP has proved to be a useful framework in mental health services, especially in primary care and community services. Many of the skills described are essential to good teamworking and should be part of ordinary professional training. VBP emphasizes respect for diversity of opinion and experience, and has been an important theoretical driver for the recovery movement.

VBP is a useful conceptual framework in psychotherapy, because it uses familiar ideas such as plurality of perspective taking and a willingness to explore different perspectives, and letting people find their own voice. Like psychotherapy, VBP assumes that the process of reflection is as important as the outcome and acknowledges that there may not always be a simple answer to a problem, nor one that is acceptable to all involved. Making conflict explicit and respecting dissent are important aspects of VBP. Personal values may also reflect conscious elements of internal working models, based on early experience with parents, and VBP may be a way that some people start to think about their valuing processes and why they value what they do.

Virtue ethics and psychotherapy

Virtue ethics is a school of bioethical thinking that emphasizes the good character of the practitioner. It is based on ideas from Aristotle that suggest that, in order to be a 'good' person, one must practise the habits of a good person and that character is formed by practice. In relation to medical ethics, virtue ethics emphasizes the character of the good doctor and argues that it is not possible to be a bad man and a good doctor, no matter how competent.

Radden and Sadler have argued that virtue ethics is crucial to the practice of psychiatry, because of the vulnerability of the patients as a result of their mental disorders. They also argued that patients become uniquely vulnerable during the psychotherapeutic process and point to boundary violations by therapists as examples of situations where therapists have exploited the intimacy of the psychotherapy process and the vulnerability of the person who shares intimate material.

Radden and Sadler argue that psychotherapists need to be good people, who practise virtuous habits (including kindness, courtesy, and compassion) and refrain from antisocial or vicious habits of mind that do harm to patients. This seems obvious but also seems to hold therapists to a high standard of practice—possibly higher than other doctors or health-care professionals.

These expectations may reflect and acknowledge the extensive training that therapists have had. Some therapists have lengthy trainings that encourage them to become more self-aware than most people and to actively self-reflect on their psychological difficulties and limitations. The training is, in some sense, equipping the therapist to deal with difficult emotions and interpersonal situations that most untrained people find hard, so that, if this training has been successful, then it might be expected that a therapist who has had such a training will be able to resist 'normal' temptations and/or handle frustrations 'better' than other people.

Most therapists would argue that they have not become 'good' people through their training, but only people who are more self-aware and willing to address uncertainty and complexity. Nevertheless, it is hard not to think that there is an aspect to therapy (including all the therapeutic trainings), which is about moral improvement, as well as technical enhancement. Just as there is an expectation that people who have therapy will not behave worse after therapy than before, there is a public expectation that psychotherapists will behave like virtuous people more often than not and that trust will be given on that basis. Perhaps this is why boundary violations by therapists (like violations by priests and teachers) cause so much alarm, distress, and outrage in the public mind.

What is good psychotherapy?

In this section, it may be helpful to think of a different sense of the word 'good'. There is therapy that is 'good' in the sense of well done or competently performed, and there is 'good' in the sense of psychotherapy being a positive or valuable process in its own right and which brings about positive or valuable outcomes (although these may not be easy to determine) (see ➜ Beneficence and non-maleficence in psychotherapy in Chapter 9, pp. 451–2).

Good psychotherapy is competently done therapy

(See ➜ Competencies framework in Chapter 3, pp. 96–9.)

All the trainings in psychological therapy aim to help trainees achieve a level of competence, so they can safely practise the technique they have chosen to offer to patients. The training and supervision process should have ensured that a trainee has both theoretical knowledge and sufficient practical experience. The different schools of therapy have professional standards and codes of ethics that practitioners must respect (see ➜ Psychotherapy protocols and codes in Chapter 9, pp. 448).

There are some general and specific principles of practice. The general principles are those of any health-care professional and include courtesy, kindness, punctuality, attention to administration, maintaining basic competencies, and a willingness to consult colleagues if unsure of how to proceed. Related meta-competencies include the capacity for self-reflection, lifelong learning, and tolerating uncertainty and the unexpected.

Specific features of a competently carried out therapy include:
- Carrying out a thorough assessment
- Not taking on a patient if they are better treated elsewhere
- Making a proper formulation and being prepared to revise it
- Offering a secure, predictable, and consistent intervention
- Setting and maintaining boundaries
- Engaging in supervision.

Psychotherapy as a 'good' practice for people: moral enhancement

It is sometimes asserted that psychotherapy makes one a better person—more self-reflective and therefore more able to appreciate the feelings of others, and more likely to give up habits of behaviour that cause unhappiness to oneself and those in one's social system. Some studies of outcomes in psychotherapy suggest that people who have positive outcomes have more coherent self-narratives and describe a sense of enhanced agency. But it is also argued that the values of the psychotherapies offered in the UK and Europe reflect Anglo-European values that privilege individual experience and personal gain, as opposed to a more relational or communitarian benefit. Individual accounts of victimization and passivity are often given high status in individual therapeutic processes, and there may be more emphasis on past hurts than forgiveness, compassion, and future responsibility for personal choices. In short, it is not at all clear what it is to be a 'good' person in therapeutic terms, yet there is some expectation that psychological therapies will not result in a patient behaving worse than before.

This is a complex area, and readers are referred to works by Alan Tjvelveit, and Holmes and Lindley.

Professional guidelines in psychotherapy

A profession is a body of people who have acquired a set of skills and a knowledge base with which to use those skills. As opposed to a trade, in which a skill is performed for money, a professional brings his expertise in his knowledge to bear on a problem; he interprets and considers different possibilities. Professional roles are generally complex ones, and they have a social structure, such that one acquires a social identity when one is admitted to the profession of one's choice.

Professions generally (but not all!) have altruism as part of their role—working for the benefit of others. For this reason, most professional bodies have guidelines about the conduct of their members. These guidelines set out what may be expected of a professional by the public and by the profession as a whole.

Professional guidelines for therapists set standards for performance and conduct of therapy. They do not have the force of law; but, if there is legal dispute which involves a professional's performance, then the courts will consider professional guidelines seriously. If unsure as to the right course of action, the professional guidelines may be a source of direction, and, when making a difficult decision in the course of a professional career, it is essential to be aware of the guidelines and what they say.

For medical psychotherapists, the GMC is the professional body that regulates entry into the profession and retention in it. Professional guidelines for doctors are set out in *Good Medical Practice* (*GMP*), which sets out the duties of doctors and what is expected of them professionally. The GMC also has specific guidance on a number of common ethical dilemmas in medicine, especially in relation to consent and refusal of treatment, the disclosure of private health information to third parties, and decisions about withholding treatment and end-of-life decision-making.

All doctors need to be familiar with *GMP* and the subspecialty documents such as *Good Psychiatric Practice* and the *Royal College of Psychiatrists Code of Ethics*. These documents are only guidelines and may not be able to offer definitive answers to all dilemmas. In complex cases, it is vital to document all thinking and reflecting processes, especially if one is going to depart from the guidelines in any significant way. It is also advised that one consults several different colleagues with experience in the issue at hand.

There is no specific professional guidance for medical psychotherapists. However, they are expected to meet the professional obligations of all doctors and psychiatrists generally, and specifically to meet the professional duties of psychological therapists, such as are set out in by the main voluntary professional regulatory bodies of psychotherapists in the UK—the UKCP and the BPC. For medical psychotherapists, there may be little difference between the therapist who is 'good' professionally and the therapist who is personally 'good'. In this sense, medical psychotherapists may be held to a higher standard than other psychiatrists (see ➔ Virtue ethics and psychotherapy in Chapter 9, pp. 445–6; Boundary setting and maintenance in Chapter 9, pp. 454–5; Boundary violations in psychotherapy in Chapter 9, pp. 455–60).

Psychotherapy protocols and codes

Protocols and codes are forms of professional guidelines. Protocols usually refer to clinical treatment regimes that have been agreed as a form of best practice, based on the available evidence. The NICE produces clinical guidelines for the treatment of common disorders, which set out the best available advice on which treatment approaches are most effective, including drug treatments.

Codes are another term for professional guidelines that relate to conduct of professionals. For example, many professional groups have codes of ethics to guide professionals in how they should behave and the standards expected of them.

Protocols and codes do not have force of law. However, if there is an established protocol for treatment of a disorder, then it is wise to use it, unless there are compelling reasons not to. If so, these need to be documented. Failure to even consider the use of a well-established treatment protocol, without good reason, could be the basis of a case in negligence.

As discussed in the section on professional guidelines, professional codes of behaviour set out standards of behaviour and may give definite advice about professional or unprofessional behaviour. As for protocols, departure from codes of practice is possible, but it needs to be justified, and evidence of reflection and discussion provided.

Clinical protocols have been criticized as being restrictive of clinical freedom and potentially biased towards certain drug treatments (especially in psychiatry). This is because protocols and clinical guidelines (such as those drawn up by NICE) rely almost entirely on meta-analyses of RCTs, which are excellent for evaluating brief, discrete treatment interventions for acute/short-term disorders, but not yet shown to be efficient for evaluating longer-term multi-aspect interventions in the treatment of chronic and complex disabilities. However, overall there is probably more benefit than harm in the use of clinical protocols, and no clinician can be made to use a treatment that she believes is inappropriate for the patient, as long as she can make a good argument for another. This is a particular issue in ethical dilemmas about resource allocation for expensive treatments (see ➔ Research in psychotherapy in Chapter 11, pp. 508–26).

Consent and psychotherapy

(See ➔ Consent in Chapter 4, pp. 113–15.)

Consent in medical practice generally

It is unlawful to carry out medical treatment without consent, which must be given voluntarily by a person who has capacity to do so. Persons who lack capacity may undergo treatment in the absence of consent, if it is in their best interests and they are not resisting treatment (see the 2007 amendment to the Mental Capacity Act, 2005). Patients who have a mental disorder and who are refusing treatment may be treated against their will, but only if they are detained under Section 3 of the MHA and if there has been a second opinion.

Medical psychotherapists are not exempt from discussion of consent, and it is good practice to document a discussion of consent at the beginning of treatment. It is especially a good idea to discuss consent to disclosure of personal information to other people, e.g. feeding back to a referring psychiatrist. It is wise to have some discussion with a new patient about consent to disclosure of information to the GP and whether there are any family members who may be involved at some point. It is also advisable to document any such discussions. Some therapists like to use consent forms, and, if so, a copy of any form should be given to the patient.

Informed consent in psychotherapy

Traditional approaches to psychotherapy have ignored the usual medical practice of warning patients about possible harmful side effects of therapy and/or discomfort during treatment. Since many therapies do entail patients either reflecting on psychological pain or giving up habitual thoughts or defences that have protected them against pain, it may be anticipated that the therapeutic process may be uncomfortable. This may be particularly so for patients with poor affect and arousal regulation, e.g. those with BPD who may also be ambivalent about therapy (see ➔ Borderline personality disorder in Chapter 8, pp. 390–6).

It may therefore be sensible to advise the patient about experiencing psychological pain or becoming more depressed during therapy. Many therapists also suggest to patients that they should not make any major life decisions, whilst they are undergoing therapy, or at least postpone them until therapy is established. Psychotherapists may like to think about what they might say to potential patients about transference issues and about any limits of confidentiality.

In general, medical law and ethics are moving away from the paternalistic stance that was essential to medicine, as Freud practised and which has influenced psychoanalytic psychotherapy. Recent case law on consent states that doctors should advise patients of the risks that any reasonable patient would want to know. This would include the limits to confidentiality described above.

Consent to psychotherapy: can therapy ever be involuntary?

There is some debate about whether it is possible to offer psychological therapy to people against their will, and even more debate about whether it should be done, even if it is possible. Some therapists argue that psychological therapy can only take place if a patient has given full and free consent to take part, so that they 'own' the process with the therapist. Forcing people to have therapy and change their mind can sound more like 'brainwashing' than an intervention designed to reduce distress.

However, the counterargument is that many people may come to therapy in ambivalent and uncertain states of mind, perhaps especially people with personality dysfunction or long-standing complex needs. They may be in divided states of mind that oscillate between positive curiosity about their minds and mental experience, and fear and hostility towards the contents of their own minds.

In these cases, the therapist may have to 'stand up for' the part of the patient's mind that does want therapy and accept the ambivalence as a problem to be addressed in therapy. When patients say they want to refuse any further therapy, it may be important for therapists to gently state that they are reluctant to accept this as the final word on the matter and suggest that the patient needs to keep coming to talk about their refusal! It may be impossible to persuade the patient to persist, but it is equally possible that patients who are apparently refusing therapy are actually making a statement about how hopeless they feel about the possibility of change.

Therapists working in secure settings or prisons may have to offer therapy within a coercive context and work with an awareness that, if the patient were not constrained to do so, they would probably not attend for therapy. However, clinical experience suggests that prisoners or forensic patients who really have no interest in therapy will not come at all, and fewer people come to therapy to 'tick a box' than might be supposed. For many such patients, the therapy they are 'forced' into is also the first experience they have had of another person being genuinely interested in them and their human situation (see ➔ Psychological therapy in secure settings in Chapter 8, pp. 428–39; Forensic psychiatry: forensic psychotherapies, applications, and research in Chapter 12, pp. 550–6).

Autonomy and psychotherapy

'Autonomy' is a Greek term which literally means 'self-rule'. The principle of respect for autonomy is an expression of the duty that health-care professionals have to respect the wishes, feelings, and values of patients. The principle became a primary ethical driver in medical ethics, as part of the more general attention to civil rights and personal liberty that occurred after the Second World War. Medical practice was included in this review and was seen as sometimes coercive of patients and as paying too much attention to professional opinion.

The concept of autonomy is complex in mental health, because psychological distress and mental disorder can compromise, or even abolish, autonomy. Individuals need capacity to exercise autonomy, and it has often been suggested that the function of mental health services is to promote autonomy and restore people to an autonomous state. The principle of using the least restrictive treatments is an aspect of the principle of respect for autonomy, as is the duty to get consent and protect personal information.

Critics of traditional accounts of autonomy have commented that it is not a unitary phenomenon and includes autonomy of will, thought, and action. They also comment that autonomy is not a purely individual phenomenon, especially for those who are dependent in some way: children, the elderly, and those living with disabilities. Feminist critics, in particular, have argued for a more relational concept of autonomy, whereby people can only exercise autonomy in the context of a network of relationships to which they belong. For example, a person with a learning disability or long-term mental illness may need a system of people around her to become autonomous and give 'voice' to her own choices.

Autonomy can be complex in psychotherapy, because people come in distress, and it may take time to work out what an autonomous state of mind means for this patient in particular. Complex personality pathology can result in people being in different self-states, e.g. people with BPD may present in childlike states of mind, with childlike wishes and feelings that seem inappropriate for adult autonomous decision-making. Many people seeking therapy do so, because they are in transitions of identity, which means that they feel unable to own their autonomy or exercise it authentically.

Psychotherapists, such as Hinshelwood, also question the concept of autonomy as a categorical state. They point out that it is common for people to have mixed feelings about choices and values, especially those seeking therapy. In addition, traditional accounts of autonomy in bioethics contain no account of unconscious feelings and motives that may also influence choices and intentions. The psychotherapeutic process requires a culture of enquiry and curiosity which does not accept wishes and choices at face value.

Such a sophisticated account of autonomy is consistent with good-quality thinking in medical ethics. Respect for autonomy does not always mean doing exactly (and only) what the patient wants but entails an analysis of the patient's values and choices at a deep level that is consistent with the analytic process. What is not acceptable is the therapist thinking they know better than the patient and deciding for them when they are uncertain. It is also ethically unjustifiable to assume that 'patients' do not know what is good for them.

Beneficence and non-maleficence in psychotherapy

'Beneficence' means 'goodness' or benefit, and the principle of beneficence in medical ethics requires health-care practitioners to act in ways that benefit patients and avoid doing them harm (non-maleficence). Both these principles need to be understood in the context of the other two ethical principles said to underpin health care, i.e. respect for autonomy (see ➔ Autonomy and psychotherapy in Chapter 9, pp. 450–1) and respect for justice (see ➲ Justice and psychotherapy in Chapter 9, pp. 443–4). The duty to benefit a patient ends at the point where it conflicts with the duty to act justly or where the benefit (or harm avoided) does not fit with the patient's own values and preferences.

Harms and benefits are complex in psychotherapy, because how people in therapy make these evaluations may change over time, as they change perspective. A classic example involves people who come to therapy to change some aspect of themselves (weight, partner, job, erotic object choice). They may have a particular beneficial outcome in mind which they see as the 'right' one for them, but this may not be the outcome that actually takes place. Alternatively, people may come to therapy seeking help, but the 'benefit' that the therapist envisages or hopes for is not one that the patient always values, e.g. patients with eating disorders may only reluctantly accept that 'their' values (in terms of weight) are not acceptable to others.

The psychotherapeutic process may cause harm in the short term when it causes pain and distress, as defences are given up or patients get in touch with painful memories that have been suppressed. It may also cause harm to use the wrong therapeutic technique for the clinical problem, and therapists may cause harm by failing to respect boundaries or other ethical duties.

Forensic practitioners may find that they are subtly coercing patients into therapy that may benefit them, in terms of making them more acceptable to society. For example, therapists working with sex offenders are working to make them behave better, not feel better. Ideally, patients may also feel better, but this may not be the main aim of the therapeutic programme (see ➲ Forensic psychiatry: forensic psychotherapies, applications, and research in Chapter 12, pp. 550–6).

A particular problem with the assessment of beneficence and non-maleficence is similar to that entailed by risk assessment. When assessing possible consequences of therapy, both good and bad, it is also necessary to consider how likely it is that these consequences will occur and over what timescale. There may be entirely unforeseen consequences of a therapeutic intervention, which cannot be evaluated ahead of time. For example, a man goes into therapy to help him drink less and finds that his relationship with his wife was predicated on his being drunk much of the time. His wife leaves him, because she cannot relate to the person he has become, and he finds himself now sober but divorced. Whether this is seen as a 'good' outcome depends on many factors, especially the therapeutic alliance with the therapist.

Confidentiality and psychotherapy

(See ➲ Confidentiality and disclosure in Chapter 3, pp. 99–100; Forensic psychiatry: forensic psychotherapies, applications, and research in Chapter 12, pp. 550–6.)

It used to be thought that psychotherapeutic spaces were secret spaces, like the priestly confessional. It is certainly true that, as a matter of law, patients own their personal information, and it cannot be disclosed to others without their consent, unless there is some compelling reason to do so. However, it is common for therapists to find themselves in situations when they feel under pressure to disclose information in ways that cause them anxiety.

There is a vast amount of professional and legal guidance that exists in relation to confidentiality and the duties of health-care professionals to disclose information in certain circumstances. Medical psychotherapists should be aware of the existing framework of professional guidance on confidentiality and disclosure from the Royal College of Psychiatrists, the GMC, and the British Medical Association. Therapists who work in NHS organizations are bound by the Department of Health's NHS Code of Practice on Confidentiality and by the policies of their employing organizations. Even those in private practice may be subject to forced legal disclosure of patient records in certain circumstances.

It is therefore wise to inform new patients that, although generally therapists are bound to keep private any information given in therapy, they may also have a duty to disclose any information they are given that indicates a significant risk of harm to an identifiable third party, especially a child. It is clear that duties of harm prevention trump duties to protect confidences; what this means is that all therapists need to think carefully about how they assess the risk of harm to others and also they need to identify peers/colleagues from whom they will get advice when they are concerned about risk and disclosure. However, although legislation may create a 'statutory gateway' to allow information disclosure, this generally stops short of creating a requirement to disclose, and therefore the common law obligations of confidentiality must still be satisfied. This means that, where psychotherapists are responsible for making information-sharing decisions, it is still the decision of the doctor or therapist to determine, on a case-by-case basis, whether this is necessary to prevent serious harm.

For therapists who are working in NHS settings, and especially those working with potentially risky patients, a good way of managing the boundary around disclosure of personal information is for the supervisor to act as an intermediary with any third parties (such as the courts or other health-care professionals). Patients need to be informed about the existence of the supervisor from the start. Therapists should be wary of taking on patients who seem to be insisting that therapy is a private secret dyadic space that no-one else can know about. Professional boundary maintenance includes the proper use of supervision, so discussion of clinical material with a supervisor is evidence of good practice, and not a breach of confidentiality (see ➔ Using supervision in Chapter 3, pp. 107–8).

It is helpful to think of patients 'owning' their own stories. It follows that no clinical work should be discussed or presented in any public forum, without the patient's knowledge and consent. It is usually relatively straightforward to explain what the forum is and why you want to present the work, and show the patient what is to be presented and how it has been anonymized and de-identified. Of course, patients will vary in how they feel about this—therapists may like to consider how they would feel if they were told that their therapist wanted to write about them or did not want to write about them! Patients with ambivalent attachment issues may find it painful to hear that they are a 'case' for their therapists. It should be obvious that, if a patient says that they do not wish their case to be discussed in any public forum, then this cannot go ahead, even if the case can be disguised.

Most journals require evidence of the patient's consent at submission. Unattributable quotes may be used without express consent, although it is good practice to inform patients that therapists (especially medical psychotherapists) are expected to participate in audit, research, and teaching, which naturally involves collection and discussion of patients' private information. In all cases, the expectation is that all and any identifying materials will be removed.

Boundary setting and maintenance

Boundaries mark out a space in which people interact. For example, the boundary line around a cricket pitch marks out an area where people play a game called 'cricket' with complex rules of engagement and terms of art. Outside the boundary, people are just hitting balls with bats.

A boundary marks out and defines a set of interactions between people. It also defines an identity, i.e. within the boundary, I am in one role; outside the boundary, I am in another role. Roles may have different duties, responsibilities, and values. For example, the GMC advises doctors not to act as therapists or doctors to their own families, and it is unwise to act like a parent at work towards one's colleagues.

Professional boundaries mark out and set the limits of professional identity. These markers may be verbal or non-verbal; they also include professional trainings and insignia such as uniform. Setting and maintaining professional boundaries is part of the duties of a professional. In general, patients are not expected to take responsibility for professional boundaries, although it is reasonable to ask patients to respect general boundaries of behaviour and language.

The function of the boundary is to keep the therapeutic space safe and the therapeutic alliance in good working order. This is especially important with those patients whose pathology means that they may be in rapidly shifting self-states involving memories and cognitions of being a child, victim, or violent adult. These patients have to rely on the therapist maintaining their professional identity in a consistent, predictable manner, no matter what states of mind the patient goes through. Maintaining the boundary is the essence of the secure base that is essential for the growth of a 'secure' mind and the development of both a coherent autobiographical narrative and 'good enough' mentalizing capacities (see ➲ Theories of personality development: attachment theory in Chapter 8, pp. 380–1).

Therapists who do not keep the boundary between their personal and professional identities run the risk of using the therapeutic space for their personal advantage, to the patient's detriment. Mild forms of boundary crossing typically involve therapists telling patients too much personal information, so that the relationship becomes more like that of friendship. More serious boundary violations involve treating the patient like a lover, partner, or parent, or a mixture of all three. Such boundary violations are usually re-enactments of episodes from the patient's (or therapist's) early life. It is well known that sexual boundary violations by therapists are commoner with patients who have been sexually abused by parents or carers; there is an argument that such patients should not be offered dyadic therapy as a first line of treatment.

Boundary setting and maintenance are full-time activities for most therapists and are best supported with regular supervision and reflection with colleagues. Although supervision will not prevent serious boundary violations, the expectation that all therapists have supervision and the explicit acknowledgement that any and all therapists are at risk of boundary violations help to establish a culture which can deter a therapist who is tempted or anxious.

Boundary violations in psychotherapy

(See ➔ Boundary setting and maintenance in Chapter 9, pp. 454–5.)

Boundary violations occur when professionals step out of their role and function and act in ways that promote their own personal values and goals. Gutheil and Gabbard distinguish between boundary crossings, which appear to have little consequence for the patient or the therapeutic work, and boundary violations which cause harm to the patient and the effective end of the therapy.

The commonest form of boundary violation in therapeutic practice is inappropriate disclosure of personal information by the therapist. Typically, this occurs when the therapist is feeling anxious about the therapeutic process, particularly if the patient is challenging or especially distressed. Therapists may disclose personal information to avoid appearing distant or aloof, or to avoid the experience of feeling as if they are being unkind or unfriendly.

It will be clear from this brief discussion that boundary violations usually arise in response to: (a) some discomfort in the therapist and (b) a failure by the therapist to either reflect on their own discomfort and/or (c) consider that such discomfort may be an aspect of the patient's clinical problems. For example, a patient who has a history of an incestuous relationship with her father may unconsciously believe that having a 'special' relationship with the therapist is inevitable and necessary. She may act in ways that invite closeness and mutuality, and resistance by the therapist may be experienced as cold or unkind. A common example is when patients ask for hugs or demand to know where therapists are going on holiday. Conversely, patients may act aggressively as a defence against the fear of closeness and being abandoned.

Boundary violations represent a failure to regulate the space between the patient and the therapist, so that they are either too close and enmeshed or too far away and distant. Both such patterns are reflections of insecure attachment styles, and they are re-enactments of toxic attachment patterns (see ➔ Theories of personality development: attachment theory in Chapter 8, pp. 380–1).

Doctors and therapists at all stages of their careers may violate boundaries, but such behaviour is commoner in more senior clinicians. However, cases where multiple offences have been committed by therapists against patients are relatively uncommon, and the majority of transgressions are committed by clinicians who experience personal and professional stress, e.g. 'burnout'. In a recent study, Gabbard and Hobday evaluated boundary violations in over 300 physicians and therapists referred to a specialized treatment centre by licensing boards, hospitals, physician health organizations, or ethics committees in the USA. They concluded that it was inaccurate to categorize physicians as simply honest or dishonest, ethical or unethical. They found that many who had been ethical practitioners tended to rationalize sexual relations with patients, stealing from professional treasuries, or lying, whilst convincing themselves that they had acted in an honourable manner. These clinicians showed a high prevalence of defensive compartmentalization, temporal splitting, and projective disavowal as means of tolerating behaviours they would generally regard as unethical.

This pattern of offence justification is similar to that found in criminal 'offenders' or social rule breakers. Most people like to think of themselves as good people, and so people who break the rules (especially if they are not habitual rule breakers) will need to reassure themselves that they are still good people, despite their rule breaking. The usual way that people do this is to generate conscious narratives that justify their rule-breaking actions and disavow any malignant intention. Distorted cognitions and immature defences help maintain the belief in one's own goodness.

Sexual relationships between therapists and patients are always violations of professional boundaries, no matter how much the patient seems keen and actively consenting. Despite the fact that every therapist knows that they must not have sexual relationships with current, or even past, patients, there are still a number of therapists who let themselves get involved with their patients in this way. When the relationship ends (as it must), the patient (nearly) always reports the therapist to their professional organization. For medical psychotherapists, this will result in automatic erasure from the general medical register for a number of years.

Readers may like to consider whether the following examples are boundary crossings or violations:

- Using financial information provided by a patient with knowledge of a share release
- Using a patient's holiday home at a reduced rate
- Attending a patient's performance at the theatre or concert
- Telling a patient what football team you support
- Telling a patient that you have children and their names/sexes/ages.

The key issue here is that whatever decision is made is not neutral, in terms of either ethics or the therapeutic work. A boundary crossing or violation by a therapist means something significant, even if not serious.

Case examples

Case one: confidentiality and boundaries
(See ➜ Confidentiality and psychotherapy in Chapter 9, pp. 452–4; Boundary setting and maintenance in Chapter 9, pp. 454–5.)

Dr Murray is a thoughtful and experienced psychotherapist. He is involved in teaching and training of local NHS staff who are working with BPD in their Complex Needs Service. In his PowerPoint training presentation, he includes a slide which has a case history on it, relating to a woman with BPD who is in treatment with him and the complexities in her treatment. He excludes any identifying details. He circulates the presentation by email. Six months later, he is told that the patient has made a complaint against him; she has seen his presentation on the Internet and recognized herself.

Issues for discussion

This case (which is based on real events) is also a good example of how boundaries in practice reflect the boundaries between minds in therapy. Boundary crossings and violations can occur, whenever the therapist stops thinking about the patient's mind as 'other', separate, and different to their own. Dr Murray's intellectual interest in his patient's case (and perhaps also his anxiety) may have meant that he was not alert to the level of his patient's interest in him and the extent to which she was looking for material about him on the Internet. Dr Murray now knows that his patient has a somewhat paranoid interest in him; if he had been aware of that before, he might have decided not to use her case in his teaching and to make up a case that illuminated the problem.

It might have made a difference if Dr Murray had asked the patient's permission, and it would have made sense if there were potential clinical benefits to others knowing about her case in the local area.

Dr Murray might have benefited from discussing the potential use of the patient's material in supervision. One possible reason that senior and experienced clinicians are so often involved in boundary violations is that they have often stopped having supervision for their work. No one is too senior or experienced for supervision, especially with complex cases.

The Internet and search engines have led to profound changes in the ways that doctors and patients relate. Psychotherapists should assume that potential and current patients will 'google' them, and therapist privacy and personal space may need particular protection. Therapists who teach may need to state clearly that their material is confidential and not to be shared outside the teaching session; increasingly, teachers are advised not to circulate actual slides, but pdf versions of their presentations.

It will clearly be important for Dr Murray to acknowledge the hurt done and apologize. Supervision will be essential for him to enhance his awareness and self-reflection about his case; it will also be essential as part of working through the relationship between himself and his patient now. Therapists might like to think about how and whether Dr Murray can work with a patient who has complained about him, both the practical and ethical issues.

Case two: confidentiality

(See ➜ Confidentiality and psychotherapy in Chapter 9, pp. 452–4; Risk assessment in Chapter 3, pp. 104–7.)

Mr Jones is a 47-year-old man who has been referred for psychotherapy following the breakdown of his marriage. His wife left him after 20 years for another man, and there was an acrimonious divorce. Mr Jones has now been divorced for 2 years, but he is still depressed, bitter, and suicidal at times. He started in therapy 6 months after taking a serious overdose.

Mr Jones comes to therapy regularly. He presents as a quiet man, who is punctual and assiduous about paying his bills. He has no history of psychiatric illness or abnormal behaviour prior to his divorce—he did have a brief previous marriage in his early 20s. In his personal history, he says his mother died when he was 14, and his father remarried soon after to a woman he did not like.

As therapy progresses, Mr Jones presents as more hostile and angry. He is belittling of his (female) therapist's comments and reflections. When he comes to therapy, he talks without stopping, and it is hard for the therapist to contribute. The content of much of his talk is about his wife's perfidy, how she has hurt him, and how she deserves to pay for what she has 'done to me'. Despite the therapist's interventions, Mr Jones seems fixed in his rage.

The therapist has to cancel a session with Mr Jones unexpectedly when a family member is ill. At the next session, Mr Jones makes no comment on the missed session but describes in detail how he has recently been to his ex-wife's new home on several occasions, watching her movements and working out how he could set fire to the house when she was in it. He seems exhilarated by his plans, and the therapist feels frightened and helpless. At the end of the session, Mr Jones says he feels better for having talked about his plans to kill his wife and says to his therapist, 'And of course, you can't tell anyone what I'm thinking'.

Issues for discussion

The obvious first issue is contained in Mr Jones's last comment. He is incorrect—the therapist is ethically empowered to disclose patient information in the 'prevention, detection and punishment of serious crime' (NHS Code of Confidentiality). She does not have to tell anyone about her concerns, but, if Mr Jones acts to harm his wife, it might be argued later that his disclosure to the therapist constituted a link to the ex-wife, which placed a legal duty of care on the therapist (and/or her employer if she has one) to protect her by warning her of the danger. In such a case, if the therapist does disclose, any complaint or legal negligence claim, with respect to confidentiality by Mr Jones, would probably fail, because of the apparent risk to the ex-wife.

Respect for patient confidentiality has never meant the upholding of dangerous secrecy, especially if someone vulnerable is at risk. The therapist could reasonably disclose her concerns to a supervisor, and possibly the police, and could justify the breach with reference to the protection of an identifiable individual and the prevention of serious harm. As a matter of good practice, the therapist should probably write a clear account of all that has happened and then urgently discuss with a supervisor, and possibly discuss with a professional regulatory body, like the GMC or UKCP, or a medical defence union.

The ethical question to be addressed is whether the potential for harm avoidance justifies the breach of confidentiality and the (possible) damage to the therapy. In terms of costs and benefits, it is possible to see the benefits of disclosure (alerting the ex-wife to the danger, protection of a potential victim, and prevention of a serious harm) and the costs (the possible end of therapy and the possibility that Mr Jones will not be so open in future about his risk, so therapy will be compromised). The current public stance in relation to information is highly risk-averse, so it is likely that the therapist would be advised that the benefits of disclosure will be seen to outweigh the costs.

A more troubling issue is the reality of the risk. Actuarially, the risk is low; Mr Jones's case has only one factor associated with increased risk of violence—he is male. The cost–benefit analysis described above assumes that what Mr Jones has said is veridically true. But the psychotherapist might think that the threats are only psychologically true; Mr Jones does want to hurt a woman who has left him for someone else, namely the therapist who cancelled his session. This disturbing material may be Mr Jones's way of expressing his anger and distress at the cancelled session; the person most in danger may be the therapist, and not the ex-wife. If this account were true, then breaching confidentiality would not have the anticipated benefits and might lead to more danger, not less.

The most troubling aspect about this case is that there is no way to distinguish between the two formulations, and there are no options that do not have costs. Doing nothing is a high-risk strategy—at the very least, the therapist must have an urgent consultation with a professional colleague and document that she has done so. Of the options, probably a discussion with the police is justifiable, both ethically and legally. From a clinical point of view, it will be important that the therapist discusses the risk issue with Mr Jones. She may need to involve another person to help her with this process such as her supervisor. There is no neat, easy solution to this process, and the costs–benefits are actually unknowable, as what the therapist does will affect them.

Psychodynamically, we may wonder at the power of the parallel process that operate between human minds—Mr Jones has managed to leave his therapist in a helpless, frightened, and somewhat humiliated state of mind, which one imagines is exactly what his internal world is like most of the time.

Case three: boundaries

(See ➲ Boundary setting and maintenance in Chapter 9, pp. 454–5; Service user involvement in Chapter 10, pp. 466–71.)

Henry was a patient who had therapy with Dr Carl, whilst he was an inpatient in a secure psychiatric hospital. Henry had made an assault on a junior doctor, whilst he was psychotic; he also had a history of assaults on family members. He made good use of his therapy and was able to continue in therapy when he was discharged. The therapy came to an end by mutual agreement, as Henry felt he was better, and he was only having psychiatric reviews twice a year in outpatients.

Five years later, Dr Carl is invited to be part of a conference run by a national organization supporting therapy and recovery for offenders with mental illness. He agrees to do this but is taken aback to find that Henry is also on the programme as an expert by experience. Dr Carl feels unsure as to whether there is a boundary issue but decides to go to the conference and see what unfolds. When he gets to the conference venue, he discovers that Henry plans to discuss the therapy they did together as part of his presentation. He also discovers that Henry is accompanied by his new wife, who was previously a staff nurse on the ward where Henry was a patient. She tells Dr Carl that she and Henry met after his discharge through their work with this national organiza-tion, and they frequently give talks and presentations to staff about how to involve service users in recovery.

Dr Carl feel uncomfortable, although he is not sure why. He mentions this discreetly to a senior colleague who says that he is old-fashioned and that his values are out of date. The colleague suggests that Dr Carl is uncomfortable because he and Henry are now on a level playing field in terms of power and authority. She also says that Henry's therapy 'belongs' to him, and he is entitled to speak about it as he wishes.

Henry's talk contains high praise of his work with Dr Carl. Dr Carl goes home, still wondering why he felt uncomfortable.

Issues for discussion

This case has no simple boundary violation to explore; rather it is a real and contemporary example of how roles and identities in mental health care are not fixed but can become blurred and ambiguous. Different pro-fessionals may feel differently about this situation—perhaps the take-home message of this case is that feelings are not always the best guide to whether a situation is right or wrong. In fact, this principle underlies many cases of boundary crossings and violations.

Dr Carl's colleague sees no problem with Dr Carl and Henry sharing a platform or discussing their work together in public. Henry sees no problem. His wife sees no problem in their change of relationship—they met in a different context and on an equal footing. Dr Carl's colleague may be right—that Dr Carl's discomfort is based on their new equality.

Hindsight bias may be an issue later on, if things go wrong. If all goes well in the future, then it may be said that there is no ethical issue at all. But if Henry assaults his wife, it is likely that someone will suggest that there was an ethical boundary violation by his wife that should have been addressed. In similar circumstances, staff members, like Henry's wife, might expect to find themselves referred to their professional regula-tor for misconduct—would this happen if she was a victim of Henry's violence?

Should Dr Carl do or say anything? What could he do? No obvious harm is done to anyone by his appearance at a conference with Henry, and possibly much good. Perhaps this case again highlights the limita-tions of relying on consequences for judging the rightness of a situation or course of action.

Recommended reading

Gabbard GO and Hobday GS (2012). A psychoanalytic perspective on ethics, self-deception and the corrupt physician. *British Journal of Psychotherapy*, **28**, 235–48.

Gutheil TG and Gabbard GO (1993). The concept of boundaries in clinical practice: theoretical and risk-management dimensions. *The American Journal of Psychiatry*, **150**, 188–96.

Hinshelwood RD (1997). *Therapy or Coercion: Does Psychoanalysis Differ from Brainwashing?* Karnac Books: London.

Holmes J and Lindley R (1998). *The Values of Psychotherapy*. Karnac Books: London.

Tjeltveit A (2003). *Ethics and Values in Psychotherapy*. Routledge: London.

Woodbridge K and Fulford KWM (2004). *Whose Values? A Workbook for Values-Based Practice in Mental Health Care*. Sainsbury Centre for Mental Health: London.

Chapter 10

The system

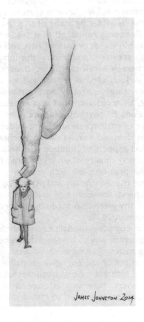

Planning psychotherapy services within psychiatric care

(See ⊃ Therapy in clinical practice in Chapter 5, pp. 154–63; Personality disorder services in Chapter 8, pp. 422–7; Psychological therapy in secure settings in Chapter 8, pp. 428–39.)

The place of psychotherapy services within mental health remains a complex area, with questions about which services should be funded becoming increasingly important in an environment beset by financial insecurity. There is an argument that this is not a new problem and is emblematic of the sometimes tenous relationship between mainstream psychiatry and psychotherapy since the very beginning of mental health services in the UK.

Historical context

(See ⊃ Medical psychotherapy modalities in Chapter 2, p. 14.)

From its early beginnings, psychotherapy could be regarded as a parallel movement, with its proponents being on the fringes of mainstream psychiatric practice in the UK. However, over the years, the influence of psychotherapy has increasingly expanded with a number of significant advances in practice and with growing impact on the delivery of care in various settings. The increase in the number of psychotherapeutic modalities offering a multitude of ways to understand the psyche of the patient helped bring it closer to psychiatry, though, at the same time, the bewildering array of choices can lead to infighting and confusion. Concerns remained over traditional psychotherapy services situated within departments of psychotherapy distant from other mental health services, underlining the long held problems of integrating psychotherapy services with psychiatry. Inter-professional rivalries between various clinical groups led to varying accusations of psychotherapy existing separately and removed from the travails of acute psychiatry, an accusation that was repeatedly responded to with words and actions by psychotherapists. One of the actions was that a broader range of patients should be considered, including those that were previously deemed unsuitable for psychotherapy treatment. Advances in technical aspects of practice also helped increase access, alongside the improving quality of interventions. Many clinicians and writers also became preoccupied with resolving antipathy between increasingly disparate psychotherapy and psychology services, with the attempt being to achieve some sort of mutual coexistence. Efforts to integrate psychotherapy were also made by the broader organization, including the NHS executive.

The emergence of cognitive modalities and their early embrace of research was an important way to bridge distances between traditional services. Addressing issues of using easily understandable language and paradigms was a strength of the cognitive modalities, which has led to increased uptake and interest by psychiatric practitioners. Some psychodynamic practitioners, however, attempted to understand these problems as defences that were used to create distances by individuals and organizations. In this way, the needs of the organization triumphed over individual needs and ensured a safe distance between the individual practitioners and the patient's pathology, whilst avoiding recognition of hidden problems within groups (Hook, 2001).

Current trends in differentiating patients at referral

The stepped-care approach has been one of the ways by which care has been made available to patients needing psychological interventions. In this model, provision is stratified, and patients are matched with the level at which they can receive the least intensive treatment likely to meet their needs. Guidance from the Royal College of Psychiatrists dictates that patients in step 1 (recognition and assessment), step 2 (treatment for mild disorders), and step 3 (treatment for moderate disorders) receive treatment in primary care settings, and only those in steps 4 and 5 (treatment for severe and complex disorders, respectively) being eligible for secondary care interventions. However, in practice, these differentiations can be much harder, and gaps in services can appear in the differing requirements that various services may have before accepting patients for a psychological intervention. The challenges of having a single point of access for patients in pathways, increasingly being delivered by multiple providers, including the private sector, third sector, and NHS services, can mean that patients end up having long waits or multiple assessments before reaching the required intervention.

Current referral streams

(See ➲ Is my patient suitable for psychotherapy? in Chapter 4, pp. 110–17.)

Referral streams to psychotherapy-based services are usually from many sources, depending on their location. Primary care referrals are usually by GPs and other staff within GP practices, referrals from services at other levels, social and other statutory or voluntary services, and by self-referral. Secondary care may receive direct referrals from primary care GPs, primary care psychology/psychotherapy services, including IAPT, secondary care CMHTs, and other service referrals, referrals from other secondary care and acute physical health settings, and third sector referrals, etc. The patient group is usually defined by the stepped-care model, with those for secondary care presenting with complex problems with difficulties in benefiting from, or making use of, services at lower levels such as within primary care. This makes their difficulties more intractable, and these patients are often harder to engage.

Improving Access to Psychological Therapies services

(See ➲ Cognitive behavioural therapy in Chapter 5, pp. 172–84.)

The IAPT programme, initiated in 2007, was one of the attempts by the government to broadly improve access to psychological therapies for moderate to severe depression and anxiety, which were recognized as being crucial and necessary to improve mental health in the wider population. The programme was implemented in phases in primary care with initial demonstration sites, followed by pathfinder trusts, leading up to its national implementation. It was initially aimed primarily at working people, with goals of returning people to work and its economic arguments built up around reducing the use of sick pay and benefits. These initial economic arguments of getting people back to work attracted criticism, with concerns also around the premise of mental illness used for the programme. Nevertheless, by 2011, 3660 new CBT workers had been trained, and over 600000 people started treatment; over 350000 completed it, and over 120000 moved to recovery, though it would seem that only 23000 came off sick pay or benefits (between October 2008 and 31 March 2011).

Over time, and perhaps in recognition of some of these difficulties, the aims and provisions in the programme broadened, whilst continuing with the theme of improving access. The programme now aims to be for all ages, including a stand-alone component for children, rather than just working-age adults. The emphasis has shifted to broaden attempts to provide a psychological service for people with physical illness and unexplained medical symptoms. IAPT is also now focusing on serious mental illness (SMI), with its plans to increase public access to a range of NICE-approved psychological therapies for psychosis, bipolar disorder, and personality disorders. Over time, there has also been much more emphasis on clinical recovery, social participation, satisfaction, and well-being for the restructured programme. However, the IAPT programme has been criticized for its unimodality (CBT) approach to its remit, with increasing arguments that an entire group of patients at the primary care level would benefit from a more inclusive range of offerings.

Secondary care

Where do the IAPT initiatives leave secondary care services? The problem could be that of a failure of demand recognition in an environment where the pressure is to provide increasingly basic services that fulfil acute need. Hence, whilst access to psychological therapies may have improved, there remains the risk of oversimplification regarding need at all levels. There seemed to be, for some time, an idea popular in the imagination of central and local commissioners that the IAPT model would become the prototype for all psychologically driven services. The seductive promise of returning patients back to work and improving their well-being offered the apparently perfect solution to the ever increasing demand reaching secondary care.

There has also been concern about the effect of the CBT-led IAPT model being to the detriment of every other modality of psychotherapy and the effect of the programme on the provision of services for more complex presentations. Some of these concerns may be valid, and there have been reports of pressures to deliver shorter-term therapies, limitations of patient choice, downgrading, and threats of closure to other psychotherapy services across England, at around the same time as the roll-out of the IAPT. Over time, the initial goals for the IAPT were modified and expanded, as real-time practice revealed problems with the vision of shorter-term interventions resolving potentially chronic issues and fulfilling the economic predictions. This has shifted the focus back on a set of patients at step 4 who have more complex and intractable presentations, for whom longer-term interventions are required.

Tertiary and specialist services

Tertiary services delivering psychotherapy-based interventions usually involve patients who have particularly severe presentations at step 5. Referral and treatment in these services is usually a longer-term process and reserved for the most complex set of patients, including services such as personality disorder, complex trauma, and eating disorders. Some of these services are now commissioned by NHS England, which arguably creates difficulties in access and local fit.

The need for a psychotherapy pathway

One of the problems is that psychotherapy itself can be viewed with a degree of reluctance by individual psychiatric staff and teams, perhaps accounted also, to some extent, by the use of the health organization of social defences against anxiety, in an effort to keep at bay more difficult feelings and experiences. In such an atmosphere, the promise of short-term treatments offering cure can be very attractive in getting rid of difficult emotions, when therapeutic pragmatism may point towards a best possible outcome of modulation, rather than a complete psychological shift. There have been identified problems with effective service delivery for psychotherapy, with concerns about organizations being prone to quick fixes with a lack of leadership and poor integration between various services, whilst demand continued to be robust. Thus, there remains a need for organizations that are less prone to revolution but more invested in evolution, as a way to improve the delivery of psychological therapies.

The many and varied attempts over the years in designing models of delivery for psychotherapy services have tried to conjure up the best fit to improve integration and delivery. These ranged from the earlier specialist psychotherapy departments' attempts to embed psychotherapy within CMHTs using hub-and-spoke designs and practice-based commissioning in primary care using the stepped-care provisions advocated by the Royal College of Psychiatrists. The range of potentially destabilizing rules introduced by the Health and Social Care Act 2012 to encourage competition present a new challenge in providing seamless care, as integration can be an easy casualty of the qualified provider model. Hence, there is an ongoing need to convince commissioners of the opportunity for a psychotherapy pathway that bridges the various steps and address current gaps in provision, as realization of unmet needs takes hold. The aim for improvements in delivery demands a longer-term perspective with commissioning keeping the vision of a specific psychotherapy pathway that accommodates stepped care and diversity of modalities, whilst remaining specific to the needs of the local population. Only such a psychotherapy pathway will address the needs of a diverse range of patients such as those with long-term frailty, physical conditions, medically unexplained symptoms (MUS), low-grade personality disorder, agoraphobia, and co-morbidity, who have arguably struggled to get a reasonable service through current provisions or take a long time to reach the right intervention.

Recommended reading

Albeniz A and Holmes J (1996). Psychotherapy integration: its implications for psychiatry. *British Journal of Psychiatry*, **169**, 563–70.
Department of Health (2011). *Talking Therapies: A Four-Year Plan of Action*. Available at: ℘ http://www.iapt.nhs.uk/silo/files/talking-therapies-a-four-year-plan-of-action.pdf.
Holmes J (1991). Psychotherapy 2000. Some predictions for the coming decade. *British Journal of Psychiatry*, **159**, 149–55.
Holmes J (1995). The integration of psychiatry and psychotherapy. *Psychiatric Bulletin*, **19**, 465–6.
Holmes J (1998). The psychotherapy department and the community mental health team: bridges and boundaries. *Psychiatric Bulletin*, **22**, 729–32.
Hook J (2001). The role of psychodynamic psychotherapy in a modern general psychiatry service. *Advances in Psychiatric Treatment*, **7**, 461–8.
Marzillier J and Hall J (2009). The challenge of the Layard initiative. *The Psychologist*, **22**, 396–9.
Menzies Lyth I (1960). Social systems as a defence against anxiety. *Human Relations*, **13**, 95–121.
Stokoe P (2014). Selling psychoanalysis to the NHS. *New Associations*, **14**, 5–6.

Service user involvement

Service user involvement can take many forms, but all types of involvement are focused on ensuring that the views of people who *use* services help to shape the way we *understand* mental health and the services provided, leading to real, sustainable changes and improvements in those services. There are many different ways of doing this, but common examples include encouraging service users to be actively involved in their own care, or to have a say or an active role in the design, delivery, and evaluation of mental health services. The principle which underpins this is that people with lived experience of mental health issues/using services have a valuable perspective; making a contribution in this way is beneficial both to that person and their development, and beneficial to the development of services.

Co-production is a term that is becoming increasingly popular. It refers to a broad range of involvement activities where staff and service users enter into a collaborative relationship, working together and recognizing one another's different skills and experience as equally valuable. This approach draws on the understanding that both staff and service users need to be empowered to be able to work in partnership together.

Types of service user involvement

In practice, service user involvement in mental health services in community settings can be applied across five main areas:
- *Service users involved in their own care*: e.g. someone's own view of their difficulties being taken into account in assessment, the service user having a say in their treatment and care plans, being listened to in care planning meetings. This may be seen as a shift from doing things *to* people, to doing them *with* people.
- *In service planning and evaluation*: e.g. giving feedback on the service, taking part in focus groups, service users working as researchers to evaluate the service, membership in clinical governance and service development structures.
- *Recruitment and training of staff*: service users sitting on staff interview panels with an equal say to other members, facilitating training, running staff inductions.

- *In-service delivery*: this might be through direct service delivery such as service users facilitating groups, working alongside staff to co-facilitate assessments, providing service inductions. Another approach is to involve service users in reflective forums for staff such as case management meetings, case formulations, complex case forums, or group supervision.

Approaches to involvement

As with any large, diverse group of people, there are widely varying views, experiences, and ways of understanding mental and personality disorders among service users. There is no single service user perspective.

To overcome this, sometimes people might ask for a *service user 'representative'*, whose role is to represent others. If you choose a representative model, it important to think about who the individual needs to represent (i.e. identify their constituency) and how they will gather the views and ideas of those they represent (e.g. through a service user group meeting or via a service user network).

Another approach to involvement is to involve those with specific experience and skills and recognize that this is valuable in itself. Sometimes people working to this model are known as *experts by experience*. Experts by experience are valued in their own right and asked to bring their own perspective to the table, rather than representing others.

There are also independent service user-led organizations which work collaboratively with those providing services in service development, evaluation, training, and so on.

Service user involvement and personality disorder

(See ⊃ Chapter 8.)

As highlighted in other chapters, many service users with a diagnosis of personality disorder have complex histories of trauma, abuse, neglect, or loss. These histories often go hand in hand with years of chronic invalidation, rejection, and simply not having their experiences or opinions heard or respected. Some service users with personality disorder have also experienced turmoil or difficulties in their relationships with others, so their interactions with mental health practitioners can often be fraught and problematic. This has often led to individuals being described as 'difficult to work with', 'attention seeking', 'manipulative' or 'untreatable', and frequently excluded from services.

Due to these kinds of experiences, many service users may mistrust authority and service providers. For some who do speak up, their feedback or opinions are often minimized or dismissed outright because of stigmatizing or discriminatory views about personality disorder; this serves to perpetuate feelings of invalidation and mistrust on both sides.

It is extremely common for people with personality difficulties to struggle with problems of identity; many people find it impossible to hold onto a sense of who they are. As people progress through treatment, this can become more pronounced; as past coping strategies are left behind, people often ask 'What's left?', 'Who am I if I'm no longer 'a self harmer' or 'an alcoholic' or 'the crazy one?'. Involvement activities can provide a space for people to begin to explore new roles and ways of relating to people. This uncertainty about identity is a core feature of the experience of personality disorder, so there is immense therapeutic potential in providing spaces where this can be experimented with.

Although the growth of authentic and meaningful service user involvement in the field of personality disorder has been problematic, there is nonetheless room for immense optimism when both the concepts of personality disorder and involvement are understood and worked with appropriately. The opportunity for service users to embark upon activities that shape and direct the services they receive promotes inclusion and therapeutic growth in itself. Many service users exceed expectations, not only in terms of their individual recovery, but in their subsequent contributions to services and their ability to sustain work and meaningful activity in the future. The social implications cover numerous areas: pathways back to work or education become realistic; appropriate use of other NHS services provides substantial financial saving; problems with housing and social services can be resolved; offending behaviour is reduced or stopped; and most importantly the quality of life for the user improves dramatically, with new-found social inclusion and a life felt to be worth living.

Principles of good service user involvement

- *Support*
  It is important not to make assumptions, but to have an open, honest conversation about what someone might need to enable them to participate. Ask yourself and those involved:
  - What support might someone need? This might be emotional support but may also be practical support.
  - Who is the best person to provide emotional support related to the involvement activity, if needed?

- *Clear expectations*
  Providing realistic expectations for involvement—both to professionals and service/ex-service users. It may be helpful to consider:
  - Why do you want to involve service users?
  - Why does the service user want to get involved?
  - What does the role entail? For example, what is the time commitment, responsibilities, details of the role? It is often helpful to write a role description to ensure that everyone has a shared understanding of the role.
  - What skills are needed? Most involvement activities require skills of some sort—if you can identify this at the beginning, you can help people decide whether they are right for the role or go through a recruitment process, to avoid difficulties later.
  - What can be changed/influenced, and what are the limits of the involvement? Be honest about the limits of service users' influence.

- *Payment*
  It is widely accepted as good practice to pay people for their involvement (except in their own care). This demonstrates that the work of service users is valued and on a more equal footing with the views and opinions of staff.

- *Who to involve?*
  Careful consideration needs to be given to the question of who to involve. It might be helpful to consider:
  - What type of personal experience is important? Some involvement activities are directed at those who are currently using a particular service; for others, it might be helpful if someone has moved on or graduated from the service.
  - Beware of 'cherry-picking' individuals, and instead identify what experience people need to have to undertake the role.
- *Diversity*
  In thinking about who to involve, ensure you consider the diversity of the population you work with, and try to ensure involvement activities reflect this. It is helpful to ask:
  - Who uses our service? Who is eligible to, but does not, access our service?
  - Consider people from minority ethnic communities; those who identify as lesbian, gay, or bisexual; gender, including those who identify as transgendered; religious groups and those with physical disabilities/sensory impairments.
  - Often it is helpful to adapt involvement activities, so they are more appealing to those who might not generally join in, e.g. consider the location, linking in culturally appropriate creative workshops, collaborating with community groups.
- *Issues of power*
  There is an inherent power imbalance between people who use services and staff that provide the service. Traditionally, most professional trainings and services were based on a view of staff as holders of knowledge and expertise, and service users as ill, damaged, and therefore incapable. On a conscious level, many staff no longer believe this, but services are usually framed with this model of 'knowledgeable professional helper' (staff) and 'person to be fixed/helped' (service user) at its core.
  - Meaningful involvement requires everyone to reconsider and try to step outside these roles.
  - Letting go of a position of 'knowing', which is so often a part of our professional identity, and inviting others to see our uncertainty are often very unsettling and can be uncomfortable. This can also be the case for service users; for some, inhabiting a position of responsibility and authority will be a new experience which challenges assumptions they may hold about their own capabilities and identity.
  - This does not mean devaluing the expertise and knowledge which staff have, but rather recognizing that service users have different forms of expertise and knowledge. The potential of involvement to deliver change and improve services arises from bringing together these two different types of knowledge and expertise.
  - Power differences can also arise from lots of other factors such as age, gender, level of education, and social class. These equally need to be attended to and carefully considered.
  - Both staff and service users benefit from reflective space where these issues can be honestly explored.

- *Feedback*
  The process of involvement does not end with the activity itself; feeding back what has happened as a result of service users' input is crucial and helps to maintain involvement in future activity.

Challenges associated with service user involvement

Some of the named challenges to involving service users in service design, development, and evaluation include:

- *They're unreliable!* Stigma and discrimination can underpin the belief that service users are 'ill all the time' and therefore unreliable. Service users do have considerable coping skills, strengths, and resources.
- *They're TOO well!* On the other hand, service users can be thought to be 'too well', 'too articulate', or 'too vocal'. Some workers are often looking for the 'typical patient', often someone who is passive and will not challenge the system or the practitioner viewpoint.
- *We can't pay them!* Does the organization have a policy in place for paying service users? If you cannot pay people, how will you reward service users for their input? There are other ways to give back, e.g. organizing a meeting around a working lunch and providing food.
- *It takes too much time!* Consulting others, working collaboratively, these do all take time, but try to think about the process, as well as the end result—involving people well is working towards therapeutic aims, as well as service development.
- *It's always the same people!* Welcome the input of regulars, whilst continuing to seek new people. Word of mouth is the best way to attract people—make people *want* to get involved.

Benefits associated with service user involvement

Involving service users in the development and running of the mental health services they use has benefits for all: service users, staff, services, and commissioners.

- *Benefits for services and staff*
  Staff can find out more about what service users want and can develop responsive services. The relationship between staff and services users will be strengthened if service users feel that their views and contributions are taken seriously. Involvement activities offer a chance to see people in a different role and to see their abilities and growth.
- *Benefits for service users*
  Service users can feel empowered by getting involved in this work, and it has been shown to strengthen self-confidence and self-esteem. Peer support from other service users can also contribute to recovery. The increase in confidence, as well developing new skills, has led many service users into paid employment. Involvement offers an opportunity to explore new roles and identities beyond that of service user.

Recommended reading

Barnes B and Cotterell P (2012). *Critical Perspectives on User Involvement*. Policy Press: Bristol.
National Survivor User Network (NSUN). 4PI Framework (a set of National Standards for Involvement). Available at: ℜ http://www.nsun.org.uk.
Staddon P (ed) (2013). *Mental Health Service Users in Research: Critical Sociological Perspectives*. Policy Press: Bristol.

Useful websites
∾ http://www.emergenceplus.org.uk.
∾ http://www.scie.org.uk.

Psychotherapeutic understanding of organizational processes

(See ➣ Group therapy and group analysis in Chapter 2, pp. 42–4.)

The conscious and unconscious processes at work

In any organization, there are conscious, less conscious, and unconscious behaviours that affect and influence the functioning or malfunctioning of the organization in its requirement to perform and service its primary task. The conscious primary task refers to the nature of its structure, management, and organization, and how these relate to dealing with the input, throughput, and output of the system. So the first issue here is whether these arrangements are suitable to carry out the task, or whether at this early stage there is already an element of an impossible task being attempted, a task that cannot be achieved. It is not the purpose of this chapter to focus on the concrete conscious structure of the organization, but it is worth remembering that organizations are at times set up to perform tasks, often more based on wish fulfilment than on a realistic expectation of achievement and results.

It also needs to be understood that an awareness of both conscious and unconscious dynamics at play in the functioning of organizations should be a requirement in all human enterprises—not only of mental health ones—and that the need for this understanding is increasingly a central plank in management and leadership programmes in business schools. It is thus somewhat of a tautology to ask for psychotherapeutic understanding (versus other understandings?). It is, however, true that work in the field of mental functioning, and individual and group processes has nowadays contributed massively to the body of knowledge available to members and leaders of organizations alike.

Organizational processes

So what are organizational processes, and why do they matter? In this regard, organizational processes refer to semi-conscious factors at play (there being a certain awareness of their presence, but an avoidance of addressing them). More important are the unconscious factors, assumptions, and states of mind that are present and can have a major disruptive effect on the functioning and well-being of the organization.

It is therefore essential that there is an acknowledgement of the existence of such unconscious factors, for only if and when the possibility of their presence and influence is acknowledged does the possibility arise that they might be addressed and their negative influence reduced or mitigated. The leader who proudly announces that no such unconscious processes exist in his or her organization is not a genius, but more likely an idiot in the grip of personal and group vanity and denial. Matters being as they are, it is obviously helpful for all members, from the top leader down to the cleaner, to have some thoughts about what else might be going on, apart from the so-called obvious, and how it affects the organization. Sadly, this in itself is not enough. The reason being that, after a matter of some months or thereabout, all concerned become more or less institutionalized and thus less open to a wider perspective on matters internal to the functioning of the organization.

What makes for the causes and persistence of unconscious underground organizational processes? There are two main factors. The first is a concrete conscious system of organization that has no clear tasks, no clear boundaries, and unclear or muddled authority structures. Whilst this may unconsciously suit the staff by helping them to avoid responsibility and accountability, it does not make for competent functioning. In effect, it makes for a breeding ground for anti-task behaviour. A garden which is uncared for will become overrun by weeds. The same happens in organizations. The second cause of the creation and growth of unconscious organizational processes has to do with the nature of the work of the organization and the effect this has on the staff, both individually and as members of a group.

The classic writings of Elliott Jaques, Isobel Menzies-Lyth, and Tom Main give full voice to the pressures that staff are under, particularly in the health services (or more realistically called the 'illness' or 'unhealth services'). Although, as mentioned, these unconscious organizational processes occur in all organizations, this chapter is specific to their occurrence in the wider human services: health, education, social services—all organizations in which human, individual, and group psychological processes are an integral part of the work. Menzies-Lyth, in particular, has focused on the nature of the anxieties arising in and from the work. The notice on a cigarette pack says 'Warning: Smoking can seriously damage your health'. There should be an equivalent warning at the foot page of contracts for workers in the health and related fields: 'Warning: Engaging in this work might seriously endanger your mental and physical health and also of those around you in your work and personal life spheres'.

Risk, fear, and defences

So what are the risk factors? In the mining industry, it is known that asbestos dust in the atmosphere causes mesothelioma—a cancer—as dust in ordinary mining causes silicosis. The same applies in our field, except that the 'dust' is of emotional, and not concrete, particles. In a recent seminar at the King's Fund, top managers in the NHS were asked what the main fears in their personal lives were; the responses were illness, insanity, divorce, madness, and death. Welcome to the health service, for these are the tasks allocated by us to the health (or illness/madness) services, to be dealt with on behalf of society. As workers in this system, it is thus our unspoken unconscious task to reduce, if not to alleviate, the risks of these conditions overwhelming us, as individuals, families, groups, and society as such.

Any element, concrete or psychic, that threatens us elicits in us defensive reactions. These take two forms—denial on an institutional level, and denial and defensive behaviour and flight on a personal level. At an organizational level, the usual form of denial is to claim that there are no particular pressures of relevance at play and to denigrate any particular individuals who point out the reality. This is particularly present in the nuclear and petrochemical industries. In our field, the fate and poor treatment of 'whistle-blowers' is well recorded and an ongoing scandal. Here energy is focused on pathologizing the whistle-blower and seeing the issue raised as having to do with the pathology of the individual, rather than of the organization. Menzies-Lyth, in her classic original paper *Social Systems as a Defence Against Anxiety*, made it absolutely clear that the major organizational response to anxiety was to unconsciously arrange the staffs' working practices and procedures to shield them from the 'psychic' painful dust arising from the work. The resulting working practices were thus designed for the benefit of the staff, rather than for the benefit of the patients. For example, tasks in a ward were allocated on the so-called basis of training and efficiency needs. Thus, one nurse would deal with 25 patient temperatures, another with 25 'bottoms', etc. This system ensured that there was minimal personal contact with the patients who were seen as 'organs in need of repair' or as numbers, and in no way as individuals. This dehumanization of the task led to poor nursing relationships and staff burnout. Another example would be difficulties in an old age home. These organizational processes, as described by Miller and Dartington, are, at their most psychological basis, warehouses en route to the cemetery, thus potentially a depressing and demoralizing job, as well as being universally poorly paid, given societal taboos about death and dying. In such places, it is not unusual for admission criteria to be developed that unconsciously sift out those most in need and to admit those that are least troublesome to the staff.

Understanding of therapeutic organizations

If we look at specifically therapeutic organizations, whether outpatient, day care, or residential, it is clear that the 'input' into the system brings with it the psychic 'dust' of pain disturbance and madness. From the staff point of view, this puts the staff constantly at risk of being affected/infected by these 'psychic particles'. A member of staff might be fairly resilient and well in themselves, but being constantly 'irradiated' by these processes from patients and immersed in the unconscious ' psychic soup' of the organization can detonate unresolved personal enclaves in the psyche of the staff, with catastrophic effects on staff, patients, and the organization. For example, it is commonly known that a disproportionately high percentage of young staff working in children's homes themselves grew up via that route, and being back in the same system, even though as members of staff, can trigger anti-task behaviour with the clients, be it sexual or drug- and alcohol-related. It needs to be understood that organizations dealing with specific issues, be they delinquency, adolescence, criminality, etc., may be thus stagnant 'psychic ponds' of pathology that can increase the risk to patients of these pathologies, as well as affect individual and group processes negatively. During the process of so-called 'rehabilitation' of the mentally ill back in to the outside world in the 1970s and 1980s, patients' personal clothes were taken away (because the laundry could not cope with diversity), and they were given uniforms. Their personal possessions were 'put into safekeeping' to protect them, thus stripping the patients of key elements of their identity. Although matters may have improved, the mechanism of arranging treatment to serve the staff, instead of the patients, is still a common occurrence.

Patient and staff relationships

(See ⮕ Consultation in Chapter 4, pp. 145–51; Balint groups in Chapter 10, pp. 484–96; Reflective practice groups in Chapter 10, pp. 497–505.)

In looking at the 'match' between client/patient and member of staff, it is therefore necessary that both the management and individual members of staff remain aware of the fact that they are in a risky business, and it is essential for them to be aware of their blind spots and 'Achilles heels', hence the requirement that staff have some elements of personal therapy, or at least regular supervision, reflective practice, and consultation in their work, whether as individuals or as part of an institutional work process. There is no doubt that, in organizations such as the ones described above, it is useful to have external consultation (from a consultant outside the institution who is not subject to its dynamic influences as readily as an insider may be). A 'visiting anthropologist' state of mind from a consultant is much more effective in highlighting problems, and thus raising the possibility of them being addressed, than to leave such processes solely to so-called 'sensitivity groups' or staff meetings. The whole purpose of such external intervention is to 'out' the institutional taboos, give the evidence for the intervention, and leave it to existing staff and management to work towards a resolution of the problems.

In looking at institutional group phenomena, it is quite common for one or other individual to be 'fingered' as the problem in the organization. This can apply equally whether it is a colleague, member of staff, or a particular client/patient. Given that training in psychiatry and many psychotherapies primarily focus on the individual, on his or her psychopathology, it is not surprising that the managerial approach derived from these trainings is either to 'therapize' the individual concerned or to arrange for the individual to be removed from the scene one way or another. Whilst this approach is understandable and does occasionally work, it usually does not.

The canary in the mine

The most effective approach is to see the individual as the 'unconscious spokesperson' or 'pit canary' in the team who represents an institutional issue that needs addressing. In nineteenth-century coal mining, a canary in a cage taken down the mine by the miners was the most important member of the team. It had been found that canaries were particularly sensitive to methane gas—a hazard in coal mines—and so, when the canary tipped over, it was time for the miners to leave the workings. The 'pit canary' therefore symbolizes the member of the team who has the greatest sensitivity to a noxious substance in the 'atmosphere', thus being the spokesperson of a dynamic in the group that needs to be aired and addressed as a group institutional issue, rather than as a personal problem.

A combination of awareness of the noxious side effects of the raw material processed in the organization (thus personal distress disturbance and madness) plus consistent questioning and modification, in line with the primary task of the organization, makes for the greatest chance for a successful organization. Most organizations also function as multidisciplinary teams, so, by definition, different professions will have specific perspectives on the nature of the work. Successful multidisciplinary teams will thus have constant debate and discussion about ways of proceeding with the work. By contrast, a team in constant agreement will be more comfortable for the staff but is likely to be less effective in dealing with the problems. It is this need to be constantly 'on one's toes' and having to think about what is going on in the less conscious regions of the organization that makes the work so exhausting. But better to be exhausted on task than burnt out and at risk.

Recommended reading

Dartington T (2010). *Managing Vulnerability: The Underlying Dynamics of Systems of Care.* Karnac: London.

Jacques E (1955). Social systems as a defence against persecutory and depressive anxiety. In: Klein M, Heimann P, and Money-Kyrle R (eds). *New Directions in Psycho-Analysis.* pp. 478–98. Tavistock Publications: London.

Main T (1989). *The Ailment and Other Psychoanalytic Essays.* Free Association Books: London.

Menzies-Lyth I (1988). The functioning of social systems as a defence against anxiety. In: *Containing Anxiety in Institutions: Selected Essays,* volume 1. Free Association Books: London (first published 1959 in *Human Relations*).

Miller EJ and Rice AK (1967). *Systems of Organization.* Tavistock Publications: London.

Psychotherapy and management

(See ➲ Psychotherapeutic understanding of organizational processes in Chapter 10, pp. 471–5.)

The context

In 1948, the NHS, the largest health-care provider in the world at the time, was established free at the point of access with Aneurin Bevan quoting a phrase from Winston Churchill—that the NHS should be provided 'from the cradle to the grave'. In 1960, the era of community care started with patients working in the community with nurses and open-door wards, a remarkable shift in paradigm from the previous culture of punitive and restrictive care. Over the years, it remained a large organization providing health as a public service, free at the point of care to people in the UK. More recently, changes in legislation introduced in the Health and Social Care Act 2012 have meant dramatic changes in the nature of health care in England, with the introduction of rules for competition, heralding a new frame for all health providers. This presents another challenge for the NHS, as its virtually autonomous foundation trusts now need to compete and survive in providing health services in competition with providers from the private and other sectors.

Management 'of and in' the NHS

For a long time, managing the health service was the prerequisite of medical clinicians, who held significant resource and influence as medical directors. In the period from the 1980s, there was increasing recognition of the balance that needed to be struck between limited resources and need. Over the 1990s, the preoccupation was with the quality of services, and numerous programmes were implemented to help improve the quality of health-care interventions in a measurable manner. The argument for trained management led to the introduction of professional managers, so that the organization could deliver on expectations. Professional management has been defined as comprising a set of skills within a person or group of people that ensure completion of tasks and so help the organization achieve its objectives, whilst continually improving its performance. One of the keys issues for management within the health service remained the problem of continual changes in the definition of objectives, which, in the NHS, seemed to shift with almost every new government that sets out a new vision for the future. However, key goals around patient safety, effectiveness of treatment, and quality were eventually defined as overarching objectives for the health service.

Management entities in NHS health-care organizations, such as foundation trusts, are represented at various levels. A typical service in a mental health foundation trust will have team leaders interacting with the local borough, holding medical and general management structures, which, in turn, are accountable to trust executives, with the board and operational management holding an overview and ultimate accountability for performance. This structure acknowledges the presence of clinical staff at various levels of the organization. More recently, the clinician manager has perhaps once again become valued, with the recognition of the added value brought by their clinical experience such as in the commissioning changes brought in by the Health and Social Care Act 2012.

What are the organization's tasks and objectives?

(See ➲ Psychotherapeutic understanding of organizational processes in Chapter 10, pp. 471–5.)

In a very straightforward manner, the health organization is continually attempting to process the health needs with which the patient presents, to help them resolve and allow the patient to get back to health. However, this relationship between those seeking care and those providing it can become easily complicated, e.g. due to more complex needs such as confusing combinations of social and health needs, intransigent issues that do not easily resolve, and also rationing of limited resources. In psychiatry, these challenges define much of the work, as patients presenting to most secondary and tertiary services have complex illnesses, often accompanied by difficulties in engaging with the care offered. Finally, from a management perspective, the average NHS foundation trust needs to engage with, and manage, the interests of many internal and external stakeholders in complex and interdependent relationships. These include patients, staff, carers, foundation trust membership, commissioners, regulators, local and central government, and the local population.

Whose needs are being addressed?

An almost constant difficulty in operational reality in the NHS has been the perceived and experienced distance between the various clinical groups and also with management. Psychotherapy has often been the subject of particular criticism within the mental health organization, with accusations of being separate and exclusive. Integration with psychiatry has brought up concerns about the difference in approaches, with psychiatry being seen as 'doing to' the patient versus 'being with' the patient in psychotherapy (Holmes, 1995). This has at times bred mutual hostility and breakdown of integration. This could be understood as various parts of the health organization feeling at risk of being deprived, and hence competing for influence, when there is an atmosphere of poverty in overall resources.

There can also be distance between management and clinical staff with problems in defining the tasks and then measuring the outcomes as those that would fulfil the objectives. There have been many recent examples where misunderstanding, or even misrepresenting, tasks and outcomes has resulted in serious consequences for patients and the health service. Amongst the many reasons identified as being responsible for the Mid Staffordshire episode, in which serious omissions of patient care occurred between 2005 and 2009, was the single-minded pursuit of foundation trust status by the trust at the behest of the Special Health Authority, which led the board to seemingly ignore all tasks that did not directly result in financial stability, whilst at the same time turning a blind eye to the ongoing difficulties in achieving its key objective of providing good-quality care. Other examples have included the consequences of the 4-hour A&E waiting times with patients being left on trolleys and 'game playing' in managing outpatient waiting lists to appear to fulfil a particular organizational diktat (Jones, 2011). There can be little doubt that these management entities (individuals or groups as boards) were trying to complete a certain task (saving money, getting patients moving, etc.) and somehow became distracted from other tasks within their organization which eventually prevented it from achieving its real objectives. Hence, there is the need to consider more deeply the setting of objectives and their understanding by the various parts of the organization.

Leadership versus management in health care

The successive, and often massive, reorganizations in the delivery of care over the past three decades have arguably challenged the provision of stable therapeutic spaces in the rapidly changing health arena. This potentially dilutes the rightful recognition of the role of attachment in a containing organization in stabilizing the unwell patient. In this context, leadership is important to separate from management, as holding a much more strategic and empowering role within large organizations. There have been links found between the style of leadership within an organization and its internal culture. The emphasis is on the capacity of the leader to form a vision that they are effectively able to communicate to better influence others and produce an integrated response, which moves beyond the narrower perspective of a manager.

Psychotherapeutic thinking around the needs of the individual versus the group can help clarify the needs of the unwell patient versus the needs of the organization. This can be especially important, as organizations are beset with primitive survival anxieties in the chaos of a competitive economic environment. The leadership of the organizations demonstrating failure of care, such as Mid Staffordshire, became blind to the needs of the patient and instead focused on revolutionary change. There was an apparent investment in remaining separate from the unwell patient, whilst the organization strove towards a narcissistically endowed foundation status. In psychiatry, this has arguably manifested in the name of financial prudence that has led to dramatic bed closures, with acutely unwell patients being sent to beds miles away from their homes (out-of-area care). Here the organization acted out its preoccupation with its own needs to survive financially by concretely withdrawing from its role to care appropriately, leading to chaos and confusion for the unwell patient.

Hence, management within health care needs not just to be about getting the tasks done, i.e. the work of the manager, but also show leadership in the sensitivity to how the task is done and remain connected to the overall objective of the organization to provide appropriate care to the patient. There are repeated examples of when organizational response and patient need become detached, with a resultant experience of poor or deficient care. There can also be the problem of not dealing with dependence and unrealistic expectations, which can create grievance and complaint.

A model of psychotherapeutic leadership in health-care management

A key contribution of psychotherapeutic thinking and practice is in making links to identify patterns that are often deep-rooted and not easily seen, which help to enhance understanding. This can make sense of the individual's problems, such as in using the care that is available, but also modulate the organization's expectations in dealing with a complex group of patients. There is benefit in aiding recognition of the limits of health-care provision and the capacity of the patient to make use of interventions, before a line is crossed to encouraging harmful dependency. Similarly, organizational dynamics using psychotherapy can help individuals and teams of staff understand their own responses to difficult patients and situations, so they are able to retain a therapeutic perspective and deliver good-quality care. Psychotherapy has been increasingly useful in training and development of staff with case-based discussions, training, and peer feedback, to help make sense of the relationships between the patient and the providers. External engagement is key to retaining the support of stakeholders. In this, psychotherapy adds particular value for the organization in moving it beyond simply being a delivery vehicle of metrics and mandatory contracted requirements. Hence, psychotherapy and its practitioners are well placed to communicate some of the difficulties in achieving individual and group objectives to clinical and managerial colleagues in secondary and primary care and also to commissioning and regulatory bodies.

Psychotherapeutic leadership within health care is important in understanding shifts in internal culture caused by envy and competition within and outside the organization. Psychotherapists and psychiatrists specializing in psychotherapy should work to use these key skills for the benefit of the patients that are served by their organizations. This will assist the larger organization and its executive leadership's engagement with its various stakeholders, whilst operating in a competitive environment. The need now is for a kind of psychotherapeutic leadership which assists in clarifying the role of tasks and continually links these to the objectives of quality. In its absence, there is a risk that the health-care organization will repeatedly get caught in anxious cycles of doing, rather than actually thinking about what it should be hoping to achieve as its objectives.

Recommended reading

Glasby J, Dickinson H, and Smith J (2010). Creating NHS local: the relationship between English local government and the National Health Service. *Social Policy and Administration*, **44**, 244–64.

Holmes J (1995). The integration of psychiatry and psychotherapy. *Psychiatric Bulletin*, **19**, 465–6.

Jones R (2011). Impact of the A&E targets in England. *British Journal of Healthcare Management*, **17**, 16–22.

Murray A (2010). *The Wall Street Journal Guide to Management*. Harper Business: New York.

National Quality Board (2011). *Quality Governance in the NHS*. Available at: ℘ https://www.gov.uk/government/uploads/system/uploads/attachment_data/file/216321/dh_125239.pdf.

Sorell T and Sorell T (1997). Morality, consumerism and the internal market in health care. *Journal of Medical Ethics*, **23**, 71–76.

Stokoe P (2014). Selling psychoanalysis to the NHS. *New Associations*, **14**, 5–6.

Teaching psychotherapy to mental health professionals

Psychotherapy is a talking treatment provided by trained professionals in a structured, boundaried, and containing manner. The focus of the treatment is on feelings, relationships, ways of thinking, and patterns of behaviour. The aim of this chapter is to offer some tips for teaching psychotherapy to mental health professionals.

Task of teaching

Whom are you teaching and why?

It is important to be clear about the task of the teaching. What are the needs and level of interest in the audience? Do the participants want to find out about the application of psychotherapeutic understanding to mental health in general, their particular patient group, and the demands of their job, or do they want to find out about psychotherapeutic practice? Usually it is the former, known as the application of psychotherapeutic thinking in general mental health practice.

Mental health professionals come from different professional backgrounds, most commonly medicine, nursing, social work, occupational therapy (OT), and clinical psychology. Therefore, most teams have a complex mix of backgrounds and experience. They will have some general preoccupations, and some that are specific to the service they work in. For example, a team working with dementia may have very different preoccupations than home treatment or crisis teams. Psychiatrists may require a different form of psychotherapy teaching from a group of social workers, as therapeutic applications in their roles are different.

Methods of teaching

The choice between lecture, seminar, workshop, or experiential teaching will vary, depending on the size of the group and the task of the teaching.

Tips for didactic teaching
Things to find out about the audience before the teaching session
- The services they are working in
- Their roles
- Their professional backgrounds
- Their level of experience of psychotherapeutic concepts
- Their preoccupations relating to their field of work
- Ascertain typical questions they may want to be addressed.

To keep the audience engaged
- If possible, ask everyone to introduce himself or herself and say which service they work in and their role.
- Check understanding with the group regularly, asking questions and allowing space for questions.
- Use case examples relevant to the group.
- Do not use too much text in PowerPoints or other visual material.
- Use as many pictures and diagrams as possible.
- Avoid using language specific to your own psychotherapy discipline.
- Get feedback afterwards verbally and formally on a feedback form.

Tips for experiential teaching
In this method, participants are encouraged to bring their own material for reflection by the group and facilitator. This can be in a workshop on a topic such as self-harm, in a less structured case discussion, or in a more structured Balint group format. The common theme in teaching in these situations is primarily in aiming for truthful emotional reflection, secondarily formulation and, in varying degrees, as this is a different task, on management of the patient.

Methods of running a case discussion or Balint group
(See ➔ Balint groups in Chapter 10, pp. 484–96; Reflective practice groups in Chapter 10, pp. 497–505.)
- Group frequency: series of sessions at regular intervals (most often weekly).
- Group size: the participant group size should not exceed 12 at any one time. Often there is a larger membership of the group but, due to the work commitments or leave plans, different participants attend on different weeks.
- Group leaders or facilitators: one or two; Balint co-leaders often include a member of the profession represented in the group.
- Presenter: there are different ways of nominating the presenter, depending on the enthusiasm and confidence of the group:
  - At the start, the facilitator can open up the group by asking, 'Who's on your mind?' and wait for a participant to come forward with some material
  - At the end of each group session, someone can volunteer, or be nominated, to present at the next group session
  - The facilitator can ask for anyone who would like to discuss a case to let them know in the week before the next session
  - A rota can be organized, so that everyone gets an opportunity to present.

- Preparation by the presenter: in general, some preparation is needed—this may range from thinking beforehand to more formalized notes (although notes are usually discouraged in Balint groups).
- Time: use a clear time boundary (generally 60 minutes).
- Discuss no more than two cases in any one session. In some groups, time is given for feedback on cases from previous weeks.
- Group leadership/facilitation: there are two main approaches:
  - The presenter talks about the case with little interruption. The facilitator then asks the group to respond to what they have heard. The group ends with a general discussion and reflection.
  - Goldfish bowl method: the presenter presents, and then the facilitator asks if there are any simple factual questions that need clarification, limiting this to two or three. He/she then asks the presenter to either literally or metaphorically 'push their chair back' and remain silent for the next 15 to 20 minutes. The presenter is then asked to rejoin the group, about 10 minutes before the end, and given an opportunity to offer their reflections on the discussion they have heard.

Topics: application

Themes of general interest

The following general psychotherapeutic themes are usually of interest and relevance to mental health professionals:
- The importance of development in relationships between mother and baby, fathers, siblings, and their influence in later years (see ➲ Theories of personality development: attachment theory in Chapter 8, pp. 380–1)
- The importance of loss and mourning and their importance in conceptualizing the development of mental illness (see ➲ Loss in Chapter 6, pp. 298–300)
- Risk, self-harm, and suicide, emphasizing the relational aspects (see ➲ Assessing and managing risk in Chapter 3, pp. 104–7; Suicide and self-harm in Chapter 6, pp. 308–11)
- Boundaries and boundary violations (see ➲ Boundary setting and maintenance in Chapter 9, pp. 454–5; Boundary violations in psychotherapy in Chapter 9, pp. 455–60)
- Understanding the meaning of psychotic states (see ➲ Psychoses in Chapter 7, pp. 331–4)
- Reflecting on the emotional responses to the patient by the mental health professional and the effects on the team (see ➲ Consultation in Chapter 4, pp. 145–51; Balint groups in Chapter 10, pp. 484–96; Reflective practice groups in Chapter 10, pp. 497–505)
- Understanding dependency and the problem of discharging patients.

As examples, here are some teaching vignettes that may help in putting together a teaching plan.
- *The importance of development in relationships*
Task: to illustrate the importance of detailed personal history in the later development of mental illness.

Teaching vignette: the relationship between the baby and the primary care-giver is very important in early life. If this goes well, the baby is loved and cared for. This relationship lays the basis for emotional stability in later life. In this case, the caregiver is attentive and thoughtful about the baby's needs and responds to them. They will then give the baby the message that life isn't pain-free, but it can be tolerated and the pain will pass. In this case, the baby is contained.

Linkage to mental illness: the baby can grow up to develop mental health difficulties in later life if they are not contained in early childhood. This can occur if the primary caregiver is not present, is suffering some disturbance himself or herself, or does not love the baby. In these cases, when the baby is upset and anxious, he or she will not be responded to and has to use primitive psychological mechanisms to psychically survive and to soothe themselves. They will then rely on these mechanisms again later in life and may develop resulting mental health problems. Some babies will not survive in these situations and will fail to thrive. (An example is Harlow's monkey experiment.)

Link to role: mental health workers function as containing relationships for patients who often have not had them in early childhood.

- *The importance of loss and mourning and their importance in conceptualizing the development of mental illness*

Task: to present a psychological model of mental illness from first principles.

Teaching vignette: loss and mourning are significant factors in all mental health difficulties. Many patients have become unwell, because they have suffered a loss event and are stuck in the mourning process. This loss event may not be easy for the patient himself or herself, or the professionals involved to see. It is often linked to other earlier losses. The stages of the normal mourning process are described by the Kubler–Ross grief cycle. An individual who gets stuck at some point in this cycle can develop a mental illness, and it is the stage they get stuck at that leads to understanding of their symptoms. For example, a patient who is suffering with clinical depression is stuck in the stage of mourning characterized by anger, blame, and guilt. The reason for getting stuck can vary, e.g. if the loss is too great or too complex or the capacity to mourn is too low.

Link to practice: understanding how this helps in conceptualizing a patient's difficulty and in choosing where to focus the therapeutic intervention.

- *Risk and suicide.*

Task: to increase understanding of the relational aspects of self-harm and suicide, and encourage open discussion.

Teaching vignette: suicide is a major preoccupation of mental health professionals. The national confidential inquiry into suicide reports that there are between 4000 and 4500 suicides a year in England. Of these, 20% to 30% have had some contact with mental health services in the last year, and around 10% of the population working with mental health services will die by suicide.

Why would an individual wish to commit suicide? They are overwhelmed by an emotional state and do not believe it will pass. Many suicides are impulsive, and often in the context of a recent loss event. The individual who takes their life may not think that they are going to die but may have a fantasy of what will happen after they die such as being reunited with a lost loved one in the afterlife or getting rid of the pain they are suffering.

Effects on health professionals: it is very stressful for the workers involved in caring for a patient who commits suicide. They can feel overwhelmed for several months, and this can interfere with their capacity to work. They can be left with complex feelings, including loss, responsibility, guilt, and shame. They may also be fearful about the challenging processes they have to face afterwards, including serious incident enquiries and giving evidence at the coroner's court. Often the response can be to withdraw and hide their feelings. However, linking and reflecting with colleagues who have had similar experiences can help with these difficulties.

Link to practice: to reduce professionals' fears of working with patients who express suicidal intent and to encourage them to ask for support that increases professional resilience and reduces 'burnout'.

Topics: practice

Why do mental health professionals need to know about psychotherapy?

This is a question that is asked occasionally. One possible answer is that psychotherapy is already part of their practice. Attendees are trained professionals providing a talking treatment to the patients they work with. They listen to their patient's feelings; they are interested in their life, and they keep them in mind. They work with their patients in addressing their maladaptive coping strategies and challenge destructive patterns of behaviour. They aim to form structured, boundaried, and containing relationships and understand why this is sometimes hard to achieve or sustain. They help their patients formulate their difficulties and come up with plans for the future. To know more about the practice of psychotherapy increases both their awareness of the resources of the psychotherapeutic approach and their confidence in the use or application of some psychotherapeutic ideas in their practice.

Teaching mental health professionals about different modalities of treatment

Keep the teaching about the different modalities of treatment straightforward and relevant. Do not spend a lot of time describing treatments that are not available in the local service. For example, it works well to compare two different, but well-recognized, treatments that are available locally such as psychodynamic psychotherapy and CBT (see Table 10.1) (see ➔ Psychoanalytic psychotherapy in Chapter 2, pp. 20–30, and in Chapter 5, pp. 163–72; Cognitive behavioural therapy in Chapter 2, pp. 30–4, and in Chapter 5, pp. 172–84).

Table 10.1 Comparison of two psychotherapy treatments.

	Psychodynamic	CBT
Treatment length	1–2 years NHS	6–25 sessions NHS
Session time	50 min	Varies
Regular	Usually once weekly or occasionally more frequent sessions	Can vary, generally weekly
Focus	Early life/past important in present difficulties and therefore important to explore past in the present and 'working through'. Patient can talk about anything on his/her mind, not focused on 'the presenting problem'	Focus on patient's current problems. Patients are taught skills to use with future problems
Therapeutic relationship	Emphasis on the therapeutic relationship and the bringing of earlier relationships into the present through exploration of transference influenced by countertransference	Collaborative emphasis
Homework	No	Yes
Coping strategies	Improve over time and exploration	Direct challenge
Formulation	Early experiences and feelings repressed in unconscious that then find expression in present day-to-day experiences. By addressing these hidden and repressed feelings, an individual is gradually freed of patterns of destructive behaviour	Uncovering dysfunctional core beliefs and automatic negative thoughts. Different adaptive coping strategies practised
Patient commitment	High	Medium to high

Recommended reading

Freud S (1917). Mourning and melancholia. In: Strachey J, ed. *The Standard Edition of the Complete Psychological Works of Sigmund Freud*, volume 14. pp. 237–60. Hogarth Press and the Institute of Psychoanalysis: London.

Holmes J (1991). *A Textbook of Psychotherapy in Psychiatric Practice*. Churchill Livingstone: Edinburgh.

Lucas R (2009). *The Psychotic Wavelength*. Routledge: London.

Peters S (2012). *The Chimp Paradox*. Random House: London.

Balint groups

What is a Balint group?

(See ➲ Michael Balint in Psychoanalytic psychotherapy in Chapter 2, pp. 25–8.)

Michael Balint was a Hungarian doctor and psychoanalyst who worked at the Tavistock Clinic in London. He started groups for GPs in the 1950s to study the doctor–patient relationship, which he described as 'training-cum-research groups'. He worked closely with his third wife Enid, who was a social worker and marriage guidance counsellor. A traditional Balint group consists of six to 12 doctors (or medical students) with one to two leaders, which meets regularly, usually weekly. Meetings usually last for one to two hours, and the group continues for one or more years. The method is that of case presentation without notes.

A Balint group is a group that focuses on a dilemma in the doctor–patient relationship relating to a feeling or an unspecified discomfort evoked in the doctor. The aim is to allow the doctor's unconscious to tell a story about the consultation. It's rather like talking with one's friends, telling them what is on your mind without using psychiatric terminology. A Balint group is about allowing oneself to open up to the possibilities of different impressions of the doctor–patient relationship by a free associative discussion within a boundaried psychoanalytic frame. It aims to open up emotional experiences usually kept outside the sphere of the doctor–patient relationship in traditional training.

The aim of a Balint group

(See ➔ Countertransference in Psychoanalytic psychotherapy in Chapter 2, p. 25.)

The aim of a Balint group is not to find a solution, but to open up a set of different impressions from different people that might enlarge the field of enquiry and introduce what Enid Balint rather wonderfully calls *suprisability*. This is by talking to the doctors' unconscious and taking it by surprise. What one is picking up is the countertransference of the doctor and trying to put that into words, because doctors are not used to, or indeed encouraged to, putting into refined words what it is they are *feeling* in the presence of a patient. The doctor tends to have to be positive and concrete about things to do with their contact with patients, and they are often pulled mainly into doing tasks such as risk management plans. The idea of taking a childhood or personal history in terms of finding patterns has become rather lost in the culture of contemporary psychiatry, and a Balint group can revive curiosity in the relevance of the past in the present.

In providing a developmental model, one frequently has to wonder with the trainees about what the person's past might be like. Not just in terms of selected facts, but in terms of how they might form patterns—unconscious patterns of how they see the world and how that might come out in the doctor–patient relationship. So one is essentially dealing with countertransference and trying to get the trainee to allow themselves to free associate a little bit and to see where it goes, introducing the idea that one can entertain difficult thoughts and feelings as part of the doctor–patient relationship.

For most doctors, the idea of *having feelings* in a doctor–patient relationship is often initially seen as unprofessional. Doctors are taught communication skills which primarily focus on how to get the patient to align themselves with the doctor's aims in offering help. The trainee often feels guilty that they have feelings about the patient and that the patient evokes feelings in them. Opening up the possibilities of free association and of dealing with feelings is potent, new material for doctors in training, and the fact that there is a discipline and a structure to this helps them. Integral to this is the psychoanalytic stance embodied not just in the psychoanalyst as a Balint group leader, but in all Balint-trained group leaders. It is essentially one of a benevolent neutrality and a sense of interest in what might be going on under the surface. It also involves accommodation of different modes of expression and different modes of communication.

A psychoanalytic lens
(See ➲ Psychoanalytic psychotherapy in Chapter 2, pp. 20–30.)

A psychoanalytic viewpoint can be helpful to the people in the group, but the aim of the Balint-trained psychoanalyst, GP, or medical psychotherapist group leader is not to teach somebody psychoanalysis or make them think psychoanalytically. It is to point out the contradictions and paradoxes, offering a different way of looking at the dilemma presented. Balint groups, when co-led by people who are psychoanalytically informed, are an important educational vehicle, e.g. of showing doctors in training the method in action. It is also important that, with all doctors, but particularly for those in foundation years and GP vocational training scheme trainees, the body can be thought about psychoanalytically as a theatre of expression in a relationship with a doctor. As Freud stated in *The Ego and the Id*, the ego is first and foremost a bodily ego. It is therefore especially important for Balint group leaders to have the body in mind, particularly when leading groups for in-psychiatry trainees where it can be forgotten. Foundation year doctors do their on call in the general hospital, and their out-of-hours work can be a fertile ground for this reminder to hold the body in mind.

The observer error
Michael Balint took the *observer error* seriously, in order to incorporate it into an understanding of a patient and his illness. This is quite central, because one is using the feelings invoked in the doctor in the service of the patient. This is good medical practice and also helps the doctor develop their self-reflection and their capacity to understand themselves as a doctor. The observer error clearly says we are not neutral or objective, but, on the contrary, the doctor is implicit in every observation and inference. The doctor's subjective viewpoint and feelings can be very useful, provided they are open to learning about, and trying to understand, the way they respond, so that they can use it to the patient's advantage. However, Balint groups are not therapy for the doctor.

Setting up a Balint group
In setting up a Balint group, there is a preliminary business meeting where the trainees or participants come and agree, as part of their learning, that they will try and attend as regularly as possible. They are told in the business meeting that:
• They will be asked to present a patient at some stage
• They will be asked to present without notes
• They will be asked to present a patient who in some way has caused them emotional difficulties, rather than one that interests them or one that they are going to present in a case conference

- The patient can be a case from A&E or any acute setting
- They are free to say whatever they want about their experience of the patient
- The normal rules of politeness and of how one might talk about a patient are in abeyance, and they know they can say what they feel and what they think if they choose to
- They have 10 to 15 minutes to do that, and then they can 'withdraw' from the Balint group (ending their presentation and listening to the other participants in the group respond to and reflect on the doctor's dilemma)
- They do not literally leave the room but are invited to be quiet. They listen to the discussion and do not intervene, and come back in 10 to 15 minutes from the end and continue to take part in the final discussion in whatever way they choose.

This is called a *push-back group* and is helpful with younger trainees. This is not the model Michael Balint originally proposed but is one that was developed in Germany, and it tends to work with people who are quite anxious about saying things and unsure what will happen in the group, and this structure seems to reassure younger trainees.

In setting up a Balint group, it is essential to be very clear about the boundaries and the structure. If the boundaries and the structure do not create the space, then the work cannot happen. This is the core of a Balint group—having a set time with a set room with a leader, and co-leader if possible, without interruptions and with clear boundaries of confidentiality. A clear stance by the leader of interest in the work of the participants, and the impartiality of not giving advice or reassurance but creating a space where anything can be said is part of this. This might be called a 'non-p.c.' stance, because, in our unconscious, we do not think in a rational 'p.c.' way. A psychoanalytic stance is that whatever comes into our mind will be of some use in thinking about the patient. It may tell us something about what the patient is doing with us or what the patient evokes in us. Therefore, creating a space where something honest can transpire is absolutely essential. Discussion and knowledge should not go outside the room, and it is the Balint group leader's responsibility to ensure and maintain that setting. It is important for continuity that breaks are notified well in advance, and people are expected to give apologies for non-attendance.

Presenting in a Balint group

The presenting doctor is always referred to as 'the doctor', and this is to help people say things they might not want to say in more direct terms, because they often all know each other from being on call and from having other overlaps. The artificial impersonality of using the phrase 'the doctor' helps this illusion of distance.

The doctor presents their case. The other doctors are allowed to have two or three questions of fact. Then the presenting doctor 'pushes back' metaphorically or literally, and the discussion can begin. At the beginning of a Balint group, there is normally a silence, and, over the course of a year, for core trainees, a pattern emerges. The Balint group leader may be more active for the first 2 or 3 months and is then able to withdraw to a less active role, as the trainees become more talkative. The silence

or abstinence of the leader in a young Balint group can be a very difficult experience for some trainees. The totally silent gnomic model of an
analyst manqué does nothing for the reputation of analytic thinking and
experience. When the trainees 'get going', the first problem becomes
stopping them speaking.

Frequently, the doctors in the group are frightened of being in a group
with a psychoanalyst or with someone who is psychoanalytically trained,
as they think they are being analysed. Balint groups are not therapy, and
the personal work of realizing how their anxieties may have something to
do with their personality is best left to them to reflect on privately. Most
good doctors learn that themselves and bring it up in an appropriate way.
The point is to create an atmosphere, so that the next time the doctor
may see the patient, he may be open to something new in observing or
relating to him or her. This then allows the doctor to be clear about his
capacity to formulate and devise a management plan.

As the trainees become attached to the experience, the second problem is in them not wanting to leave the group.

Theory

Balint groups and seminars are guided by simple and elegant concepts. As
Michael Balint observed: '*This (group) is to examine the relationship between
the doctor and the patient to look at the feelings generated in the doctor as
possibly being part of the patient's world and then use this to help the patient.
If these feelings do not seem to belong to the patient but to the doctor it helps
to know that too, to be a participant in a relationship and its observer is fraught
with difficulties and potential bias. The aim is to study this (bias) carefully. As a
consequence, the doctors can take the feelings that arise from their work seriously and pay attention to much that would otherwise be disregarded.*'

A theory is needed to explain how the feelings evoked in a doctor
may be of use in understanding a patient's dilemma as re-enacted in the
relationship, and/or a doctor's propensity to get drawn into certain
types of relationships. Something is being re-enacted with feelings that
the patient may use to create an impact that will alter the content of the
outcome of the consultation. Therefore, a method is needed to reflect
both with a theoretical base that allows the doctor not to blame the
patient and not to feel blamed himself, but to take a scientific stance on
what might be happening.

The Balints (Enid and Michael) were the first to introduce the idea of
the participant observer into the arena of clinical medicine. There are
various psychoanalytic constructs which underline this precept theoretically. '*Whenever doctors use their feeling as a tool, as a personal internal
barometer, they open themselves to the kinds of error to which any instrument
is prone. What troubles the patient may be obscured as the doctor picks up
other sounds, they may arise from inside the doctor patient interaction or they
may be extraneous.*' (Michael Balint).

The doctor–patient relationship

The basis of the Balint group is the *doctor–patient relationship*. When
Michael Balint set up groups in the Tavistock Clinic with GPs, he thought
it might be helpful for doctors to have a space to reflect and think about

their work with patients and the difficulties they got into with them. Over the course of several years, he ran a number of groups. Balint groups became very popular in general practice training but has gradually died out in recent years, although the Balint group has become an established part of psychiatry training in the UK and even more so in Ireland.

When a patient meets a doctor, there is a relationship between them, in which it is not just *what* is said, but *how* things are said and what else is communicated beyond the presenting problem that is important. The doctor metabolizes this data in a complicated conscious and *unconscious* way to lead to a formulation of the person and their illness. The core of what doctors do is to formulate patients and then come to a conclusion on how to manage them. This formulation contains internally complicated dynamics and mechanisms. The Balint group is there to help the doctor to look at how these dynamics work. Some doctors would disagree, seeing themselves and their role as being technical dispensers of rational advice and medication.

Balint and his colleagues looked at the data and began to observe certain facets to the doctor–patient relationship which he described. Balint came at these observations from psychoanalytic theory. This is a body of theory that started with Freud and puts emphasis on unconscious mental processes that are not logical or rational, but that are set up almost instantly between two people. Certain dynamics may be re-enacted that may have nothing to do with the ostensible purpose of a visit and may lead to all sorts of feelings.

Most times, the doctor–patient relationship works relatively well, and we do not have to question it. When it goes wrong, then we do have to sit back and think 'What happened there?' or 'How did I get into that tangle?' or 'Why is it I get into this sort of mess with this sort of patient?'.

Some doctors never reflect on this at all; they just think they are right. An observation of Balint groups is that one does not need to be steeped in psychoanalytic theory to do this, but it is helped by having someone with some experience of listening in a psychoanalytic way to the unconscious undercurrents. This involves creating a space and a setting where doctors can feel free to say what they actually think and most importantly, feel.

Balint terminology

One of the first things Balint talked about was the '*Apostolic function of doctors*'. The religious connotations of Apostles might make some hesitate to think about it or use it. What he is talking about is what he calls a '*fallacy of common sense where a doctor has a set view which is unconscious, unstated and unformulated as to how a patient should be and how a doctor's role should be*'. These assumptions may never be brought into contrast, until you meet a patient who does something with you that causes dissonance in that view of yourself as a doctor or how the patient should be. Balint proposed that it was almost the doctor's *givens* (the bias mentioned earlier) that they bring unconsciously or out of their awareness to every consultation and to their sense of being a doctor. It also has what he called a function of trying to *convert* patients to agree with that function, so our patients learn to either adapt to our way of being or to move on and go to another doctor. This becomes more difficult in psychiatry where patients cannot 'doctor-shop', as they do with GPs. Once a Balint group goes beyond a year, it begins to become central, as the doctor suddenly begins to realize and think that 'There are these patients I struggle with, this is the sort of reaction I have to them, and this leads to this outcome or that outcome'. This frequently has to do with negative feelings, and it is where Balint groups can be really helpful.

This may help to challenge the *tyranny of positivism* which is currently prevalent. If doctors cannot be free to use their negative feelings as communication about the patient's difficulties, then they are going to feel burdened by being bad doctors or become cynical and detached. However, if the feelings they have can be used for reflection as something that is happening as part of the consultation, then it can be very helpful in understanding what the patient might be communicating and doing with the doctor. It helps if the doctor's feelings become data and something of intellectual interest, rather than a burden or failure. It also helps if the doctor is struggling with a particular reaction to a patient to think it is something that gets in the way. In psychiatry, simple diagnoses do not always work. Difficulties are multi-factorial, and an essential task for everyone is understanding how one's personality interacts with an illness. Perhaps now that the power differential has changed in psychiatry, negotiation and compromise in finding ways of dealing with patients has become more and more part of our job.

For example, patients come with some distress which can be correctly labelled as anxiety or depression and treatment prescribed. However, it might also be important to the patient to get a glimpse of what is causing that anxiety or depression. This does not mean that the doctor has to give psychotherapy or counselling, but finds a space in their mind for a formulation that recognizes that the patient is depressed or anxious because they are this sort of person and they are reacting to this sort of life event in this way. That can then help the patient to begin to think about themselves as a particular type of person with a particular way of dealing with things.

Another important phenomenon that Balint identified was what he called '*elimination by appropriate physical investigation*'. This is, when presented with bizarre, obscure, and worrying symptoms, the doctor or psychiatrist's default position is physical investigations.

This leads to another facet where a patient is referred on in the hope of clarifying something, but instead it can lead to something else which Balint termed the '*collusion of anonymity*'. Patients who have either multiple diagnoses or a personality disorder interacting with specified diagnoses may frequently end up seeing many different professionals in different services. Despite all the care programme meetings and the professionals meeting, somehow central decisions are taken, and nobody really has any responsibility or central thinking about the patient—this is what Balint meant by the collusion of anonymity.

The bad doctor–patient relationship
Michael Balint noted that *some patients seemed to be determined to have a bad doctor–patient relationship*. This is the doctor–patient relationship

that most disturbs and is commoner in psychiatry. Where there are elements of a dissatisfied, aggrieved, threatening, confrontational, hateful, or envious doctor–patient relationship, these are hard to bear and metabolize. This happens both by the nature of the illness and by the nature of the person with personality disorder. This may also be linked with the increase in expectations and ideas that people have on how they should be made well, and concomitant change in the context of the doctor–patient relationship. The idea of somebody having to mature into, and deal with, their own difficulties has shifted whereby people now insist on being independent but, at the same time, demand that they are looked after in a particular way. The old standby of reassurance, advice, and guidance does not work the more a personality disorder is involved. A rational logical explanatory model of the doctor–patient relationship works with quite a lot of patients, but it breaks down the more the personality is vulnerable. Frequently, doctors are left feeling helpless, despairing, furious, angry, and resentful of the demands that patients make upon them. It is important that these negative feelings and impressions are recognized, as they may give us a clue about what is going on in the doctor–patient relationship. These belong not just to the doctor, but also to the patient.

This is linked with Balint's idea of the *apostolic function*, which is that every doctor creates the unique atmosphere by way of his/her individual way of practising medicine and tries to convert his/her patients to accept that. This includes an unconscious attitude that a doctor brings to medicine that is the result of their personality interacting with their teaching and their anxiety. A Balint group may help the doctor come to terms with his/her *valency*—a term Balint borrowed from chemistry. It is one's predisposition to react with certain compounds more quickly than with others, and certain patients will spark this off or deaden us. It is important to have a clue about how this comes about in each individual case, because it will influence the formulation and the treatment.

Enid Balint wrote about *surprisability in the doctor–patient relationship*, in that there can be such an accumulation of the doctor thinking 'It is this sort of patient, so I know what will happen' that it shuts the doctor down and stops him being open and wondering. This can be due to something deadening or something too intense in the relationship or consultation. It does not falsify what we know about the patient, but other things might be going on, so how do you keep yourself open to being surprised when you have very busy clinics and are under pressure?

We also use our intuition as a short cut to formulate patients and to manage them, but sometimes it gets in the way. A famous analyst was once supervising an analyst in training who said she intuited a truth about her patient because 'I knew it in my guts.' The famous analyst replied 'That is just indigestion my dear.' There is a place for intuition, but it needs to be linked with what is actually happening, observed, and processed. Otherwise, this may result in something wild which is a parody of a psychoanalytic approach.

The theory of Balint groups and the way they are applied in Balint groups in Britain today is essentially psychoanalytic. It does not have the trappings of theoretical frameworks or controversies that might lead to dissonance, but it does share the commonalities of a psychoanalytic endeavour that all psychoanalysts would agree upon. It is about the operation of the dynamic unconscious and its impact on the doctor–patient relationship, and it attends to the intermingling of the life and death instincts and infantile sexuality.

Cradle to grave Balint groups

(See ➲ Psychotherapeutic medicine: thinking cradle to grave in Chapter 2, pp. 8–12.)

The doctor at different stages of their development may use a Balint group in a way that involves the same emotional tasks in relationship with their patients but experienced at different levels because of context, complexity, and culture, as follows:

• *Nascent: medical students*

The conflict here seems to be with an apostolic function that develops in medical school where a good doctor–patient relationship leads to the patient doing what you want them to do because that is what is best for them. One of the educational Trojan Horses to facilitate this fantasy of a doctor–patient relationship is training in *communication skills* which seem almost magically to open the door to a good doctor–patient relationship. The other medical cultural idea is of *becoming a professional* which means being neutral in terms of feelings and seeing it as a personal failure that a patient has provoked personal feelings in one. In a sense, this means that the nascent doctor is left identifying with a projection, and many may feel guilty and ashamed about unvoiced 'unprofessional' feelings. They then become registered junior doctors.

• *New: foundation and core trainee doctors*

Certain aspects of the doctor–patient relationship appear to have changed and have become more difficult in NHS settings. The fact that one can realize that having feelings about a patient is not unprofessional, but that it is potential data that is in itself useful is something very new for junior doctors. In the foundation and core trainee years, Balint groups, offering a space for feelings, seems to free some of them up. Once they begin to realize that there is something emotional that happens in their relationship with a patient that may help their understanding of the patient, they can relax and begin to explore a less affectively strait-jacketed view of the psychiatric task. The harsh medical student superego means they fear they will be judged and assessed to be failing, and, once the doctor realizes that they are not going to be persecuted (or worse, analysed), the doctors seem to take to the sense that their feelings are legitimized and do not make them unprofessional, illegitimate bad doctors.

• *Nostalgic: advanced trainees and consultants*

One of the striking features of advanced trainee and consultant groups in the UK is the absence of using literature, books, films, or art to metabolize one's experience in psychiatry. In the lack of these cultural references, what may be suppressed, or even killed off, is the capacity to free associate or to use one's unconscious and other aspects of one's life to help one metabolize what patients are presenting. Medicalization, protocols, and policies seem to play a large part in the suppression of this creative freedom to think, free associate, and 'play at work.'

For the higher (advanced) trainee, a leitmotif of the Balint groups is a conflict in the transition to becoming a consultant in bearing feelings of limitation of self, other, and the system, whilst being expected to *know*. In the face of not knowing, the advanced trainee and the consultant bring an unspoken doctor–patient relationship that the Balint group can help them intellectually *formulate* their patients' problems, and, by knowing the *formulation*, they can then manage all the risks and burdens they have to bear. As responsible medical officers, psychiatrists are often in an invidious position of being left with the risk of being told that they will not be blamed for mistakes, but actually knowing they will. Underneath these constraints, in Balint groups for consultants and advanced trainees, there can be a sense of disempowerment and paralysis almost, as if they are under siege from both their patients and their organizational policies, and yet none of them feel able to take a stand. It is clear at times that senior clinicians do not feel it is possible or safe for them to say anything about their experience to the people in charge. They seem both battered by relentless institutional changes and a very real dismissal of their skills, but at the same time feeling they have to go along with it. Despite this disempowering context, senior clinicians and trainees on the threshold of becoming senior clinicians do keep attending and have some very lively discussions about disturbing patients.

It may be part of running a Balint group to try to work through the context and return to what is happening in the doctor–patient relationship, because the leader can be invited in these groups to join in the external pressures and embattled organizational stuff and nonsense. Notwithstanding this, what emerges is a sense of shame in the service the senior clinicians are obliged to offer, as they know it is not enough or it is not what they would do if 'they had their say'. This leads them to blind themselves to the real doctor–patient relationship in front of them, as it will carry obligations, demands, and pleas which frequently go back to more policy/protocol-driven ways of relating. Occasionally, in these Balint groups, there is a nugget that comes out that allows one to get back to the doctor–patient relationship through the clouded strains of the organizational context—through a glass darkly experience, some affective light is glimpsed. Keeping one's eye on the internal world of affective subjectivity is important, if not vital, particularly when external changes are so rampant, unpredictable, and destructive at the present time in the NHS.

These cradle to grave descriptions offering a developmental view of the different uses medical students, foundation trainees, core trainees, advanced trainees, and consultants psychiatrists make of Balint groups are derived from UK experience of medical education and the NHS.

Vignette

This is a Balint group from another European country, composed of a mixture of general physicians, psychiatrists, and psychologists.

One of the general physicians said she would like to present a case if that was okay, rather hesitantly, and the leader said that was fine. She said, 'I would like to talk about a patient of mine who is a 34-year-old man whom I saw last week and whom I have seen three or four times and will continue to see. He followed me from the public hospital to my private clinic. I am not really sure why he comes. We have very pleasant consultations, and we go over the same things a lot, but he seems quite happy and settled with that. Whenever I see him, he comes with his MRI scan, we review his antiepileptic medications, and we get on very well. He has a wife, and she has come in once or twice, and she asks really difficult questions. I get the impression they are a really happy couple and that she is not intruding but is just asking questions that perhaps they have both thought about but that he doesn't ask or isn't as bothered about as she is. In his medical background, he had an aneurysm that was unnoticed, as most of them are, that burst, and he had a brain bleed followed by an epileptic fit. He recovered from this, and we put him on antiepileptic medication, and his fits settled. He has not had any major seizures since, nor any absence seizures.' (She explained what these were to the group.) She continued, 'He has had two procedures to try and tie off, or block, the aneurysm, but they have only been partially successful. This time when he came, his MRI scan showed that it was slightly improved, I thought, but it was a different consultation in that he asked if his wife could come in, and when she did she was very intense. I don't know why she was so disturbed, because they have asked me the same questions before. They wanted to know whether he could drive and that it had been over 18 months since he has had this aneurysm and the treatment, that he had not had a fit and he was doing fine on medication. In the law here, it's one of those grey areas, in that he really shouldn't drive, it's illegal, but people do, and if they do and have an accident, then it is their responsibility. It is quite difficult, but I could see his point because he hasn't had a fit and he is not likely to have a fit.'

The doctor said to the group, 'You may wonder why I am presenting this case. I felt very confused during this consultation, because he and I get on fine, and we have answered these questions before, and I didn't know why she was asking them now. At the same time, I could see how she might want to know because she asked me whether they could have a second child—they have got one child—and she seemed really anxious and worried about it all. We had a good discussion, and they seemed happier, but they wanted me to tell them definitely, and I kept trying to say to them it's a grey area, I can't say. Eventually the woman asked whether it would help if they went to see a neurosurgeon. I let them see a neurosurgeon colleague, but I am not sure whether I should keep following him up, as I don't have the expertise in this. He is doing really well with his medication, and he is not on a drug that is known to cause difficulties with babies' development.' She stopped there.

There was a couple of questions from a psychologist—what is an aneurysm?—which the Balint leader thought was very helpful, and one of the psychologists had not heard the man's age and was struck by how young he was. Then the doctor withdrew by literally pushing her chair back and sitting out until 10 minutes from the end. Part of the culture of this group was that the presenter did not say a lot about what feelings struck them but that this was more for the group to speculate. The group piled in with questions about why the patient kept asking the same question and what was going on for him, wondering about his past and about why the wife came in and asked questions. There was a discussion about how the wife seemed to represent the part that needed to ask the hard questions and what was going on there. Then another physician who was a very straightforward woman said, 'This is a grey area, he can't drive, but it seems that he can't accept that this is a grey area.' They all wondered what the grey area was, and she said it was about driving. The leader came in a couple of times to help them to think about what might be the reason for the wife being anxious and upset. There was an absolute consensus that, at age 34/35, it would be time to have a second child and how hard it must be for the wife to have a husband who is impaired. Then it became clear that she would have to drive him everywhere and what that would mean in terms of work. One female psychologist wondered what that would mean for him in terms of being seen as a man in this country where the man does the driving. They laughed, and the women agreed in some ways, but not in others. The child psychiatrist said that it was around that time when people have to try and think about what they are going to do with their lives. The physician came in again about being asked about whether he could drive and repeated that it was a grey area.

The leader said, 'Well, I thought it was a grey area in more than one sense, the doctor had mentioned that the aneurysm wasn't totally tied off and that might be something in the patient's mind as well as in his brain.'

There was a pause, and the physician said, 'Oh I just thought that everybody knew that the blood vessel could burst at any moment.' The psychologists all looked a bit disturbed and asked, 'So this man is carrying something around in his brain that could at any moment just pop?', and the physician and the child psychiatrist said, 'Well yes of course and that was really straightforward.' The psychologists replied, 'Well it's not, of course, because that's a huge thing that you are saying—he has got an aneurysm, he has got to get used to it—actually what does that mean? At any moment he could be driving along and it could pop and he could die.' Then they began to talk really seriously about what it would be like having this on his mind, and the physician came in again and said, 'What's intriguing is that the doctor and patient, it's all very warm and calm and comfortable, and then the wife has to come in and introduce reality and that she is anxious, but the doctor and the patient are quite happy just talking about the same things and not really thinking about any of this.'

The child psychiatrist went back to this idea of what it would be like for this man's wife to have a husband whom she clearly loved but to whom something could happen, that he had been lucky the last time but asked why he might be lucky. He said that the presenting doctor had mentioned there were no deficits. The psychologists said they thought she had been referring to financial matters or they had not lost anything, and he said, 'No, she meant when she examined him neurologically there was no weakness, there was no loss of sensation, he didn't seem cognitively impaired, he seemed all right, and that's really lucky.' One of the psychologists said, 'Gosh, you'd think if you'd been lucky once, you are not going to be lucky again, and if it happens what would you do? I don't know how you would live with that.' The physician said, 'I just think you have to get on with it', but then she stopped and said, 'Actually when I think about it, I think that's what we do in medicine, we go: you've got this, you need to get on with it. It is a huge thing. I don't know if they have ever grieved for what's happened to them.'

It was time for the presenting doctor to come back in. She talked about how she had been surprised by all the things she had taken for granted and that, hearing the psychologists' and other people's responses, she suddenly thought of the things that she does not really take into account, 'That of course for a man who has got a weakness in a blood vessel that could pop at any moment, I don't know how you could live with that, but you have to. What's the best way to live with it? For them, it was just going along as if nothing was wrong and saying you can get on with it, but actually this question—can you drive?—is where it all comes into focus. Because that's where they have to face that something could still happen and something has happened.' She thought they were so insistent on him being able to drive it was as if they wanted to say, 'Well this is never going to happen again and this is over with now'. She felt she had not been clear enough in saying to them. 'Well it isn't over yet'. She now said that she felt quite sad that the relationship they had was quite comfy and that maybe she should send him to a psychologist. The other group members were all in general agreement with this. The leader said that perhaps the patient *was* doing the work with the doctor and that it seemed that nowadays we want to send people off for emotional treatment when actually there was already a doctor–patient relationship to which the patient was bringing his difficulties. The presenting doctor said that it would be hard for her, as she does not know how to even think or talk about those things, but then revealed that, when she sent the patient to the neurosurgeon, he said, 'I have booked in to see you again in 3 months, and I will come back'. Another group member said she thought he was saying 'This is where I do the work.'

The idea of there being an unspoken concern that the husband would die if they had sex was not addressed. This is a good example of the work of a Balint group, as the next time the doctor sees this patient, this anxiety might be addressed if it struck her from the reflections emerging in the opening up of the discussion which continue to reverberate.

Recommended reading

Balint M (1957). *The Doctor, His Patient and the Illness*. Churchill Livingstone: London.

Balint E (1984). The history of training and research in Balint groups. *Psychoanalytic Psychotherapy*, 1, 1–9.

Balint E, Courtenay M, Elder A, Hull S, and Julian P (1993). *The Doctor, the Patient and the Group: Balint Revisited*. Routledge: London and New York.

Das A, Egleston P, El-Sayeh H, Middlemost M, Pal N, and Williamson L (2003). Trainees' experiences of a Balint group. *Psychiatric Bulletin*, 27, 274–5.

FitzGerald G and Hunter MD (2003). Organizing and evaluating a Balint group for trainees in psychiatry. *Psychiatric Bulletin*, 27, 434–6.

Reflective practice groups

What are reflective practice groups?

Mirror mirror on the ward …

Running reflective practice groups for professionals in mental health settings is like going to look at the reflection of one's mind in a broken mirror, a sometimes fragmented conversation about a patient stirring a dull narcissistic echo in the professional. Because such mirrored experiences are unconscious, it may not be obvious what the emotional echo of the patient in the professional is, but it might be revealed by professional behaviour, including how this is manifest in trying to contain anxiety. For example, in a psychiatric ward, the decision as to how closely observed the patient needs to be may also contain the professional worry about the institutional impact of their death.

… Who is the unfairest of them all?

Patients admitted to psychiatric wards sometimes feel aggrieved, because they are subject to unfair treatment, being detained in the 'brick mother' against their will. The enforced treatment of a patient against their will is an external manifestation of unfairness; conversely, for some patients, not being admitted to the brick mother is a source of grievance, because they are excluded from the resource of concrete containment, feeling abandoned to the responsibility for their mind and problems in the community. The experience of unfairness, whether resenting being admitted or not admitted, frequently echoes a sense of being treated unjustly in earlier life, an unspoken echo of a childhood feeling of resentment and bitterness enacted in the here and now. The echo of this unfairness for the patient lies in professionals feeling they too are treated unjustly by the organization, e.g. in cuts to services, in downgrading posts, generally feeling uncared for, ignored, and hurt in devaluing reorganizations, etc.

Reflective practice as a form of chronic consultation

(See ➲ Consultation in Chapter 4, pp. 145–51.)

Reflective practice might be seen as a long-term or chronic observation in the ward or team, in which a series of consultations about patients whose pain and conflict and the dilemmas they pose to professionals become part of a cumulative history of emotional themes and patterns.

Difference from staff support groups

Unlike a staff support group, in which the conscious primary task is to focus on the relationships between team members, the patients and the professional experience of being with patients is the conscious primary task of a reflective practice group. The patient offers an unconscious Trojan Horse for staff to relate with each other—a 'patient buffer' who cushions the unconscious task of indirectly exploring the impact of their experiences of each other through reflection about a patient.

Difference from individual or group therapy

Unlike group analysis or therapy, interpretation of individual or team behaviour or the matrix of the group is not the aim; a different language from being with patients in therapy has to be found. The main aim is to allow the team members a safe enough space to say honestly what they feel about the patient, the work, and each other.

Difference from consultation
(See ➲ Consultation in Chapter 4, pp. 145–51.)

Unlike consultation with particular colleagues about particular patients, open-ended reflective practice work is about consulting with some members of the team who turn up on the day wanting to discuss some patients, but on a more long term-basis and more randomly and partially than in the acute focused, and often intense, encompassing consultation. This gives reflective practice a potential lightness of touch which is not easy to find in consultation but prepares the ground in the culture of the organization for receptivity to, and meaningful use of, consultation.

Running a reflective practice group
(See ➲ Psychotherapeutic understanding of organizational processes in Chapter 10, pp. 471–5; Psychotherapy and management in Chapter 10, pp. 475–9.)

Running reflective practice groups needs preparation, for you, the team, and the environment, all of which can take longer than you expect. Meeting the team and their manager, attending a couple of the team meetings gives you a sense of some of the problems and challenges they face in their daily work, as well as insight into the overall culture, team dynamics, and whether they support the idea of reflective practice.

Issues to agree upon include:
• What will be the day, time, duration, frequency, and venue of the reflective practice group?
• Will the group have an overall time limit or be open-ended?
• Will the reflective practice group be closed or open?
• Can people come in late or leave early?
• Are groups totally confidential to whoever attends each week, or shared with others?
• Are any records or notes kept?

Aims of reflective practice
The aim of reflective practice is to try to evoke an ordinary resonance or echo in the experience of professionals about the kinds of problems the patient is struggling with, without it becoming personal therapy. The idea is to foster empathy and shared humanity, but also to try to allow a more discomforting identification to allow more difficult feelings to emerge. This takes time and varies, depending on the disturbance in the patient, the experience of the staff, their status in the hierarchy, their degree of comfort with one another, and who is present in the room.

The primary task of the reflective practice group
The primary task of the reflective practice group is to think about the work with patients. The relationship with the patient has to lie at the heart of the reflective practice group and the distraction of institutional criticism respected but considered in the context of the work with patients.

Reflective practice groups where the primary task migrates

A reflective practice group can easily draw together around an embattled view of the institution, locating conflicts and paranoid tension beyond the team, especially as there are often many actual hooks in the running of the organization on which to hang grievances. However, a reflective practice group which settles comfortably into a spirit of furious impotence about the latest inept or careless changes management has inflicted on them will have a short shelf life in the institution.

Internal versus external reflective practice group leadership

The internal leader (an insider who works in the same organization as the reflective practice group) is more challenged by managerial migration than the external leader (an outsider who is not part of the organization) who can, to a degree, offer the 'Emperor seems to be naked' type observation, as they have the benefit of separateness. Conversely, the internal leader can identify more closely with the problems faced in the organization and is intimate with the culture. When the group has stopped reflecting on patients and migrates to critique the latest managerial ignominy, the aim is to draw the group's attention to wondering how this particular experience, e.g. of perceived neglect or cruelty, might relate to what is happening or not happening with the patients.

The big finger of guilt, the blame game, and shame

Clinicians can at times feel they are treated in an unfair way by managers, especially after a serious incident, citing a 'blame culture'. The big finger of guilt and blame often reveals a downward percolation of shame from unfair and mortifying exposure passed as if through a shame infusion from the senior management into the veins of clinicians—no one wanting to be exposed and found wanting. The unfairness in the lives of so many patients seems to find an echo in the professionals, the blind eye turned to the patient, as professionals fret about being exposed as negligent, becoming a poignant repetition of neglect; an ironic echo of the blind eye turned to the patients in their childhoods, a past quotidian obliviousness in parent figures finding a present partner in oblivion in the worried preoccupied professional.

Membership dynamics

When more senior staff are present in the group (managers or consultants), there is a tendency for those more junior to remain quiet and observe and to say more when senior staff are absent. This is particularly so for medical staff, and for nurses who are not managers who will say more about their feelings in the absence of doctors, including differences between the ways the doctors think about their patients. Managers are rarely seen as 'the fairest of them all', and it is very hard not to be drawn into discussion about management failures or incompetence or the experience of unfair treatment of staff. However, non attendance of team managers and senior doctors undermines the work of the reflective practice group as a devalued entity not integrated in the leadership dynamics of the team.

Through a glass darkly

Be prepared to hear, and to have to respond to, the dark side of providing acute and community psychiatric care. Reflective practice group leaders need personal robustness and the ability to stay grounded in their own reality. Additionally, emotional regulation skills to manage in the moment the anxiety, a sense of outrage, or not knowing what to say or do, that running a reflective practice group can evoke in the leader, are also required. Certain aspects of working on a psychiatric ward are very stressful and disturbing, with no easy option or solutions.

Examples of what you might hear include:

- Being responsible for the ward as the only permanent member of staff on duty working with bank staff
- Rarely having a meal break because mutual protection becomes more important than taking a break
- The pervasive fear of a patient committing suicide or attacking someone and the parallel fear of being blamed by the organization if this happens
- The perception that 'out there' does not care about, or value, the team
- Racial harassment, sexual harassment, deeply hurtful personal insults about personal appearance, or patient-perceived character flaws
- Threats and intimidation, threats of assault when leaving work at night, threats against children or other family
- A constant 'background noise' of verbal abuse, hostility, demand, and non-cooperation from a minority of patients
- Witnessing or receiving physical aggression and assault, often serious enough to warrant hospital treatment
- Aggrieved feelings that managers do not take violence and harm to staff seriously enough
- Feeling powerless, but also compelled to step in and do something, when a very violent patient needs restraining.

Reflective practice group supervision

All of these issues can evoke powerful feelings in reflective practice group leaders, especially if they are part of the same organization and share some of the same fears that the staff hold. Reflective practice group leaders need to find a way to handle the feelings stirred up in them, and seeking supervision with colleagues running groups is helpful. The use of supervision lies in trying to process the feelings of the group leader in receiving the projections of the professionals.

Vignette A: reflective practice group in an inpatient psychiatric ward

This once-weekly reflective practice group on a female psychiatric ward had been running for 9 years. The foundation year doctor on the ward began to discuss a woman in her forties who, she said, had created a dispute in the team about whether or not to treat her. The doctor said it felt as if they had to *endure* treating her and indicated a worry about harming her, making her worse. The patient dressed in an animal costume, known as a 'onesy', with replaceable animal tails to signify different animals she wanted to represent—tigers, leopards, etc.

The onesy was like the 'all-in-one' suit of a baby. Despite the onesy, this patient, however, seemed far from integration or being 'all in one'. The woman felt the staff were treating her like an animal in treating her against her will on a section and so dressed like one. She was said to have delusions of abuse, that she had been forced to take harmful drugs, such as cocaine, and on two separate occasions abducted and forced into being a prostitute in mainland Europe.

The doctor presenting thought there was a dispute in the team about treating her, and another doctor said that it was not a question of a dispute about diagnosis, more a doubt and concern about causing her to be damaged by treatment, to be made worse. Along with concern about iatrogenic harm, the nurses voiced a profound sadness, feeling despondent and empty when with the patient.

The team manager felt the staff experienced their treating the patient with a depot against her will as abuse. The woman was described as being held down to receive the injection and going floppy, not being angry or resistant; they simply had to support her, whilst they injected her. After the injection where they had cut her 'onesy' to give the depot, she walked around with the opening showing, as if displaying the stigma of where she had been violated. The nurses felt a keen sense of guilt. There was a debate, as had happened before, about letting her go untreated; this dilemma—to leave her deluded or to 'cure' her, yet damage her—seemed a manifestation of an unfair, or even cruel, treatment.

The consultant psychiatrist said in a way that was uncharacteristic of him, that she has a schizophrenic illness, and, if they left her untreated, there was a serious risk she would kill herself. This unambiguous statement met with an immediate response from the team manager of 'Well, that's cheered everybody up!' She patted his arm. He smiled, looking uncomfortable. There was a tension between them, and in what was witnessed at that moment the eye of the dispute was in sight.

Causing harm to the patient and a split being along medical and nursing lines emerged in the discussion, including the sense of stewing in their guilt, leaving the nurses feeling powerless. The patient had taken a large paracetamol overdose on the first day of her depot and had let the staff know she had done so, and so could be treated medically for the overdose. This communication of her distress, her increasing despondency, and the atmosphere of despair led the team to want to take her off her section and discharge her from the ward. The consultant psychiatrist, the resident medical office (RMO), however, was clear in asserting the need to treat her, but the nurses seemed to resent having to do his dirty disturbing work.

At this point, a therapist who specialized in dissociation arrived on the ward to see the consultant and team manager, and they were called out of the reflective practice group, full of apology saying that another patient who was seeing the dissociative identity disorder (DID) therapist on the ward had left the ward and was now in the West Indies, no longer their responsibility, and they could not keep the dissociation specialist waiting. It felt to the reflective practice group leader that the parental couple had left the team to this guilty, conflicted, and dirty discussion, dissociating from it.

After the consultant and team manager left the group, the theme of guilt about harming the patient was explored with an emerging idea that what the foundation doctor had described as *enduring* treating her was right, that rather like a parent establishing an attitude of 'being cruel to be kind,' there was a painful doubt about treating the patient in a state of painful uncertainty about whether this would help or harm her. In the absence of the team manager, who had asked the team to let her know what the outcome of the discussion was, there was a sense of futility and confusion, not knowing what to do. The nurses and junior doctors left behind seemed abandoned, left at sea and facing an emotional tsunami.

The reflective practice group leader explored the feelings of guilt and the patient not having contact with her children whom she had become estranged from, and her own early life history of her parents separating when she was small. One of the nurses said that the patient may have been exposed to a couple fighting before they separated when she was 2 years old. One of the doctors seemed to ignore this painful picture of infancy and, with potency, asserted the robust ontology of psychiatry, saying 'On paper this woman is ill and she needs to be treated; this is what psychiatrists do, we have to treat people against their will.'

But what was unspoken, and then named by the reflective practice group leader, was that this is a flesh-and-blood live problem of facing doubt and guilt about causing harm; it is painfully *not* a paper exercise.

Reflective practice reflections
The reflective practice group leader raised a question about what the group would feed back to the team manager, and, when he asked, the team said they did not know; they were still left uncertain, confused about whether or not to treat the patient. The group leader said it seemed the RMO, the consultant psychiatrist, was asking for support to treat this patient, but rather like a father saying to a mother, *you* leave our baby to cry, *you* do the hard emotional work, the nurses feeling left to hold this baby burden. The sense of disavowal was being enacted in the parental couple leaving the group to go to the dissociative therapist, whom the reflective practice group leader thought of as a therapist who helps people to dissociate. The dissociation of responsibility from painful feelings of guilt and loss was projected into the nurses. The patient was splitting off her feelings of guilt and projecting mental pain, doubt, and guilt about harm done into the professionals, leading to splitting within them and between them.

The reflective practice group leader was reminded of the reflections of Hannah Segal and John Steiner, psychoanalysts who had seen patients with psychotic illnesses in analysis and who described the painful feelings of sadness in the countertransference of the professional who has to bear split-off feelings of loss and guilt on behalf of the patient. Freud saw psychosis as an inadequate attempt to repair a breach in a damaged ego, and what was evident in this team was that they felt not only that their repair of this patient's damaged ego was not enough, but it was adding to her damage. They had aligned their view with hers, that they were abusers, not healers, causing a profound sense of painful dissonance with grave doubts about their identity and primary task.

Vignette B: reflective practice group in a crisis team

This once-weekly reflective practice group in a crisis team had been running for 7 years at the time of this vignette. As the group was forming, with people arriving, the reflective practice group leader noticed some positive feedback written on the team whiteboard about a senior male worker present. The man, a nurse, laughed and said he tended to mainly receive negative feedback, as he was often called in to see patients for whom it was important to tell them the truth, which they may not like and would sometimes lead to complaints about him.

When asked if anyone had a case, another senior female team member, an occupational therapist (OT), said she had done an assessment a few weeks ago of a woman from whom the colleague who had just spoken had received a complaint, which troubled her. The patient was a woman whom she thought was not mentally ill but was struggling with rumination and guilt about an affair which she had not disclosed to her husband. Her adolescent daughter was not her husband's, and he did not know. The daughter wanted her mother to be admitted to hospital, but the worker thought there was no need for admission.

The theme she wanted to explore was the problem of holding a line not to admit, which is then undermined by colleagues who take a line of less resistance, an approach of taking less therapeutic risk and admit. The senior male colleague had supported the view not to admit when he saw the patient the day after the OT, but the patient had afterwards drunk, had crashed her car, and was admitted to the psychiatric ward, albeit on seemingly spurious diagnostic grounds. The patient and her daughter had made a complaint that she had not been admitted earlier. The clinical team manager had suggested the nurse complained about would not be supported by senior managers in not having admitted her, and she wondered about removing him from seeing patients to a purely middle managerial role. The presenting OT felt vexed and upset by the fact that her colleague was subject to this unfair complaint. The OT added that she felt stressed, and she had really needed her yoga at the weekend to try to clear her mind of all this horrible stuff.

Another patient was then discussed under the umbrella theme of trying to hold a line not to admit and this being undermined by colleagues, which was seen as a cynical covering one's back, as opposed to having integrity and taking therapeutic risks. Another team member then discussed a man who had been in the army and had a forensic history of violence; he was an alcoholic released from prison and accepted through baptism into the local church. The priest felt threatened by the man when drunk, but the patient forgot his threats of violence towards the priest the following day. The presenter was critical, concerned that the priest and the church absorbed the man's problems and absolved him of taking any responsibility for himself. He went on to describe a very difficult 'overwhelming' assessment in which it was very hard to know what to believe about the man's history of heroism and conflict in the army; but, in the confusing maelstrom of trauma, one selected fact stood out, the sense of betrayal the man had felt by his parents in allowing his uncle into his bed to sexually abuse him at the age of 6.

This feeling of betrayal seemed to act as an orientating emotion for the reflective practice group discussion. The presenter described an episode of violence in which the man had felt put down by a man in a shop and he had 'decked' him, knocking him unconscious and pulling him out of the shop by his feet. When the presenting nurse who described this

overwhelming, violent assault of an assessment was asked if he felt vulnerable by the group leader, he laughed and said he did not do yoga and
was playfully dismissive of the notion he might feel disturbed—'You've
just got to move on,' he said, looking flushed and exposed. Another
member of the team then diffused the sense of shame in stress and said
she managed stress with horse riding and drinking.

The reflective practice group leader said he hoped not at the same
time. He went on to say that the idea of a reckless fall or a dangerous
out-of-control animal instinct was in the room.

The nurse who was being complained about said he wondered
whether he might have tried to challenge the violent man with the truth
of what he was doing, that is not absorb his problem like the priest or
church forgiving him, colluding with him, reinforcing 'anti-responsibility.'

The reflective practice group leader thought the staff felt that the
Trust in which they were working might be experienced like the church
in absolving patients of guilt and locating the blame for the problem in the
professional. However, there was a potential masochism in challenging
someone like this man, in drawing the fire of hatred and humiliation in
asserting a demand for conscious cognizance of the damage he did which
he evidently needed to split off, forgetting his responsibility and guilt, and
using drink to disavow his violence.

The reflective practice group leader felt assailed by fragmented images
of patients and workers feeling helpless. The disturbing image of violence in which a man was knocked unconscious and pulled by his feet
from a shop pressed itself forward as a selected fact, as a potential link
with betrayal in the painful associations to staff feeling exposed to abuse
and filled with doubt, trying to do the right thing but feeling attacked
for doing so. The unfairness of all this seemed to link with the issue of
the senior nurse who had been warned that he may be knocked out of
the team, removed with his feet pulled from under him like the victim
of violence. The reflective practice group leader wondered about him
being presented by the OT colleague as an innocent victim of an unjust
organizational assault, pulled out of the door of the crisis team by his feet
unconsciously.

The theme of the organization not 'having your back', as is said in the
army, was discussed—not supporting the clinician in trying to do more
meaningful work in holding therapeutic risk with integrity and not colluding with inappropriate admission. The painful experience of unfairness
and betrayal lies in finding they collide with an organization which seems
to collude with the patient against them and more cynical colleagues who
know this and protect their own backs in 'boundary skirmishes' by passing the buck from service silo to service silo, maintaining disintegration at
all costs, because facing integration and the painful realities of limitation
and responsibility are too costly.

Reflective practice reflections

The demand to be admitted as a concretization of the evacuation of guilt
was a theme; taking responsibility is not supported in the culture, and
the clinician is left wondering about the dilemma about losing integrity
and becoming cynical, simply admitting without thought; or holding a

thoughtful therapeutic line and feeling isolated and not supported by their parent figures in the organization, their leaders colluding with evasion of responsibility by the patient while they shouldered the responsibility. It seemed they felt that their feet had been pulled out from under them by a managerial assault on the terra firma of clinical truth.

Recommended reading

Kets de Vries MFR (2003). *Leaders, Fools and Impostors: Essays on the Psychology of Leadership.* iUniverse, Inc.: New York, Lincoln, and Shanghai.

Lemma A and Patrick M (2010). *Off the Couch: Contemporary Psychoanalytic Approaches.* Routledge: London and New York.

Main T (1989). *The Ailment and Other Psychoanalytic Essays.* Free Association Books: London.

Racker H. (1968). *Transference and Countertransference.* Maresfield Library: London.

Searles HF (1999). *Countertransference and Related Subjects: Selected papers.* International Universities Press Inc.: Madison.

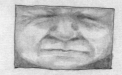

JAMES JOHNSTON 2014

Chapter 11

Psychotherapy research

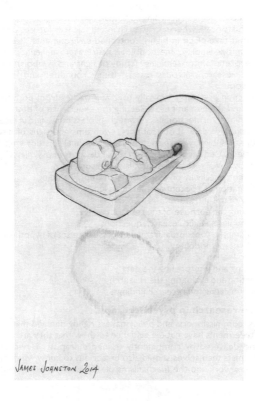

James Johnston 2014

Research in psychotherapy

What is research?

Research is a systematic process of inquiry leading to new knowledge or new ways of thinking about a concept. It usually involves the collection and analysis of information or data to establish, confirm, or refute hypotheses, as well as to support known theories and to generate new theories.

Approaches to research vary according to *epistemology*, or theory of knowledge, usually split between the sciences and the humanities. *Scientific* research tests theories that generate explanations of the nature and properties of the world. Scientific research is broadly *empirical* in the sense of measuring and gathering data that are observed by the researcher. In contrast, research in the *humanities* is more conceptual in nature and is based on detailed exploration of argument, counter-argument, and the analysis of the strengths and weaknesses of argument. Research in the humanities tends to focus on issues and questions that change according to human context (e.g. social, political, cultural, historical), whereas research in the sciences focuses on experiments that take place in highly controlled environments. Research in the humanities employs methodologies such as *hermeneutics* (study of text interpretation) or *semiology* (study of signs and symbols), whereas scientific research favours categorizing, counting, and statistical comparisons.

Research in psychiatry typically uses approaches from both the biosciences and the humanities, reflecting the experience of both patients and psychiatric professionals. Although professionals find it useful to gather objective data about patients' symptoms and signs of disorder, the patients' subjective experience is also essential to study empirically. Humanities-based research is also crucial because of psychiatry's theoretical cross-over with philosophy, law, and sociology.

Research typically involves a number of steps, including:
- Identification of a potential research issue
- Review of the literature
- Specifying the purpose of the research
- Determining specific research questions
- Specifying the conceptual framework, usually a set of hypotheses
- Choice of methodology
- Data collection
- Analyzing and interpreting the data
- Reporting and evaluating the research
- Communicating the research findings.

Why do research in psychotherapy?

Patients, commissioners, and policymakers rightly demand that psychological treatments have robust evidence to show that they are effective, safe, and delivered by competently trained therapists. However, psychotherapists themselves should also be curious to know whether their treatments work and the mechanisms of how change occurs. Although a therapist's individual experience may convince them of the validity and efficacy of their treatment method, their views may be biased by the support of like-minded colleagues, a limited sample of patients seen and clinical problems posed, and the particular modality or setting in which they work. Research provides a necessary external, more objective perspective; an opportunity to validate or disprove hypotheses; and a reflective space in which new ideas may be generated.

Research in psychotherapy is essential to address the following questions:

- Does change occur in therapy? Is it 'therapeutic' change? Does it bring about a good outcome for the patient?
- What happens in therapy? How does the process of change occur?
- Are the psychological therapies offered safe and of high quality? How will we assess quality?
- What is the patient's experience of therapy?
- Are the psychological therapies that are offered cost-effective?
- Are our therapies outmoded or based on unproven theories and practices?
- Can we use research to communicate better with colleagues, commissioners, and patients?
- Can we refine existing therapies and develop new therapies for specific patient groups and settings?
- How can we improve and protect the professional reputation of psychotherapists?

Research in psychotherapy: a historical overview

The history of research into psychological therapies can be divided into the following phases (see Orlinsky and Russell, 1994):

- **Phase I (c.1927–54): establishing a role for scientific research**

The earliest research focused on trying out modifications to the psychoanalytic method, and theoretical discussions of Freud's concepts. The earliest research on psychoanalytic methods were published as early as 1924. The single-subject case study was the main research method at this time used to document and communicate evolving theory; however, psychoanalysts in the 1930s, such as Otto Fenichel in Berlin, Ernest Jones in London, and Franz Alexander in Chicago, also published larger-scale outcome reports of patients being treated in their local institutes.

An important technical development was the application of psychoanalysis to groups during the Second World War. The first experiments in group analysis were carried out by Wilfrid Bion, Harold Bridger, and Tom Main in the context of their work as military psychiatrists. Later in the same period, Maxwell Jones introduced the concept of social therapy for soldiers with war neuroses, and SH Foulkes developed group analysis as a method in the late 1950s. Research methods remained confined to before-and-after assessments of patients, often with crude measures of outcome (see ➔ Group therapy and group analysis in Chapter 2, pp. 42–7; Therapeutic communities in Chapter 2, pp. 75–80).

Other challenges to Freudian psychoanalysis came from Carl Rogers' client-centred therapy (1942), which proposed that the change process came from the patient's potential for self-healing within a positive therapeutic relationship characterized by warmth and empathy, rather than from the therapist's theoretically based interpretations. This was followed by the growth of learning-based approaches which focused on behavioural change, a more active stance of the therapist than that of the traditional psychoanalyst, and briefer treatments lasting weeks or months, rather than years. From the outset, both the Rogerian and learning-based approaches were actively interested in evaluating their therapies—Rogers' research groups audio-recorded therapy sessions, and learning-based therapists tried to link outcomes to therapist interventions. Such methodology was, for the most part, disapproved of by the psychoanalytic community, due to their belief that it interfered in the treatment process by disrupting the therapeutic relationship and transference.

- **Phase II (c.1955–69): searching for scientific rigour**

In 1952, the British psychologist Hans Eysenck reviewed 24 studies of psychoanalysis. He found that patients in these studies improved no more than untreated controls, and famously declared that psychoanalysis was less effective than no treatment. This provocative claim spurred a dramatic increase in the quantity and quality of scientific research in psychotherapy over the next two decades, including more studies comparing treated patients to control subjects and techniques to reduce bias such as randomization and blinding of outcome measurements.

- **Phase III (c.1970–83): expansion, differentiation, and organization**

This period was marked by the development of more formal and systemic research endeavours, including the establishment of scientific organizations devoted to psychotherapy research and increased sophistication in conceptualization and methodology. By 1980, Eysenck's conclusion that psychological therapies were ineffective had been refuted by many well-controlled studies and meta-analyses, which showed the effectiveness of such therapy, compared to untreated controls. Many of these studies were in cognitive therapy, advocated by Ellis and Beck, which emerged in the 1970s, partly from the disillusionment with psychoanalytic treatments, but also due to concerns that learning-based therapies focused too much on behaviours, rather than cognitions (see ➔ Cognitive behavioural therapy in Chapter 2, pp. 30–4).

- **Phase IV (1984–94): consolidation, dissatisfaction, and reformulation**

Although empirical research methods in psychotherapy continued to advance, doubts began to emerge regarding their relevance to the study of human psychology. The field became split between those advocating empirically based objective or quantitative methods drawn from medicine, psychology, and other scientific disciplines and those advocating more subjective or qualitative methods of inquiry. Other discourses, such as the sociological, hermeneutic, and relational, became popular and were offered as more suitable alternatives to the scientific paradigm in exploring subjectivity and meaning. The rapid proliferation of the many different modalities of therapy led to competition and fragmentation of the field, and a preoccupation in demonstrating which specific modalities were superior in efficacy to other less 'evidence-based' therapies (see ➔ Medical psychotherapy modalities in Chapter 2, pp. 17–8).

- **Phase V: contemporary psychotherapy research—from evidence-based practice to practice-based evidence**

Within most of the UK, NICE makes recommendations for evidence-based practice in health care by reviewing research into treatments for specific disorders and publishing recommendations in the form of clinical guidelines to determine the types of treatment available in the NHS (Scotland has a similar body, the Scottish Intercollegiate Guidelines Network or SIGN). Commissioners are increasingly requesting that the health services that they fund, including psychological therapy services, adhere to NICE guidelines.

No practising psychotherapist can therefore escape the imperative to ensure that the treatments they deliver have a sound evidence base which demonstrates their efficacy, safety, and cost-effectiveness. Psychotherapists who avoid engagement in the evidence base discourse risk specific therapies and services being decommissioned, leading to a decrease in patients' choices of the range of therapies, especially in the public sector, and the risks of a one-size-fits-all approach. Some psychological therapists have questioned NICE's 'top–down' approach in which therapeutic practice is expected to change according to the evidence produced from meta-analysis of RCTs, rather than patient-based data. They complain that evidence based on quantitative studies and statistical analyses seems disconnected from individual therapy encounters concerned with the subjective, experiential, and relational.

Although NICE guidelines are meant to enhance, not replace, clinical judgement, its approach has been controversial. In its choice of the type of evidence reviewed for any particular treatment, NICE prioritizes evidence from RCTs, which is the standard means of looking at treatments in other branches of medicine. However, in mental health, there are many therapies and therapeutic techniques that are established and accepted in clinical practice but have not been subject to RCTs. Furthermore, it is hard to see how many psychological therapies that rely on patient engagement and commitment could be assessed using randomization methods that undermine autonomy and choice. Barkham has suggested that the historical discourse in psychotherapy has progressively shifted from (a) *justification* (is psychotherapy effective?) to (b) *specificity* (which psychotherapies are effective?), then to (c) *efficacy and cost-effectiveness* (can therapies be made more effective within limited resources?), and on to (d) a current focus on *effectiveness and clinical significance*. Many therapy practitioners today challenge the claim that the RCT is the optimal source of evidence to address clinical significance. Instead they promote *practice-based evidence* in which evidence is created from within the therapeutic setting, rather than outside of it.

Practice-based research is more pragmatic and enables therapists to adopt a research-oriented approach within their naturalistic environment, leading to a sense of ownership of outcomes that seem more meaningful to their work. In practice-based research, using patient-based data routinely will not only improve the quality of local day-to day psychotherapy practice, but will filter upwards to enhance the scientific evidence for the effectiveness of that therapy.

An active current example of practice-based evidence is the routine administration of outcome measures in psychotherapy services. These may be clinician-rated outcome measures (CROMs) or patient-rated outcome measures (PROMs), which are administered either pre- and post-intervention or on a session-by-session basis to provide real-time feedback on patient progress. Most commissioners now expect routine outcome monitoring with performance feedback to be embedded within service delivery to enhance the quality of the service and patient care. Practice-based networks in which practitioner–researchers pool data from disparate settings have developed to produce large data sets that may make significant contributions to the evidence base. *Benchmarking* allows similar services to compare outcomes with each other. One measure, the Clinical Outcomes in Routine Evaluation (CORE), developed by a multidisciplinary group of practitioners and researchers, has been prominent in offering a cost-free practical system of psychotherapy service quality evaluation and support for service quality development (see ➲ Assessing the outcome of therapy in Chapter 4, pp. 142–5).

Research methodology

A basic knowledge of research terminology and methodological approaches is needed to negotiate the psychotherapy research literature, and to understand and communicate the main findings of research in psychotherapy.

- *Efficacy* measures how well an intervention or treatment works in clinical trials designed to show internal validity, so that causal inferences may be made.
- *Clinical effectiveness* is the extent to which an intervention or treatment improves the outcome for patients in everyday clinical practice. There is often a gap between efficacy and effectiveness.
- *Effect size* refers to the difference between treatment and control groups, expressed in standard deviation units. An effect size of 1.0 indicates that the average patient receiving the treatment under consideration is one standard deviation healthier on the normal distribution than the average patient receiving no treatment. An effect size of 0.8 is considered a large effect; 0.5 is considered moderate, and 0.2 is small.
- *Meta-analysis* is a widely accepted method used in medicine and psychology to strengthen the evidence about treatment efficacy. It refers to the statistical analysis of a collection of results for the purpose of summarizing and integrating the findings of independent studies of a specific treatment that, in themselves, are too small or limited in scope, to come to a conclusion about treatment efficacy.

Quantitative research

Quantitative research is the systematic measurement of observable phenomena via statistical, mathematical, or numerical data or computational techniques. These phenomena are typically manipulated or observed under different types of controlled environmental conditions, and comparisons made between different data sets. This is the main approach to research used in the biomedical sciences.

It begins with a hypothesis which generates data through measurement, which, following analysis, allows a conclusion to be drawn by deduction. Quantitative studies typically involve the collection of many forms of data from large numbers of experimental subjects. Data are analysed using statistical manipulations that describe trends, compare groups, and relate variables, as well as compare results with past research.

Qualitative research

Qualitative research also develops hypotheses and utilizes an empirical approach to data. However, in qualitative research, it is assumed that the data to be gathered are context-dependent and subject to different levels of interpretation, depending on perspective. The numbers of research participants is smaller, and the subjective nature of the data is not controlled experimentally. It is assumed that there is not an infinite number of potential measurements, but that an in-depth investigation of a small number of human responses can yield a wide range of data, which will be generalizable to other similar contexts. Typically, different kinds of data are collected from different sources.

Qualitative research is most often used to gather an in-depth understanding of human behaviour and the reasons that govern such behaviour. It focuses on subjective experiences, collecting data from people in their natural environments, and investigates how social, cultural, and other factors influence experience and behaviour. Data collection may involve interviews (structured, semi-structured, guided, or unstructured), focus groups, telephone interviews, and observation (direct observation by researcher; indirect, e.g. via video-recording of sessions). In qualitative research, samples tend to be smaller and more focused than in quantitative research, and results are typically reported in words, rather than in numbers. Conclusions are drawn from induction.

Qualitative methodologies

- *Grounded theory*: a research method used most commonly in the social sciences employing a 'bottom–up' or inductive approach in which theory is developed from data, moving from the specific to the more general. As data are progressively collected and reviewed, repeated ideas are tagged as *codes*, which may then be grouped into *concepts*, and finally into *categories*, which may become the basis for new theory.
- *Thematic analysis*: focuses on identifiable themes and patterns of lived experience or behavior, e.g. identifying patterns of experience from transcribed conversations in a therapy session.
- *Content analysis*: word frequency count in transcribed conversations/ therapy sessions, assuming that the words most mentioned reflect the greatest concerns.
- *Discourse analysis*: analysis of the underlying social structure contained in conversations.

Quantitative and qualitative research are not mutually exclusive but should be viewed as complementary. *Mixed methods research* employs both quantitative and qualitative methods and aims to investigate the phenomena in more depth. *Triangulation* involves the application and combination of several different methodologies in the study of the same data source or sample, so that the area under investigation is looked at from different perspectives, and intrinsic bias is reduced.

Outcome versus process research

Research in psychotherapy is traditionally divided into outcome research and process research:

- *Outcome research* looks at the results of psychotherapy, how much a particular therapeutic intervention has helped or benefitted the patient, i.e. is it effective? The term 'outcome' refers to all aspects of change that patients can make in psychotherapy. Outcomes chosen to measure will depend on the perspective of the person assessing change (e.g. patient, therapist, commissioner), as well as the goals of treatment and treatment model. Outcome research, also described as 'efficacy' or 'evaluation' research, usually involves quantitative methods (see ➲ Assessing the outcome of therapy in Chapter 4, pp. 142–5).

- *Process research* looks at what goes on within the psychotherapy process, i.e. how does it work? Process research may involve quantitative methods, such as questionnaires or rating scales completed at the end of sessions by patients or therapists, or using external researchers to independently rate processes occurring in transcripts or video-recordings of therapy sessions, or may involve qualitative methods such as grounded theory analysis of the patterns of discourse in the transcripts of therapy sessions or interviews with patients and therapists.

- *Process–outcome research* looks at the relationship between process and outcome in attempting to identify the specific ingredients or technique of therapy (process) responsible for therapeutic change (outcome) using a correlational approach. Such studies tend to assume a 'drug metaphor' logic, in that effective treatments should contain large amounts of the therapeutic ingredient (strength); be delivered in a pure manner (integrity); and that causality is linear and runs in one direction from process variable to influence outcome. Psychotherapy, however, involves complex interpersonal interactions which may not be a linear process but involves bidirectional, reciprocal, relational influences, as both the patient and therapist respond to each other in complex ways.

Psychotherapy study designs

The investigation of clinical problems in psychotherapy may draw on a range of different methodologies and study designs, depending on the stage of investigation of a therapy or the specific research question of interest. The types of study design are ranked below, from strongest to weakest, according to the *hierarchy of evidence* reflecting their relative validity or the strength of their findings in the evaluation of the effectiveness of clinical interventions.

- *A randomized controlled trial (RCT)* is a trial comparing two or more groups constituting different treatment conditions to which patients or participants have been randomly assigned, as a means of minimizing bias. Any differences in outcome (the dependent variable) that emerge between the treatment groups may be attributed to the effects of therapy (the independent variable), as all other factors should have remained constant or 'controlled' via the randomization process, given a large enough sample size and power calculation. The RCT is widely held to be the 'gold standard' of study designs used in empirical research, as it is the most reliable method of demonstrating causality.

However, the RCT may be more suited to drug trials than studies of psychotherapy, in which the administration of the therapy under investigation may vary widely in practice according to the experience and characteristics of the therapist. For this reason, methods to standardize psychotherapeutic treatments are employed, such as treatment manuals and assessing therapist competence and adherence to the specific therapeutic model of interest. RCTs have high internal validity and are the most reliable method of determining the *efficacy* of a therapy. However, this is often at the price of sacrificing external validity, in that the narrowly defined participant entry criteria and tightly controlled trial conditions may not reflect everyday clinical practice where clinical populations and therapeutic interventions are less clearly defined and categorized.

- *Dismantling studies* form part of process–outcome research and attempt to identify the specific components of therapeutic change in a treatment package. Two or more therapies that are identical, except for the inclusion of one or a few specific techniques, are compared, e.g. a group of patients with BPD receiving psychodynamic therapy with a high frequency of transference interpretations per session is compared to a group of similar patients receiving psychodynamic therapy with a lower frequency of transference interpretations.

- *Quasi-experimental* designed studies are studies comparing similar groups of patients in which there was no random assignment, but who were assigned to different treatments on some other basis than randomization. For example, patients suffering from a similar condition, such as depression, may be allocated to different treatments available at different sites. These studies may be more feasible to conduct in practice than RCTs but will always contain variables which will not be controlled for, and therefore confounded with the variable of interest, so that causality cannot be assumed.

- *Naturalistic, observational, or practice-based studies* provide a means of gathering information on outcomes of therapy that is more faithful to everyday conditions. They focus on real clinical settings and tend to examine uncontrolled groups or cohorts of patients, who are not usually preselected and who are given treatments which are not manualized. These studies have high external validity in being more representative of routine clinical practice, but internal validity is weaker, and therefore causal inferences should be treated with more caution. Naturalistic studies may be *cohort studies* in which a group of patients who are linked in some way (e.g. diagnosed with depression) and exposed to a particular variable (the therapy under investigation) are followed over time. This group may then be compared to a similar group that has not been exposed to the variable.

- *Case control studies* compare people with a certain health problem, such as BPD, or outcome (cases) and a similar group without the problem (controls), and seek associations between the outcome and exposure to a particular risk factor (e.g. childhood sexual abuse). These studies are usually retrospective and concerned with elucidating the causes of disease or health condition.

- *Clinical case studies* were the standard medical research tool in Freud's day and, for some psychotherapists, remain the standard research approach for investigating psychotherapeutic theory and practice. Although an accessible means of communicating ideas, they are limited methodologically. Case report construction is subject to the individual practitioner's selective bias for recalling or distorting clinical data to fit the author's views, and/or excluding important information that does not fit. There are also important ethical issues about the ownership of clinical information; it is now deemed to be ethically and legally unjustifiable to publish a case history of a patient without their consent. Nevertheless, single case studies may be a valid starting point in researching a particular therapy, technique, or clinical situation, in which hypothesized ideas may be initiated and explored through clinical observation and theoretical inference. In recent years, there has been a resurgence of interest in the value of clinical case studies in offering a meaningful source of evidence to confirm a clinical theory. Single or small-sample case studies may be better able than larger-scale studies to examine the complexities of the therapeutic process and track how changes unfold over time. Contemporary systematic case study research employs a formal set of principles, including the construction of a data set from different sources and analysis of the data set by a team of researchers (which may include the therapist and/or patient).

Difficulties in doing research in psychotherapy

Many psychotherapists have been reluctant to embrace a research agenda. This may be due to a variety of reasons, including suspicion of research methodology and fears that it may interfere with effective and ethical clinical practice; viewing narrowly defined trial criteria and research conditions as non-representative of clinical practice (the gap between efficacy and effectiveness); and a reluctance to give up beliefs about theory and technique based on selective experience, and accept empirical findings which may challenge established practice.

Although we believe that empirical studies of psychotherapy are essential for its survival as credible forms of treatment, it is important to be aware of some of the problems and limitations inherent in psychotherapy research which include the following:

- *The gap between efficacy and effectiveness*: the strictly controlled conditions of an RCT may be hard to apply in routine clinical practice where patients and treatments delivered are less well defined
- *Research yields generalities or probabilities, rather than specifics or certainties*: the results of a trial may predict that, on average, the

treatment under investigation is effective in the population studied, but this does not mean that any individual patient will definitely improve with this specific treatment

- *Positive correlations do not always confirm causality*, due to undetected confounding factors
- *Splits between academics who do research and clinicians who do therapy*: much of the psychotherapy research is generated by academics based in universities, and may not be easily accessible or appear relevant to therapists in practice
- *Splits between therapists/modalities who have embraced research and those who have not*: there are ten times more RCTs of CBT than of psychoanalytic psychotherapy, and many of the latter are of poor quality. However, lack of evidence does not equate with lack of efficacy
- *Allegiance effect*: researchers and clinicians inevitably have assumptions and agendas, including a loyalty for the therapy that they are researching, which may lead to significant bias in the interpretation and dissemination of results. Any allegiances should be declared in publications
- *Therapeutic change is not linear*: progress in therapy is unlikely to proceed in an orderly constant manner but involves a more complex trajectory involving periods of progress, followed by regression; shifting and reciprocal changes in affect regulation, impulse control, and awareness of self and others; and a deepening of insight and reflective capacity
- *Medical model/categorical diagnoses*: research often focuses on 'pure' categories of mental disorder according to a medical model which assumes that discrete conditions have different aetiologies and warrant different treatments. However, such categories may not reflect the types of patients and problems, particularly in the relational realm, seen in everyday clinical practice. Moreover, co-morbid conditions and more complex psychopathology, particularly personality disorders, tend to be excluded from such studies
- *Manualization*: promoting strict adherence to a prescribed model of therapy may not reflect how therapy is more flexibly and responsively delivered according to the vicissitudes of everyday practice. Manualization may also inadvertently lead to therapists refusing to discuss themes or issues that are 'not in the manual', which may be clinically dangerous and distorting of the therapeutic process under study
- *Limitations of measures*: measures are more easily designed to identify overt symptomatic or behavioural change but may fail to capture more complex intrapsychic or interpersonal processes that underlie personality difficulties and relationship problems. This is a particular issue with self-report measures
- *Research methodology may interfere with the treatment model under investigation*: for example, the recording of sessions or administration of patient-completed measures during therapy may influence the transference–countertransference dynamics between the patient and therapist which are the focus of psychodynamic psychotherapy

- *Length of treatment studied*: most studies focus on brief treatments which are easier to research, rather than longer-term therapies, and do not study long-term follow-up
- *Variation in quality and standards of training in psychotherapy*: this may be an impediment to research if it is not known how good the therapists are in delivering the treatment under investigation.

Outcome research in psychotherapy

(See ➲ Assessing the outcome of therapy in Chapter 4, pp. 142–5.)

Does psychotherapy work?

There is now extensive evidence that psychological therapies produce positive change, compared to untreated controls, and are effective for a number of different disorders and clinical problems. The use of meta-analyses in pooling the results of outcome studies has been conclusive in demonstrating the efficacy of psychotherapy in general. One of the first most influential meta-analyses was published by Smith *et al.* (1980), which summarized the results of 475 outcome studies of psychotherapy giving an effect size of 0.85 for treated patients, compared to untreated controls.

In 1991, McNeilly and Howard disproved Eysenck's assertion that psychotherapy was no more effective than spontaneous remission, using Eysenck's original data. Since then, hundreds more meta-analyses have been published, summarizing the positive outcomes of therapy in general, as well as results for specific therapies, specific disorders, and specific treatment settings. Therapies appear to be equally effective for adults, young people, and children, with outcomes as good as, and sometimes superior to, medication. Many studies have also demonstrated the cost-effectiveness of psychotherapy, as well as convincing evidence that positive gains can last years after the termination of treatment.

However, a proportion (20% to 40%) of patients in these studies do not improve with treatment, and a minority (5% to 10%) deteriorate. Evidence also suggests that, in routine clinical practice, patients do not fare as well as those in formal clinical trials, with deterioration rates reported as high as 14% with adults, and 24% in children, treated with psychotherapy. Not all such deterioration can be accounted for by therapist activities but may depend on individual patient characteristics such as patients who are already on a negative trajectory at the time of entering treatment. Nevertheless, in general, therapists tend to overrate their patients' progress, and may miss signs of patient worsening and do not take the necessary actions to address this. Where negative patient change is due to therapist factors, this is usually due to therapist actions within the therapeutic relationship of a rejecting nature.

How much therapy is needed?

Researchers have also looked at the length of therapy necessary for positive change to occur. 'Dose effectiveness' studies and meta-analyses of such studies have suggested that around 50% of patients improve after 20 sessions of therapy, and 75% after 50. Moreover, different levels of functioning respond differentially to treatment, with symptomatic and behavioural change responding more quickly than personality difficulties and interpersonal functioning, which may need longer and more intensive treatments.

Are some therapies more effective than others?

(See ➲ Medical psychotherapy modalities in Chapter 2, pp. 17–8.)

As well as demonstrating the efficacy of psychotherapy in general, researchers have also investigated the differential effectiveness of different modalities, such as CBT, and psychodynamic and humanistic therapies, in comparative studies. Here, however, results have been consistently inconclusive, in that no therapy has been convincingly shown to be superior in effectiveness to any other. This has been termed the *equivalence paradox*, or dodo bird effect, after the dodo's pronouncement 'Everyone has won, and all must have prizes' in Lewis Carroll's story *Alice in Wonderland*.

Early meta-analytic reviews showed some evidence that CBT was more efficacious than psychodynamic and interpersonal models of therapy, but later more sophisticated meta-analyses which controlled for investigator allegiance and case severity suggested that there were no significant differences between CBT and other therapies in terms of outcome, thus supporting the equivalence verdict.

Critics of such meta-analyses assert that they are not comparing like with like, that studies should be conducted by genuinely independent bodies to eliminate allegiance bias, and that the dodo effect is due to a failure to measure real differences that exist between different therapies but have eluded detection because our measures are inadequate. However, others have concluded that, although different therapeutic modalities overtly differ in theory and technique, these are, in fact, less important than 'common factors', i.e. techniques and mechanisms common to all therapies, which may go unnoticed but which constitute the real agents of change.

Process research in psychotherapy

How does psychotherapy work?

Process research looks at what happens in psychotherapy and whether therapies differ in their processes, and tries to identify the effective ingredients or mutative agents, how they effect change, and how change develops and is experienced by patients as they progress through treatment. The process research field has been marked by a proliferation of thousands of different instruments, measures, and classification systems catering to different theoretical orientations, treatment modalities, target populations, measurement and data formats, and communication channels, which may appear bewildering to the uninitiated. Nevertheless, consistent findings regarding both common and specific therapy factors have emerged which are summarized below.

Common factor research

It has been estimated that modality-specific factors account for as little as 8% of positive outcome for psychotherapy, and that the majority of change processes in therapy are due to 'non-specific' or 'common' factors. Various attempts have been made to define and quantify these, based on theoretical considerations, studies of the literature, surveys, and empirical findings, and may be summarized as:

- Therapy relationship factors
- Patient characteristics
- Individual therapist characteristics
- Placebo effect
- Extra-therapeutic factors.

- *The therapeutic relationship*
(See ➔ Therapeutic alliance in Chapter 3, p. 99).

Most of the research into common factors has investigated aspects of the therapeutic relationship, including the treatment alliance, and therapists' attitudes and behaviours towards the patient. Such research has consistently shown that the quality of the therapeutic relationship is a crucial determinant of positive outcomes in psychotherapy and can also mitigate against premature dropout from therapy. These results hold true for both therapies that are overtly relationally oriented (e.g. psychodynamic, interpersonal) and therapies that are not primarily relationship-focused (e.g. CBT).

The therapeutic alliance may be defined by the extent to which therapists and patients agree and collaborate on the tasks and goals of therapy, as well as the existence of a positive affective bond between the patient and therapist. The strength of the alliance is strongly related to positive outcome in therapy and should be established before more challenging interventions are introduced (e.g. interpretation of the negative transference). Addressing, within the therapeutic frame, disruptions or ruptures in the alliance that are generated from patients' negative reactions to the therapist and/or treatment process is critical to the repair and maintenance of a positive therapeutic alliance and is more likely to lead to better therapeutic outcome.

Generic relational skills or attitudes linked to positive outcome include therapists' levels of empathy, positive regard, and levels of congruence (also referred to as 'genuineness', 'authenticity', or 'openness'). More specific therapist relational skills and techniques, such as the capacity to repair alliance ruptures, the ability to manage countertransference reactions, giving modest, rather than high, levels of self-disclosure, giving positive feedback, and making fewer, rather than more, frequent, transference interpretations per session, have also been shown in empirical studies to be associated with positive therapeutic outcome.

- *Patient characteristics*
Research on common factors related to the patient or client show that those who are more motivated to engage in therapy and are motivated to change, and those with a clear sense of goals and focus of therapy tend to have better outcomes. Patients who are able to frame their problems in psychological terms and have faith in the possibility of change through therapy, but also have realistic aims and recognize that therapy can be difficult, also tend to do better. Other factors, such as secure attachment style, supportive social network, and previous positive relational experiences, have also been demonstrated as correlating with positive outcomes of therapy.

Demographic characteristics, such as age, gender, sexual orientation, socio-economic class, and ethnicity, have not been shown to substantially influence therapy outcome, although there is some evidence that patients from black and minority ethnic backgrounds and those of lower socio-economic class may not access psychotherapy services so often, as well as have higher rates of premature dropout when they do engage in therapy.

• *Therapist characteristics*

Many studies have found that marked differences exist in therapeutic success with patients between therapists of the same theoretical school or orientation, even amongst therapists delivering manualized treatments. Much of this variation appears to be related to the therapist's ability to form a positive therapeutic alliance with their patients. Where the quality of the alliance is poor, this is more likely to be due to factors associated with the therapist than with the patient, and is associated with poorer outcome than where there is a stronger therapeutic relationship. Therapists' characteristics which may account for the capacity to form a strong therapeutic alliance, or are independently associated with good outcome, are not clear—there is some evidence that therapists with higher levels of psychological well-being and those demonstrated to have more secure attachments, as well as those with more professional experience as a psychotherapist, have better patient outcomes, although the effect sizes observed in studies are small. Age, gender, a therapist's personal experience, and personality traits appear to have little influence on therapy outcome.

• *Patient–therapist matching* (see ➲ Choice in Chapter 4, p. 113)

Patients sometimes request therapists with particular characteristics such as gender, ethnicity, or sexual orientation. However, the research findings on 'patient–therapist matching' are inconclusive. Matching of patient and therapist by sex does not appear to influence outcome. There is some evidence that patients who identify themselves as lesbian, gay, bisexual, or transgender report better outcomes, when matched with therapists who have a similar sexual orientation. Similarly, there is some evidence that therapist–patient matching on ethnicity does contribute to better outcome, as well as to lower dropout rates. Regarding age, there is no strong evidence that matching of patient and therapist by age affects outcomes, although a couple of studies have indicated that therapists who are 10 years or more younger than their patients may have less good results than those who are within 10 years of their patients' age. Studies have also shown that matching of specific attachment styles between therapist and patient may predict psychotherapy process and outcome. For example, patients who have a therapist who is opposite to them on the preoccupying to dismissing dimension of attachment on the AAI tend to have better outcomes than patient–therapist pairs who do not (see ➲ Theories of personality development: attachment theory in Chapter 8, pp. 380–1).

• *Placebo effect*

The placebo effect in psychotherapeutic research is less easy to determine than in pharmacological trials where it is more feasible to construct placebo control conditions that do not contain the putative curative substance (i.e. the drug under investigation). However, as psychological factors are assumed to account for the placebo effect in any trial, it is less easy to disentangle these from psychological factors that may constitute some of the 'common factors' accountable for positive outcome in psychotherapy. Placebo factors have been defined as the generation of belief in the treatment, the expectancy of positive outcome, the installation of hope, a decrease in demoralization, and an increase in experience of self-efficacy.

Many studies have been conducted to explore the relative benefits of therapies, compared to placebo controls. Recent meta-analyses have concluded that, although placebo conditions do contribute to positive outcome, the effects of these factors are smaller than those of therapy-specific factors, and it is difficult to disentangle which placebo-specific factors are responsible for any positive change.

• *Extra-therapeutic factors*

Finally, unexpected positive and negative life events that occur during therapy may lead to change that is not connected to specific therapy factors, but may account for some of the variance found in common factor research.

Research into therapy-specific techniques

Thousands of studies have examined the effects of specific techniques (i.e. a defined therapeutic procedure designed to bring about a specific goal) and have shown that many techniques are linked with psychological improvement, compared to control or placebo conditions. As well as having a direct impact, certain techniques have also been shown to strengthen the therapeutic alliance and therefore offer an important mediating effect on positive outcome.

However, as noted above, researchers have estimated that specific technique and psychotherapy orientation factors account for only a small proportion of the overall outcomes of psychotherapy, and studies comparing the outcomes of different modalities (which assume the delivery of modality-specific techniques) rarely yield significant differences. Studies asking patients to describe what they found most helpful in therapy have found that factors associated with a positive relationship (e.g. 'the therapist was warm and caring') are reported more frequently than technological factors. Dismantling studies rarely find that the presence or absence of specific techniques makes much difference to overall outcome, and studies comparing one technique with another also seldom find significant differences.

Nevertheless, there is some evidence that specific techniques are effective, the strongest being for cognitive behavioural techniques, particularly exposure-based interventions for anxiety. For psychodynamic therapy, carefully worded interpretations embedded in a strong therapeutic relationship have been consistently linked to positive therapeutic outcomes, and more specifically transference interpretations at moderate, rather than high, levels or 'doses'. Both directive and non-directive approaches in therapy have been shown to be beneficial, although extremes of either are associated with poorer outcome. Generic techniques and practices, such as listening, paraphrasing, and encouraging, are usually experienced by patients as helpful, whereas the therapist asking questions or giving advice is less frequently experienced by patients as positive.

More recent innovative research has demonstrated that giving therapists feedback about their patients' progress may produce dramatic improvement in patients exhibiting distress, at risk of deteriorating, or disengaging from therapy. Such feedback is generated by systems that track patient progress on a session-by-session basis, by giving patients a brief outcome measure at every therapy attendance. The results are then computer-processed and fed back to the therapist before the next session. If the patient is 'not on track', the therapist is expected to proactively respond by, for example, focusing attention on repairing therapeutic alliance ruptures.

Finally, although research into therapies delivered by different modes of communication is in its infancy, a growing body of studies indicates that telephone and Internet-based therapeutic interventions may be as effective as face-to-face therapies.

What constitutes good therapy?

Lambert and Bergin have identified and integrated many of the factors and interventions that are empirically associated with positive outcomes into a useful phasic model of what constitutes good therapy by dividing common factors into support, learning, and action factors. 'Support factors' are mainly concerned with aspects of the therapeutic relationship and should be present in all therapies before change may occur. Support factors include catharsis/release of tension, identification with the therapist, mitigation of isolation, reassurance, release of tension, provision of a safe and structured environment, therapeutic alliance, therapist/client active participation, therapist warmth, and trust/open exploration. 'Learning factors' include interventions and strategies that facilitate changes in belief systems and attitudes and emotional regulation, and may be specific to particular therapies. Learning factors include advice, affective experiencing, cognitive learning, correctional emotional experience, exploration of internal frame of reference, feedback, insight, rationale, and reframing of self-perceptions. Learning factors, in turn, lead on to behavioural changes subsumed under 'action factors'. Action factors include behavioural/emotional regulation, cognitive mastery, facing fears, mastery efforts, modelling, practice, reality testing, success experiments, taking risks, and working through.

New ways forward

As in any evolving and creative area of research, researchers in the psychotherapy field generate as many questions as they answer. One of the most pressing and affectively charged questions remains that of the dodo bird—are all therapies equally efficacious, or are some therapeutic orientations and specific techniques more effective than others? At the same time, many other research questions regarding common factors warrant further exploration: How do the therapist, the patient, and the therapeutic relationship variables influence each other? How are they related to outcomes in specific disorders and settings? Which kinds of patients do best in which types of therapies? How do cultural and social factors influence patients' responses to therapy?

The following list represents some of the most promising areas that future researchers might wish to focus on in attempting to address these and the multitude of other questions and challenges posed by contemporary psychotherapy research:

• *More integrative approaches*

Competing epistemological discourses (e.g. outcome/process, subjectivity/objectivity, qualitative/quantitative, scientific/hermeneutic, positivism/relational, specificity/pluralism) should be replaced by more collaborative and integrative approaches to avoid further unnecessary fragmentation; elucidate common methodologies, mechanisms, and areas of interest; and engender respect and enquiry for real differences where they are found.

• *Neuroscience* (see ➲ Neuroscience and psychotherapy in Chapter 11, pp. 526–42)

One of the most exciting and fertile interdisciplinary areas in recent years has been the collaboration between psychotherapy and neuroscience researchers in exploring how the psychological biochemical workings of the mind are linked to the anatomical structures and biochemical processes of the brain. Psychological experiences are no longer viewed as solely the products or epiphenomena of brain function, but are now known to directly alter brain structure and function via neural plasticity, synaptic rearrangement, and genetic expression.

• *Attachment paradigm* (see ➲ Theories of personality development: attachment theory in Chapter 8, pp. 380–1)

Attachment theory is one of the most promising and convincing theoretical paradigms guiding contemporary psychotherapy treatment and research. It provides a coherent model in which the findings on the influence of the therapeutic alliance and the effects of other psychotherapeutic techniques may be conceptualized, integrated, and further empirically tested. The developmental perspective of attachment theory provides a framework for psychotherapy, in which the therapist is experienced as a secure base and temporary attachment figure for the patient (a strong therapeutic alliance), enabling him to explore past and current relationships, external to and within the therapy, with the opportunity to revise internal working models, leading to better adaptation and interpersonal relating. Although certain specific psychodynamic psychotherapies, such as IPT, transference-focused therapy, and MBT, have developed as explicitly attachment theory-based interventions, one can argue that attachment theory implicitly guides all psychotherapies in improving the patient's capacity for mentalization or self-reflective functioning, which is dependent on the person's early developmental attachment experiences, and is a key component of all psychotherapies.

• *Transdiagnostic methods*

Psychotherapy research is moving from single disorder-focused manualized approaches towards 'transdiagnostic' treatments which focus on similarities amongst disorders, particularly in a similar class of diagnoses (e.g. anxiety disorders). Transdiagnostic treatment protocols have been pioneered by CBT-oriented researchers but are also relevant to other therapeutic modalities such as psychodynamic psychotherapy, as they focus more on the core underlying processes of mental conditions in general, an understanding of which may be more easily applied to the less well-defined diagnostic categories and co-morbidities seen in clinical practice.

• *Challenging the supremacy of the RCT paradigm*

On the one hand, as long as influential bodies, such as NICE, prioritize RCT evidence, more RCTs evaluating the efficacy of non-CBT therapies are needed to ensure that a wider range of effective therapies are commissioned and available for patients to choose. On the other hand, the dominance of the RCT paradigm marginalizes other research methodologies, such as single case studies and qualitative research, which may be more suited to exploring essential components of the therapeutic process and are easier to apply in clinical practice.

• *Closing the gap between research and practice*

Not all practising psychotherapists will have the opportunity or be inclined to engage in formal research, but we should aim for a situation in which the majority of therapy practitioners are not only 'research-aware', but are also more confident, inspired, and excited by the findings of research and what they can offer to clinical practice. To some extent, this has been achieved by translating more research ideas into practice-based therapy, but further work needs to be done to embed research teaching in psychotherapy trainings, establish more research-practitioner networks linking academics with clinicians, and apply competency frameworks without losing therapeutic flexibility and expertise gained from clinical experience.

• *Involving service users* (see ➔ Service user involvement in Chapter 10, pp. 466–71)

More involvement in psychotherapy research of service users or 'experts by experience' with lived experience of psychological distress and its therapeutic treatment may help bridge the gulf between research and practice. The service user perspective is increasingly recognized as valuable and influential in all stages of research, including study design, testing proposed measures, data collection, and the analysis and interpretation of findings. Patients participating in research trials may be more amenable and reliable to having measures administered by service users than by research assistants, and a growing number of service user organizations are able to offer training in research methodology and skills.

Recommended reading

Aveline M, Strauss B, and Stiles WB (2006). Psychotherapy research. In: Gabbard GO, Beck JS, and Holmes J (eds). *Oxford Textbook of Psychotherapy*. pp. 449–62. Oxford University Press: Oxford.

Cooper M (2008). *Essential Research Findings in Counselling and Psychotherapy: The Facts are Friendly*. Sage: London.

Eysenck HJ (1952). The effects of therapy: an evaluation. *Journal of Consulting Psychology*, **16**, 319–24.

Lambert MJ (ed) (2013). *Handbook of Psychotherapy Behaviour and Change*, sixth edition. John Wiley & Sons: Hoboken, NJ.

McNeilly CL and Howard KI (1991). The effects of psychotherapy: a re-evaluation based on dosage. *Psychotherapy Research*, **1**, 74–8.

Orlinsky DE and Russell RL (1994). Tradition and change in psychotherapy: notes on the fourth generation. In: Russell RL, ed. *Reassessing Psychotherapy Research.* pp. 185–214. Guildford Press: New York.

Reeves A (2014). Research in individual therapy. In: Dryden W and Reeves A, eds. *The Handbook of Individual Therapy,* sixth edition. pp. 577–602. Sage: London.

Smith ML, Glass GV, Miller TI (1980). *The Benefits of Psychotherapy.* John Hopkins University Press: Baltimore, MD.

Neuroscience and psychotherapy

Almost 15 years ago, Glen Gabbard wrote in the *British Journal of Psychiatry* that 'advances in neuroscience research have led to a more sophisticated understanding of how psychotherapy may affect brain functioning. These developments point the way towards a new era of psychotherapy research and practice in which specific modes of psychotherapy can be designed to target specific sites of brain functioning'. A few years later, Eric Kandel and colleagues wrote that 'with the advent of neuroimaging techniques with high spatial and temporal resolution, the ability to probe the biological consequences of psychotherapeutic interventions has begun to come within reach, and with it the ability to document psychotherapy's effectiveness, to follow its course, and to refine its appropriate applications for selected patients and disorders. Psychotherapy is a controlled form of learning that occurs in the context of a therapeutic relationship. From this perspective, the biology of psychotherapy can be understood as a special case of the biology of learning'.

Freud originally practised as a neurologist in Vienna, whilst developing his interest in understanding all aspects of mental functioning more fully. He wanted to be able to integrate his knowledge of brain functioning with his evolving interest in mental phenomena and with the new evolving science of psychoanalysis. Unfortunately, the available knowledge of the brain and the means to explore this further at the end of the nineteenth century were not adequate for this task. Freud therefore resolved to concentrate his efforts on understanding mental functioning more fully and left it for posterity to attempt to integrate this understanding with a fuller understanding of brain development when the time and the means of investigation were right.

Since the early 1990s, a variety of imaging technologies have revolutionized brain research. These technologies let scientists see what is happening inside subjects' brains without having to open up their skulls. Researchers can ask subjects to perform specific mental tasks, then 'watch their brains think' as they perform these tasks in real time.

There have been major advances also in our knowledge of genetics since the discovery of the double helical structure of deoxyribonucleic acid (DNA) by Watson and Crick in 1953. Molecular biology is a hybrid discipline of genetics and biochemistry that attempts to understand life processes at the level of the macromolecules of the cell and at the level of their structure and function.

Our genes are seen to have two functions. 'The template function' allows our genes to replicate and make copies that are passed from generation to generation. 'The transcription function' refers to a gene being turned on to make a new protein that alters the structure and function of the cell. This transcription function is influenced by what we do or think. Information inherited through encoding on DNA can be activated or suppressed by other genetic or environmental elements. Information is also remembered through the actions of messenger ribonucleic acid (mRNA) but is not transmitted genetically to other generations in this way.

The practical applications of this knowledge to our clinical work are varied. When psychotherapy changes people, it does so through learning. It produces changes in gene expression that alter the strength of synaptic connections. In an exciting link to attachment theory, polymorphism in the serotonin transporter gene (5-HTTLPR) has been typed and is seen to be clinically relevant. Attachment patterns in infants were explored on the basis of the genetic expression of the serotonin transporter gene. For short allele (ss/sl) infants, low responsiveness in the mother predicted a particularly high risk for insecure attachment, and high responsiveness offset that risk. For infants homozygous for the long allele (ll), there was no association between responsiveness and attachment organization. Homozygous infants were securely attached, whatever the responsiveness of the mother (see ➔ Theories of personality development: attachment theory in Chapter 8, pp. 380–1).

The complexity of the molecular biology of the neuron is illustrated by the intricacies of chemical transmission of impulses across synaptic gaps between neurons and by the impact of the chemical involved in the biochemistry of the post-synaptic neuron. There are nine different types of classical neurotransmitters and more than 50 types of neuroactive peptides. Most neurons produce multiple neurotransmitters, which act on very different timescales. Genes are activated within the cell nucleus to start producing new proteins. These proteins facilitate excitability of previously activated synapses and enhance the production of neurotrophins that lead to the formation of additional synapses around previously activated synapses.

Freud would probably be very happy to be alive in our age of advancing knowledge of brain development and mental functioning. There has been a massive expansion in knowledge about the development and functioning of the brain and body, about the sensorimotor and autonomic nervous systems, about the neurodevelopment of attachment and of personality, and about experiences that lead to likely disorders of functioning. This paradigmatic shift in understanding when linked with an active awareness of communicating styles leads to effective clinical interventions with particular patient groups.

The brain

Brain structure and function

The concept of the *triune brain* has evolved over the past 50 years. According to this theory, the following three distinct brains emerged successively in the course of evolution and now co-inhabit the human skull:

- The *reflex* or *reptilian* brain is the oldest of the three and consists of the structures of the brainstem and the cerebellum. It controls the body's vital functions such as heart rate, breathing, body temperature, and balance. The reptilian brain is reliable but tends to be somewhat rigid and compulsive in function.

- The *feeling* or *limbic* brain emerged in the first mammals and consists of areas of brain cells and their connections known as the hippocampus, the amygdala, and the hypothalamus. It records memories of behaviours that produce agreeable and disagreeable experiences. It is responsible for what are called emotions in human beings. The limbic brain is the seat of the value judgements that we make, often unconsciously, that can exert such a strong influence on our behaviour.
- The *thinking* brain or the *neocortex* first assumed importance in primates. It culminated in the human brain with its two dominant large 'cerebral hemispheres'. These hemispheres have been responsible for the development of human language, abstract thought, imagination, and consciousness. The neocortex is flexible and has almost infinite learning abilities. Learning is a process that will modify a subsequent behaviour. Memory is basically nothing more than the record left by a learning process. The neocortex is what has enabled human cultures to develop.

These three parts of the brain do not operate independently of one another. They have established numerous interconnections through which they influence each another. The neural pathways from the limbic system to the cortex, for example, are especially well developed.

Experiences arriving at areas of our brains through our senses are laid down as 'memories' in specific areas of the brain, and integrated through neural connections across a number of functional systems in our brains. We gain sensory experiences through our senses of vision, hearing, touch, taste, and smell. Each motor experience is likewise registered in specific parts of the brain and integrated across a number of brain areas and functional systems necessary for the finer control of movement and actions. An infant learns to control head movements, turn over, sit up, crawl, walk, run, control hand movements, develop precise hand coordination, vocalize, make words, link words, make sentences, and make verbal sense all in the first 3 years of life. All such progress is registered in neural networks of the brain.

The blueprint for brain development is genetically mediated. Genetics determine the form and structure of our brains, especially what we understand as our reptilian brain. Our limbic brain is likewise to a great extent genetically determined, but it is also directly influenced by experiences we have as infants. Such experiences are laid down in neural networks within the limbic structures, and in the neural networks that connect to the limbic structures. The timing of patterns of brain growth and development is genetically determined, but it is also influenced by experiences and by environmental factors.

The building blocks of the brain are *neurons*, nerve cells that each makes thousands of connections with other nerve cells. Chemicals, known as *neurotransmitters*, make connections across the gaps between cells, known as *synapses*. Small electrical impulses are transmitted quickly down long fibre-like outgrowths, known as axons, from the body of the nerve cell, which connect with thousands of other neurons. These mechanisms of neuron development and action are genetically laid down in

DNA, the genetic material of the neurons. Neurons are supported, in turn, by other cells in the brain, which ensure the presence of the correct environment and the correct nourishment for neural growth and activity. Some of these supporting cells coat the axon of the neuron with a protective covering that quickens the transmission of nerve impulses down the axon. This process is known as myelinization and makes for more effective and more efficient nerve impulse transmission.

The capacity of neurons and neuronal networks to respond to the environment is genetically determined. When neurons fire (are activated), they fire off neighbouring neurons connected via axons, synaptic gaps, and neurotransmitters. Repeated firing of particular neurons makes future firing more likely. Neurons that fire together are primed to repeatedly further fire together, forming networks of neurons. These neural networks, if repeatedly activated, continue to develop further connections with other neurons and with other neural networks. 'Neurons that fire together wire together'. Such connections are the forerunners of memory systems in the brain.

The human brain is a very complicated three-pound mass of matter. It contains over 100 billion neurons and another one trillion support cells. There are up to 10000 synapses on each neuron. Each neuron contains the entire genome, and approximately 35000 genes can have a direct impact on brain development. The size of our brains, and those of our primate cousins, correlates with both the length of our juvenile period and the complexity of our social structure. Long childhoods and complex societies make for larger brains.

Likewise, relational experiences, emotional experiences, verbal experiences, and thinking experiences are both registered in, and made possible by, brain activity. All this activity represents growth and development in our brains made possible through our genetic potential and made actual by our experiences in life. It is a clear example of a process where both nature and nurture are seen to be essential elements for normal growth and development to occur.

The right hemisphere generally processes non-verbal communication; it allows us to recognize faces and read facial expressions, and it connects us to other people. It thus processes the non-verbal visual cues exchanged between a mother and her baby. It also processes the musical component, or tone, of speech by which we convey emotion. Our right hemisphere dominates the activity of the brain for the first 2 years of our lives. Brain scans show that, during the first 2 years of life, the mother principally communicates non-verbally with her own right hemisphere to reach her infant's right hemisphere.

The left hemisphere generally processes the verbal linguistic elements of speech, as opposed to the emotional musical ones, and analyses problems using conscious processing. The left hemisphere dominates activity in the brain from 2 years onwards, whilst language is actively developing.

Periods of brain growth and development
Whilst the evolution of the structures of the brain has happened over millions of years, an individual's brain develops over a lifetime of about 85 years. There are three stages of particularly rapid brain growth and

development during this time. The first stage is the time spent in the womb, when we develop from the joining of two cells at fertilization, to a very complex living organism at birth 9 months later. The second rapid stage of brain growth and development occurs during the first 3 years of life. The third stage of significant brain development occurs during our adolescent years. The brain, however, continues to develop throughout life.

The brain continues to mature during our 'adult years'. All activities become much easier with practice. This is reflected in the degree of activity measurable in the brain. Many areas of the brain are seen to 'light up' on neuroimaging when we attempt something new. With practice, the areas and neural networks in the brain that are activated to achieve the same result become more defined and refined. Sometimes, as when motor movement and activity are involved, the necessary brain functioning takes place mostly in non-cortical brain areas such as areas in the brainstem and cerebellum. When some 'higher executive functioning' uses areas of the prefrontal cortex (PFC) to achieve a desired result, the area of the PFC used by adults is smaller to achieve the same result than that used by adolescents. Brain functioning becomes more efficient with practice.

Throughout adult life, a small region of the hippocampus, the dentate gyrus, continues to generate new differentiated nerve cells from stem cells. Antidepressants may exert their effects on behavior, in part, by stimulating the production of neurons in the hippocampus.

How does this apply to clinical practice?

Memory and learning
Understanding memory as a representation and record of altered brain functioning is helpful in the context of learning. A child's brain functions very differently to an adult's brain. Memories and emotional reactions early in childhood are based on a more 'immature and primitive' mechanism of brain functioning. Brainstem reflexes and limbic activity organize much of the infant's experiences. Development of more primitive brain structures precedes the development of later evolving ones. Early experiences influence the wiring that is installed in the brain, whilst later adult learning usually influences how already established wiring fires. Once neural networks are established, new learning often relies on the modification of these established patterns.

The basic feature of the intercellular memory process is the pairing of neurons with each other. When two connecting neurons fire at the same time, they are more likely to fire together again in the future, because the strength of the connections between them will be greater. When two connected neurons fire frequently together, they develop new synaptic connections. These memory processes seem likely to be the basis for what is known as *implicit (procedural, non-hippocampal) learning* (see ➔ Memory and emotions in Chapter 11, pp. 531–3).

Simple repetition can effect change, even in the absence of reasoning or logic to support the change. The development of associations between events and emotions is an example of non-hippocampal learning based on simple pairing, even in the absence of awareness and insight.

Non-hippocampal learning will not readily change despite the presence of new insight. When implicit memory associations weaken, they are likely to do so slowly and incrementally over time. Memory is highly influenced by affect.

Explicit (sometimes called declarative or autobiographic) memory (see ➔ Memory and emotions in Chapter 11, pp. 531–3) is based in the hippocampus and affiliated structures. When two neurons both innervate a third neuron, the process of long-term potentiation can, in effect, form a bond between them, even though they are not directly connected. Pyramidal cells are neurons that receive input from extremely high numbers of other neurons. They are structured in a way that facilitates development of such new connections. These cells occur in high numbers in the hippocampus, as well as in the outer surface layers of the cerebral cortex.

Connections between the hippocampus and frontal cortical areas appear to support conscious processing and decision-making, and the area as a whole is particularly well suited to establish novel connections supporting new learning. Hippocampal learning coincides with declarative and explicit conceptualizations of learning, whilst non-hippocampal learning coincides with implicit memory formation. Hippocampal learning supports efficient processing of incoming information and integration of new information with information previously stored in the brain. It also supports flexible retrieval of stored information.

The concept of the *'remembered present'* suggests that much of what we take to be perception is, in fact, memory. We adults project our expectations onto the world all the time. We largely construct, rather than perceive, the world around us. Memory traces may be unconsciously activated all the time. One does not have to explicitly retrieve a memory for it to be active and for it to influence cognition and behaviour.

Memory and emotions

The early sensory–motor and emotional memories of infants and toddlers are mediated via the amygdala, thalamus, cerebellum, and orbital medial prefrontal structures. This system organizes and retains primitive vestibular–sensory–emotional memories of early care taking, rendering them of permanent psychological significance. These early implicit memories come to serve as the emotional background against which subsequent psychological development takes place. Implicit memory is usually non-verbal, non-symbolic, and is not available for conscious reflection. Implicit memory can be understood as 'knowing how', rather than 'knowing what'. Its content involves emotional responses, patterns of behaviour, and skills. As the brain matures, the hippocampus, temporal lobes, and lateral prefrontal lobes begin to organize the systems of explicit memory. Hippocampal–cortical networks need to be functioning for the conscious recollection of the learning process. This usually happens somewhere between the ages of 3 and 4 years old. Explicit memory can be consciously retrieved, reflected upon, verbalized, and symbolic, and contains information and images.

The distinction between explicit and implicit, as outlined above in relation to memories, can be applied also to other mental processes such as learning, emotions, emotional regulation, motivation, action control, and interpersonal behaviour. Implicit processes are independent of the capacity limitations of working memory. Many implicit processes can happen simultaneously, without interfering with one another. They typically happen quickly and without effort, are not error-prone, and do not require attention and conscious awareness. They are typically linked to a specific sensory modality. They cannot easily, if at all, be controlled volitionally. They are typically learnt more slowly than explicit mental processes. They need many repetitions to be learnt. It is difficult to change them, once they are well ingrained.

Lack of recall in adults of details of their childhood experiences strongly suggests high levels of anxiety during childhood that mitigate against the consolidation of long-term memory. A lack of recall is associated with attachment styles that are anxious, ambivalent, and dismissing. Insecure and traumatized children have a difficult time self-regulating their emotions and suffer from anxiety, depression, and a variety of other symptoms. What the mind forgets, the body often remembers in the form of fear, pain, or physical illness.

The amygdala is a key component of emotional memory throughout life. The direct and rapid neural connections of the amygdala with the hypothalamus and limbic–motor circuits rapidly translate the rapid appraisal of threat into bodily states and action. The primary role of the amygdala is to modulate vigilance and attention in order to gather information, remember emotionally salient events and individuals, and prepare for action. The emotionally expressive face is an increasingly important transmitter of information across the social synapse. The amygdala networks with circuits throughout the brain to 'read' information from the eyes, direction of attention, gestures, body postures, and facial expressions. The amygdala becomes activated to both sad and happy faces but appears to be vital for recognizing fear. Faces judged to be untrustworthy, as well as verbal and written threats, automatically activate areas of the amygdala.

The amygdala and orbitomedial prefrontal cortex (OMPFC) are major players in the regulation of our experience of safety and danger. The amygdala connects negative experiences with autonomic arousal, generating anxiety, fear, panic, and flashbacks. The OMPFC assesses the reality of the danger and is capable of inhibiting the amygdala activation when a fear response is deemed unnecessary. The OMPFC and amygdala have a reciprocal regulatory relationship.

Evolution seems to be far more interested in keeping us alive than keeping us happy. Overall, negative emotions trump positive ones and weigh more heavily on our evaluation of people and situations. A single highly charged affective moment may predispose any of us to be anxious for the rest of our lives. Learning not to be afraid can take years of struggle. The amygdala is quick to learn and slow to forget. Learnt fears are tenacious and tend to return when we are under stress. Based on our neurobiology, fear outranks and outwits love in a number of ways. Fear is faster, automatic, unconscious, spontaneously generalized to other stimuli, multisensory, and resistant to extinction. Whereas the hippocampus is constantly remodelled to keep abreast of current environment changes, the role of the amygdala is to remember threat, generalize it to other possible threats, and carry it into the future.

Memory and attachments
(See ➲ Theories of personality development: attachment theory in Chapter 8, pp. 380–1.)

Memory is intimately connected with the development of attachment patterns and behaviours. Communication between individuals occurs via smells that influence identification, attraction, and repulsion; via sounds such as grunts, groans, sighs, and laughter, and vary according to volume, tone, prosody, rhyming, and song; via touch that influences affection, nurturance, grooming, sex, support, soothing, and calming; and via visual stimuli such as facial expressions, smiling, gestures, pupil dilation, and blushing. The activation of networks of the brain by these multiple streams of information occurs in the internal systems facilitating interpersonal connection and regulation.

Louis Cozolino, in his book *Attachment and the Developing Social Brain*, notes that, even though we cherish the idea of individuality, we live with the paradox that we constantly regulate each other's internal biological states. Our interdependence is a constant reality of our existence. The individual neuron or single human brain does not exist in nature. Without mutually stimulating interactions, people and neurons wither and die. He helpfully describes the human brain as a social organ criss-crossed with neural networks dedicated to receiving, processing, and communicating messages across what he terms the social synapse—or the space between us as individuals.

Positive social interactions result in increased metabolic activity, mRNA synthesis, and neural growth. Relationships can create an internal biological environment supportive of neural plasticity. Early neglect, stress, and trauma all impact on developmental processes in negative and destructive ways. Neglect and abuse decrease the growth of experience-dependent neural circuits, especially of the OMPFC, anterior cingulate, and insula cortex. We are individuals, but the architectural structures of our brains are records of our interpersonal histories.

Mirror neurons are neurons that fire when observing others performing a task. They are most likely involved in the learning of manual skills, the evolution of gestural communication, spoken language, group cohesion, and empathy. Thus, we can learn by observation. Mirror neurons were first discovered in the 1990s by recording the firing of single neurons in monkeys' brains, whilst they were awake, alert, and interacting with other monkeys. Specific neurons in the PFC were seen to fire when a monkey was both observing an action in another and when the monkey itself performed the same action. Non-invasive scanning technologies have been used to extend these findings to human brains. Brain regions involved in perceptual action mirror systems are now thought to include the premotor cortex, motor cortex, cerebellum, basal ganglia, somatosensory cortex, parietal lobe, Broca's area, amygdala, and the frontal lobe. Observing becomes a way to rehearse. Resonance behaviours, triggered by mirror systems, are automatic responses that are reflexive, implicit, and obligatory. Reflexively looking up or yawning when we see others do the same are examples. Therapists unconsciously mirror the facial expressions, tone of voice, and body postures of their clients. Resonance reactions occur before we are consciously aware of them. Fears, anxiety, and phobias can all be passed from one person to another, especially from parents to children, through observation of their behavioural manifestations in the other.

The ability to link feelings and words does not come automatically but relies on relationships to build connections between separate neural networks dedicated to affect and language. Language, in combination with emotional attunement from primary caregivers, creates the opportunity to support neural growth and network integration. The normal development of the mind is dependent on the intersubjective process of emerging psychological awareness between the child and his primary caregivers in the context of a secure attachment. The caregiver's empathic ability to reflect on the infant's state of mind facilitates the infant's capacity to understand his own mind and that of others (theory of mind). The child becomes increasingly aware of his own mind through his growing awareness of the mind of his mother via her capacity to demonstrate to him that she thinks of him as a separate person with his own distinct intentions, beliefs, and desires. The capacity to ascribe meaning to human behaviour ultimately shapes our understanding of others and ourselves, and develops through experiencing our internal states being understood by another mind.

The most important aspects of child rearing are, firstly, love and attachment, and secondly, being curious about who your children are. In this way, you learn how to play with them and how to encourage their imaginations. Every child is an experiment of nature. Children need their parents' curiosity about them as an avenue of self-discovery. Attunement, secure attachment, curiosity, and affect regulation go hand in hand with neural plasticity in the brain.

Memory and early trauma
(See ➔ Trauma-related conditions in Chapter 7, pp. 355–9.)

Early trauma, especially at the hands of caretakers, may begin a cascade of effects that result in a complex post-traumatic reaction. Some abused children learn not to look at faces and are less skilful at decoding facial expressions. When they do look at faces, they are hypervigilant to any signs of negativity or criticism. In the face of early interpersonal trauma, all of the systems of the social brain may become shaped for offensive and defensive purposes. Regulatory systems become biased towards arousal and fear, and prime our bodies to sacrifice well-being in order to stay on full alert at all times. Reward systems designed to make us feel good by contact with loved ones are manipulated with drugs, alcohol, compulsive behaviours, and self-harm.

The development of theory of mind, or a capacity to mentalize, is compromised when children are abused and neglected. Both neural growth and integration are impaired, leading to the abnormal development of experience-dependent structures such as the cerebral cortex, corpus callosum, and hippocampus.

Some antisocial or 'psychopathic' individuals seem to have less activation to aversive stimuli when either they or others are experiencing it. They react with abnormally low autonomic activation to social stimuli such as faces and expressions of emotions. These individuals demonstrate only superficial amygdala activation in response to faces and are less accurate in recognizing fearful faces. Antisocial patients do have a theory of mind of the other, but, instead of using it to connect empathically, they may use it to manipulate others to get their way. General damage to the PFC at any time during life can result in a loss of empathic capacities (see ➲ Antisocial personality disorder in Chapter 8, pp. 396–401).

Consciousness

Consciousness may be understood from a neural perspective. We experience as conscious only those processes that occupy working memory for at least a few seconds. Working memory has a very limited capacity, is localized in the PFC, and works in close collaboration with the anterior cingulate cortex, which plays a key role in the internal control of attention. The stream of consciousness is characterized temporally by continuity and simultaneously by consistency, because the current content of working memory largely determines what will enter into working memory next. External events that enter the focus of attention also influence working memory. All forms of consciousness are linked to the associative cortex where internal connections far outweigh those that it has to and from the outside (by about five million to one!). The close interconnections of neurons and networks within the associative cortex are the main neuroanatomical bases for our subjective experience of consciousness and allow us to generate internal states that rely very little on external input. Unconscious processes that are beyond our conscious control precede our conscious acts of will in many instances.

The left hemisphere usually takes the lead in semantic and conscious processing, whilst social and emotional processing happens mainly in the right hemisphere. Mammals are characterized by a right hemispheric bias in the control of emotion, bodily experience, and autonomic processes in the cerebral cortex, subcortical, and brainstem structures. The right cortex is far more densely connected with subcortical regions than the left. Right brain functions are similar to Freud's notion of the unconscious. They develop earlier and are guided by emotional and bodily reactions, and their non-linear mode of processing allows for multiple overlapping realities akin to Freud's conception of primary process thinking. The right brain responds to negative emotional stimuli prior to conscious awareness. Thus, unconscious emotional processing based on past experiences invisibly guides our moment-to-moment thoughts, feelings, and behaviours. The phenomena of projection and transference are generated through these networks. The dominance of the right hemisphere for bodily and emotional functioning and its ability to process this information reflexively and unconsciously have freed the left cortex to attend more to the environment and to engage in logical and abstract reasoning.

Learning throughout life

The plasticity of the brain leads to a continuing capacity for learning throughout our lives. As we learn, our individual neurons alter their shape and strengthen the synaptic connections between them. When we form long-term memories, neurons change their anatomical shape and increase the number of synaptic connections they have to other neurons. Appropriate spacing of learning is a key factor in developing long-term memory. For short-term memories to become long-term, a new protein has to be made. The more we use a skill like playing the piano, the more space and brainpower it gets. Repetition alone is not enough, however, for plastic change to occur. Close attention is also necessary.

Brain-derived neurotropic factor (BDNF) plays a critical role in triggering the brain's ability to absorb and learn. When a child's body releases a lot of BDNF, keeping the brain constantly stimulated to absorb new information, the child's brain remains engaged and absorbent. At the end of a critical period, release of increased quantities of BDNF triggers an effective shutdown of the critical period. We are designed to stop effortlessly learning past a certain point in adulthood, as it would be difficult to function if we were constantly distracted by new learning and therefore unable to determine priorities and 'accumulate wisdom'.

The brain's ability to grow new nerve cells, forge plastic change, and learn new skills is not completely shut off in adults. There are three steps required to effect change in the brain. Firstly, considerable focus and attention are required to activate the nucleus basalis to produce acetylcholine and choline acetyltransferase, which, in turn, instructs the brain to fix the memories being formed. Secondly, a mental challenge that leads to a sense of satisfaction and reward is also needed for the brain to produce dopamine, the second ingredient required for plastic change. Thirdly, targeted training is then required. Acetylcholine and dopamine prompt the growth of new nerve cells in the dentate gyrus of the hippocampus and create conditions under which the brain can change. The way in which the brain actually grows and changes depends on what we are doing to stimulate that growth. Training exercises that strengthen and improve core brain functions can generate lasting improvements in our mental ability.

Many everyday activities stimulate neural growth and help us stay mentally fit. Studying a new language, tackling puzzles and brain teasers, or learning a new skill, however, is not as directed and effective as that produced by a carefully designed brain training programme. The practical applications are many and varied. Learning specialists use brain training software to help children reverse learning deficits. Senior centres offer brain training resources to their customers, reversing memory loss and delaying or preventing the onset of Alzheimer's symptoms and dementia. Progressive school systems have introduced brain training to help optimize classroom study. Individuals have taken to brain training as a way to maintain and improve their mental agility. The factors that can influence and train the brain to engage in, and to gain maximally from, psychotherapy now remain to be explored more fully.

Learning of new information, whether by students, trainees, or patients, is more likely to be effective when:

- Their degree of vigilance, alertness, attentiveness, and concentration is sufficient to engrave information into memory
- Their interests, strength of motivation, and needs all enhance learning
- Noticeable affective values are associated with the informational to be memorized, and the individual's mood and intensity of emotion at the time facilitates memory. If an event is very upsetting, a vivid memory of it is likely to be formed
- The location and accompanying light, sounds, smells, and entire context are recorded, along with the information being memorized. One can very often recall information by first recalling its context. Forgetting rids the brain of information that will not be needed in future
- Perceptions are consciously experienced to the degree that attention is devoted to them. It is so much easier to learn things that we actually desire to learn.

Getting information across well

- Keep it simple
- Do not present a lot of information at one go
- Alternate information giving with activity
- Structure the information to make it meaningful
- Connect with what already exists
- Exploit beginnings and endings.

Applications to the practice of psychotherapy

Psychotherapy as a learning experience

Psychotherapy is fundamentally a learning experience for patients and for therapists, and involves the triggering of structural changes in specific neurons and neuronal pathways. Whatever the modality, there are a number of patterns associated with change in psychotherapy. *Clarification of meaning* addresses the causation and presentation of psychological difficulties. *A sense of mastery* develops from the concrete experience of learning to cope with situations previously experienced as very difficult or anxiety-provoking. The patient's problems can be changed most effectively through being *activated, experienced, and understood in the present*, and within the transference and countertransference relationship in psychoanalytic psychotherapy. *The activation of resources in the patient* can be harnessed to support change.

The therapeutic relationship

(See ➔ Therapeutic alliance in Chapter 3, p. 99; Common factor research in Chapter 11, pp. 519–22.)

The work of psychotherapy depends on the development of a therapeutic relationship between a therapist and a patient. The therapist provides consistency and reliability in setting, in behaviour, and in attitudes; warm, caring, positive regard, and an ability to see value in what the patient offers; repeated opportunities to develop a positive therapeutic alliance; and optimal circumstances to facilitate fresh learning. The patient brings her difficulties and her strengths as part of who she is; some difficulties she wants to address in her life; some preparedness to risk involving herself in a therapeutic relationship; some recognition of her part in the development and continuation of these difficulties; and some wish to seek an understanding of why these difficulties continue to impact directly on her life.

Concepts of change arising from the neurosciences

Changes in mental functioning resulting from the practice of psychotherapy include structural changes evidenced by rigid mental functioning becoming more flexible; conflictual internal object relationships becoming less concrete, less highly charged, more complex, and more highly differentiated; and a gradual assimilation of conflict. From a psychodynamic point of view, conflicts become accessible to consciousness; conflictual internal object relationships are increasingly understood to be part of the self; there is increasing acceptance of the loss of ideal images; losses are mourned, and guilt is worked through; ambivalence is tolerated, and a capacity for concern develops; in Klein's terminology, 'paranoid schizoid functioning' shifts to become predominately 'depressive functioning'; change occurs as a result of a process of containment and interpretation (see ➲ Psychoanalytic psychotherapy in Chapter 2, pp. 20–30, and in Chapter 5, pp. 163–72).

How may these therapeutic changes observed clinically be understood and translated into changes in the brain's function and structure?

- *Psychotherapy helps people put their unconscious procedural memories and actions into words and into context, so they can better understand them.* In the process, they plastically retranscribe these procedural memories, so that they become conscious explicit memories, sometimes for the first time. Patients then no longer need to 'relive or re-enact' them. Repetition or working through is required for long-term neuroplastic change.

- *New ways of relating have to be learnt through wiring new neurons together.* Old ways of responding have to be unlearnt through the weakening of neuronal links. Emotions and the patterns we display in relationships are part of the procedural memory system. When such patterns are triggered in therapy, it gives the patient a chance to look at them and change them. Positive bonds appear to facilitate neuroplastic change by triggering unlearning and dissolving existing neuronal networks, so the patient can alter his existing intentions.

- *Psychotherapy can result in detectable changes in the brain.* Brain scans done before and after psychotherapy show that the brain plastically reorganizes itself in treatment. The more successful the treatment, the greater is the resultant change.

- *Implicit mental processes have both advantages and disadvantages.* They are independent of the capacity limitations of working memory; they can happen simultaneously without interfering with one another; they typically occur quickly and without effort; they are not error-prone and do not require attention and conscious awareness; they are linked to a specific sensory modality and cannot easily, if at all, be controlled volitionally; they are learnt more slowly than explicit memory contents; they need many repetitions to be learnt, and it is difficult to change them once they are well ingrained.

- *The explicit mode of functioning is better for relearning.* The most important function of conscious awareness is the facilitation of new learning. The qualities linked with the explicit mode of functioning, such as conscious reflection, intention formation, planning, volitional control, and verbal communication, can all be viewed as resources for therapeutic change. The formation, facilitation, and maintenance of appropriate goals and intentions in the patient are important therapeutic tasks.

The plasticity of the brain

The brain responds to injuries and stimuli with a great deal of adaptability. Very well-developed brain structures that are not used over a long period of time begin to atrophy. With sufficiently intensive stimuli and experiences, new self-sustaining structures emerge in the brain, which then become the foundation for enduring changes in experience and behaviour. The intensity, duration, and mode of delivery of therapeutic interventions have a significant bearing on the development of structural changes in the brain. Intense new learning in psychotherapy associated with structural changes in the brain requires conscious, volitional, self-motivated patient collaboration, and functioning in the explicit mode. Structural changes in the brain occur only as the result of intensive and long-lasting influences.

Implications for psychotherapy technique

(See ➔ Chapter 5; What constitutes good therapy? in Chapter 11, p. 523.)

- The therapeutic relationship is central to positive change, regardless of the theoretical orientation of the therapist. A safe and trusting relationship with an attuned, resonant, empathic therapist reactivates attachment circuitry in a patient and makes it available to neuroplastic processes. Training of therapists might usefully emphasize the development of resonance, attunement, and empathy as central to the relationship we have with patients.
- The more the dialogue follows the patient's patterns, the more easily the patient will engage in meaningful communication with the therapist; however, the patient needs to be challenged in addition for long-term changes to occur at the neuronal synapses.
- Change requires the intense, frequent, repeated activation of synaptic connections that are not yet well established; this opens up the *N*-methyl-*D*-aspartate (NMDA) receptors and kicks off a second messenger cascade, particularly if dopamine receptors are simultaneously activated.
- The activation of cognition and emotion together allows frontal systems to re-associate and re-regulate the various neural circuits that organize thinking and feeling—those very circuits that are most vulnerable to dissociation.
- The maintenance of moderate levels of arousal maximizes the biochemical processes that drive protein synthesis necessary for modifying neural structures.
- Therapy is most effective when it is focused only for a short time on the identification and activation of problems and then predominantly on altering the problem and on facilitating new thoughts, behaviour patterns, and emotions.

- This activation of new neural connections must be repeated as often as possible.
- Permanent facilitation of new patterns of experience and behaviour on the neural level requires a concentrated and long-lasting effort to establish and maintain these new experiences and behaviour patterns.
- Using the concept of inhibition of something problematic, rather than extinction, shifts the focus from that which is problematic to that which should be put in its place instead.
- Seeking to shift the brain towards a state that is maximally incompatible with fear involves developing a secure attachment relationship with a therapist who conveys competence, understanding, and personal engagement.
- The therapist should provide the patient with intense and varied perceptions that support his therapeutic goals and should structure the therapeutic situation to utilize a patient's own resources.
- The construction of narrative that reflects a positive, optimistic self creates an evolving language for experience that can modify self-image, aid in affect regulation, and serve as a guide for positive behaviour.
- The malleability of memory and the potential to rewrite history can be extremely helpful in psychotherapy. As long as patients are capable of understanding the difference between accurate history and therapeutic co-constructed narratives, many patients may be able to transform their oppressive memories into healing stories.
- Differing and multiple inputs can influence the brain in complementary and additive ways. Therefore, using more than one modality simultaneously in a way that is complementary and cohesive, such as concurrent group work, family work, or psychosocial nursing work with individual therapy, creates opportunities for further learning and experimentation by the patient. Patients may be actively encouraged to be physically active and aware of their physical condition. Medication may also be used judiciously to support the work of psychotherapy. The use of lifestyle changes, relaxation exercises, yoga, or medication reduce levels of arousal and maximize neuroplastic potential.
- Educating patients about their brains—teaching them about how the brain works, explaining to them the impact of early learning on the brain and on the body, explaining the workings of memory and the biases of the amygdala, discussing vulnerabilities to prejudice and to phobias—can create a common less-threatening language between the patient and therapist within the working relationship.
- Therapy, at times, necessitates the teaching of new skills and competencies to patients. This may mean that psychotherapists may themselves need to learn a range of new skills and competencies centred on teaching and educational skills.

Table 11.1 gives some examples of how psychodynamic concepts may be understood in terms of brain development and functioning.

Table 11.1 Exploring psychodynamic concepts using the language of brain development and brain functioning

Psychodynamic principles	Alternative understanding using brain developmental language	Examples and explanatory notes
Unconscious	Unconscious Not conscious Preconscious Implicit or procedural memory and functioning	Examples: 1. 'Social brain' functioning involving: 　Perception of danger, 　Recognition of facial expressions, 　Determinants of relationships 2. 'Non-hippocampal' memory systems
Transference	Implicit relating	Explanatory notes: Initially a 'conversation' between areas of 'right social brain functioning' in patient and therapist Worked with to make it explicit and available to the higher executive brain functioning (HEBF) of therapist and patient
Countertransference	Implicit pressure to react and relate in complementary ways	Explanatory note: There is value in understanding the pressure, making it explicit and available to HEBF of the therapist and patient
Defence mechanisms (DMs)	Usually the less mature DMs are active in situations where fresh learning is not achieved or is not possible	Explanatory note: Generally DMs are functional and healthy, whether 'depressive' or 'paranoid schizoid' in nature
Psychotic/immature or primitive DMs: Denial Splitting Idealization Dissociation Projection Projective identification Introjective identification	Old implicit neuronal pathways are stimulated, strengthened, and reinforced Fight/flight limbic system functioning is dominant	Explanatory note: There is activation of the limbic system with little explicit HEBF in the patient

(Continued)

Table 11.1 (Contd.)

Psychodynamic principles	Alternative understanding using brain developmental language	Examples and explanatory notes
Neurotic/more mature DMs: Repression Identification Reaction formation Regression Conversion Restriction Intellectualization	These DMs involve mainly implicit limbic functioning but include some implicit cognitive processing in the PFC	Explanatory note: Activation of HEBF, alongside some manageable limbic influences, make these mechanisms explicit and open to influence by the HEBF of the PFC
Mature/ healthy DMs: Sublimation Art Humour	New fresh learning is usually present alongside use of mature DMs	Explanatory note: HEBF is linked with manageable limbic functioning and leads to fresh learning
Focusing on the interpretation of DMs seems increasingly less central to the current practice of psychoanalytic psychotherapy	Focus on situations and conditions that make fresh learning possible Avoid stimulating fear and overwhelming limbic activity, as this is incompatible with learning Create circumstances conducive to new learning	Explanatory note: It may be possible to bypass DMs by finding non-threatening ways to contain, think, and talk about the underlying issues that stimulate them
Working through	Frequent repetition leads to new learning, via the laying down of new pathways (hard wiring) by a process of 'neurons that fire together wire together'	Explanatory notes: This is hugely important. Old ways of coping are never fully relinquished and may come into play again at times of particular pressures and stress

Recommended reading

Cozolino L (2010). *The Neuroscience of Psychotherapy: Healing the Social Brain*. WW Norton & Co: New York.

Gabbard GO (2000). A neurobiologically informed perspective on psychotherapy. *British Journal of Psychiatry*, **177**: 117–22.

Ogden P, Minton K, and Pain C (2006). *Trauma and the Body: A Sensorimotor Approach to Psychotherapy*. WW Norton & Co: New York.

Schore A (2012). *The Science of the Art of Psychotherapy*. WW Norton & Co: New York.

Siegel DJ and Solomon M (eds) (2013). *Healing Moments in Psychotherapy*. WW Norton & Co: New York.

Psychiatric specialties: medical psychotherapies, applications, and research

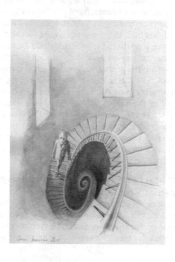

General adult psychiatry: medical psychotherapies, applications, and research

History of medical psychotherapy

(See ➔ Medical psychotherapy: what is it? in Chapter 1, pp. 2–8.)

Medical psychotherapy was only described as 'medical' psychotherapy for the first time in 2010. In obtaining a Certificate of Completion of Training (CCT) today, Medical Psychotherapy is the title on the GMC Specialist Register. The reasons for this change of name from being a Psychotherapy Faculty in the Royal College of Psychiatrists to becoming a Medical Psychotherapy Faculty are connected with asserting the medical identity of the psychiatrist whose distinct training in medicine and psychiatry offers a unique foundation for bridging the gap between psychology and psychiatry.

The culture from the 1950s, 1960s, and 1970s of psychotherapy offered in psychiatry was predominantly of psychoanalysts. However, in the last three decades, there has been a development of an array of therapies which have been launched from the mother ships of psychoanalysis, CBT, and systemic therapy, many of these therapies described in this book. The psychotherapy training undertaken by psychiatrists in the 1970s was a development within general adult psychiatry in the newly formed Royal College of Psychiatrists in 1971. Many of the psychoanalytically trained psychiatrists went into specialist NHS psychotherapy settings, such as the Tavistock Clinic in London, which meant the integration of therapeutic thinking in mainstream psychiatry was impoverished by fewer therapeutically trained psychiatrists remaining in quotidian psychiatry.

There are many notable exceptions of psychoanalysts and psychoanalytic psychotherapists remaining in mainstream psychiatry, and it is their contribution which has built the most significant foundation for the applications of medical psychotherapy, which include both providing therapeutic thinking in day-to-day acute and community psychiatry in practice and also in offering a different vantage point on the mind from organic psychiatry in the UK. The CBTs have tended to become more integrated in mainstream psychiatry, though the model remains one associated with clinical psychology in the UK, again with notable exceptions of medical psychotherapists at the research vanguard where CBT has tended to be on the whole more active until recent years than psychoanalytic evidence. The systems therapies have tended to be reserved for family work within child and adolescent psychiatry, but with important developments into organizational consultancy.

General adult psychiatry roots of medical psychotherapy

General adult psychiatry is the ultimate foundation for medical psychotherapy with the longest history dating back to the days of origins of the Bethlem Royal Hospital (Bedlam) in 1247. The word 'general' in the current description of the specialty of adult psychiatry is misleading, as it implies non-specialist. It refers, however, to the all encompassing nature of the patient population of general adult psychiatrists, between the ages of 18 and 65. All problems of life and mind present to the general adult psychiatrist.

There was an epoch in which it might have been said that schizophrenia was the clinical heartland of adult psychiatry, but this is no longer the case. Whilst psychosis may be at the eye of the clinical storm, the broader non-psychotic problems of people with personality disorder have become the daily bread of psychiatry. This diagnostic tension, between deciding who is and who is not psychotic, who can be treated with antipsychotic medication and who should be managed with applications of therapeutic thinking, managing splitting, or referred for psychological treatment, to a personality disorder service or specialized therapeutic setting, are a leitmotif of the decision-making process for the adult psychiatrist.

There has been a cultural shift in adult psychiatry away from a language of phenomenology towards a language of risk. The shibboleths of the 1980s were 'care in the community', 'close the asylum', and a vague subversive anti-psychiatry debate about the restrictive and dehumanizing aspects of the old with an idealized view of the possibilities of a non-medical model. The realities of closing the asylums, some of which have now become housing estates, is that care in the community has not been as caring or as effective as once was hoped. The inevitable demands for increased containment in the patient without the security of the walls, because of limited beds in the brick mother, have meant that the shibboleths of the twenty-first century are 'risk' and 'responsibility' and 'moving the service user on'.

This shift from phenomenology to risk in psychiatry has gone hand in hand with a reduction of time with the patient, as increasing pressure on teams, with increasing turnover of patients and professionals, has contributed to a challenge to the ontology of the psychiatrist, whose function can be reduced to that of prescriber in the team, their social and psychological functions withering as they are painted into a biological corner which reduces the medical model to a solely organic perspective of mental illness. Psychotherapy or psychological treatments in general adult psychiatry are now the preserve of others, not the general adult psychiatrist. The identification of a patient who might benefit from some form of therapeutic intervention would usually lead to a referral to a service offering a range of time-limited therapies. The shibboleth of moving the service user on has also influenced psychotherapies.

The risk of not having time or training to offer psychotherapy means that the general adult psychiatrist can come to feel ill-equipped to deal with that large population of people with personality pathology, who, since the influential Department of Health document *Personality Disorder: No Longer a Diagnosis of Exclusion* (2003), present and do not benefit from medication alone. A tension here can be played out in trying to fit round pins in square holes, as psychiatrists inevitably look in their toolkit and, finding a hammer, continue to see nails where there are screws. The diagnoses of bipolar affective disorder, depressive disorder, or treatment-resistant depression are the moving diagnostic feast of the smorgasbord of disturbance demanding to be legitimized with an illness worthy of a psychotropic. People with personality disorder may no longer be excluded from services, but they recognize the diagnosis excludes them in a different way, as they are not perceived as ill legitimate patients, becoming illegitimate patients who do not belong. There is therefore a pressure to receive a diagnosis of illness and to be validated in being mentally ill, a strange cultural inversion of the shame of stigma when people sought to hide and deny mental illness.

As a response to securing a place and identity in the diversity of the multidisciplinary team, some psychiatrists have embraced new ways of working, becoming a pair of psychiatric hands in the team, rather than leaders. This has had the effect for some of reducing their contribution to a narrow brain-spotter caricature, in which their utility is in diagnosing and treating psychosis, rather than in fostering a culture in which medicine in mind is part of a whole person understanding in the context of a social, cultural, and economic perspective, without which psychiatry becomes a technical, weakly neurological, and marginal impoverished profession. Hence, it is unattractiveness to doctors and the recruitment crisis facing psychiatry today. One of the important aspects of psychotherapy in psychiatry is to challenge the reductionism of psychiatry to hold recognition of relationships and reflection where there is a valency towards risk and restriction.

Psychotherapy experience in training psychiatrists
(See ➲ Training in Medical psychotherapy: what is it? in Chapter 1, pp. 2–8; Balint groups in Chapter 10, pp. 484–96.)

In their training, psychiatrists are exposed to psychotherapy in Balint groups in their first year and in seeing a couple of therapy cases, one a shorter therapy case, up to 20 sessions in any model, and one longer case over 20 sessions in any model. The aim of this psychotherapy experience is not to train psychiatrists to become psychotherapists, but to train them to become therapeutically minded psychiatrists. The experience of seeing someone in psychotherapy is not about developing a detailed technical understanding of the theory and practice of the model, but aims to foster an experience of a relationship with a patient in which the psychiatrist can get beyond the desire to treat and can begin to learn to listen. Psychotherapy is sometimes called a talking cure, after the first psychoanalytic patient of Freud's colleague Josef Breuer gave it this name, though the patient Anna O also called it chimney sweeping. We no longer need as many chimney sweeps these days, and the term talking cure is equally anachronistic, as it is primarily about listening and not about cure. A better description of psychotherapy than talking cure might be *listening curiosity*.

Psychiatry as a cross-bearing
The psychiatrist and psychoanalyst Tom Main wrote of psychiatry as a cross-bearing. What he did not mean was bearing the cross in the religious sense with its echo of Christ, though he may have intended to leave this ambiguity in the phrase. He was using cross-bearing in the nautical sense of being at sea and taking one's bearings using different ways of thinking from different directions as guides in a storm.

Main wrote in 1967, 'The general psychiatrist, without being an expert in any, needs a wide range of fairly good skills derived from three viewpoints, for in his professional work he will meet with a variety of disorders, upsets of material process, biological and behavioural reactions to disturbances in the human environment and internal psychical disturbances. He will need training in these viewpoints by several experts who will aim to make him, not a material scientist, or a biologist or a psychoanalyst, but a *psychiatrist* who can apply all three viewpoints appropriately to the particular setting in which he works. Like a sailor who needs to seek not only bearings but cross-bearings to find out the truth, he will welcome material science, biology and psychoanalysis, as offering three different but non-contradictory viewpoints yielding different kinds of truth, with each always available and legitimate. Sometimes one viewpoint will be important for him, sometimes another. Which one will be decided not only by the enthusiasms of his teachers but by the facts before him. The most we can hope for is that he should be trained to notice them.'

In the language of research, Main is arguing for a position of equipoise, in which a balanced capacity in the psychiatrist to have a mind of their own but value different contributions is proposed. Main's outline of the stance of the psychiatrist precludes the quotidian problem of none of the available theories or treatment paradigms offering a resolution for chronic and irreparable mental pain.

Psychiatry as bearing limitation
The underlying theme in the work of the general adult psychiatrist today is one of a silent leadership in subversion of the shibboleth of 'moving the patient on' and sometimes painfully bearing patients who cannot be accommodated in any framework of remediation in which their chronic and enduring disturbance can be mitigated. In these cases, the other unspoken meaning of Main's ambiguous use of the phrase cross-bearing applies.

Medical psychotherapy practice
In keeping with its roots in general adult psychiatry, there is no single model of therapy which defines medical psychotherapy. In practice, the three main modalities are psychoanalytic, CBT, and systemic therapy, and, of these, most psychiatrists tend to major in psychoanalytic psychotherapy, as reflected in the GMC quality assurance small specialties thematic review of medical psychotherapy in 2012 which showed that, of the 48 trainees in post at that time, 46 majored in psychoanalytic psychotherapy and two in CBT. Medical psychotherapists vary from being focused solely on one model of therapy to being more towards the eclectic. However, medical psychotherapy trainings, unlike clinical psychology trainings, are not usually eclectic in nature, tending to focus on one therapeutic model, whilst also ensuring an ability to assess for, and deliver, at least two other models. This allows for cross-bearing in using the different therapeutic lenses of medical psychotherapy.

What do medical psychotherapists do?
(See ➲ What does the medical psychotherapist do? in Chapter 1, pp. 5–6.)

Because it is a broad church, there is a welcome diversity in what medical psychotherapists do, but what they usually have in common is an active therapeutic practice which acts as the hub of a variety of spokes of other functions and roles which include:

- Medical Psychotherapy Tutor leading the Royal College of Psychiatrists core psychotherapy training in psychiatry
- Training Programme Director leading the Royal College of Psychiatrists advanced medical psychotherapy scheme
- Leading a specialist therapeutic service
- Leading a personality disorder or tier 4 service
- Leading a complex case consultation service
- Medical management role
- Trainer on multidisciplinary psychotherapy courses
- Supervisor of various professions and levels
- Medical psychotherapy applications (see next section).

Medical psychotherapy applications

Direct therapeutic applications

The notion of 'a therapeutic application' stems from describing the therapy offered to patients itself as one application, such as five times weekly psychoanalysis, which can be applied in a translated form in other settings, e.g. as psychoanalytically informed, less intensive therapies in once-weekly or twice-weekly form which are more typical of NHS practice. To offer the spokes of indirect therapeutic work, the hub of direct active therapeutic practice is necessary to inform and keep alive the model of therapy in its applied form.

Indirect therapeutic applications

(See ➋ Consultation in Chapter 4, pp. 145–51; Reflective practice groups in Chapter 10, pp. 497–505.)

When a theoretical model of therapy is offered outside the direct provision of therapy, this can take many forms, such as consultation and reflective practice, and the principle informing the application is that the primary task is different from the task of therapy but derives principles from therapy to assist in the task.

Relationship with psychiatry

As it is derived from psychiatry, and medical psychotherapists are trained as psychiatrists, they have an understanding of the challenges of the task of psychiatry, but more importantly they have a feel for the ontology and role of the general adult psychiatrist. This relationship, embodied in the advanced dual medical psychotherapy training with general adult psychiatry, reflects one particular way in which medical psychotherapists can maintain and develop psychotherapeutic psychiatry. They can do so through consultation, training, and offering Balint groups for advanced trainees in psychiatry and consultant psychiatrists.

Training in medical psychotherapy

The history of medical psychotherapy training has been closely linked with extinction anxiety. The worry that medical psychotherapy posts were being lost led to anxiety that psychotherapy would disappear from psychiatry. The introduction of dual medical psychotherapy training with general adult psychiatry in Yorkshire in 2008, and since then in other parts of the UK as well, and its ratification by the GMC as a CCT in 2012, has meant that there is a greater sense that psychotherapy has a chance not only of surviving, but thriving within psychiatry. Dual training can be integrated with the psychotherapy and psychiatry trainings in parallel, e.g. with one specialty being a major for 2 years, then the other for 2 years, and spending the fifth year in an area relevant to future career aspirations. Some dual trainees seek to work in acute psychiatry settings, such as inpatient wards, early intervention in psychosis or liaison psychiatry, whilst others want to work as medical psychotherapists.

The single CCT in medical psychotherapy is a vehicle for psychiatrists who want to specialize in psychotherapy and not work at the interface with general adult or other psychiatric subspecialties. The advantage of single CCT training is that it allows an immersion in the psychotherapeutic experience in a more limited time frame of 3 years, whereas the dual training over 5 years allows more time, but this is with therapeutic time spread out and in dialogue with the acute and chronic emotional demands of psychiatry training.

Personal therapy is a requirement of psychoanalytic training as a major, and this can be as much as a full five times weekly analysis for some trainees. This is usually partially, rather than fully, funded by the trainee's local Deanery and/or Trust, as the personal investment in therapy, as well as its value for training, means that the commitment should be reflected out of the pocket, as well as the heart. For trainees in other models of therapy, alternative vehicles of self-reflective development must be negotiated with their Training Programme Director.

The GMC requirement that only psychiatrists with a CCT in medical psychotherapy can lead core psychotherapy training means that consultant posts will be available, and it is further specified in the Royal College of Psychiatrists curriculum that the consultant should be providing a clinical service. This is so they are practising what they teach and also means the medical psychotherapist does not write the obituary of their specialty by only teaching it and becoming less and less credible, as an increasing distance from meaningful contact with patients corrodes their clinical acumen.

Medical psychotherapy research

(See ➋ Research in psychotherapy in Chapter 11, pp. 508–26.)

Within the body of medical psychotherapists, there are individuals who have contributed to developing the evidence base for therapy and have also developed new models of therapy. The three mother models—the CBT evidence base, the psychoanalytic evidence base, and the systemic therapy evidence base—have all been informed by medical psychotherapists. However, in recent years, as with the delivery of psychological therapies, the field of psychotherapy research has become increasingly dominated by psychologists who are conversant with the language of research methodology and trained from an early stage to conduct empirical research. Many medical psychotherapists, however, may feel inadequately equipped to design and implement research studies, or sceptical of the mantra of 'evidence-based treatments', which may not appear to reflect their clinical practice or the needs and choice of their patients. Further work is needed to both prioritize research teaching and experience in the training of medical psychotherapists and to meaningfully engage practising medical psychotherapists in empirical research by harnessing the therapeutic curiosity and passion in their everyday work, so that evidence-based practice may become practice-based evidence.

Recommended reading

Department of Health (2003). *Personality Disorder: No Longer a Diagnosis of Exclusion. Policy Implementation for the Development of Services for People with Personality Disorder.*

General Medical Council. *Small Specialties Thematic Review: Quality Assurance Report for Medical Psychotherapy 2011–2012.* Available at: % http://www.gmc-uk.org/Medical_psychotherapy_ _report__FINAL.pdf_51696150.pdf.

Main T (1989). Psychoanalysis as a cross-bearing. In: *The Ailment and Other Psychoanalytic Essays.* Free Association Books: London.

Royal College of Psychiatrists and Royal College of General Practitioners (2008). *College Report CR151: Psychological Therapies in Psychiatry and Primary Care.*

Royal College of Psychiatrists (2006). *Council Report CR139: Role of the Consultant Psychiatrist in Psychotherapy.*

Forensic psychiatry: forensic psychotherapies, applications, and research

The field of *forensic psychotherapy* is a relatively recently created discipline that can be broadly defined as the application of psychological understanding to the assessment, management, and treatment of mentally disordered offenders. It emerged from the adaptation and application of the psychoanalytic body of knowledge to the related disciplines of psychiatry, psychology, criminology, sociology, and ethology. Forensic psychotherapy's emphasis is on psychoanalytic psychotherapy, although other modalities of psychotherapy are increasingly included under the rubric of forensic psychotherapy today.

In the UK, the roots of forensic psychotherapy grew from the pioneering efforts of psychoanalytically trained psychiatrists who were mostly working in the public health sector in forensic mental health or the prison system. Some, such as Arthur Hyatt-Williams, Murray Cox, and Leslie Sohn, worked in prisons and secure hospitals; others worked in outpatient settings, notably the Portman Clinic in London, an NHS outpatient clinic that provides psychoanalytically informed treatments for violence, criminality, delinquency, and sexual deviancy. Initially founded in 1931, the Portman Clinic had on its staff prominent psychoanalysts, such as Edward Glover, John Bowlby, and Wilfred Bion, and became a centre for training forensic practitioners in psychoanalytic thinking, with notable contributions from Mervyn Glasser, Adam Limentani, Estela Welldon, and Donald Campbell.

These psychoanalysts, working first-hand with violent and antisocial patients, laid the foundations for the field of forensic psychotherapy. The discipline has rapidly expanded over the last 30 years to produce a multitude of clinicians from many different core professional backgrounds, including psychiatry, psychology, social work, art and music therapy, nursing, and probation, working in a variety of inpatient and community forensic settings. Forensic psychotherapy has also been heavily influenced by group psychoanalytic and TC ideas and practice (see ➔ Group therapy and group analysis in Chapter 2, pp. 42–7, and in Chapter 5, pp. 188–94; Therapeutic communities in Chapter 2, pp. 75–80, and in Chapter 5, pp. 243–50.)

In 1991, the International Association for Forensic Psychotherapy (IAFP) was founded, bringing together a growing group of professionals, trainees, volunteers, experts by experience, and others with an interest in the psychodynamic understanding of offending and its treatment from a variety of countries, including the UK, Germany, Austria, Italy, the Netherlands, Sweden, New Zealand, and the USA. In 1995, the first Consultant Psychiatrist in Forensic Psychotherapy was appointed in the UK at Broadmoor High Secure Hospital, and, in 1999, forensic psychotherapy was approved by the GMC and Royal College of Psychiatrists in the UK to become a formal subspecialty of higher psychiatric training. The Forensic Psychotherapy Special Interest Group (SIG) was established within the Royal College of Psychiatrists in 2007 and aims to promote practice, training, and research in forensic psychotherapy within psychiatry and other disciplines.

Principles of forensic psychotherapy

Forensic psychotherapy is based on psychodynamic principles and is primarily concerned with: (a) understanding both the conscious and unconscious aspects of all forms of antisocial behaviour and criminal offending, and (b) offering treatment to offenders in the context of their individual history and personality development. A central tenet of forensic psychotherapy is that violence and antisocial behaviour are not senseless, incomprehensible acts, but are communications that are meaningful, although the meaning may not be obvious or conscious to either the perpetrator or the victim. Forensic psychotherapy promotes the exploration of the meaning and significance of offence behaviours, focusing on the internal world of the offender, whilst taking account of the interactions and influence of the external world, both past and present.

Forensic psychotherapy differs from the dyadic nature of traditional psychotherapy where the relationship between the patient and therapist offers a private confidential space. In forensic psychotherapy, there are always at least three parties—the patient, the therapist, and some form of representation of the criminal justice system (e.g. police, the courts, probation). This triangulation necessarily brings in a third into the patient/therapist dyad, which alters notions of confidentiality, disclosure, risk, and containment. If handled well, this can be thought of psychodynamically as the bringing in of a third perspective or paternal function (in contrast to the more maternal function of the therapist), to form a 'parental couple' who may think about the patient in a helpful way. This parallels the way in which a good parental couple will promote the best interests of their child, an experience that is lacking in many forensic patients who have childhood histories of neglect, abuse, and abandonment.

Forensic psychotherapy also includes contributions to theory and practice in the management and dynamics of institutions where offenders live and work with the professionals who have to balance duties of care and custody. Other areas in which the forensic psychotherapist may be involved and offer a particular viewpoint include risk assessment and medico-legal work. Forensic psychotherapists are increasingly active in both criminal and family courts where judges often welcome a more nuanced psychodynamic understanding of the defendant's behaviour linked to their personality and history, rather that the terse conclusion common to traditional forensic psychiatric court reports that 'there is no evidence of mental illness'.

What does the forensic psychotherapist do?

As there are few specialist institutions which provide forensic psychotherapy such as the Portman Clinic, most forensic psychotherapists work in mainstream forensic services, including high secure institutions and prisons, medium secure units, and community forensic teams. As the forensic psychotherapist works primarily from a psychodynamic perspective to facilitate the understanding and management of the forensic patient, this may raise tensions within services that offer predominantly CBTs and may be unfamiliar with, or even antagonistic to, a psychodynamic approach. The forensic psychotherapist must therefore have the capacity to work as part of a multidisciplinary team where a variety of modalities of treatment are offered.

The forensic psychotherapist can contribute to the therapeutic work in forensic institutions in a variety of ways. Direct clinical work may involve the assessment of patients to see if they might benefit from psychotherapeutic treatment, or to provide a formulation to assist in the patient's overall therapeutic and risk management plan. The forensic psychotherapist may also be involved in treating patients in individual therapy, or in running psychotherapy groups. Supervisory work is also important, with the forensic psychotherapist supervising therapists and trainees who are providing psychodynamic therapy to patients, as well as clinicians who are using other treatment modalities. The forensic psychotherapist may also be available to speak to individual nurses about their patients, to regularly attend ward rounds and case conferences, and to participate in the discussions about the treatment and progress of patients.

One of the most important types of work which the forensic psychotherapist can provide is institutional supervision or consultation (see ➔ Psychotherapeutic understanding of organizational processes in Chapter 10, pp. 471–5). This involves thinking about the forensic setting in its entirety and offering a psychodynamic overview which addresses the complex dynamics provoked within staff groups and institutions by the disturbed patients that they contain. Forensic patients will often have diagnoses of both psychotic illness and personality disorder and tend to unconsciously employ primitive defence mechanisms that distort their perception of the world and interactions with others, including the staff looking after them. The latter may unwittingly become the recipients of the patients' projections and unconsciously respond by mobilizing unhelpful defensive reactions, which may diminish the therapeutic potential of the treatment offered and erode the containing environment.

A key role of the forensic psychotherapist is therefore to facilitate and promote reflective forums, such as reflective practice groups (see ➲ Reflective practice groups in Chapter 10, pp. 497–505), in which staff can come together in a non-threatening and creative way to think about their conscious and unconscious emotional reactions to patients and how these are enacted within the organization. The Royal College of Psychiatrists recommends that all secure services, as part of the quality standards, should have access to an accredited psychotherapist with a psychodynamic or psychoanalytic training and forensic experience once a month as a minimum who is available to support assessment, supervision, consultation, training, and reflective practice.

Forensic psychotherapies for offender patients

(See ➲ Psychological therapy in secure settings in Chapter 8, pp. 428–39.)

Most psychological interventions available for offenders in the UK derive from a cognitive behavioural paradigm, and are delivered within the Criminal Justice System, rather than the NHS. These include relapse prevention programmes, programmes combining cognitive skills with social skills and problem-solving, such as 'Reasoning and Rehabilitation' and 'Enhanced Thinking Skills', anger and violence management programmes, SOTPs, and treatments for psychopathic individuals on RNR principles. Psychoanalytic or psychodynamically oriented forensic psychotherapies are less commonly available, although there is provision within some prisons and in some secure forensic mental health settings within the NHS in the UK. Community-based psychological therapies for offenders of all modalities are particularly scarce, due, in part, to the difficulties in engaging such individuals in treatment.

Many violent and antisocial individuals do not fulfil conventional suitability criteria for psychoanalytic psychotherapy, such as psychological mindedness and ego strength, so the normal threshold for offering such therapy may need to be lowered. Most forensic psychotherapists working from a psychoanalytic perspective advocate modifications of technique in both the individual and group treatment of violent and antisocial offenders. These include actively fostering the therapeutic alliance by avoiding silence and free association, focusing on affect and interpretations of the 'here and now', rather than interpretations of unconscious conflicts and fantasies or the transference, and using mentalization techniques, such as helping the patient to connect internal states of mind to his behavioural actions. Modifications in technique takes time and skill, and forensic psychotherapists assessing and treating offender patients should have sufficient training, expertise, support, and supervision. Consideration of the setting in which the patient is seen forms an essential part of the treatment in providing adequate containment and risk management, so that specific therapeutic interventions can take place safely.

Group therapy may be the treatment of choice for many violent and antisocial patients, who may feel more contained in a group setting where the multiple transferences offer more than one target for their aggressive and sexual impulses. Engaging in a therapeutic group and seeing one's own difficulties reflected in others can be effective in reducing antisocial behaviour and bring about therapeutic change (see ➲ Group therapy and group analysis in Chapter 2, pp. 42–7, and in Chapter 5, pp. 188–94).

Training

Until very recently, formal specialist training in forensic psychotherapy was limited to medically qualified professionals. Since 1999, after completing core psychiatric training, psychiatrists may do a 5-year advanced dual training in forensic psychotherapy, which integrates training provision in the two psychiatric sub-specialties of medical psychotherapy and forensic psychiatry. Trainees have to meet the competencies for each curriculum of the two sub-specialties to qualify on the Royal College of Psychiatrists' specialist register with two Certificates of Completion of Specialist Training (CCT) recognized by the GMC as a medical psychotherapist and as a forensic psychiatrist. There are currently ten training posts in forensic psychotherapy in the UK.

Until now, there has not been a well-defined clinical training route for non-medical forensic psychotherapists, who historically gained their forensic experience through working in forensic settings and completed parallel psychoanalytic, psychodynamic, or group psychotherapy trainings which did not specialize in forensic work. However, in 2014, the BPC formally approved two new clinical trainings in forensic psychotherapy: the Forensic Psychodynamic Psychotherapy (D59F) at the Tavistock and Portman NHS Foundation Trust; and a similar training offered by the Forensic Psychotherapy Society (FPS) which is a new national organization for the study, development, and application of psychoanalysis and psychodynamic psychotherapy in forensic and complex needs mental health settings. Both courses last 2 years and require trainees to see patients under supervision, as well as having their own personal psychotherapy. For further details, see ℛ http://www.bpc.org.uk.

Research

Forensic psychotherapists may be engaged in many different areas of research specific to their field of interest. Two notable areas are the investigation of the efficacy of psychodynamic therapies in the treatment of offenders and the elucidation of aetiological factors in the genesis of violent and antisocial behaviour from a psychodynamic developmental perspective.

Research in specific psychotherapies for offenders

Forensic psychotherapy has promoted the application of specific therapies to antisocial offenders that have been developed and empirically supported in recent years for the treatment of personality-disordered offenders. DBT has been evaluated for use with women in prisons in England and Wales, and schema-focused therapy has been used to treat distorted antisocial cognitions in personality-disordered offenders as part of a multi-modal treatment programme in the TBS system in the Netherlands (see ➲ Dialectical behavioural therapy in Chapter 2, pp. 63–6, and in Chapter 5, pp. 220–9). Trials of MBT have included patients with ASPD (see ➲ Mentalization-based treatment in Chapter 2, pp. 66–70, and in Chapter 5, pp. 229–34). In a trial comparing MBT with structured clinical management (SCM), which included problem-solving and social skills, MBT was found to be more effective than SCM in patients with ASPD, but the effectiveness of both was reduced when compared with patients without ASPD. MBT for ASPD targets the mentalizing problems thought to underlie violent behaviour through a programme of group and individual psychotherapy. A recent pilot project of MBT for violent men with a diagnosis of ASPD has shown that treatment leads to a reduction in aggressive acts, and plans for a multi-site RCT in the UK are under way.

Studies have also investigated the efficacy of TCs for general offenders in institutional (including prospective and retrospective cohort studies for prisoners treated in the TC at HMP Grendon, UK) and community settings but found little evidence to suggest that TCs were effective for general offenders (see ➔ Therapeutic communities in Chapter 2, pp. 75–80, and in Chapter 5, pp. 243–50). These studies have been criticized for their weak design. Subsequently, three well-designed RCTs have been conducted in institutional settings, evaluating the evidence for TCs in substance misuse offenders, which all found a relatively large reduction in re-offending. These findings have led to the conclusion by NICE that TCs are only effective for ASPD and offender populations if they are targeted specifically at those individuals with co-morbid drug misuse (NICE, 2009), and that there is insufficient evidence to apply these findings to TCs targeting general offenders who do not abuse substances. However, given that many of the previous studies were based on weak methodology, it is premature to suggest that the TCs are ineffective. Enthusiasm for this therapeutic model persists, and, in the UK, there are currently plans to extend the availability of TC treatment of high-risk offenders in prisons as part of the National Personality Disorder Offender Strategy (see ➔ Psychological therapy in secure settings in Chapter 8, pp. 428–39).

The developmental roots of violent and antisocial behaviour
(See ➔ Violence and aggression in Chapter 6, pp. 304–8.)

In recent years, there has been much interest in the genetic contribution to antisocial behaviour, particularly in those children showing 'callous and unemotional traits', thought to be the precursors of psychopathy in adulthood. Aggressive and antisocial behaviour in such children shows a strong heritability, suggesting that such behaviour is 'hard-wired' into the brain from an early age. However, recent sophisticated adoption studies demonstrate significant gene environment interactions and evidence that children who are genetically vulnerable to behaving in an antisocial manner are also more likely to suffer from harsh and inconsistent parenting.

There is increasing empirical evidence to support the hypothesis that ASPD is a developmental disorder rooted in attachment pathology (see ➔ Theories of personality development: attachment theory in Chapter 8, pp. 380–1). There is now a considerable evidence base of studies showing higher levels of insecure attachment in violent offenders than in the normal population. This evidence is supported by studies which show that offenders in prison or secure forensic institutions are more likely to report having experienced separations, abuse, and neglect from their early caregivers than in the general population.

Moreover, emerging evidence that links psychopathic tendencies in children with disorganized attachment relationships, maladaptive interactive patterns in families, and severe institutional deprivation challenges the view that constitutional factors are dominant in the development of psychopathy.

Recommended reading

Cordess C and Cox M (eds) (1996). *Forensic Psychotherapy: Crime, Psychodynamics and the Offender Patient.* Jessica Kingsley: London and Philadelphia.

McGauley G, Yakeley J, Williams A, and Bateman A (2011). Attachment, mentalization and antisocial personality disorder; the possible contribution of mentalization-based treatment. *European Journal of Psychotherapy and Counselling,* **13**, 1–22.

Welldon E (2012). *Playing with Dynamite: A Personal Approach to the Psychoanalytic Understanding of Perversions, Violence and Criminality.* Karnac: London.

Yakeley J (2010). *Working with Violence: A Contemporary Psychoanalytic Approach.* Palgrave Macmillan: London.

Yakeley J and Adshead G (2013). Locks, keys and security of mind: psychodynamic approaches to forensic psychiatry. *Journal of the American Academy of Psychiatry and the Law,* **41**, 38–45.

Child and adolescent psychiatry: child and adolescent psychotherapies, applications, and research

Historical links

Child and adolescent psychiatry in the UK is a relatively new speciality. It has developed from a variety of rich sources of thinking, research, and clinical practice, including many links to psychoanalytic psychotherapy. Historically, child and adolescent psychiatry grew from the child guidance movement in the 1920s and 1930s; these were clinics staffed by three key disciplines: social workers, psychologists, and child and adolescent psychiatrists.

John Bowlby (see ➔ Psychoanalytic psychotherapy in Chapter 2, pp. 25–8; Theories of personality development: attachment theory in Chapter 8, pp. 380–1) was a key figure in the history of child development research. He studied psychology, worked with deprived young people, and later became an adult psychiatrist and psychoanalyst. He was deeply influenced by Anna Freud's work with children separated from their parents during the Second World War. Bowlby developed the theory of attachment and held that children's real experiences were as important as their internal world phantasies.

Another link to psychoanalysis was Donald Winnicott (see ➔ Psychoanalytic psychotherapy in Chapter 2, pp. 25–8), who first trained as a paediatrician and then as a psychoanalyst. He advocated that child psychiatrists should follow the same route in their training. His influential ideas included the '*good enough mother*' which refers to the 'ordinary devoted mother'—an example of the way in which the foundations of health are laid down by the ordinary mother in her ordinary loving care of her own baby. Winnicott wrote about the '*transitional object*' (security blanket or teddy), the '*holding environment*', and *play* as important aspects of child development. He also wrote about the 'anti-social tendency', not as something intrinsic within a child, but rather as a child's expression of having needs that were not being met in their family, thus often leading the child to search outside the home to find the missing stability.

Other important contributions to child and adolescent psychiatry in the UK came from adolescent inpatient units. These were often run as TCs and offered longer-term, containing experiences to disturbed adolescents and their families (see ➜ Therapeutic communities in Chapter 2, pp. 75–80, and in Chapter 5, pp. 243–50).

In the 1960s and 1970s, family therapy (see ➜ Systemic family and couple therapy in Chapter 2, pp. 34–42, and in Chapter 5, pp. 184–8) became a highly stimulating arena. A number of social workers, child and adolescent psychiatrists, and other clinicians became fully trained family therapists. Many of the early founders in family therapy had psychoanalytic backgrounds, including the Milan group (Palazzoli and colleagues) and Salvador Minuchin, who developed structural family therapy. Other influences included cybernetics and systems theory from the USA and British object relations ideas.

As the research base developed in genetics, a keen interest grew in the heritability of mental illness and developmental difficulties. In the 1980s and 1990s, Michael Rutter's research, a more epidemiological and biologically based approach, became influential. As genetic knowledge grew, so did ideas about how genetic contributions to a child's temperament became accepted, and the idea of *epigenetics*—psychological development as the result of an ongoing, bidirectional interchange between heredity and the environment—became influential.

Current role of the child and adolescent psychiatrist

Child and adolescent psychiatry work is primarily carried out in community CAMHS teams, inpatient units, and some more specialized teams such as early intervention in psychosis, adolescent outreach teams, and paediatric liaison services.

The role of the child and adolescent psychiatrist may be seen most helpfully as holding in mind the multitude of perspectives from which a patient can be viewed: individual, family, school, wider culture/environment, as well as through the lens of biological, psychological, and social aspects. Taking account of these complexities allows a clinician to arrive at a formulation about where the problem/s lie. Following this assessment process, consideration can be given to the best form of treatment—this may involve physical input, such as medication or OT, psychological input (individual, family, or group work), or assistance in placing the young person in the right environment (e.g. home or school). The role of the psychiatrist also includes keeping up-to-date with the evidence base for treatment, as well as developing one's own internal understanding of 'what works for whom'—and in what circumstances. Decisions about treatment have to be made depending on the availability of local resources, and child and adolescent psychiatrists should engage with leadership and service development in order to ensure the best allocation of resources.

Despite the shift to a more biological focus in child and adolescent psychiatry, many of the traditional psychotherapy skills, in applied form, remain relevant and useful. For instance, the 'holding' function of containing the anxiety of parents is often a key task for the child and adolescent psychiatrist, as is the ability to listen and simply 'be with' parents who are coming to terms with a diagnosis. These parents may need time and space to process the diagnosis, accept the child that they do have, and mourn the child that they expected to have but did not get.

Child and adolescent psychiatrists need to be able to discuss difficult situations such as parents who scapegoat a child or who may have little reflective capacity and use their child as a container for their own projections or to meet their own emotional needs. The child and adolescent psychiatrist needs to be able to withstand the parent's almost inevitable initial rejection and anger at the suggestion of these ideas. Child and adolescent psychiatrists also need to be able to tolerate thinking about the significant harm that children may have experienced, whether neglect, or physical, emotional, or sexual abuse. To be able to not turn a blind eye, to take forward safeguarding concerns, whilst still working with a family, is a challenging task that tests the emotional resilience of the clinician.

Child and adolescent psychiatrists may undertake further study in therapy, e.g. family therapy (see ➔ Systemic family and couple therapy in Chapter 2, pp. 34–42, and in Chapter 5, pp. 184–8), psychodynamic psychotherapy (see ➔ Psychoanalytic psychotherapy in Chapter 2, pp. 20–30, and in Chapter 5, pp. 163–72), CBT (see ➔ Cognitive behavioural therapy in Chapter 2, pp. 30–4, and in Chapter 5, pp. 172–84), or MBT (see ➔ Mentalization-based treatment in Chapter 2, pp. 66–70, and in Chapter 5, pp. 229–34), or they may become interested in academic research. The majority of child and adolescent psychiatrists will work in a community setting where the focus is on meeting with families and dealing with the distress/problems they bring, collaborating with the family, the multidisciplinary team, and the wider network of school, social care, and other professionals to determine how help can best be offered.

Ideally, a wide range of treatments should be available for a young person, with treatment being targeted at where the problem lies, i.e. if the conditions of development have caused a child to remain stuck in one of the earlier psychosexual stages, or if a child has suffered a severe trauma (e.g. physical, emotional, or sexual abuse), then child psychotherapy focusing on his/her inner world and unconscious difficulties may be needed. If the problem is located more generally in family relationships, then family therapy should be provided. For children whose difficulties are internal but more available to their conscious mind, CBT (see ➔ Cognitive behavioural therapy in Chapter 2, pp. 30–4, and in Chapter 5, pp. 30–4), IPT (see ➔ Interpersonal therapy in Chapter 2, pp. 52–5, and in Chapter 5, pp. 203–7), or supportive counselling CBT (see ➔ Counselling in Chapter 2, pp. 91–94, and in Chapter 5, pp. 274–81) in a school setting are likely to be effective, particularly for children who have had ordinary good care in their early life and good attachment relationships.

Parent–infant psychotherapy

This is a fairly recent therapeutic treatment which recognizes that the early interactive experiences of a child and its caregivers are at the heart of a child's developmental trajectory. Treatment models bring together findings from developmental psychology, neuroscience research, attachment theory/research, and the psychoanalytic tradition of infant observation.

The development of secure attachments depends on parents/carers recognizing and understanding their baby's behaviour, containing their baby's feelings, and responding in a sensitive and timely manner to their baby's needs. In attachment research, this capacity is known as *reflective function*. Many factors can impair the capacity for reflective function in parents (e.g. mental illness, high anxiety, low mood, lack of support, socio-economic pressures). The risk is that a preoccupied or distressed parent will be less able to tune into, and respond to, the baby's needs (see ➔ Theories of personality development: attachment theory in Chapter 8, pp. 380–1).

Parent–infant psychotherapy involves having the parent and infant in the consulting room together, the relationship being seen as 'the patient'. Parents with traumatic pasts may find that the arrival of a baby stirs up unresolved feelings that 'haunt' them and interfere with the bonding process. The therapist will explore these 'ghosts' from the parent's past, hoping that understanding will bring resolution. The aim is to free the baby from displaced projections from the parent's past.

The therapeutic focus may shift to here-and-now behavioural interactions with the baby which are used to feed back the observable effects that a parent has on a child (and vice versa). Drawing parents' attention to the detail of their dynamics with their baby can encourage greater parental curiosity and sensitivity to the child's emotional experience which, in turn, facilitates more timely and appropriate responses from the parent such as holding, soothing, etc. Of particular importance is attention to the baby's repertoire of attachment-seeking behaviours. For example, does the baby who bumps his head communicate his distress effectively by crying, or does the baby stay quiet, having learnt it is safer to deal with distress on its own? The therapist will highlight the parent's repertoire of attachment-giving behaviours, i.e. noticing the baby's need for comfort, using physical touch, voice, and gaze. The therapist will also note when parents minimize or reject the baby's need for help. It is in the subtle detail of parent–infant interactions that a baby's attachment style develops.

Attachment and mentalization

(See ➔ Theories of personality development: attachment theory in Chapter 8, pp. 380–1; Mentalization-based treatment in Chapter 2, pp. 66–70.)

It has been postulated that, as children grow and develop, they will continue to have a similar attachment style as seen in babyhood. Attachment styles are categorized as: secure, insecure avoidant, insecure anxious, and disorganized, according to the child's reactions in Mary Ainsworth's *strange situation procedure*, in which the child is observed playing for 20 minutes and caregivers and strangers enter and leave the room. Linked to the understanding of attachment style is the idea of the capacity of an individual to reflect on their own mental state. Securely attached individuals find it easier to undertake this, whilst insecurely attached people, in particular when their area of difficulty with attachment becomes stimulated, find it much harder to have reflective capacity or the ability to mentalize, and they tend to lose the reflective capacity they do have when feeling emotionally overwhelmed. MBT has developed from these ideas. Originally used for adults, there is now evidence beginning to accumulate that MBT is helpful for adolescents as well.

Child and adolescent psychotherapy

For children with complex, unconscious difficulties, as a result of experiences of trauma or abuse, child and adolescent psychotherapy may be indicated. The first recorded treatment of a child being given a form of psychotherapy is of Freud's account of 'Little Hans', a child who had a phobia of horses. Freud understood that Han's symptoms represented something more complicated, i.e. Hans' Oedipal feelings towards his father. Freud treated the child indirectly, by helping Han's father to understand what Little Hans was experiencing internally and unconsciously (see ➜ The Oedipus complex in Chapter 2, p. 22).

Anna Freud (Freud's daughter) and Melanie Klein (see ➜ Key contributors in Psychoanalytic psychotherapy in Chapter 2, pp. 25–8) developed the psychoanalytic theoretical ideas from which child psychoanalysis and child psychotherapy grew. Child psychotherapy works with children by examining their inner world through play. For instance, a child may express violent feelings with toy animals or by tearing up carefully made drawings. The therapist puts words to the feelings being expressed through behaviour and play, building the child's capacity to understand and link feelings with actions and enabling him or her to feel understood and contained. It helps a child to be with an understanding 'other' who can bear the intensity of what is being expressed. The aim is for a child to be able to make sense of feelings that may be experienced as unmanageable or unknowable. The regularity of therapy and the experience of holiday breaks are all part of the 'frame' of the therapeutic work. Most practitioners, particularly in the NHS, would work with a colleague who would see the parents regularly and whose goal would be to help the parents understand that their child's behaviour is an attempt at communication, and decode the message. In particular, this work aims to help parents contain a child's conscious or unconscious anxieties.

In addition to therapeutic work with individual children and parents, child and adolescent psychotherapists also work within schools, with social care, including foster carers and social workers and may offer group work, consultation to the network and 'state of mind' assessments which are a way of understanding the inner world of a child and the child's ability to use a therapeutic intervention. The research base for child psychotherapy has been gathering strength and there is evidence for the effectiveness of psychoanalytic therapy for children and young people.

Parent work alongside direct treatment for the young person has been found to be an important aspect in order to achieve a positive outcome. A large multicentre randomized controlled trial is currently underway in the UK evaluating the effectiveness of short term psychoanalytic psychotherapy as a treatment for adolescent depression (see ✍ https://www.ucl.ac.uk/psychoanalysis/research/impact-me).

Family therapy
(See ➔ Systemic family and couple therapy in Chapter 2, pp. 34–42, and in Chapter 5, pp. 184–8.)

There are a variety of different types of family therapy, but, in the UK, systemic family therapy is the most common. This therapeutic approach locates the problems not within any one person within the family, but in the family system. The focus is often on the present difficulties in communication, and the therapeutic stance is one of positive reframing of difficulties. Where possible, a family therapy team works together, with one therapist in the room with the family, whilst another sits behind a one-way screen observing the process and giving feedback.

A psychodynamic family therapy model is used in some specialist centres and focuses on the way that unconscious feelings and the intergenerational transmission of difficulties can be preventing the family from functioning well in the present.

Consultation and applied work
(See ➔ Consultation in Chapter 4, pp. 145–51.)

In addition to direct work with young people and families, another important way of helping understand the communications of children is based on a consultation model. This is frequently offered to groups of staff in children's homes or adolescent inpatient units, as well as to foster carers, social workers, or teachers who are supporting young people. In this model of applied work, a highly trained therapist can support other professionals to develop their skills and thus disseminate a way of working with children and adolescents that emphasizes that behaviour is communication and facilitates workers in providing not only containment and appropriate boundaries for young people, but also support for staff who may struggle to understand the feelings that disturbed children can elicit in them.

Recommended reading
Bradley E and Emmanuel L (2008). *What Can the Matter Be?: Therapeutic Interventions With Parents, Infants, and Young Children (The Tavistock Clinic Series)*. Karnac Books: London.

Carr A (2014). The evidence base for family therapy and systemic interventions for child-focused problems. *Journal of Family Therapy*, **36**, 107–57.

Fraiberg S, Adelson E, and Shapiro V (1975). Ghosts in the nursery: a psychoanalytic approach to the problems of impaired infant-mother relationships. *Journal of the American Academy of Child Psychiatry*, **14**, 387–421.

Midgley N and Kennedy E (2011). Psychodynamic psychotherapy for children and adolescents: a critical review of the evidence base. *Journal of Child Psychotherapy*, **37**, 1–29.

Rossouw TI and Fonagy P (2012). Mentalization-based treatment for self-harm in adolescents: a randomized controlled trial. *Journal American Academy of Child Adolescent Psychiatry*, **51**, 1304–13.

Psychiatry of intellectual disability: psychotherapies, applications, and research

(See ⬀ Intellectual disability in Chapter 7, pp. 368–71.)

Psychiatrists working with people who have a learning disability need to have a wide range of clinical skills, as this population have higher rates of mental health problems than the general population, because they experience more biological and psychosocial risk factors. People with intellectual disability often have concurrent physical problems, such as epilepsy and cerebral palsy, along with communication problems and challenges in accessing services. It is essential to consider the system around the person (such as family, support staff) to understand clinical problems and deliver effective interventions. A wide variety of treatments are available, as in mainstream psychiatry, including pharmacology, psychological (including psychotherapy), social, and educational interventions. Much work has been done in recent years in applying psychotherapeutic and systemic approaches to working with people with learning disability.

Training in psychotherapy for adults with intellectual and developmental disorders

The delivery of various types of psychotherapy to adults with IDDs is mainly provided by clinical psychologists or counsellors specifically employed by community intellectual services in the UK. However, psychiatrists may also be interested in delivering a specific therapy as part of their clinical work. Psychiatrists gain experience in psychotherapy during their core training before they go on to specialize further, and often trainees are encouraged to provide some forms of psychotherapy to persons with IDD, whilst in placement. Such work is supervised either by a psychologist or the consultant psychiatrist clinical trainer. Generally, if a psychiatrist wishes to deliver a psychological therapy, she/he will be required to obtain specialist training, in order to acquire specific skills in the treatment modalities, and can then apply the treatment to different populations, including those with mild to moderate intellectual disability.

Clinical practice

In some instances, e.g. where the person with IDD does not have regular contact with the community intellectual disability services, he or she may be referred to the general practice counselling service or to IAPT services (see ⬀ Improving Access to Psychological Therapies services in Chapter 10, pp. 463–4). Depending on the presenting problem, a low-intensity therapy may lead on to a higher-intensity therapy. In cases where the patients may need to be referred outside the community intellectual disability service, a model of shared care operates whereby either the patient is seen by the specialist service with regular joint reviews or the therapist supervises a professional from the intellectual disability service who then delivers the psychological treatment.

Patients who are identified as being willing to talk about their difficulties and may have a capacity for reflection are referred to the professionals in psychiatry or psychology, with the view of being assessed for commencing psychological therapy. Usually, there are several (up to five) introductory sessions in order to explore the person's understanding of therapy, the setting and format of therapy, and the tasks associated with it. Practicalities to consider include an appraisal of the person's communication skills, his/her commitment to therapy, co-morbid problems such as substance misuse or aggression, attending appointments, and support with homework tasks. Therapies are adapted to simplify language and to include pictorial representations. Patients are usually able to concentrate for the duration of the session, which usually lasts for 60 minutes and often for longer, and therefore the offer of breaks is not necessary, although it is advisable that the therapist keeps this in mind. Setting a framework around acceptable and non-acceptable behaviour during treatment is very important, as is the flexibility around the use of free association which many people with IDD find very difficult to manage. It is recommended that the therapist focuses on the person's reasons for being in therapy and the problems they are experiencing currently. Although the principles of psychodynamic psychotherapy are to be observed, a more direct approach may be more helpful in allowing the person to use the session to reflect on their difficulties and ways in which they can address those (see ➲ Psychoanalytic psychotherapy in Chapter 2, pp. 20–30, and in Chapter 5, pp. 163–72).

Behavioural interventions may be delivered by specially trained behavioural therapists who are either embedded in a community intellectual disability service or are situated in a specialist behaviour service which specifically receives referrals for people who present with challenging behaviour.

The issue of a person with IDD making an informed choice about receiving psychological treatment is an important one and should not be underestimated. Most individuals will be referred by their paid or family carers and thus may have little or no motivation to carry on with the therapy. Therefore, it is essential for the therapists to take time at the beginning to ensure that the person is willing to commit to several weekly sessions and that she/he understands what they will be asked to do during the therapy. A note of how the individual with IDD has responded to questions about consenting to treatment or whether a best interests decision has taken place should be made. In addition, the therapist should provide information about the goals of therapy and how they will be achieved and monitored (see ➲ Consent in Chapter 4, pp. 113–15).

Applications

Several types of psychotherapies have been described for the treatment of people with IDD and mental disorders. CBT and individual psychodynamic counselling are the most widely used, but other treatments, such as mindfulness for challenging behaviour, motivational interviewing for substance misuse, MBT or DBT in those with BPDs, are also available (see ➔ Cognitive behavioural therapy in Chapter 2, pp. 30–4, and in Chapter 5, pp. 172–84; Counselling in Chapter 2, pp. 91–94, and in Chapter 5, pp. 274–81; Mentalization-based treatment in Chapter 2, pp. 66–70, and in Chapter 5, pp. 229–34; Dialectical behaviour therapy in Chapter 2, pp. 63–6, and in Chapter 5, pp. 220–9; Substance misuse in Chapter 7, pp. 338–45; Borderline personality disorder in Chapter 8, pp. 390–6).

For adults with more severe IDD who are likely to lack verbal communication ability and present with challenging behaviour, differential reinforcement of other behaviour (DRO), differential reinforcement of alternate behaviour (DRA) and differential reinforcement of incompatible behaviour (DRI) may promote pro-social behaviour, as well as reducing undesirable behaviours. Positive behaviour support, sensory integration, music therapy, or snoezelen (usually provided in a specially designed multisensory room and facilitated by a therapist) have also been used in this population.

Research evidence

The evidence base for most psychological therapies in people with IDD is limited at best. The best researched treatments are behavioural interventions, followed by individual and group CBT. The literature mostly comprises single case studies and case series. A high proportion of the published studies are uncontrolled, and there is little exploration of other outcomes, such as quality of life, carer burden, or costs. Despite sophisticated meta-analyses which suggest significant effect sizes of these interventions, caution should be exercised in interpreting the findings, given that randomized controlled designs are likely to produce more conservative treatment estimates.

In recent years, there has been an increase in the efforts of the international research community to improve the evidence base of psychological interventions, and this has led to an increasing number of clinical trials of interventions for children and adults with IDD. These studies address methodological problems of previous research, including longer follow-up, investigation of secondary outcomes, and economic evaluation. When people with IDD themselves have been asked about their experience of therapy, both psychodynamic psychotherapy and CBT, they have, in the main, expressed positive views and appear to have made some gains in becoming more resilient and reflective.

Recommended reading

Hassiotis A, Serfaty M, Azam K, et al. (2012). *A Manual of Cognitive Behaviour Therapy for People with Mild Learning Disabilities and Common Mental Disorders.* Available at: ℜ http://www.ucl. ac.uk/psychiatry/cbt/downloads/documents/cbt-id-manual.

Vereenooghe L and Langdon PE (2013). Psychological therapies for people with intellectual disabilities: a systematic review and meta-analysis. *Research in Developmental Disabilities,* **34**, 4085–102.

Willner P, Rose J, Jahoda A, et al. (2013). A cluster randomised controlled trial of a manualised cognitive behavioural anger management intervention delivered by supervised lay therapists to people with intellectual disabilities. *Health Technology Assessment,* **17**, 1–173.

Psychiatry of old age: psychotherapies, applications, and research

(See ➲ Dementia in Chapter 7, pp. 372–6; Later life in Chapter 6, pp. 291–3.)

Clinical practice

Old age psychiatry is not a new specialty. It is, however, a specialty of two parts, in that services are provided separately for dementia and for the so-called 'functional psychiatric disorders'—everything that is not dementia. This separation in practice is never so clearly cut, particularly as cohorts of referrals nowadays include people well into their nineties. Extreme old age may bring with it MCI—a state of decreased memory, but not of function, and not meeting the criteria for a diagnosis of dementia. Psychotherapy with older people, by contrast, is newer but has become firmly established as a rational and expected part of both the assessment as well as the treatment of the older person with mental health problems. Having cognitive impairment is not a barrier to receiving psychological treatment, although frank dementia precludes many different modalities. Creative therapies, such as art, music, and dance movement therapies, are useful in managing some patients in distress who also have an established dementia, although empirical evidence for this is lacking, mainly due to the tiny numbers of people who end up in any of these therapies. More importantly perhaps is the growth of the psychological approach to dementia care in the consideration given to imparting the diagnosis, post-diagnostic counselling, and cognitive stimulation therapy. The latter is an evidence-based treatment which, in clinical trials, has been demonstrated to be equal in efficacy to anti-dementia drugs. In addition to the above is the important work done mainly by the British Psychological Society on psychological approaches to BPSD. This approach is particularly focused on the experience of the person with dementia and helps them and us make sense of their experiences in the context of their lived lives and of their current disabilities.

For people with functional psychiatric disorders, every effort should be made to offer older people the same opportunities to receive similar psychological therapies services to younger adults. As long as the effects of ageing and sometimes physical health problems are taken into account, most older adults should benefit from a psychological approach to their condition, whether this is depression or personality disorder. Simple one-to-one counselling is well taken up by older people in the context of bereavement counselling, and yet there are still very low numbers of older people being seen in the primary care settings of IAPT and psychology. People are not being routinely referred by their GPs (clearly a situation that will need to change urgently), but also the services may not be well suited to older peoples' needs. Difficult-to-access venues, late afternoon sessions, and long waiting lists all mitigate against older people taking up psychological treatments in a primary care setting.

Secondary care services dedicated to treating older people with mental health problems are likely to have the expertise required, as well as the flexibility, e.g. providing home treatments and offering therapy groups for older patients. Sadly, these too are subject to the 'postcode lottery' and may well be missing from parts of the UK.

Applications

Older people can manage and may be offered a range of psychological therapies. Unfortunately, numbers offered are relatively low. Counselling (see ➲ Counselling in Chapter 2, pp. 91–94, and in Chapter 5, pp. 274–81), bereavement work, and group therapies (see ➲ Group therapy and group analysis in Chapter 2, pp. 42–7, and in Chapter 5, pp. 188–94) are well documented as providing a forum for people to share their feelings and gain support. More in-depth psychodynamic work tends not to be available on the NHS in a practical way, and many seek help from private and voluntary sector organizations. There is a body of descriptive work using case studies to demonstrate practice and outcomes. There is no technical difference in working with older than with younger adults, although transference and countertransference (see ➲ Psychoanalytic psychotherapy in Chapter 2, pp. 20–30) feelings will include intergenerational elements perhaps more than with younger adults. Anecdotally, older patients may feel less safe with young therapists but can use the fact of therapist youth and inexperience to offset painful feelings of personal decline and decrepitude. Narcissistically wounded patients, suffering indignities of late life, may be challenging for the less experienced practitioner. In practice, there has to be a senior person within a GP consortium or a consultant psychiatrist or psychologist within a service who endorses a psychological approach in older people as a viable alternative to physical medication, before this becomes readily available.

CBT (see ➲ Cognitive behavioural therapy in Chapter 2, pp. 30–4, and in Chapter 5, pp. 172–84) and IPT (see ➲ Interpersonal therapy in Chapter 2, pp. 52–5, and in Chapter 5, pp. 203–7) are particularly useful alternatives or adjuncts to medicinal treatments for mood disorders. As with much younger adults, children, and adolescents, older people can lose their independence through illness or by being very old and mildly cognitively impaired. In these situations, families become more powerful and often have a greater say in an older person's treatment than when that older person was working or bringing up the family themselves. Practitioners should be cautious about who is asking for treatment and about maintaining confidentiality. Family therapy, using a systemic approach, can benefit the whole family system, as well as the older person, and can reinforce progress, as well as improvements, made in mental state (see ➲ Systematic family and couple therapy in Chapter 2, pp. 34–42, and in Chapter 5, pp. 184–8). Goals for therapy need to be clearly defined by potential patients, and therapists should be realistic about what their patient can manage.

Research

Most of the research evidence available on efficacy centres on CBT. Since anxiety disorders are so prevalent in older people, psychological management of these conditions is available in most places. There is less evidence for CBT and DBT in this age group, although the mantra 'absence of evidence of efficacy is not evidence of absence of efficacy' applies here. IPT is, by contrast, well researched in the younger old age group, particularly in relation to adjunctive treatment with antidepressant medication. Enthusiastic proponents of a psychodynamic approach or systemic therapy model have written about the perceived usefulness of interventions using these different modalities, but none meets the standard of an RCT. The task at present is to ensure equality of access. It is disheartening that a decade of health service changes, including the unchecked introduction of so-called 'ageless services', has done little to change the situation that was described in a survey of psychological treatments for older adults (Evans, 2004). Equality of service does not mean the same service, as in ageless services, but refers to equality of access, so that services can be tailored to the needs of older people. Ignoring difference is not only perverse, but it is excluding and iniquitous.

Training

In the Royal College of Psychiatrists' core curriculum, there are guidelines relating to having a knowledge of healthy ageing and the particular psychosocial aspects of old age. With respect to psychotherapy, trainees should be aware of the applications of psychological treatments in older people and their efficacy. In some examples of good medical practice, core psychiatry trainees may take on an older patient for CBT or short-term psychodynamic therapy under supervision. This is especially helpful when trainees are in old age psychiatry placements, so that their clinical time is used to address issues that come up in their own service. Supervision may be offered by a consultant medical psychotherapist or psychologist trained in that modality. Elderly patients may also benefit from family therapy, but training and supervision are dependent on a local lead, as well as support from the head of service. Higher trainees and consultants in old age psychiatry can and do take on private psychotherapy trainings to become psychoanalysts, psychoanalytic psychotherapists, or group analysts, and CBT, family therapy, or IPT practitioners. Work is being done within the Royal College of Psychiatrists to support old age trainees to do dual trainings, e.g. in old age psychiatry and medical psychotherapy, or to gain accreditation in their modalities.

Recommended reading

Evans S (2004). What works for whom? A Survey of provision of psychological therapies for older people in the NHS. *Psychiatric Bulletin*, **28**, 411–14.

Evans S and Garner J (eds) (2004). *Talking Over the Years: A Handbook of Dynamic Psychotherapy with Older Adults*. Brunner Routledge: Hove.

Hinrichsen GA and Clogherty KF (eds) (2006). *Interpersonal Psychotherapy for Depressed Older Adults*. American Psychological Association: Washington DC.

Pachana N, Laidlaw K, and Knight B (eds) (2010). *Casebook of Clinical Geropsychology: International Perspectives on Practice*. Oxford University Press: Oxford.

Quinodoz D (2009). *Old Age: A Journey of Self-Discovery*. Routledge: Hove and New York.

Spector A, Thorgrimsen L, Woods B, et al. (2003). Efficacy of an evidence-based cognitive stimulation therapy programme for people with dementia: randomised controlled trial. *British Journal of Psychiatry*, **183**, 248–54.

Rehabilitation and social psychiatry: psychotherapies, applications, and research

Clinical practice

Rehabilitation and social psychiatrists provide clinical services for people with psychosis, mainly schizophrenia, where there are additional complexities such as substance misuse, trauma, communication difficulties, or neurodevelopmental disorders. Social psychiatry involves the study of social factors and their influence on mental health problems and, when integrated with psychotherapeutic understanding concerning the individual's development, their response to their immediate environment, and interpersonal relationships, is a potent force for change. The provision of interventions to address this includes a broad scope, from attending to the needs of an individual patient with disability and distress arising from mental health problems to the promotion of recovery, including changes in social and environmental influences. Rehabilitation and social psychiatrists also extend their efforts to challenge stigma against mental illness in society.

Patients coming under the care and treatment of rehabilitation services usually have complex presentations of psychosis which are treatment-resistant (see ➔ Psychoses in Chapter 7, pp. 331–4). They may experience psychotic perceptual disturbances such as auditory hallucinations, often in the form of voices which torment and insult them. The nature of their disorder is long-term, and, in addition to mental health problems, secondary disabilities in the form of social stigma and exclusion occur. They will often be socially isolated, performing poorly, or excluded from work and educational environments and experience low self-esteem, distress, and isolation, living on the fringes of society. Risky behaviours, such as self-neglect and suicidality, are common and worrying, but less common is the risk of harm to others.

Treatment approaches centre on value-based recovery principles which recognize the important contribution hope and optimism make to a positive direction in life. Central to this is the principle that the right to a fulfilling life should not be denied by illness, that patients can be helped to utilize their own resources, and in order that this is successful a long time frame is required. Positive risk taking is an important component of treatment, decisions being taken as far as possible in collaboration with the patient and a key worker and supported by the multidisciplinary team.

The intensity of treatment is determined by the needs of the patient. Ideally, there will be an umbrella reaching across services in the form of a managed clinical network which takes a whole-system view of the care pathway. This will encompass specialist rehabilitation inpatient units, assertive outreach offering high-intensity community interventions, community forensic, community rehabilitation, and community mental health services, which may be provided alongside supported community living arrangements. This network provides consistency across the care pathway, enshrining a value base which respects the individual's autonomy, works towards empowerment, uses recovery principles, and has pathways to mainstream community activities, including education, training, and opportunities for employment. In services which are functioning well, there is a strong ethos of teamworking, bringing together different skills to ensure the patient has access to biological, psychological, and social interventions, and that these are integrated in a care and treatment plan.

The multidisciplinary team provides an essential containment function for the inevitable frustrations experienced by both staff and patients, given the long time frame and slowness of change. This provides a supportive matrix for the treatment programmes, the whole team becoming more than just a group of individuals working together.

A small proportion of this patient group has very high needs. Such patients are experienced by staff as eroding therapeutic optimism. This occurs, e.g. when they have been admitted to an acute inpatient ward and prove difficult to discharge, resulting in long admissions with little therapeutic benefit. The acute inpatient ward does not provide an optimal recovery environment for this population. Instead, they benefit from specialized inpatient rehabilitation of high intensity. This takes the form of a structured environment with an intensive therapeutic programme where the patient may stay for between 1 and 3 years. Biological treatments in the form of medication are supported by psychological therapy and social interventions, including healthy living programmes, e.g. focusing on diet and exercise to minimize the adverse impact of some medications which can cause weight gain.

Many patients are treated out of area, at considerable distance from their home and family networks, thus adding to the experiences of social isolation and stigmatization which are part of the challenges faced. Rehabilitation psychiatrists consistently advise that treatment should be provided close to home, which also facilitates a graduated supported transition to community living.

It is central to the recovery process that the individual patient begins to express their personal wishes and likes, along with recognition of their strengths, so their journey in life can be personally owned. Empowerment is at the core of this, and hence it is essential to fully involve the individual in shaping their own future and recovery journey. Increasingly, the positive impact of empowerment is leading to service users becoming active as peer workers, supporting others in their recovery journey and advising on the delivery of services (see ➲ Service user involvement in Chapter 10, pp. 466–71).

Applications

Psychotherapy has an important contribution to the recovery of this population; however, to be effective, it needs to be integrated into a wider plan for care which takes into account the nature of the internal disorder, alongside the challenges of external reality faced by the patient. This requires modifications in the way psychotherapy is conducted, adaptations to take into account the setting of the work, and specific techniques to assist with common symptoms.

Psychotherapy can be applied at different stages of recovery, in assessment, care planning, treatment, and maintenance in psychosis. It can also be utilized across a range of intensities of services, from inpatient to community.

As part of a comprehensive assessment, it is essential to understand what the patient experiences and what they make of these experiences. The first stage of this involves working with the patient in a one-to-one setting to develop a narrative account. The central strand of this is a developmental history, including gaining understanding of their psychological journey, social and interpersonal experiences, and education. The development of a narrative account, or patient journey, is a common approach used in psychotherapy; however, in rehabilitation services, it is adapted to take account of the patient's problems which typically include low motivation and consequently difficulty with engagement. The pace of this therefore is slower than in other settings, taking place over a number of sessions and in an atmosphere of support and encouragement. The role of the therapist is to listen closely to the patient's experiences, as in all forms of therapy, paying attention to their verbal and non-verbal behaviour, conveying a sense of value to the patient that they are worth listening to which, in turn, has a beneficial impact, enhancing trust and motivation. The therapist will employ an adapted approach to history taking, e.g. being more structured and supportive, taking care about how challenges are put, whilst being able to provide a different perspective to the patient.

Communication with the team is important throughout this process; the narrative and concerns shared in therapeutic exploration will usually be more open to the team than in other forms of therapy. This aids in ensuring that the aspects of treatment are joined up and also assists with ongoing risk assessment and management.

A narrative assessment gathers together past and present experiences, leading to the development of a formulation, which aims to make sense of the individual's beliefs and experiences. Psychotherapeutic approaches focus on collaboration with the patient to facilitate the expression of their fears, hopes, and values; hence, the formulation should also be collaborative, leading to the next step—the development of a treatment plan which places at its centre the patient's hopes and desires for change.

There are a number of specific psychological interventions that are utilized in psychosis, both for positive symptoms, such as hallucinations and delusions, and for negative symptoms such as withdrawal (see ➔ Psychoses in Chapter 7, pp. 331–4). CBT, specifically targeting positive symptoms of schizophrenia, such as hallucinatory and delusional experiences, is well established and integrated into intensive treatment programmes (see ➔ Cognitive behavioural therapy in Chapter 2, pp. 30–4, and in Chapter 5, pp. 172–84). There are also variations of this such as cognitive therapies and behavioural therapies widely used in practice. It should be noted that, as with all treatment approaches, these interventions, when applied with this patient group, require an extended duration of therapy which will usually continue throughout a 1- to 3-year inpatient stay and be further extended as the patient moves into the community.

Other psychological interventions include an application of mindfulness in which there is a focus on actively paying attention to the internal world, accepting this, and finding a way to live alongside it. In psychosis, this includes attending to hallucinations and is increasingly being used as a technique to manage psychotic experiences, to reduce the impact, rather than obliterate the perceptions (see ➜ Mindfulness-based interventions and therapies in Chapter 2, pp. 73–5, and in Chapter 5, pp. 239–43).

Family therapy, especially behavioural family therapy, is also widely used. This can assist family members and carers in understanding and appreciating the difficulties their relative experiences and in ensuring the environment is not too challenging or stressful, as this may provoke a relapse. Interventions include psycho-education about psychosis, development of skills in negotiation, problem-solving, and managing crises. As recovery is attained, there may also be family interventions to aid the detection of early warning signs and to assist with risk management in the community. The family are often an important point of contact and able to report concerns and improvements to staff, e.g. following periods of home leave during an inpatient stay (see ➜ Systemic family and couple therapy in Chapter 2, pp. 34–42, and in Chapter 5, pp. 184–8).

Exploratory therapies are generally used with caution in this group of patients, as they can provoke decompensation, though there are applications which take an approach more suited to the treatment of psychosis. Here it is important to adapt for a patient population who, as part of their condition, have challenged reality testing, as some exploratory approaches may be experienced as overly stressful and, as a consequence, cause deterioration in emotional state.

Negative symptoms of schizophrenia have proved difficult to treat with conventional approaches. However, there are promising outcomes emerging from art therapy, which historically has been part of a structured treatment programme, in assisting the recovery of negative symptoms of schizophrenia (see ➜ Art psychotherapy in Chapter 2, pp. 81–83, and in Chapter 5, pp. 188–94).

In addition to specialized inpatient rehabilitation treatment units, there are also some TCs which specialize in the treatment of psychosis. In these settings, in addition to a structured treatment programme, there is a more democratic management of the whole unit, in which patients take an active role on behalf of the community members, often chairing meetings, organizing crisis support, and developing a social microcosm in which interpersonal learning can take place. This includes group interactive therapies, in which patients provide feedback to each other, resolve conflicts and tensions which emerge when people live together, learn how to negotiate with others, listen to different views, and empathize with others. This social milieu is a central part of therapy and can be continued with beneficial effects into community and shared accommodation settings (see ➜ Therapeutic communities in Chapter 2, pp. 75–80, and in Chapter 5, pp. 243–50).

In addition to active treatment episodes, it is also effective to have access to 'top-up' treatments for those who need support, especially when they have progressed through a treatment programme and are living in local communities. This can help prevent relapse or minimize the severity of relapse, especially when the therapeutic approach is consistent with previous therapy.

Research

There is a long history of social and rehabilitation research demonstrating improvements in social and psychological functioning and reduced distress and disability, dating back to the era when psychiatric asylums began opening their doors in the 1950s. This was a time when the full deleterious impact of institutionalization began to be recognized, in response to which institutional authority was lessened and personal empowerment began to be valued as a positive outcome. In turn, this has led to enhanced levels of personal responsibility, improvements in family relationships, and improved capacity to work. Economically, this is beneficial, as the level of support required by an individual lessens as they progress down the recovery route and become contributing members of society. There is a high financial and emotional cost of placing patients out of area which continues to happen in excess numbers; however, this is increasingly being challenged with a drive to bring patients into treatment closer to home.

The research demonstrating positive outcomes from CBT in early intervention services is very convincing (see ➜ Psychoses in Chapter 7, pp. 331–4). However, disentangling the impact of psychological interventions from other approaches in an integrated intense treatment programme is a complex task, and, although clinically there are recordings of improvement, this continues to be a research challenge.

Training

Training in rehabilitation and social psychiatry is undertaken through placements with specialist rehabilitation teams providing care for patients with severe chronic disability. This would usually include experience across a range of services from inpatient to community settings, including supported residential placements.

Assessment of complex patients requires a multifaceted narrative that describes and makes sense of the individual in relation to their development, family history, sociocultural background, and present day networks. Medical psychotherapy training, which continues throughout core and specialist training, assists in making meaningful linkages between present day experiences and developmental processes, the psychotherapeutic approach in rehabilitation services enhancing the personal narrative. This takes place through therapeutic interviewing in which the relationship between the trainee doctor and patient is established often over several meetings. Psychotherapy supervision of the assessment process helps the trainee to maintain their active listening stance and curiosity. This enhances the formulation of the patient's problems and planning of collaborative care and interventions.

Specific interventions require skills in individual, family, and group therapies. The rehabilitation and social psychiatrist will work with patients who may self-harm and be a risk to others; therefore, it is important to work with the patient to develop prevention strategies such as those based on psychological and emotional awareness. Training in mindfulness for both the doctor and patient may assist this process. Individual therapy in rehabilitation psychiatry is often focused on specific symptoms, and it follows that the trainee will need to develop skills in approaches, such as CBT, to reduce the impact of auditory hallucinations. This should be individual therapy supervised by a trained and competent therapist. Family and group therapies provide excellent opportunities for training, as the doctor can become a co-therapist, observing and participating in the therapy. The learning experience is strengthened by live supervision of these interventions.

Most importantly, the trainee will develop knowledge and skills to ensure psychological interventions are integrated into a comprehensive treatment and care plan, recognizing the contribution these make to the overall recovery of the patient. This also requires the capacity to work within a team. Supervision on team approaches often takes place with the whole team such as a reflective practice session where differing perspectives can be expressed and understood (see ➔ Reflective practice groups in Chapter 10, pp. 497–505). Through this, the trainee is able to develop wider understanding about the processes of splitting which can occur in teams and ways in which this can be addressed to the benefit of the patient.

In relation to patients who are resistant to treatment, including those with co-morbid personality disorders, further interventions, including MBT, CAT, and DBT, are helpful, and opportunities to develop training in these areas are a valuable addition to the toolbox of the rehabilitation psychiatrist.

Training in psychotherapy should ideally be overseen by a medical psychotherapist who will ensure that supervisors are appropriately equipped as therapists, supervisors, and teachers. The medical psychotherapist will generally be more effective if they are an accepted part of the service, often in the form of a visiting clinician, working with their rehabilitation psychiatry colleagues, modelling and reinforcing the need for psychotherapy to be integrated into the care of patients.

Recommended reading

Al-Khudhairy N, Smith E, Saxon C, Handover K, and Tucker S (2000). *A Therapeutic Community Approach to Care in the Community: Dialogue and Dwelling.* Jessica Kingsley: London and Philadelphia.

Davidson L and Strauss J (1992). Sense of self in recovery from severe mental illness. *British Journal of Medical Psychology,* **65**, 131–45.

Kingdon D and Finn M (2006). *Tackling Mental Health Crises.* Routledge: London.

Mace C and Margison F (1997). *The Psychotherapy of Psychosis.* Gaskell: London.

Wolfson P, Holloway F, and Killaspy H (eds) (2009). *Enabling Recovery for People with Complex Mental Health Needs: A Template for Rehabilitation Services.* Faculty report FR/RS/1, Royal College of Psychiatrists, Faculty of Rehabilitation and Social Psychiatry. Royal College of Psychiatrists: London.

Psychiatry of addictions: psychotherapies, applications, and research

(See ➲ Substance misuse in Chapter 7, pp. 338–45.)

Addiction psychiatrists are medical doctors who have completed extensive training in psychiatry (including the use of mental health legislation) and addiction. They have expertise in the management of addiction problems in complex cases, particularly co-morbid mental health problems. The substances involved may include alcohol, illicit drugs, prescribed or over-the-counter medication, and volatile solvents. Expertise requires knowledge in all aspects of addiction, including individual brain mechanisms, the impact of the addictive behaviour on the family and society, as well as knowledge of the criminal justice system. Addiction psychiatrists offer a holistic approach that considers how biological, psychological, and social factors impact on a person's life and recovery journey. Dealing with patient needs may involve other health-care professionals, such as GPs, hospital-based specialists in liver disease and HIV, as well as in mental health. Social problems, legal problems, housing, and employment may also require help; thus, addiction psychiatrists work in teams with other professionals and disciplines.

Training in psychotherapies in addictions

Most of the therapists delivering psychological treatments within addiction services are non-medically trained and are from disciplines, such as psychology or nursing, or may be experts by experience. However, all psychiatrists specializing in addictions are expected to have some training and expertise in psychological therapies. In the UK, addiction psychiatry is a sub-specialty of general adult psychiatry. Following their training in core psychiatry (CT1–3), psychiatrists specializing in addictions need to have undertaken 2 years of higher training (ST4–6) in general adult psychiatry and 1 year of sub-specialty training in addiction psychiatry to have an endorsement in addiction.

The selection of psychological therapy cases in advanced training in general psychiatry and substance misuse psychiatry takes account of the experience relevant to the trainee's future practice as a consultant in a substance misuse service. For example, trainees in addiction psychiatry should gain experience in motivational enhancement therapy and relapse prevention interventions. Higher trainees also have the opportunity to undertake further psychotherapy training during specifically designated special interest sessions for gaining additional psychotherapy under supervision. In addition to the required psychotherapy training in the core and higher psychiatry training programmes, clinicians can undertake further specialist postgraduate courses in specific psychotherapy interventions such as CBT or psychoanalytic psychotherapy. These types of training tend to be self-funded though, in some instances, might be part-funded by the trainee's employer through local agreements.

Applications

There are a range of treatment options for people with substance misuse problems, from advice and information to psychological and pharmacological treatments, which may include drug substitution or detoxification regimes. Specific therapies for addictions include:

- *CBT*: CBT for addictions incorporates different elements (e.g. behavioural in contingency management, cognitive in relapse prevention, etc.) and different styles of delivery (e.g. using maps, homework, self-help, computerized manuals), and is delivered in different settings (e.g. group or individual). Relapse prevention incorporates CBT principles, as well as, more recently, mindfulness (see ➲ Cognitive behavioural therapy in Chapter 2, pp. 30–4, and in Chapter 5, pp. 172–84; Mindfulness-based interventions and therapies in Chapter 2, pp. 73–5, and in Chapter 5, pp. 239–43)
- *Motivational interviewing* (MI): developed by Miller and Rollinick, is a therapy which encourages and strengthens the motivation to change in a skilled, non-confrontational way (see ➲ Motivational-based approaches in Chapter 7, p. 342)
- *Behavioural couples therapy* (BCT): involves joint therapy with the patient's partner and aims at improving the substance misuse, as well as the quality of the relationship. BCT has been shown to reduce drug use and provide greater relationship satisfaction
- *Contingency management*: may also be considered a variant of CBT, as it works on operant conditioning theory
- *Psychoanalytic or psychodynamic psychotherapy*: may be useful to explore the patient's unresolved conflicts which may underlie the drug-seeking behaviour. However, it is not commonly offered in addictions, as psychodynamic therapy services often require the patient to be abstinent from substances before such therapy may be embarked upon. This is due to the increased risk of escalation of drug or alcohol misuse, as the patient's distressing thoughts and feelings are made conscious and explored in therapy, which may destabilize his or her mental state (see ➲ Psychoanalytic psychotherapy in Chapter 2, pp. 20–30, and in Chapter 5, pp. 163–72).

A key issue, however, is the application of specific psychotherapy interventions in clinical practice within core addiction services. A mixed picture of access to psychotherapy services exists across the UK, with some areas better resourced than others. One of the initiatives in the UK to increase availability of psychological treatments is IAPT (see ➲ Improving Access to Psychological Therapies services in Chapter 10, pp. 463–4). This scheme provides training in evidence-based short-term psychological interventions, largely based on CBT principles. Following the training, IAPT therapists are affiliated to GP practices to offer first line to patients with mental health problems. The National Treatment Agency for Substance Misuse (now part of Public Health England) has recently published guidance for IAPT workers to be able to work effectively with patients with substance misuse, as many of the general cognitive and behavioural techniques used within IAPT are transferable to working with drug or alcohol use. A recent study in York has shown that IAPT therapists working in an addiction service managed to have good results regarding engagement, attendance, and outcomes with dual diagnosis patients. Addiction-specific services also adopt the Drug and Alcohol National Occupational Standards (DANOS) competencies framework to increase levels of knowledge and skills in a number of workers. DANOS is a national workforce strategy aimed at developing a competent workforce with an improved knowledge base and increased range of skills.

Research

Overall, psychosocial interventions have been shown to be effective across a range of addictive disorders. The most researched and commonly used therapies in addictive disorders are CBT and MI. CBT, in combination with pharmacotherapy, has shown robust outcomes. CBT, MI, and relapse prevention appear to be effective across the treatment of many drugs of abuse. Recent research also shows good outcomes in addiction treatment with DBT and mindfulness therapy. However, research on optimal psychological therapies for particular substances and particular matching effects has not shown any specific advantage of particular therapeutic interventions over others and highlight that individual therapist factors have an important role to play in positive outcomes in clinical settings (see ➔ Research in psychotherapy in Chapter 11, pp. 508–26).

Recommended reading

Manual JK, Hagedorn HJ, and Finney JW (2011). Implementing evidence-based psychological treatment in specialty substance use disorders care. *Psychology of Addictive Behaviors*, **25**, 225–37.

McHugh RK, Hearon BA, and Otto MW (2010). Cognitive-behavioural therapy for substance use disorders. *Psychiatric Clinics North America*, **33**, 511–25.

Pilling S, Heskethand K, and Mitcheson L (2010). *Routes to Recovery: Psychosocial Interventions for Drug Misuse. A Framework and Toolkit for Implementing NICE-Recommended Treatment Interventions*. British Psychological Society: Leicester.

Royal College of Psychiatrists (2008). *Specialist Module in Addictions (Substance Misuse) Psychiatry*. Royal College of Psychiatrist: London.

Witkiewitz K, Bowen S, Harrop EN, Douglas H, Enkema M, and Sedgwick C (2014). Mindfulness-based prescribing to prevent addictive behaviour relapse: theoretical models and hypothesised mechanisms of change. *Substance Use and Misuse*, **49**, 513–24.

Liaison psychiatry: psychotherapies, applications, and research

Clinical practice

Liaison psychiatry is principally concerned with the assessment, diagnosis, treatment, and management of people with co-morbid physical and mental health problems. Most liaison services are based in acute hospitals and provide mental health services for patients who attend A&E departments or who are admitted to general hospital inpatient wards. However, there is also great diversity across liaison services, with some liaison teams providing specialist outpatient clinics, support and liaison with primary care, input to services which operate across the secondary and primary care sector (e.g. GP-led rheumatology services), and the provision of mental health services to cancer hospitals, maternity units, other specialist hospitals, specialist pain centres, and specialized units. Liaison psychiatry also overlaps with neuropsychiatry services and perinatal services.

Psychotherapy or psychological treatments in liaison psychiatry services are usually provided by specialist nurses, counsellors, or clinical psychologists. They may be delivered on an individual basis or as part of a multidisciplinary approach (e.g. as part of a pain management programme). Liaison psychiatrists may be interested in delivering a specific therapy as part of their clinical work, but the scope to do this is limited. However, understanding the processes involved in adjusting to physical illness or living with MUS is an essential requirement of liaison work, and training in a psychological therapy (e.g. cognitive therapy or psychodynamic therapy) can enhance skills in this area.

Psychiatrists gain experience in psychotherapy during their core training, but some form of additional training in psychotherapy during their higher training should be encouraged. It is important that liaison psychiatrists have a good understanding of both CBT and psychodynamic treatment approaches. More specifically for liaison psychiatry, however, it is important to be aware of the common psychological models of adjustment to illness, which have been developed within the field of health psychology. An understanding of existential psychotherapy is also helpful, as life and death issues are extremely common in liaison psychiatry, and some issues that people struggle with cannot be explained by conventional CBT models. An understanding of group dynamics is also invaluable, as much of the work in liaison psychiatry involves close working with medical and nursing teams on general hospital wards. It is quite common for staff to become embroiled in dynamics, such as splitting, without being aware of this, in relation to specific patients under their care.

Psychotherapy in liaison psychiatry, no matter the modality, usually starts with a focus on the client's physical symptoms/illness and how this has affected his/her life. Most people are keen to talk about their problems and receive some kind of help. However, some patients may be more ambivalent about involvement with psychological treatment services, and any worries or concerns about this may need to be discussed at an early stage of the therapy. If a person's illness is life-threatening, it may result in some form of existential concerns about the meaning or value of life. If the person has young children, the focus of therapy may be about their concerns for their children and the effect the illness is having on them.

Physical illness itself may impede people's ability to participate in treatment, if their concentration or memory is impaired, or they are nauseous or in acute pain. Noxious side effects of treatment (e.g. chemotherapy) may also interfere with therapy, and there may need to be some flexibility about scheduling sessions.

Perhaps more than any other specialty within psychiatry, therapists need to be aware that some clients who are being seen for psychotherapy may die during treatment, or shortly after psychotherapy has been completed, because of their physical condition. This can be very distressing for therapists, particularly if there has been some identification with the client (e.g. they have children of a similar age to those of the therapist) or a close bond has been formed during the treatment.

Applications

There is a wide range of different ways that psychological therapies are used within the liaison setting. These will be discussed according to the main type of problem presentation.

Long-term conditions

Most work in this area involves low-intensity interventions, including self-management, psycho-educational initiatives, and brief behavioural programmes. All have the main aim of improving patients' ability to cope with their physical health problems and improve function. Liaison psychiatrists are not usually involved in the delivery of such interventions but may be involved in managing a team in which such interventions are delivered. Knowledge of, and familiarity with, these techniques are important. Some hospital-based liaison services may offer brief psychological treatment or counselling to help people who are having difficulty coping with, or adjusting to, their illness. Psycho-oncology services are a good example of this and usually will have a nurse therapist, counsellor, or clinical psychologist as part of the team.

The availability of psychological treatment services for people with LTCs is very variable both at a local and national, and international level. In England, there has been a recent initiative to provide a national psychological treatment service for people with depression and anxiety. This is called the 'Improving Access to Psychological Treatment' programme (IAPT) (see ➜ Improving Access to Psychological Therapies services in Chapter 10, pp. 463–4). It provides psychological treatment at different steps of intensity, depending upon the nature of people's problems. There are plans that IAPT should also provide psychological treatment services for people with LTCs, although exactly how this is done will vary. Liaison psychiatrists are unlikely to be directly involved in this work but are offering training and supervision to some IAPT services.

Medically unexplained symptoms

(See ➜ Medically unexplained symptoms in Chapter 7, pp. 359–63.)

Liaison psychiatrists have historically been involved in the development of psychological treatment services for people with MUS. These may be generic services but are more often condition-specific such as services for people with CFS or IBS. Liaison psychiatrists often play a major role in the overall supervision of staff and management of patients. As with psychological services for people with LTCs, IAPT has been given a major role to develop services for people with MUS and will be taking on greater responsibility for such patients in the future.

Services for people with persistent and disabling physical symptoms

Liaison psychiatrists are often referred patients at the very severe end of the physical/mental health spectrum who either have LTCs or MUS or both. These people require multidisciplinary team treatment and management, utilizing both pharmacological and psychotherapeutic interventions. Such treatment may be offered as part of an outpatient service or day-programme treatment or, in very severe cases, inpatient specialized treatment.

Self-harm services

(See ➔ Suicide and self-harm in Chapter 6, pp. 308–11.)

Liaison psychiatry services are principally responsible for the assessment and initial treatment of people who present to hospital following self-harm. There are a small number of specialist psychological treatment services that have been set up across the UK for self-harm. The treatment is usually provided by specialist nurses who have been trained in either CBT (see ➔ Cognitive behavioural therapy in Chapter 2, pp. 30–4, and in Chapter 5, pp. 172–84) or PIT (see ➔ Psychodynamic interpersonal therapy in Chapter 2, pp. 56–61, and in Chapter 5, pp. 207–14). A good example of such a service is the SAFE team in Manchester, which offers four sessions of brief PIT for people who have self-harmed. The team also run primary care clinics, so that GPs can refer patients who they feel are at high risk of self-harming, before they actually self-harm.

Alcohol services

(See ➔ Substance misuse in Chapter 7, pp. 338–45.)

Alcohol problems are very common in the general hospital setting, and there is evidence that people who are developing an alcohol problem often present with a physical health problem secondary to alcohol (e.g. head injury, fit, gastric problem) many years before their problem with alcohol is officially recognized. Many liaison services therefore offer screening, earlier diagnosis, and brief interventions for problem drinking.

Working with specialized units

Liaison work to a specific unit, such as, e.g. the renal unit, the liver unit, or the critical care unit, may involve working in a different way to that demanded as part of a busy conventional general hospital liaison service. Usually, there will be more time to work with staff and patients and a greater focus upon prevention and healthy adjustment to illness, rather than the 'fire-fighting' approach of liaison psychiatry teams in a general hospital. Many general hospital staff are interested in psychological issues and are keen to learn more about psychological problems and develop skills in this area. Brief behavioural activation techniques can be learnt easily by general hospital staff, provided they receive supervision and support.

Types of psychological treatment

CBT, and its many variants, is the most widely used form of intervention in liaison settings. Other approaches, such as psychodynamic therapy, PIT, IPT, and CAT, are also used, and mindfulness is becoming increasingly popular. Counselling is also offered by some services.

Research evidence

There is a strong evidence base for the efficacy and effectiveness, as well as the cost-effectiveness, of psychological therapies for MUS (see ➔ Medically unexplained symptoms in Chapter 7, pp. 359–63). This includes cognitive therapy, behavioural interventions, and PIT. The evidence base for mindfulness is growing, and other treatment approaches, such as hypnotherapy, may also be helpful for certain conditions (e.g. IBS). Multi-component treatment approaches and behavioural-based interventions are helpful for chronic pain management.

There is a good evidence base for the efficacy of psychological treatments for self-harm. This mainly applies to CBT and PIT. There is also evidence supportive of brief interventions for problem-drinking in the general hospital setting.

The evidence base for the effectiveness of psychological treatments for people with LTCs is patchy and limited, and there are a relatively small number of studies that have evaluated the benefits of individual psychological treatment approaches. The majority of interventions which have been evaluated for people with LTCs usually involve treatment packages of care, such as collaborative care or stepped care, which involve low-intensity cognitive behavioural interventions coupled with antidepressant treatment or some other appropriate intervention. Collaborative care was pioneered and developed by the liaison psychiatrist Wayne Katon in Seattle, and there is now a substantial evidence base for the benefits of collaborative care-type interventions for people with LTCs (e.g. diabetes, heart disease).

Cancer deserves a separate mention, due to the relatively large number of evaluations of psychological treatment for people coping with this form of disease. There is little evidence that psychological interventions prolong life or alter the disease course in cancer, despite some early studies of group therapy which appeared to show this. There is, however, good evidence that brief psychological interventions, including CBT and counselling and group work, can be helpful for treating depression and other psychosocial problems related to cancer. Recent work from the UK has also demonstrated that cancer specialist nurses can be trained to deliver brief CBT interventions plus antidepressant medication, supervised closely by liaison psychiatrists, for the treatment of depression in cancer sufferers.

The evidence base for the efficacy and effectiveness of psychological treatment interventions is continuing to grow in liaison psychiatry. There has been recent interest in developing ever more efficient low-intensity treatments. These include telephone CBT and Internet-based CBT, or Internet-based psychodynamic therapy, for certain MUS-type conditions. Preliminary evaluations suggest that such interventions may be very helpful, although it is unlikely they will have a significant impact for people with very severe MUS, who are generally referred to liaison psychiatry.

Recommended reading

Guthrie E and Sensky T (2007). The role of psychological treatments. In: Lloyd GG and Guthrie E, eds. *The Handbook of Liaison Psychiatry.* pp. 795–817. Cambridge University Press: Cambridge.

Marks M and Murray M (2011). *Health Psychology. Theory, Research and Practice.* Sage Publications: London.

Rosenbaum E (2012). *Being Well (Even When You are Sick): Mindfulness Practices for People with Cancer and Other Serious Diseases.* Shambhala: Boston and London.

Sage N, Sowden M, Chorlton E, and Edeleanu A (2008). *CBT for Chronic Illness and Palliative Care: A Workbook and Toolkit.* John Wiley and Sons Ltd: Chichester.

White C (2001). *Cognitive Behaviour Therapy for Chronic Medical Problems.* John Wiley and Sons Ltd: Chichester.

Key UK-based psychotherapy organizations

Accrediting Organisation for Medical Psychotherapy: AcOMP, London, SW1X 8PG. Tel: 020 7235 2351.

Anna Freud Centre: 12 Maresfield Gardens, London, NW3 5SU. Tel: 020 7794 2313.

Arbours Psychotherapy Service: 6 Church Lane, London, N8 7BU. Tel: 020 8340 7646/ 020 8348 6466.

Association of Child Psychotherapists: Suite 7, 19–23 Wedmore Street, London, N19 4RU. Tel: 020 7281 8479.

The Association for Cognitive Analytic Therapy: PO Box 6793, Dorchester, DT1 9DL. Tel: 0844 800 94 96.

Association for Family Therapy and Systemic Practice: 7 Executive Suite, St James Court, Wilderspool Causeway, Warrington, Cheshire, WA4 6PS. Tel: 01925 444414.

Association for Group and Individual Psychotherapy: 1 Fairbridge Road, London, N19 3EW. Tel: 020 7272 7013.

Association of Jungian Analysts: 7 Eton Avenue, London, NW3 3EL. Tel: 020 7794 8711.

Association of Medical Psychodynamic Psychotherapists: c/o BPC, Suite 7, 19–23 Wedmore Street, London N19 4RU. Tel: 020 7561 9240.

Association of Psychodynamic Counsellors: c/o BPC, Suite 7, 19–23 Wedmore Street, London, N19 4RU. Tel: 020 7561 9240.

Association for Psychoanalytic Psychotherapy in the NHS: Unit 7, 19–23 Wedmore Street, London, N19 4RU. Tel: 020 7272 8681.

Association for Psychodynamic Practice and Counselling in Organisational Settings: 60 Lordship Park, London, N16 5UA. Tel: 020 7690 8849.

Awaken School of Outcome Oriented Psychotherapies: Awaken House, Northallerton, DL7 8SE. Tel: 0845 873 2036.

Bath Centre for Psychotherapy and Counselling: 1 Walcot Terrace, Bath, BA1 6AB. Tel: 01225 429 720.

Beeleaf Institute for Contemporary Psychotherapy: Beeleaf House, London, E3 5AX. Tel: 020 8983 9699.

The Berne Institute: Berne House, Kegworth, DE74 2EN. Tel: 01509 673 649.

The Bowlby Centre: The John Bowlby Centre, London, E1 6BJ. Tel: 020 7247 9101.

British Association for Behavioural and Cognitive Therapies: Imperial House, Hornby Street, Bury, Lancashire, BL9 5BN. Tel: 0161 705 4306.

British Association for Counselling and Psychotherapy: BACP House, 15 St. John's Business Park, Lutterworth, Leicestershire, LE17 4HB. Tel: 01455 883300.

British Association for Psychoanalytic and Psychodynamic Supervision: 35 Manor Road, Potters Bar, EN6 1DQ. Tel: 01234 771 595.

British Society of Couple Psychotherapists and Counsellors: 70 Warren Street, London, W1T 5PA. Tel: 020 7380 1979.

British Psychodrama Association: 33 Princes Road, Cheltenham, GL50 2TX. Tel: 07582 842 231.

British Psychotherapy Foundation: 37 Mapesbury Road, London, NW2 4HJ. Tel: 020 8452 9823.

British Psychoanalytic Association: 37 Mapesbury Road, London, NW2 4HJ. Tel: 020 8452 9823.

British Psychoanalytic Council: Suite 7, 19–23 Wedmore Street, London, N19 4RU. Tel: 020 7561 9240.

British Psychoanalytical Society – The Institute of Psychoanalysis: Byron House, 112A Shirland Road, London, W9 2BT. Tel: 020 7563 5000.

Cambridge Body Psychotherapy Centre: 28 Ditton Walk, Cambridge, CB5 8QE. Tel: 01223 214 658.

Cambridge Society for Psychotherapy: PO Box 620, Cambridge, CB1 0GX. Tel: 01223 335 377.

Canterbury Consortium of Psychoanalytic & Psychodynamic Psychotherapists: 51 Archers Court Road, Dover, CT16 3HS. Tel: 01227 761 310.

Caspari Foundation: Gregory House, London, WC1N 2NY. Tel: 020 7923 6270.

Centre for Counselling and Psychotherapy Education: Beauchamp Lodge, London, W2 6NE. Tel: 020 7266 3006.

Centre for Freudian Analysis and Research: Suite 56, London, NW3 7BN. Tel: 0845 838 0829.

Centre for Transpersonal Psychology: 17 West View Road, St. Albans, AL3 5JX. Tel: 01727 761 947.

Chiron Association for Body Psychotherapists: 14 Bryony house, Bracknell, RG42 1PH. Tel: 01223 240 815.

Confederation for Analytical Psychology: Forest Hill, London, SE23 3QY. Tel: 020 7515 2012.

College of Sexual and Relationship Therapists: P.O. Box 13686, London, SW20 9ZH. Tel: 020 8543 2707.

Counsellors and Psychotherapists in Primary Care: Queensway House, Bognor Regis, PO21 1QT. Tel: 01243 870 701.

Forensic Psychotherapy Society: c/o Room 18/02/47, Learning and Development Dept, E block, St. Bernard's Hospital, Uxbridge Road, Southall, UB1 3EU.

Forum for Independent Psychotherapists: 11 Genotin Terrace, Enfield EN1 2AF. Tel: 020 8367 4359.

Foundation for Psychotherapy and Counselling: 5 Maidstone Buildings Mews, 72–76 Borough High Street, London, SE1 1GN. Tel: 020 7795 0315.

Gestalt Centre London: 96–100 Clifton Street, London EC2A 4TP. Tel: 020 7247 6501.

Gestalt Psychotherapy Training Institute: P.O. Box 2555, Bath, BA1 6XR. Tel: 01225 482 135.

Group Analysis South West: 12 Sydenham Road, Bristol, BS6 5SH. Tel: 0117 942 3343.

Guild of Analytical Psychologists: 4 Ennerdale Road, Reading, RG2 7HH. Tel: 0118 922 2993.

Guild of Psychotherapists: 47 Nelson Square, London, SE1 0QA. Tel: 020 7401 3260.

Hallam Institute of Psychotherapists: P.O. Box 4253, Sheffield, S10 9BY.

Independent Group of Analytical Psychologists: P.O. Box 22343, London, W13 8GP. Tel: 020 8933 0353.

Improving Access to Psychological Therapies: See the website http://www.iapt.nhs.uk for a list of services by area.

Institute for Arts in Therapy and Education: 2–18 Britannia Row, London, N1 8PA. Tel: 020 7704 2534.

Institute for Psychotherapy and Disability: Kirton Lindsey, DN21 4LX. Tel: 01652 648 335.

Institute of Family Therapy: 24–32 Stephenson Way, London, NW1 2HX. Tel: 020 7391 9150.

Institute of Group Analysis: 1 Daleham Gardens, London, NW3 5BY. Tel: 020 7431 2693.

Institute of Psychosynthesis: 65a Watford Way, London, NW4 3AQ. Tel: 020 8202 4525.

Institute of Psychotherapy and Social Studies: Endeavour House, Enfield, EN1 2AF. Tel: 0845 271 3303.

Karuna Institute: Natsworthy Manor, Newton Abbott, TQ13 7TR. Tel: 01647 221 457.

London School of Biodynamic Psychotherapy: Bickerton House, London, N19 5JT. Tel: 020 7263 4290.

Matrix College of Counselling and Psychotherapy: Lavender Cottage, Hethersett, NR9 3DB. Tel: 01603 812 479.

Metanoia Institute: 13 North Common Road, London, W5 2QB. Tel: 020 8579 2505.

Minster Centre: 20 Lonsdale Road, London, NW6 6RD. Tel: 020 7644 6240.

NAFSIYAT Intercultural Therapy Centre: Unit 4, Clifton House, Clifton House, London, N4 3JP. Tel: 020 7263 6947.

National College of Hypnosis and Psychotherapy: P.O. Box 5779, Loughborough, LE12 5ZF. Tel: 0845 257 8735.

The National Register of Hypnotherapists and Psychotherapists: 1st Floor, Nelson, BB9 7JS. Tel: 01282 716 839.

Neurolinguistic Psychotherapy and Counselling Association: NLPtCA admin, c/o Changeworks Communication, St. Albans House, St. Albans Road, Stafford, ST16 3DP. Tel: 0870 241 3276.

North of England Association of Psychoanalytic Psychotherapists: Claremont House, Off Framlingham Place, Newcastle Upon Tyne, NE2 4AA. Tel: 0191 282 4547.

Northern Guild for Psychotherapy and Counselling: 83 Jesmond Road, Newcastle-Upon-Tyne, NE2 1NH. Tel: 0191 209 8383.

Northern Ireland Association for the Study of Psychoanalysis: 8b North Parade, Belfast, BT7 2GG.

Personal Construct Psychology Education and Training: 44 Park Road, Coventry, CV1 2LD. Tel: 020 8994 7959.

Philadelphia Association: 4 Marty's Yard, London, NW3 1QW. Tel: 020 7794 2652.

Psychosynthesis and Education Trust: 92–94 Tooley Street, London, SE1 2TH. Tel: 020 7403 2100.

Refugee Therapy Centre: London, N4 3RF. Tel: 020 7272 2565.

The Regent's School of Psychotherapy and Psychology: Regent's Park, NW1 4NS. Tel: 020 7487 7584.

Research Society for Process Oriented Psychology: Hampstead Town Hall Centre, NW3 4QP. Tel: 020 7435 0756.

Re-Vision: 97 Brondesbury Road, London, NW6 6RY. Tel: 020 8357 8881.

Scarborough Counselling and Psychotherapy Training Institute: 1 Westbourne Grove, Scarborough, YO11 2DJ. Tel: 01723 376 246.

Scottish Association of Psychoanalytical Psychotherapists: c/o The Administrator of SAPP, 3F2, 41 Bruntsfield Gardens, Edinburgh, EH10 4DY.

School of Infant Mental Health: 27 Frognal, London, NW3 6AR. Tel: 020 7433 3112.

Severnside Institute for Psychotherapy: 11 Orchard Street, Bristol, BS1 5EH. Tel: 0117 923 2354.

Sherwood Psychotherapy Training Institute: Thiskney House, 2 St. James Street, Nottingham, NG1 6FW. Tel: 0115 924 3994.

Site for Contemporary Psychoanalysis: 35 Manor Road, Potters Bar, EN6 1DQ. Tel: 01707 649 788.

Society of Analytical Psychology: 1 Daleham Gardens, London, NW3 5BY. Tel: 020 7435 7696.

Society for Existential Analysis: BM Existential, London, WC1N 3XX.

South Trent Training in Dynamic Psychotherapy: c/o Dynamic Psychotherapy Specialty, Lincoln, LN2 5RA. Tel: 01522 512 000.

Spectrum: 7 Endymion Road, London, N4 1EE. Tel: 020 8341 2277.

Tara Rokpa Therapy Association: 15 Rosebery Crescent, Edinburgh, EH12 5JY. Tel: 0131 313 0304.

Tavistock and Portman NHS Foundation Trust: The Tavistock Centre, 120 Belsize Lane, London, NW3 5BA. Tel: 020 7435 7111.

Tavistock Centre for Couple Relations: 70 Warren Street, London, W1T 5PB. Tel: 020 7380 1975.

Tavistock Society of Psychotherapists: The Tavistock and Portman NHS Foundation Trust, 120 Belsize Lane, London, NW3 5BA. Tel: 020 8938 2344.

Terapia: P.O. Box 25295, London, N12 9YQ. Tel: 020 8201 6101.

The Portman Clinic: 8 Fitzjohn's Avenue, London, NW3 5NA. Tel: 020 7794 8262.

Royal College of Psychiatrists: 21 Prescot Street, London, E1 8BB. Tel: 020 7235 2351.

The UK Association for Humanistic Psychology Practitioners: BDM AHPP, London, WC1N 3XX. Tel: 0845 766 0326.

United Kingdom Association for Transactional Analysis: Suite 3, Broadway House, Cambridge, CB23 7QJ. Tel: 01954 212468.

UK Council for Psychotherapy: 2nd Floor, Edward House, 2 Wakley Street, London, EC1V 7LT. Tel: 020 7014 9955.

Universities Psychotherapy & Counselling Association: UPCA Administration Office, P.O. Box 3076, Reading, RG1 9YF. Tel: 07806 804 508.

Wessex Counselling: Fairfield House, King Street, Frome, BA11 1BH. Tel: 01373 453 355.

West Midlands Institute of Psychotherapy: 36 Harborne road, Birmingham, B15 3AF. Tel: 0121 455 7888.

Westminster Pastoral Foundation: 23 Magdalen Street, London, SE1 2EN. Tel: 020 7378 2000.

Index